PATHOPHYSIOLOGY OF DERMATOLOGIC DISEASES

NOTICE

Medicine is an ever-changing science. As new research and clinical experience broaden our knowledge, changes in treatment and drug therapy are required. The editors and the publisher of this work have checked with sources believed to be reliable in their efforts to provide information that is complete and generally in accord with the standards accepted at the time of publication. However, in view of the possibility of human error or changes in medical sciences, neither the editors nor the publisher nor any other party who has been involved in the preparation or publication of this work warrants that the information contained herein is in every respect accurate or complete. Readers are encouraged to confirm the information contained herein with other sources. For example and in particular, readers are advised to check the product information sheet included in the package of each drug they plan to administer to be certain that the information contained in this book is accurate and that changes have not been made in the recommended dose or in the contraindications for administration. This recommendation is of particular importance in connection with new or infrequently used drugs.

PATHOPHYSIOLOGY OF DERMATOLOGIC DISEASES

SECOND EDITION

EDITORS

Nicholas A. Soter, M.D.
Professor of Dermatology
New York University School of Medicine

Medical Director
Charles C. Harris Skin and Cancer Pavilion

Attending Physician
Tisch Hospital, The University Hospital of New York University
New York, New York

Howard P. Baden, M.D.
Professor of Dermatology
Harvard Medical School

Dermatologist
Massachusetts General Hospital
Boston, Massachusetts

McGraw-Hill, Inc.
Health Professions Division

New York St. Louis San Francisco Colorado Springs Auckland Bogotá
Caracas Hamburg Lisbon London Madrid Mexico Milan Montreal
New Delhi Paris San Juan São Paulo Singapore Sydney Tokyo Toronto

One of the editors (N.A.S.) dedicates this book to his mother, Mildred Elizabeth Soter, and the other editor (H.P.B.) dedicates this book to his family.

PATHOPHYSIOLOGY OF DERMATOLOGIC DISEASES

1234567890 HALHAL 9876543210

ISBN 0-07-059747-2

This book was set in Palatino by Monotype Composition, Inc.; the editors were William Day and Lester A. Sheinis; the production supervisor was Clare Stanley; the cover was designed and the project was supervised by M 'N O Production Services, Inc.
Halliday Lithograph Corporation was printer and binder.

Library of Congress Cataloging-in-Publication Data

Pathophysiology of dermatologic diseases / [edited by] Nicholas A. Soter, Howard P. Baden. — 2d ed.
p. cm.
Includes bibliographical references.
Includes index.
ISBN 0-07-059747-2
1. Skin—Pathophysiology. I. Soter, Nicholas A. II. Baden, Howard P.
[DNLM: 1. Skin Diseases—physiopathology. WR 140 P297]
RL96.P37 1991
616.5—dc20
DNLM/DLC
for Library of Congress 90-6646
CIP

Contents

Section 3 Disorders of the Epidermis

Section 4 Disorders of the Epidermal Appendages

Section 5 Disorders of Melanocytes

Contributors

Honnavara N. Ananthaswamy, Ph.D.
Associate Professor, Department of Immunology, The University of Texas M.D. Anderson Cancer Center, Houston, Texas

Howard P. Baden, M.D.
Professor of Dermatology, Harvard Medical School; Dermatologist, Massachusetts General Hospital, Boston, Massachusetts

Donald V. Belsito, M.D.
Associate Professor of Dermatology, New York University School of Medicine; Attending Physician, Tisch Hospital, The University Hospital of New York University, New York, New York

Timothy Berger, M.D.
Assistant Clinical Professor, School of Medicine, University of California at San Francisco; Chief of Dermatology, San Francisco General Hospital, San Francisco, California

Jeffrey D. Bernhard, M.D.
Associate Professor of Medicine and Associate Dean for Admissions; Director, Division of Dermatology and Director, Phototherapy Center, University of Massachusetts Medical Center, Worcester, Massachusetts

Peter Buchan, Ph.D.
Head, Pharmacokinetics and Metabolism Group, Centre International de Recherches Dermatologiques Galderma, Sophia Antipolis, Valbonne, France

Richard A.F. Clark, M.D.
Professor and Chairman, Department of Dermatology, School of Medicine, State University of New York at Stony Brook; University Hospital of Stony Brook, Stony Brook, New York

Clay J. Cockerell, M.D.
Assistant Professor of Dermatology and Pathology, Associate in Dermatopathology, University of Texas Southwestern Medical Center, Dallas, Texas

Marcus A. Conant, M.D.
Clinical Professor of Dermatology, School of Medicine, University of California at San Francisco, San Francisco, California

Luis A. Diaz, M.D.
Professor and Chairman, Department of Dermatology, Medical College of Wisconsin, Milwaukee, Wisconsin

Richard L. Edelson, M.D.
Professor and Chairman, Department of Dermatology, Yale University School of Medicine; Yale New Haven Hospital, New Haven, Connecticut

Michael J. Fazio, M.D.
Research Instructor of Dermatology, Jefferson Medical College; Chief Resident, Department of Dermatology, Thomas Jefferson University Hospital, Philadelphia, Pennsylvania

Jo-David Fine, M.D.
Associate Professor of Dermatology, The University of North Carolina at Chapel Hill; Attending Dermatologist, North Carolina Memorial Hospital, Chapel Hill, North Carolina

George B. Fitzgerald, Ph.D.
Research Associate, Department of Dermatology, Harvard Medical School, Boston, Massachusetts

Thomas B. Fitzpatrick, M.D., Ph.D.
Edward Wigglesworth Professor Emeritus of Dermatology, Harvard Medical School; Massachusetts General Hospital, Boston, Massachusetts

R. William Gange, M.D.
Associate Professor of Dermatology, Harvard Medical School; Attending Dermatologist, Massachusetts General Hospital, Boston, Massachusetts

Barbara A. Gilchrest, M.D.
Professor and Chairman of Dermatology, Boston University School of Medicine; Chief, Department of Dermatology, University Hospital, Boston, Massachusetts

Ernesto Gonzalez, M.D.
Assistant Professor of Dermatology, Harvard Medical School; Chief of Dermatology Associates II, Massachusetts General Hospital, Boston, Massachusetts

Jon M. Hanifin, M.D.
Professor of Dermatology, Department of Dermatology, The Oregon Health Sciences University, Portland, Oregon

Harley A. Haynes, A.B., M.D.
Associate Professor of Dermatology, Harvard Medical School; Director, Dermatology Division, Brigham and Women's Hospital; Chief, Dermatology, West Roxbury Veterans Administration Medical Center, Boston, Massachusetts

Peter W. Heald, M.D.
Assistant Professor of Dermatology, Yale University School of Medicine; Attending Dermatologist, Yale New Haven Hospital, New Haven, Connecticut

Karen A. Holbrook, Ph.D.
Professor of Biological Structure, Adjunct Professor in Medicine (Dermatology), Associate Dean, Scientific Affairs, School of Medicine, University of Washington, Seattle, Washington

Jean-Claude Jamoulle, Ph.D.
Head, Pharmaceutical Sciences, Centre International de Recherches Dermatologiques Galderma, Sophia Antipolis, Valbonne, France

William D. Ju, M.D.
Postdoctoral Biotechnology Fellow, National Cancer Institute, National Institutes of Health, Bethesda, Maryland

Margaret L. Kripke, Ph.D.
Professor and Chairman, Department of Immunology, University of Texas M.D. Anderson Cancer Center, Houston, Texas

Joseph C. Kvedar, M.D.
Instructor of Dermatology, Harvard Medical School; Assistant Dermatologist, Massachusetts General Hospital, Boston, Massachusetts

James J. Leyden, M.D.
Professor of Dermatology, University of Pennsylvania School of Medicine; University of Pennsylvania Hospital, Philadelphia, Pennsylvania

Henry W. Lim, M.D.
Associate Professor of Dermatology, New York University School of Medicine; Chief, Dermatology Service, New York Department of Veterans Affairs Medical Center, New York, New York

Douglas R. Lowy, M.D.
Chief, Laboratory of Cellular Oncology, National Cancer Institute, National Institutes of Health, Bethesda, Maryland

Ronald Marks, M.D.
Head, Section of Dermatology, Department of Medicine, University of Wales College of Medicine, Cardiff, Wales, United Kingdom

Richard Masters, M.D., Ph.D.
Assistant Clinical Professor of Dermatology, Harvard Medical School; Assistant Dermatologist, Massachusetts General Hospital, Boston, Massachusetts

Minoru Ohtsuyama, M.D.
Postdoctoral Associate, University of Iowa College of Medicine, Iowa City, Iowa

Arthur R. Rhodes, M.D.
Assistant Professor of Dermatology, University of Pittsburgh School of Medicine; Attending Dermatologist, Presbyterian Hospital, Pittsburgh, Pennsylvania

Mary Ann Robledo, M.D.
Postdoctoral Research Fellow, Medical College of Wisconsin, Milwaukee, Wisconsin

Fusako Sato, M.S.
Research Assistant III, Department of Dermatology, University of Iowa College of Medicine, Iowa City, Iowa

Kenzo Sato, M.D., Ph.D.
Professor of Dermatology, Department of Dermatology, University of Iowa College of Medicine, Iowa City, Iowa

Daniel N. Sauder, M.D.
Professor, Division of Dermatology, University of Toronto; Chief, Division of Dermatology, Sunnybrook Medical Centre, Toronto, Canada

Robert J. Scheuplein, Ph.D.
Director, Office of Toxicological Science, Center for Food Safety and Applied Nutrition, Food and Drug Administration, Washington, D.C.

Arthur J. Sober, M.D.
Associate Professor of Dermatology, Harvard Medical School; Associate Chief of Dermatology, Massachusetts General Hospital, Boston, Massachusetts

Richard D. Sontheimer, M.D.
Professor of Dermatology and Internal Medicine, Vice Chairman of Dermatology, University of Texas Southwestern Medical Center; Parkland Memorial Hospital; Zale-Lipshy University Hospital, Dallas, Texas

Nicholas A. Soter, M.D.
Professor of Dermatology, New York University School of Medicine; Medical Director, Charles C. Harris Skin and Cancer Pavilion; Attending Physician, Tisch Hospital, The University Hospital of New York University, New York, New York

John S. Strauss, M.D.
Professor and Head, Department of Dermatology, University of Iowa College of Medicine; Chief of Dermatology, University of Iowa Hospitals and Clinic, Iowa City, Iowa

Yuichi Suzuki, Ph.D.
Associate Professor, Department of Dermatology, Yamagata University School of Medicine, Yamagata, Japan

Jouni J. Uitto, M.D.
Professor and Chairman of Dermatology; Professor of Dermatology, Biochemistry, and Molecular Biology, Jefferson Medical College; Thomas Jefferson University Hospital, Philadelphia, Pennsylvania

Michael M. Wick, M.D., Ph.D.
Associate Professor of Dermatology, Harvard Medical School; Associate Physician, Dana Farber Cancer Institute; Clinical Associate, Massachusetts General Hospital; Associate in Medical Dermatology, New England Deaconess Hospital, Brigham and Women's Hospital, and Beth Israel Hospital, Boston, Massachusetts

Preface

In its second edition, *Pathophysiology of Dermatologic Diseases* remains a concise text on the biological basis and pathophysiology of selected skin disorders. This new edition represents a major revision incorporating the great expansion of basic scientific knowledge and its impact on cutaneous biology and dermatologic disease.

Although the book is aimed primarily at medical students and physicians-in-training in dermatology and dermatopathology, it retains its value for physicians interested in refreshing their knowledge of the pathophysiology of the skin and for scientists in industry whose work requires a knowledge of physiology of the skin. We believe the book creates a firm basis for further study into the particular problems with which the reader is concerned.

Section 1, "Structure, Development, Aging, and Function of the Skin," includes certain basic physiological processes, such as temperature regulation and the skin as an organ of protection. Sections 2 through 8 discuss cutaneous disorders based on anatomic areas, such as the epidermis, dermoepidermal interface, dermis, and subcutaneous tissue. The cutaneous disorders selected as illustrative examples are those in which recent advances in research have occurred, an approach that allows insights into pathophysiology. Sections 9 through 12 consider certain specialized topics that are particularly important in the skin, including photobiology, infections, carcinogenesis, and the psyche.

New chapters have been added on percutaneous absorption, the skin as an immunologic organ, the pathophysiology of wound healing, and the pathophysiology of the acquired immunodeficiency syndrome.

The original basis of this book was a long-running course on pathophysiology of the skin taught at Harvard Medical School. For the second edition, the roster of contributing authors has been expanded to comprise new authors, including members of many different departments in the United States, Canada, France, Japan, and the United Kingdom. The contributing authors are all individuals who have made major contributions to the basic and clinical understanding of skin diseases.

The authors express appreciation for the secretarial dedication of Nellie Malave and Laurie Fitts.

Nicholas A. Soter
Howard P. Baden

PATHOPHYSIOLOGY OF DERMATOLOGIC DISEASES

SECTION ONE

STRUCTURE, DEVELOPMENT, AGING, AND FUNCTION OF THE SKIN

1

Structure and Development of the Skin

Karen A. Holbrook

The skin is the largest organ system of the body. It includes all of the tissues except bone and cartilage and has several types of cells organized to subserve unique functions. The skin is an organ of protection, forming a tough but pliable covering, a barrier between the body and the environment. It functions as a sensory receptor, has a role in temperature regulation, and is involved in immunologic surveillance.

EPIDERMIS

Layers of the Epidermis

Different cellular layers of the stratified epidermis correspond to progressive stages of differentiation (Fig. 1-1). The names of the layers in order of increasing differentiation are the stratum germinativum (basale), stratum spinosum, stratum granulosum, and stratum corneum. The stratum corneum consists of dead, terminally differentiated keratinocytes; the keratinocytes of all other layers are viable.

Stratum Germinativum

The stratum germinativum is a single layer of columnar cells attached to a basement membrane (Fig. 1-1). The layer is named for the ability of the basal keratinocytes to proliferate. The progeny of these mitoses move

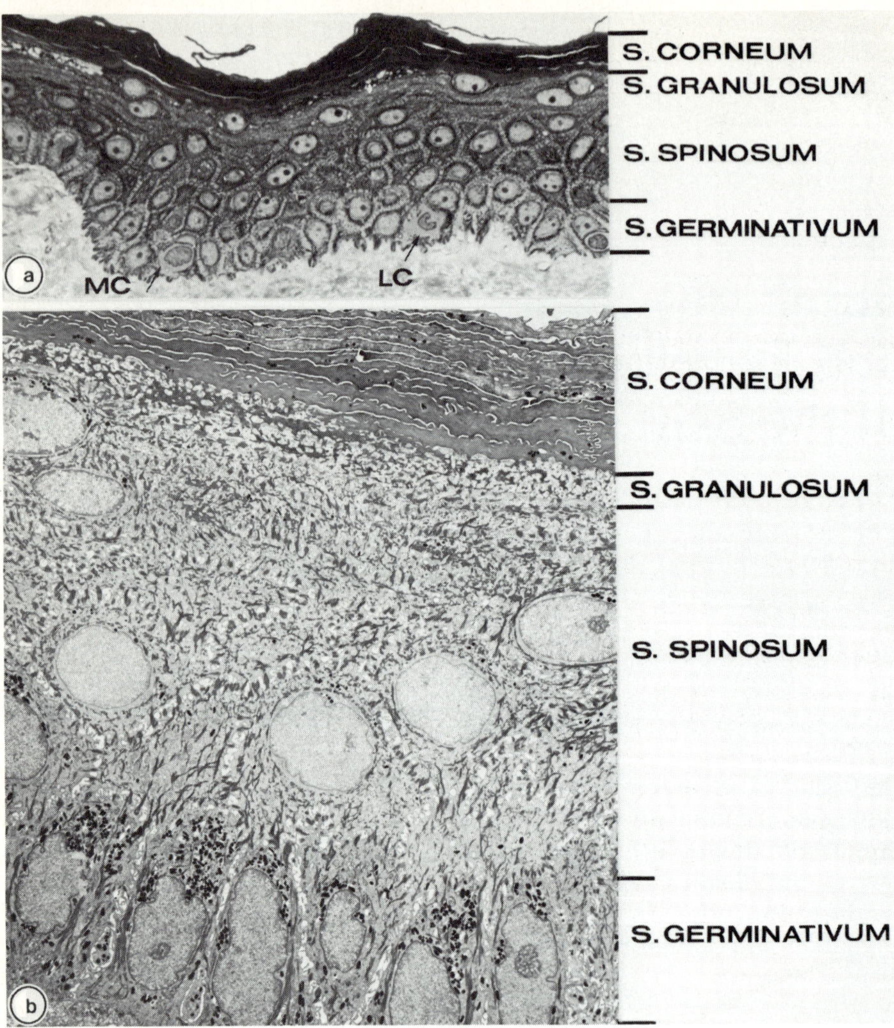

Figure 1-1 (*a*) Light microscopy of full-thickness epidermis. ×200 in the original magnification. (*b*) Transmission electron microscopy of full-thickness adult epidermis from a black individual. Note the particular abundance of melanosomes in cells of the stratum germinativum. ×2800 in the original magnification. MC = melanocyte; LC = Langerhans cell.

upward within the epidermis and replenish the cells lost at the surface during normal epidermal turnover. Typical basal keratinocytes have an oval nucleus, prominent nucleolus or nucleoli, and little heterochromatin. They contain the cellular organelles and enzyme systems responsible for synthetic and maintenance metabolism; melanosomes within membrane-bound vacuoles (melanosome complexes); and cytoskeletal structures including keratin intermediate filaments, microfilaments, and microtubules. The keratin filaments are organized in fine bundles that extend between the plaque regions of desmosomes. Desmosomes are structurally and biochemically complex junctions specialized to join adjacent epithelial cells in all layers of the epidermis.[1] Glycoproteins present on the surface of the epidermal cell are also important in cell-cell adhesion.

The biochemistry of the keratin polypeptides in all layers of the epidermis correlates with the state of keratinocyte differentiation. A low molecular weight keratin pair (one acidic and one basic) is characteristic of basal cells.[2]

Although basal cells are relatively uniform in morphology, they are heterogeneous with regard to their proliferative potential. Unlabeled and labeled cell populations exist in the basal layer when the skin is exposed continuously to ^{3}H-thymidine for several days longer than the cell cycle. Labeled cells belong to a cycling population, while unlabeled cells are a noncycling or slowly cycling population, possibly equivalent to epidermal stem cells. Stem cells are slowly cycling cells that are thought to regulate proliferation. In the skin, such cells divide infrequently producing one daughter cell that will enter the cycling pool, undergo augmentation divisions, and then differentiate. The other daughter cell remains in the basal layer as a stem cell. It has been suggested that noncycling cells can be induced back into the cycling population as needed or in diseases where there is epidermal hyperplasia.[3] Except for specialized regions of the skin such as the thick, ridged skin of the palm and sole, these populations of basal cells are indistinguishable.[4]

The cell bodies of melanocytes, Merkel cells, and, occasionally, Langerhans cells are present among keratinocytes in the basal layer. Dendritic cells processes of both the melanocytes and Langerhans cells insinuate among cells of the spinous layer.

Stratum Spinosum

Daughters of basal cell mitoses move into the first suprabasal layer of the stratum spinosum, a zone of two to four layers in which cells become progressively differentiated as they move outward (Figs. 1-1 through 1-3*a*). Adjacent cells join by abundant desmosomes. The retraction of the cell borders between desmosomes gives a spiny appearance to the cells in histologic preparations, hence the name of the layer.

Cells of the deepest spinous layer are at first polyhedral (Fig. 1-2) and then become flattened as they move toward the skin surface (Figs. 1-1*b* and 1-3). Spinous cells contain typical cellular organelles (rough endoplasmic reticulum, Golgi, mitochondria, etc.), microfilaments, and melanosome complexes, but have a greater quantity of keratin filaments (by volume density) that are organized into prominent bundles often called tonofibrils. The pairs of keratin filament-forming polypeptides synthesized in spinous cells are higher in molecular weight than those of basal cells and are referred to as the differentiation- or keratinization-specific pair.[2]

Cells of the uppermost one or two layers of spinous cells and the

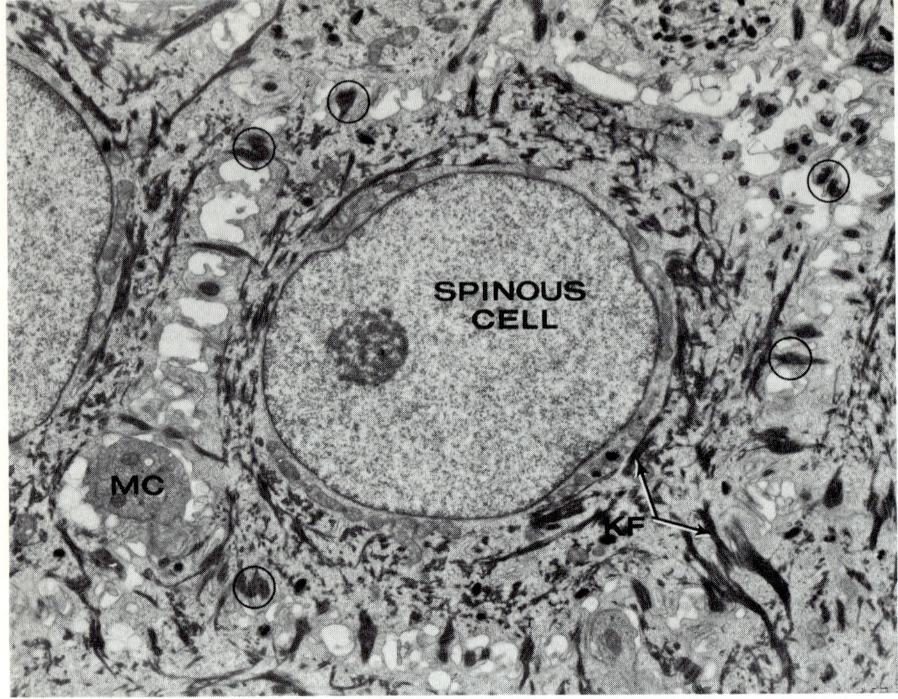

Figure 1-2 Spinous cell in a lower layer of the stratum spinosum. The process of a melanocyte is seen in cross section (MC). KF = keratin filaments. The circles enclose desmosomes. ×8800 in the original magnification.

granular layer contain small (100- to 500-nm), oval-shaped, membrane-bound organelles called lamellar granules (Fig. 1-3). They are also referred to as membrane-coating granules, keratinosomes, and Odland bodies. The internal compartment of the granule is organized into a series of complete and incomplete alternating, electron-dense and lucent membranes.[5] Lamellar granules are formed in the Golgi region and then migrate to the periphery of upper spinous and granular cells, where they release their contents into the intercellular space (Fig. 1-3*a* and *b*).

Stratum Granulosum

The granular cells are the most highly differentiated cells of the viable epidermis. They are flattened polyhedrons that appear as elongated rectangles in sectioned specimens (Figs. 1-1*b* and 1-3). The major distinguishing feature of the granular cell is the keratohyalin, seen light microscopically as a granule but resolved ultrastructurally as an electron-dense substance accumulated in the interstices of keratin filament bundles, thus forming irregularly shaped structures (Fig. 1-3). Profilaggrin is the richly phosphorylated polymeric protein of the keratohyalin granule.[6] It is thought to function in the aggregation of keratin filaments during the

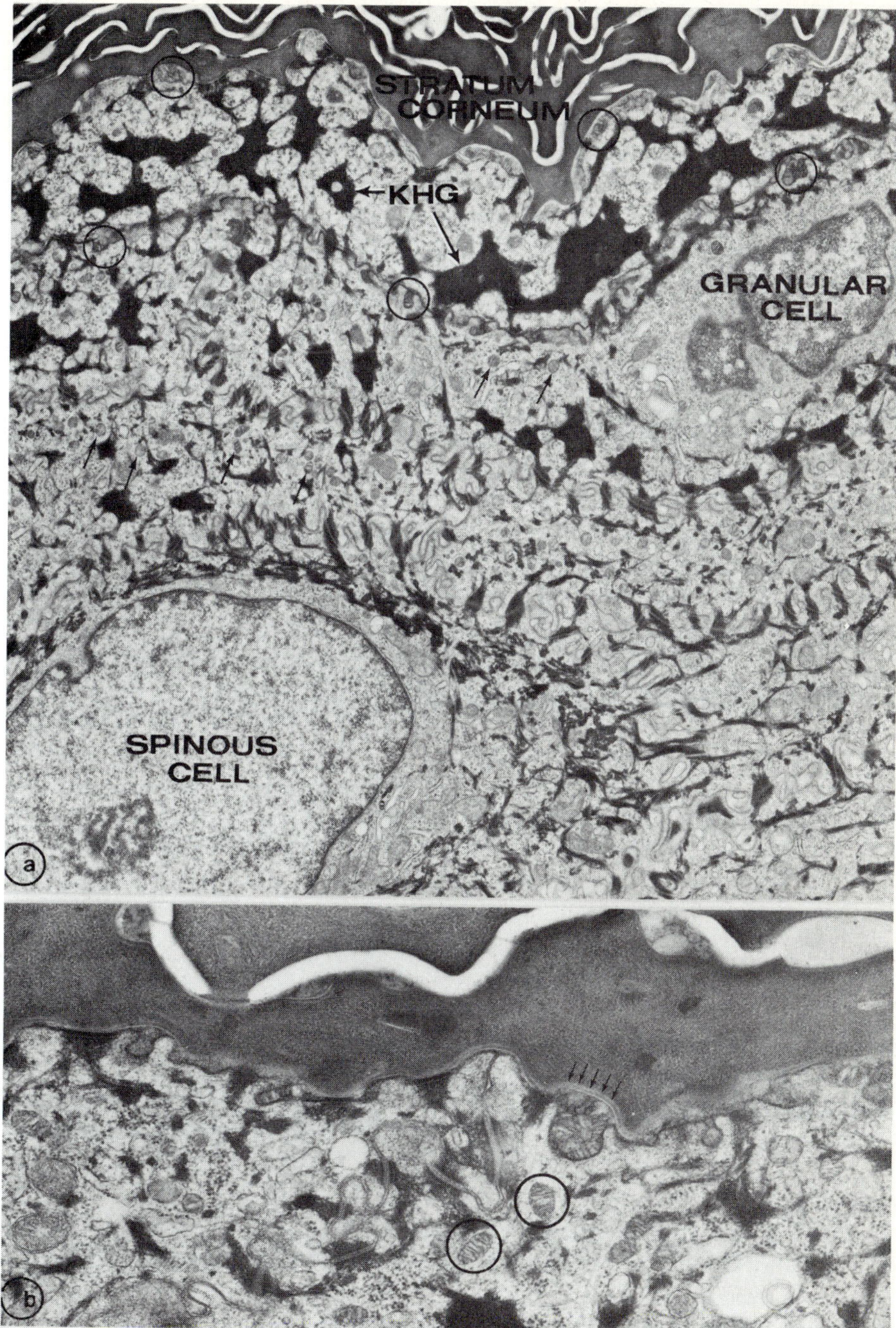

Figure 1-3 (*a*) Spinous granular and lower cornified cells of the epidermis. The arrows point to lamellar granules in the cytoplasm, and the circles enclose lamellar granules at the cell margins. ×10,000 in the original magnification. (*b*) Uppermost granular cell and first cornified cell. Lamellar granules are circled and arrows point to the cornified cell envelope. ×23,300 in the original magnification. KHG = keratohyalin granules.

granular-cornified cell transition and to serve as the interfilamentous "matrix" of the cornified cell.[7]

The lamellar granules first formed in spinous cells aggregate beneath the plasma membrane of granular cells. The membranes of the lamellar granules fuse with the granular cell plasma membrane, opening a channel for the release of granule contents into the spaces between granular cells and cells of the granular and first cornified layers (Fig. 1-3*a* and *b*). Lamellar granules contain complex polysaccharides, glycoproteins, several acid hydrolases, and "probarrier" lipids.[8] Once released into the extracellular space, the polar lipids are remodeled into hydrophobic, neutral, lipid-rich lamellae that form an effective barrier. Hydrolases of the granule may play a role in this process and may facilitate desquamation.[9]

Changes in the plasma membrane become apparent in some granular cells and in all cornified cells (Fig. 1-3*b*). A 12- to 15-nm-thick, dense layer of highly cross-linked protein is deposited inside the inner leaflet of the membrane. Together with the membrane, this boundary is referred to as the cornified cell envelope.[10] It is a rigid structure that resists degradation by keratinolytic agents, organic solvents, and denaturing agents.

Granular cells are a curious contradiction of simultaneous synthetic and degradative events. The cells still contain the typical organelles suggestive of biosynthesis (Fig. 1-3*a*), but they also possess numerous lysosomal proteases and nucleases indicative of degradative activity.[11] The abrupt transition between granular and cornified cells, with the loss of nearly every cellular organelle and the nucleus, clearly indicates that degradative events must be in progress. Nuclei of the granular layer flatten, condense, and cease to direct RNA synthesis. They show an increase in heterochromatin content and, ultimately, the breakdown of nucleoprotein. Remnants of the nucleus can be recognized as dense, fibrillar material.[11,12] A decrease in DNA content accompanies the morphologic changes. DNase, RNase, proteases, and serum plasminogen activator have all been shown to contribute to the breakdown of the nucleus and organelles under certain conditions. Other changes in desmosomes and cell surface glycoprotein adhesion molecules have been noted. The mechanism for final dissolution that brings about a loss of approximately 45 to 86 percent of the dry weight of the granular cell is not fully understood. Keratins, profilaggrin/filaggrin, and the cornified cell envelope are passed on to the cornified cell.

Transitional Cells. Transitional cells[13] are a small population of cells recognized sporadically within the granular layer by their large, dense keratohyalin and filament aggregates, a pyknotic nucleus or nuclear fragments, and a cornified cell envelope. They retain some of the features of viable cells, including organelles or organelle remnants.

Stratum Corneum

The stratum corneum contains the most cell layers and has the largest cells of any zone of the epidermis (Fig. 1-1). It ranges from approximately

15 layers in thickness, in thin areas such as the face, to 25 or more on the arm.[14] In specialized regions, such as the palm or sole, 100 or more cell layers are present. Cells of the stratum corneum are large, flattened, and polyhedral-shaped. Those near the surface have more exaggerated flattening than the deeper ones (Fig. 1-4). Adjacent cornified cells overlap at the margins and associate with cells of underlying and superficial layers through interlocking ridges and modified desmosomes.

The contents of a cornified cell are limited primarily to disulfide-bonded keratin filaments and filaggrin. The filaggrin is electron-dense in electron micrographs of the stratum corneum and outlines the electron-lucent profiles of the filaments. The organization of these proteins is compact in the deepest (first) cornified layers but becomes looser toward the outer epidermal surface. It is thought that breakdown of the filaggrin to its constituent amino acids in the outer cell layers accounts for the greater water-holding capacity of the cells and the more diffuse organization of the keratin filaments.[15]

Epidermal Architecture

The epidermis (in many regions) has an intrinsic pattern of organization consisting of vertical columns of stacked cells. This was first observed in frozen sections of skin that were allowed to swell in alkali or hypotonic buffer solutions. The stacks are most prominent in the stratum corneum but can be followed into the deeper epidermal layers in some species. The

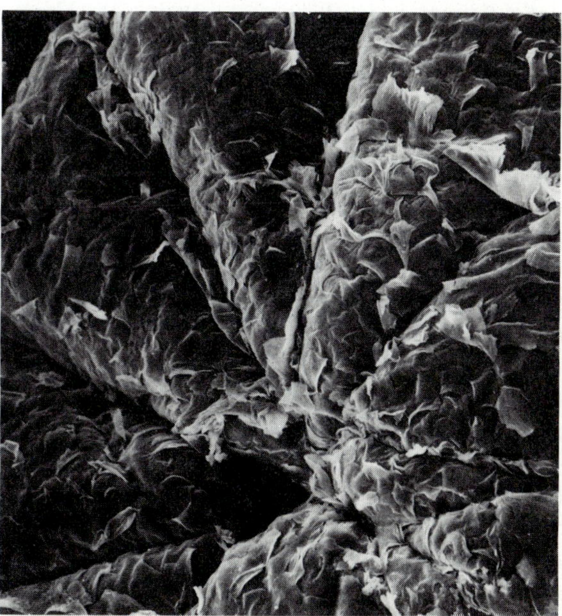

Figure 1-4 Surface view of the epidermis shows loose squamae and the patterns of ridges and grooves. ×310 in the original magnification.

borders of stacked cells of one column overlap and interdigitate with those of adjacent columns; thus, upward movement of one column influences, to some extent, movement of all the others. The mechanism of column formation is largely unknown, although there is a clear correlation between epidermal columns, epidermal thickness, and the rate of cell production. Only an epidermis that is *normal* in thickness and has a slow rate of cell production possesses columnar-type organization. The cells of greatly thickened epidermis of the palms and soles, and thickened epidermis at sites of early wound repair of hypertrophic diseases, are organized at random and have higher rates of mitosis. Cell stacking may influence ordered cell movement during differentiation and desquamation, as well as the extent of transepidermal water loss; regions that lack the stacked pattern permit water loss to a greater degree.[16]

Nonkeratinocytes of the Epidermis

Three populations of cells migrate into, or originate and differentiate within, the epidermis during embryogenesis. They become established as permanent residents of the tissue and augment its functional properties.

Melanocytes

Melanocytes are pigment-synthesizing cells derived from the neural crest. They migrate into the skin during the second month of embryonic development.[17] Melanocytes are nearly always confined to the basal layer, although processes of melanocytes extend among keratinocytes of at least the first layer of spinous cells (Figs. 1-1*a* and 1-5). They are frequently seen in histologic sections as pale, rounded cells bulging downward from the epidermis (Fig. 1-1*a*). Although they do not form desmosomes with adjacent cells or hemidesmosomes along the dermal-epidermal boundary, they maintain a rather uniform distribution relative to a specific number of keratinocytes.[18] This is accomplished even though both keratinocytes and melanocytes are dividing cell populations. The nucleus of the melanocyte is rounded, and the cytoplasm contains typical cellular organelles, vimentin intermediate filaments, microfilaments, and microtubules.

Melanin pigment is synthesized in membrane-bound organelles called melanosomes through a series of enzymatically catalyzed reactions stimulated initially by binding of the peptide hormone melanocyte-stimulating hormone (MSH) to the melanocyte cell surface. Keratinocytes appear to phagocytize processes of melanocytes, thus incorporating melanosomes in vacuoles within their own cytoplasm. This provides a uniform distribution of pigment to absorb light across the basal layer of the epidermis.

Langerhans Cells

Langerhans cells are a second population of cells that migrate into the epidermis of the embryo and become established among keratinocytes of

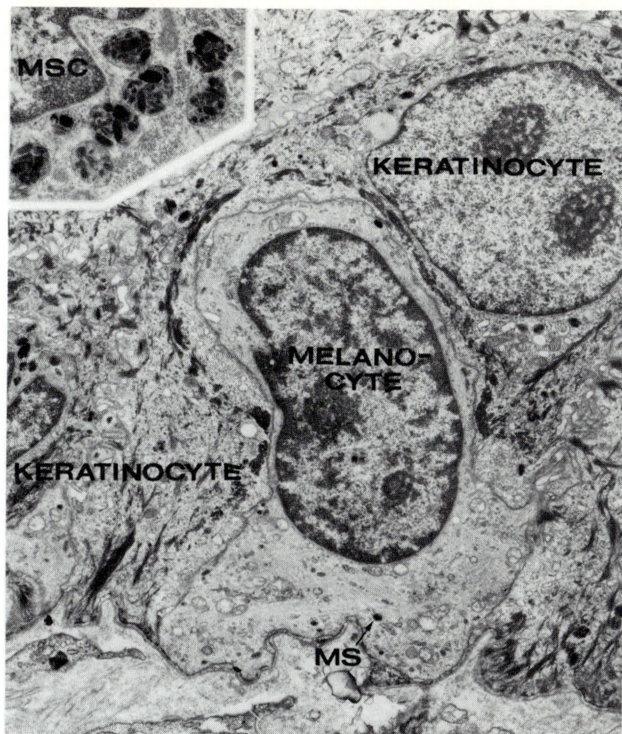

Figure 1-5 Melanocyte bordered by two keratinocytes. Compare the filaments of the two cell types. Melanosomes (MS) are sparse in the melanocyte but abundant in the melanosome complexes (MSC) within keratinocytes (see inset). ×7750, inset ×10,500 in the original magnification.

the suprabasal layers (Fig. 1-6). They account for approximately 4 to 7 percent of the cells in a square millimeter of adult epidermis. Langerhans cells are derived from, and continually repopulate the epidermis from precursor cells originating in the bone marrow.[19] Like melanocytes, Langerhans cells have pale cytoplasm and extend dendritic processes among keratinocytes, but the two cell types are easily distinguished from one another by the convoluted nucleus in the Langerhans cell and the distinctive cytoplasmic organelles in each type—the melanosome in the melanocyte and the Langerhans cell granule (Birbeck granule) in the Langerhans cell (Fig. 1-6).

The Langerhans cell granule can assume a variety of shapes in three dimensions, but it most often appears cuplike or disclike, with one edge expanded into a vesicle.[20] In sections the granules appear racket-shaped. The "handle," a trilaminar rod with a central striated linear density (Fig. 1-6, inset), is equivalent to a section through the flattened portion of the disc. The "racket" portion of the sectioned granule is a profile of the expanded region of the disc. Langerhans cell granules are found in both

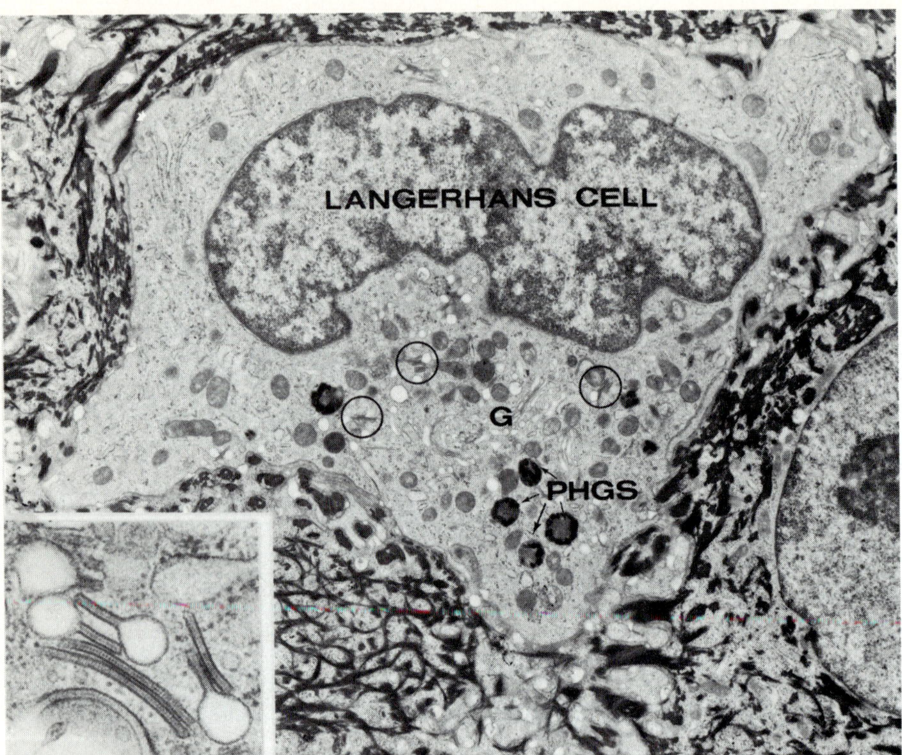

Figure 1-6 Langerhans cell surrounded by keratinocytes of the spinous layer. Note the absence of desmosomes between the Langerhans cell and keratinocytes. Langerhans cell granules are circled and are enlarged in the inset. Numerous phagolysosomes (PHGS) are seen within the cell. G = Golgi region. ×8370, inset ×45,600 in the original magnification. (*Inset courtesy of Susan K. Anderson.*)

the main body of the cell and the dendritic process. They are thought to be formed either in the Golgi region or by endocytosis of the plasma membrane with bound antigen.[21]

The antigenic phenotype of the epidermal Langerhans cell has been well characterized.[22] It expresses the major histocompatibility class I and II antigens, CD45 (the leukocyte common antigen), CD1a, and the Fc IgG and C3b receptors. Other membrane and cytoplasmic markers of Langerhans cells include S100, T200, and membrane ADP and ATPase. The role of Langerhans cells in the epidermis is related to the expression of these cell surface components. Like cells of the monocyte-macrophage lineage, Langerhans cells are involved in the uptake, processing, and presentation of antigen to immunocompetent T lymphocytes to initiate an immune response. Their location in the skin suggests that they serve in the first line of immunologic defense to protect against environmental antigens.

Langerhans cells contain the typical organelles associated with cellular metabolism, vimentin intermediate filaments, and microfilaments. In some instances, the rough endoplasmic reticulum is dilated, suggesting secretory activity by the cell. It is uncertain what substances are synthesized for extracellular transport, but there is some evidence that the Langerhans cell may be an important source of prostaglandins in the skin. Phagolysosomes containing particulate matter, including melanosomes, are often evident in the cytoplasm (Fig. 1-6).

Merkel Cells

Merkel cells (Fig. 1-7*a* and *b*) appear first in the basal epidermal layer of thick skin (palmar/plantar), primarily during fetal development. They are the only nonkeratinocyte that forms desmosomes with keratinocytes and contains keratin intermediate filaments. Because of these similarities, it is hypothesized that they are derived from ectoderm, possibly from keratinocytes. Experimental evidence for an in situ origin supports this contention,[23] even though the keratins in the Merkel cell are not the same as

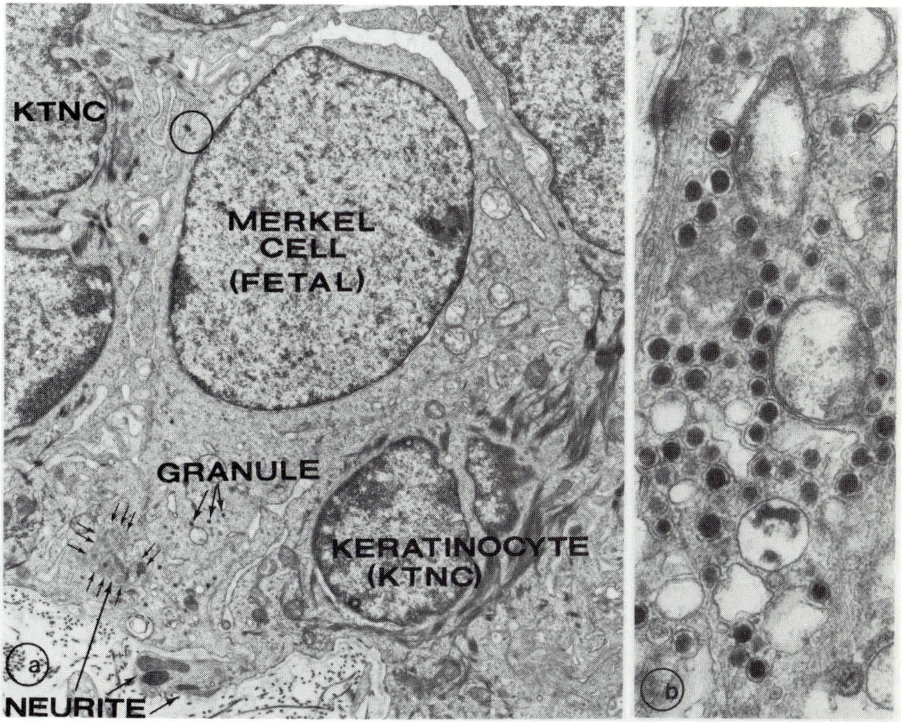

Figure 1-7 (*a*) Merkel cell found in fetal skin (26 weeks gestational age). The circle encloses a desmosome between the Merkel cell and an adjacent keratinocyte (KTNC). A neurite is evident as it penetrates the basal lamina and within the epidermis (surrounded by a series of arrows). Only a few Merkel cell granules are apparent in the cell. ×7900 in the original magnification. (*b*) The structure of the granule is shown in an enlarged portion of a Merkel cell. Note the desmosome between the Merkel cell and a keratinocyte. ×39,900 in the original magnification.

those in keratinocytes but are equivalent to keratins in simple epithelial cells.

Other features of the Merkel cell, however, tie them to the diffuse neuroendocrine tissue of the body. This supports an alternative origin from the neural crest or by differentiation of ectodermal cells within the epidermis along a neuroendocrine pathway. Merkel cells are often associated with an intraepidermal neurite, and they contain a population of 80- to 200-nm dense-core granules localized opposite the Golgi region, proximal to the neurite (Fig. 1-7*b*). These granules resemble the neurosecretory granules and contain neurotransmitter-like substances including met-enkephalin, vasoactive intestinal peptide (VIP), chromogranin A, neuron-specific enolase, and synaptophysin.[24,25]

Merkel cells are recognized in histologic preparations by pale cytoplasm and a lobulated nucleus. Electron microscopy shows that the cytoplasm contains sparse amounts of intermediate filaments and rough endoplasmic reticulum, as well as abundant polyribosomes, Golgi, mitochondria, lysosomes, and glycogen.

Merkel cells in mammals are found primarily in glabrous skin in specialized touch receptors where, complexed with the neurite, they function as slowly adapting type I mechanoreceptors, receiving stimuli from the deformation of epidermal cells. Although the structure of the contact between the Merkel cell and the neurite appears to resemble a chemical synapse, it has not yet been documented to function in this manner.[26]

THE DERMAL-EPIDERMAL JUNCTION

Structure of the Basement Membrane Zone

The basement membrane zone (BMZ) is a complex of structures that involves cells and extracellular matrix of both the dermis and epidermis. It serves as a boundary and as a mechanical linkage that integrates these two regions of the skin (Fig. 1-8*a* and *b*). Components of the BMZ are both epidermal and dermal in origin. In histologic sections, the zone is visible light microscopically as a single periodic acid Schiff (PAS)–positive band. It is resolved ultrastructurally into several planes: the basal portion of the basal layer keratinocytes, a narrow clear zone called the lamina lucida, the basal lamina (lamina densa), a continuous feltlike layer between the epidermis and dermis, and the sublamina densa region of the papillary dermis (the subepidermal band or reticular lamina). Each of these planes can be a zone of mechanical weakness that can separate in blistering disorders.

Hemidesmosomes join the basal membrane of epidermal basal cells with the lamina densa. They consist of intracellular (a dense plaque and related keratin filaments) and extracellular structures (subbasal dense plate and anchoring filaments) that connect the keratinocyte to the lamina densa. Bullous pemphigoid antigen has been localized to the hemidesmosome.[27]

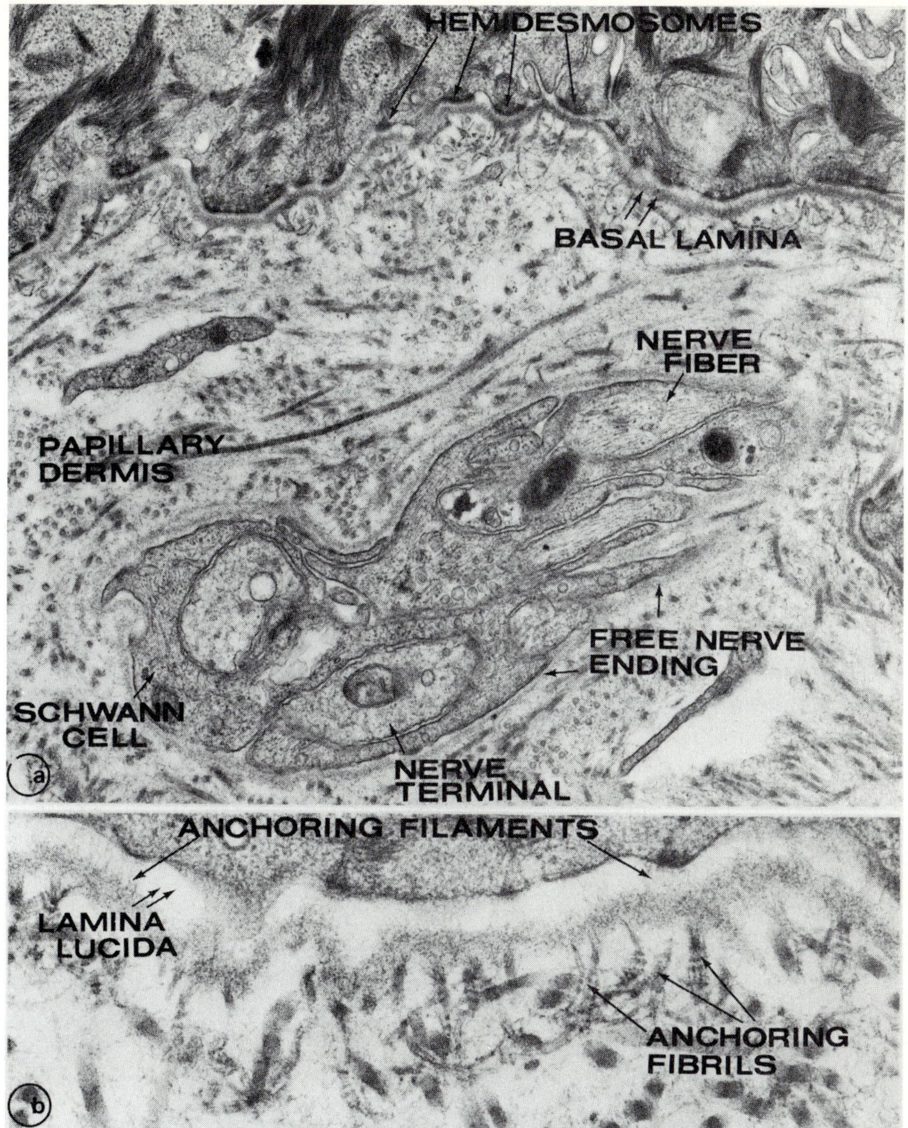

Figure 1-8 (*a*) Structures of the BMZ between the epidermis and dermis. Note the free nerve ending in the papillary dermis proximal to the epidermis. ×20,000 in the original magnification. (*b*) Detailed structure of the components of the BMZ. Note particularly the structure of the anchoring fibrils. ×69,650 in the original magnification.

The basal lamina, in turn, is anchored to the connective tissue matrix of the papillary dermis by 200- to 750-Å-diameter banded anchoring fibrils and by bundles of microfibrils (oxytalan fibers) that belong to the elastic connective tissue network.[28] Anchoring fibrils are composed (at least) of type VII collagen molecules.[29] They originate in the basal lamina and extend into the dermis, where they terminate freely in brushlike termini, are embedded in anchoring plaques of lamina densa–like material, or loop back to reinsert in the lamina densa (Fig. 1-8*b*). The microfibrils extend to the approximate boundary of the papillary and reticular dermis, where they join with fibrils of the horizontal elastic network.[28]

Biochemistry of the BMZ

The biochemical and antigenic composition of the BMZ is complex.[30] The basal lamina is composed of type IV collagen molecules thought to be arranged in a honeycomb-patterned meshwork. Heparan sulfate proteoglycan is assembled in this structure with the collagen. The presumed organization of the type IV collagen and proteoglycan explains the ultrastructural appearance and would impart qualities of tensile strength and elasticity. The lamina lucida is the primary site of several noncollagenous glycoproteins: laminin, fibronectin, and bullous pemphigoid antigen. Laminin is an attachment factor that binds epidermal cells to type IV collagen of the lamina densa.

In addition to its structural role, the BMZ serves as a size- and charge-selective filter. As in the glomerular basement membrane, heparan sulfate proteoglycan of the cutaneous basement membrane accounts for the anionic sites within the basal lamina. These are important in inhibiting permeability by repelling anionic macromolecules and blocking their passage.[31] Inflammatory and neoplastic cells, circulating pemphigus and pemphigoid antibodies, immigrant cells, and neurites, however, can penetrate the BMZ. These cells, therefore, must possess some mechanism to degrade or disrupt the organization of the lamina densa.

EPIDERMAL APPENDAGES

Plates, scales, nails, teeth, hair, and glandular structures are elaborated by cells of the epidermis. In humans, these are restricted to the teeth, nails, pilosebaceous apparatus, and eccrine and apocrine sweat glands. The appendages are distributed over the body with regional variability and, in some cases, specificity.

The Pilosebaceous Apparatus

The hair follicle and the sebaceous gland are a structurally and functionally integrated unit that forms during development from a cluster of basal epidermal cells and a specialized related population of mesenchymal cells.[32] Regions of the follicle proximal to the epidermis have the same basic layers of cells as the interfollicular epidermis and include all of the immigrant cells. Modifications in the pattern of epidermal layers occur below the level of the sebaceous gland, where the inner and outer root sheaths are organized and where synthesis of the hair and sheaths is initiated. The terminus of the follicle, the bulb, encloses a collection of mesenchymal cells called the dermal papilla.

Few structures of the skin can have as much variability as the pilosebaceous apparatus. The type of hair, density, and rate of growth are all regionally variable; sex, age, and race influence the amount of hair, hair shape, patterns, color, and growth. Genetic and hormonal control and receptor properties of the structures account for the marked variation among individuals. A single hair can show variation in color, size, and structure at different phases of follicle growth.

Hairs are classified as terminal, vellus, and lanugo. Terminal hairs are coarse, relatively long, pigmented hairs found in the most visibly hairy areas of the body, such as the scalp, beard, eyebrows, axilla, and pubis. A medulla (central core of the hair; see below) of varying diameter is present in some scalp hairs and is characteristic of beard, axillary, and pubic hairs.

Vellus hairs are short, soft and fine, nonmedullated, small-diameter, nonpigmented hairs present in nonhairy areas of the body. Some vellus hair follicles (beard region in prepubertal males) respond to hormones at puberty and begin to produce terminal hairs.

The first product of the hair follicle is the lanugo hair, formed in utero on the scalp and face in the mid-second trimester and over all the body toward the end of that period. Lanugo hairs are replaced in the child and adult by terminal and vellus hairs. New follicles are not formed after birth.

Gross Structure of the Follicle and Hair[33]

Follicles in the fetus and adult extend into the dermis at an angle. The hairs on the arms and legs project laterally and downward from the midline of the body, downward on the back and sides, and whorled on the scalp and over the sacrum. Terminal hair follicles in their most elongated state end in the subcutaneous fat; vellus hairs terminate within the dermis. Regions of the follicle are defined by anatomic landmarks (Fig. 1-9). The infundibulum lies between the sebaceous gland and the epidermis; the isthmus is between the sebaceous gland and the insertion of the arrector pili; and the "lower follicle" is the region between the attachment of the arrector pili muscle and the bulb. The lower follicle undergoes growth or atrophy, depending upon the stage of the hair cycle.

Histologic and Fine Structure of the Lanugo Follicle and Hair

The structure of the anagen follicle is equivalent to that of a late-stage, actively growing lanugo hair except for the absence of a medulla in the latter (Figs. 1-9 through 1-11).

The follicle is surrounded by connective tissue sheaths composed of oriented layers of collagen and elastic fibers and fibroblasts (Figs. 1-10*a* and 1-11). The sheaths surround the end of the bulb, enclosing cells of the dermal papilla within its concavity.

Growth of the follicle and the hair relies upon cells of the germinal matrix. These cells are positioned close to the cells of the dermal papilla, although separated from them by a basal lamina. This relationship is

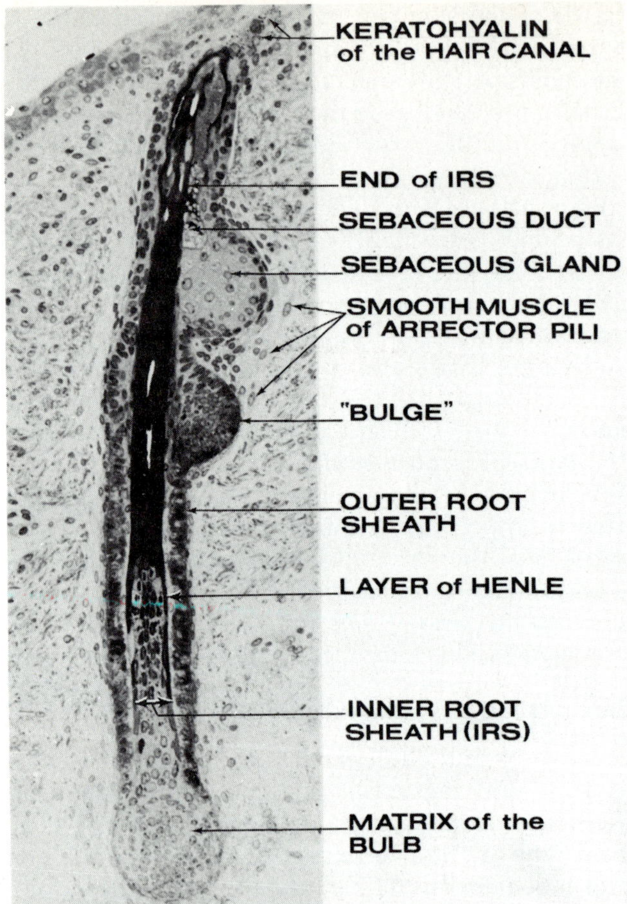

Figure 1-9 Full-length lanugo follicle. ×100 in the original magnification.

important because dermal papilla cells regulate the size and rate of growth of the hair.[34] Cells of the matrix are spatially organized such that mitoses at particular sites give rise to concentric layers of cells (Fig. 1-10*a*) that form the inner and outer root sheaths and the hair. Melanocytes present among the matrix cells (Fig. 1-10*a* and *b*) transfer pigment to the cells that enter the hair cortex. Melanin synthesis and extension of dendritic processes are influenced by the activity of matrix cells throughout the hair cycle.

The outer root sheath is derived from the deepest cells of the matrix (Figs. 1-9, 1-10*a*, and 1-11). It consists of at least two layers of keratinocytes. These cells do not keratinize at any level of the follicle (Fig. 1-11). The outermost layer of cells attaches to a thick basal lamina that, because of its appearance in histologic sections, is called the glassy membrane (Figs. 1-10*a* and 1-11).

Immediately within the outer root sheath are the three layers of the inner root sheath. These layers originate from matrix cells found at an

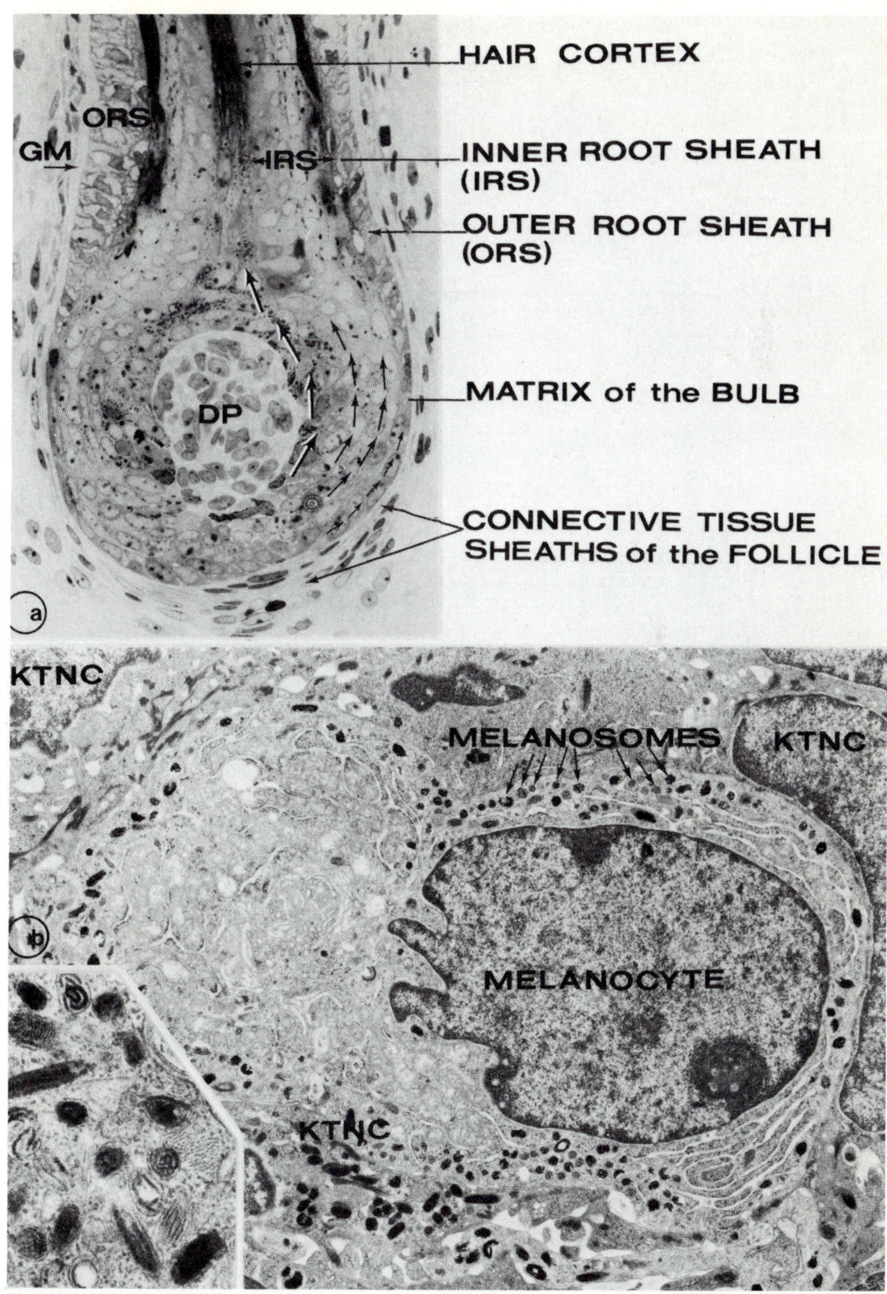

Figure 1-10 (*a*) The bulb of a lanugo hair showing the layers of matrix cells. The shaded arrows indicate cells of the presumptive hair cortex. Medium-sized arrows indicate cells of the presumptive layers of the inner root sheath, and small arrows point to the matrix cells of the presumptive outer root sheath. The thickened clear zone external to the outer root sheath is the basal lamina, called the glassy membrane (GM). Note the pigmented cells of the presumptive cortex. DP = dermal papilla. ×550 in the original magnification. (*b*) A melanocyte enlarged from the matrix of the hair cortex. Note the various stages of pigment formation in the melanosomes (inset). KTNC = keratinocyte. ×7900, inset ×29,550 in the original magnification.

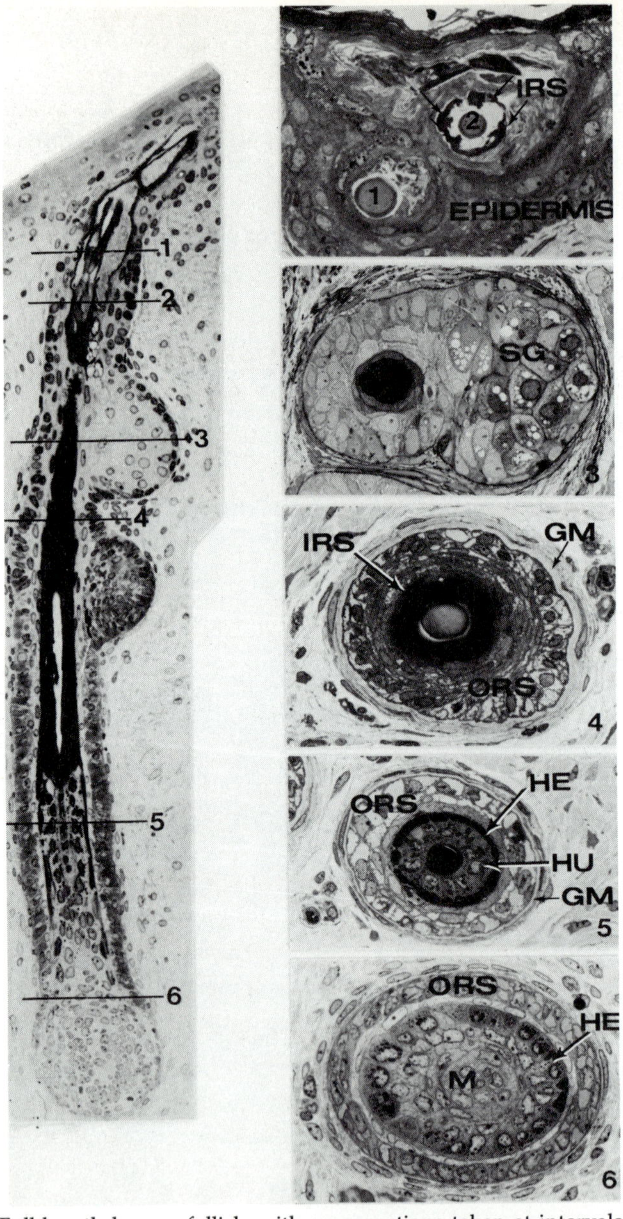

Figure 1-11 Full-length lanugo follicle with cross sections taken at intervals and identified by numbered lines. IRS = inner root sheath; SG = sebaceous gland; GM = glassy membrane, ORS = outer root sheath; HE = Henle's layer; HU = Huxley's layer; M = matrix. ×100 (whole mount), ×300 (cross sections) in the original magnification.

intermediate level of the bulb (Fig. 1-10*a*). Henle's layer is the most external of the three (Figs. 1-9 and 1-11). Huxley's layer is the middle layer, and the cuticle of the inner root sheath is the most internal layer (Figs. 1-9 and 1-11). Cells in each of these layers have abundant keratin filaments and synthesize trichohyalin as they undergo differentiation. Each layer keratinizes but at different levels within the follicle. Henle's layer keratinizes at the lower (first) level in the follicle, followed by the cells of the inner root sheath cuticle and the cells of Huxley's layer. All the layers are keratinized around the mid-level of the lower follicle, forming a keratinized tube that persists to the level of the infundibulum, where it begins to disintegrate, shedding cells into the infundibiulum of the follicle (Fig. 1-11). Some of the squamae remain adherent to the hair as it grows outward. It is important to point out that cells of the basal epidermal layer and the follicle matrix both divide and give rise to cells that differentiate. The process of keratinization, however, involves different sets of keratin and matrix proteins in the suprabasal epidermal keratinocytes and the cells of the inner root sheath and hair.

The hair organizes from matrix cells positioned centrally in the bulb. The outermost layer of the hair is the cuticle, a series of overlapping, shinglelike, cornified cells that interdigitate with cells of the cuticle of the inner root sheath; thus the two move toward the surface as a unit (Fig. 1-10*a*). The cuticle encloses the cortex of the hair, the substance of all or most of the hair shaft. Cortical cells arise from matrix cells directly above the deepest cells of the dermal papilla (Fig. 1-10). They contain melanin granules and large, dense bundles of longitudinally oriented filaments enmeshed in an electron-dense material that does not appear to be equivalent to either keratohyalin or trichohyalin. Cortical cells keratinize later than cuticle cells. Their nuclei persist after the organelles are no longer visible and until the cells are fully keratinized approximately one-third of the distance between the tip of the follicle and the epidermal surface. The thickness of the cortex varies with the type of hair. A medulla, when present, is usually a poorly keratinized single or discontinuous strand of cells separated by a large amount of intercellular space.

The infundibulum of the follicle opens to the surface. The cell layers of this region are continuous with those of the interfollicular epidermis and, in all respects, are equivalent structurally and biochemically.

Arrector Pili Muscle

Most hairs of the body can be elevated by an arrector pili muscle, which consists of a bundle of smooth muscle cells that originate beneath the epidermis, in association with elastic connective tissue fibers, and terminate on a collection of follicular cells, termed the *bulge,* located distal to the sebaceous gland (Fig. 1-9). When the muscle contracts, the angulated follicle is pulled vertically, thus elevating the hair.

The Sebaceous Gland and Sebaceous Follicles

Sebaceous glands develop during fetal development from keratinocytes of the elongating follicle. They are small in the child and produce little sebum; in the adult, their size and development depend upon the body region. The scalp, face, upper back, and chest are sites of large sebaceous glands; they are sparsely distributed on the dorsal surface of the hands and feet, and are absent on the palms and soles. The gland is composed of multiple acini separated by connective tissue partitions (Figs. 1-12 and 1-13); the cells of each acinus exhibit a hierarchy of differentiation. The peripheral cells divide mitotically to produce daughter cells that move

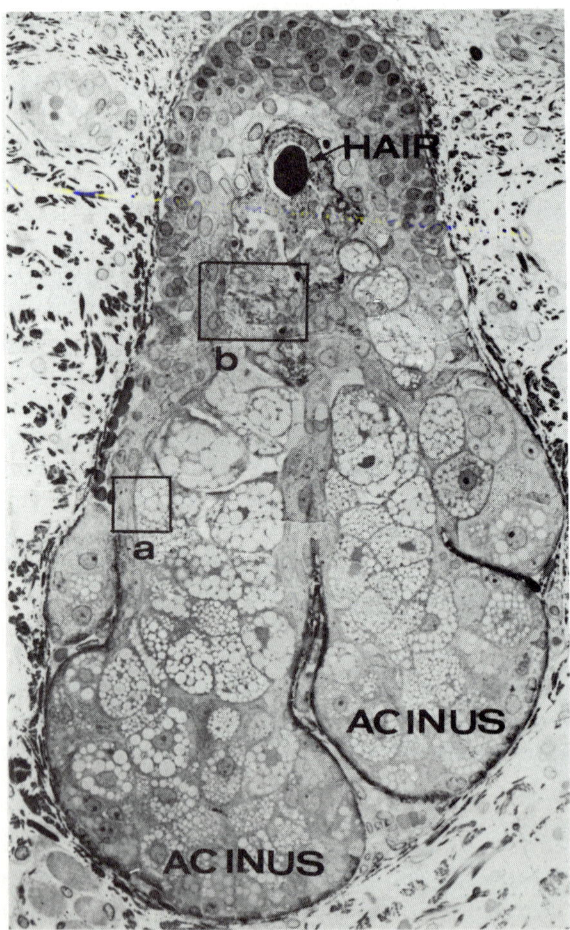

Figure 1-12 Sebaceous gland associated with a follicle from the scalp of a newborn infant. Note the multiple acini separated by connective tissue partitions and the progressive filling of cells with lipid toward the center of the gland and the hair. The two boxed areas are enlarged in Fig. 1-13. ×300 in the original magnification.

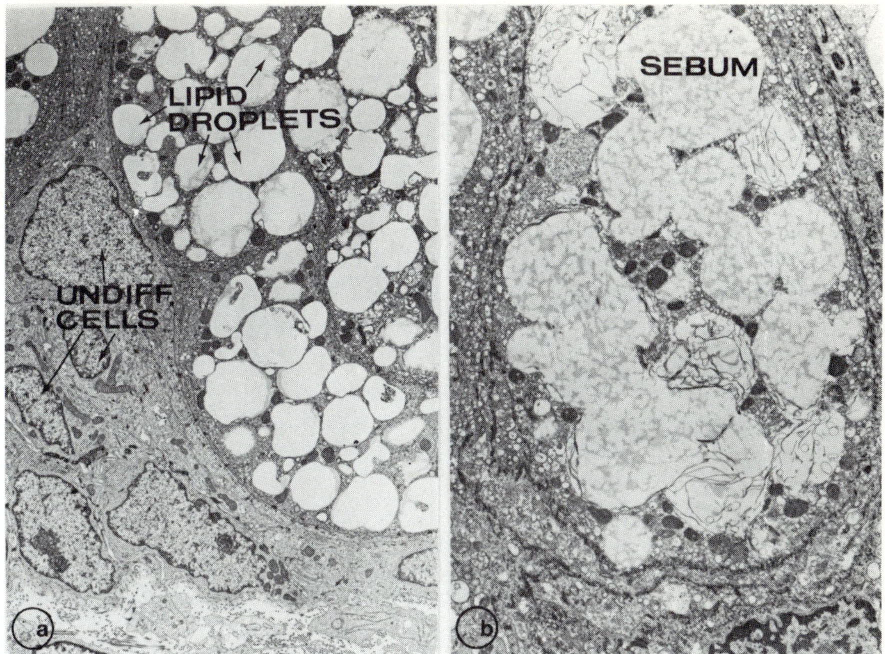

Figure 1-13 (*a*) Cells from the periphery of an acinus indicated on Fig. 1-12. Note the undifferentiated cells and the lipid vesicles in more central cells. ×3400 in the original magnification. (*b*) Most of the cell has disintegrated as it has filled with lipid. ×6200 in the original magnification.

toward the interior of the gland, accumulating lipid-rich droplets in the cytoplasm that increase in size and coalesce, ultimately disintegrating into lipid-rich cellular fragments that collect in a short sebaceous duct that empties into the infundibulum (Fig. 1-13). Lysosomes within the cell may be responsible for the programmed autolysis that accompanies holocrine secretion by this gland.

Secretion begins early during intrauterine life and contributes to the oily coating on the surface of the fetus known as vernix caseosa.[35] Growth and secretory activity of the gland in both the fetus and the pubertal-postpubertal individual are stimulated directly and primarily by androgenic hormones; other hormones (e.g., from the adrenal gland, thyroid gland, anterior pituitary gland) influence sebaceous gland activity indirectly.

While all follicles have an associated sebaceous gland, there are some follicles that are little more than sebaceous glands and therefore are referred to as sebaceous follicles. They lack a hair or have only a tiny vellus hair, are large and multilobulated, and have a wide piliary canal. Sebaceous follicles are found on the face, back, and chest; specialized cutaneous glands on the eyelid, lip, nipple, glans penis, prepuce, and buccal mucosa are modified sebaceous glands.

The Eccrine Sweat Gland

The eccrine sweat glands are simple tubular glands that are important in secretion of water and electrolytes; excretion of heavy metals, macromolecules, and other organic compounds; and thermoregulation.[36] Two-thirds of the tubule forms the coiled secretory end piece (Fig. 1-14). A straight or undulating duct conveys the secreted sweat toward the epidermis, where it penetrates the tissue and opens via the sweat pore opening at the skin surface (Fig. 1-15*a* and *b*). Eccrine sweat glands are typically located in the deep reticular dermis or subcutaneous fat and are often embedded in fat and other diffuse connective tissues surrounding the terminal portion of a hair follicle. They are distributed over all the body surface, with different regional densities; high concentrations of sweat glands are found on the palmar and plantar surfaces (where they also develop first) and the forehead.

The Secretory Segment

A single layer of columnar or pyramidal cells forms the wall of the secretory segment (Figs. 1-14 and 1-16). Basophilic, mucin-secreting "dark" cells and pale, sweat-producing "clear" cells border the lumen of the gland. The dark cells present a greater surface area to the cavity than the clear cells. Both cell types are modified at their apical borders by microvilli and seal the cellular compartment from the lumen by tight junctions. Myoepithelial cells are located at the periphery of the gland inside the basal lamina (Fig. 1-16).

Dark cells contain large (1- to 2-μm-diameter), membrane-bound mucous granules that are slightly irregular in shape and variable in density. Mitochondria are dispersed among the granules; a nucleus lies along the basal border of the cell, capped by a supranuclear Golgi apparatus. Rough endoplasmic reticulum, intermediate filaments, lysosomes, and other typical cytoplasmic organelles are also evident in the cytoplasm. Dark cells join with clear cells by desmosomes.

Clear cells are serous fluid–secreting cells that produce sweat (water and electrolytes). They have a pale cytoplasm, lack granules, and are characterized by intricate cell margins (canaliculi) and large stores of glycogen (Fig. 1-16). Intercellular canaliculi are complex tubular channels, lined by long, densely packed, interdigitating microvilli, organized between two or more adjacent clear cells. They convey the secretion into the lumen of the gland (Fig. 1-16, segment). Clear cells also interdigitate with dark cells by microvilli, but these borders are not as extensively developed as those between clear cells.

A discontinuous layer of myoepithelial cells lies external to the secretory cells. They are aligned with a slightly helical turn relative to the long axis of the gland and have morphologic and mechanical properties of smooth muscle cells (Fig. 1-16). Bundles of myofilaments with intermittent densities are present within the cytoplasm, glycogen is distributed about the nucleus,

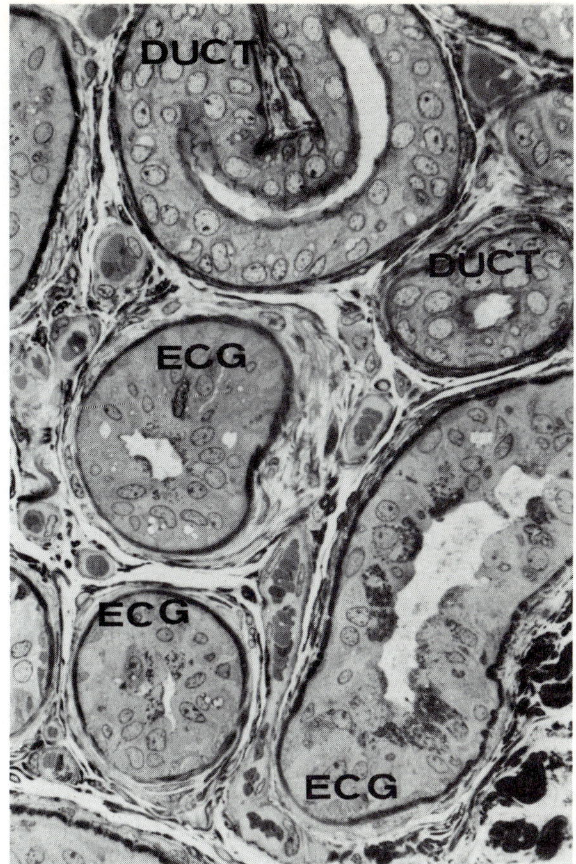

Figure 1-14 Light micrograph through the secreting end piece of an eccrine sweat gland. Three coils of the gland (ECG) and two sections through the duct are evident. Granules within dark cells are apparent adjacent to the lumen of the gland. Note the rich supply of vessels surrounding the glandular coils. ×400 in the original magnification.

and dense plaques and micropinocytotic vesicles are evident at intervals along the plasma membrane. Although myoepithelial cells are capable of contraction, this action may not be related to the propulsion of sweat. These cells are thought, instead, to provide support to the secretory segment and prevent swelling of the gland when sweat accumulates in the lumen, thus forcing the sweat upward into the duct.[37] Dark cells abut myoepithelial cells and project processes between them to attach to the basal lamina; neither type of secretory cell forms junctions with the myoepithelial cells.

The eccrine sweat gland is surrounded by a broad, regular zone of collagen fibrils interspersed with elastic microfibrils and small amounts of elastin matrix (Fig. 1-16). Long, circumferentially arranged processes of fibroblastic cells form an external boundary to the sheath.

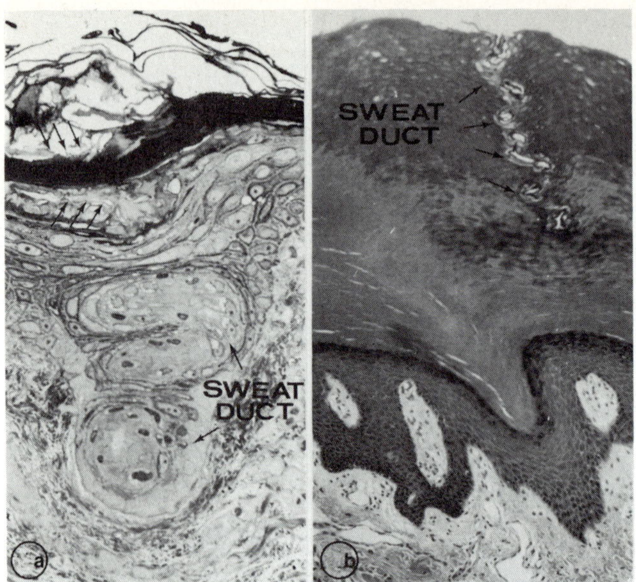

Figure 1-15 (*a*) Coiled sweat duct penetrating the epidermis of the arm. The disorganized area of the epidermis near the surface is the approximate position of the sweat pore (*arrows*). ×450 in the original magnification. (*b*) The path of the coiled intraepidermal sweat duct is evident in the thickened stratum corneum of the plantar epidermis. ×170 in the original magnification.

Most nerve fibers supplying the sweat gland are cholinergic, although adrenergic fibers have also been recognized. There is evidence that sweating can occur in response to stimulation of both types of fibers, although it is likely that cholinergic stimulation is the major stimulus for visible sweating.

The Eccrine Sweat Duct

The eccrine sweat duct is the site of resorption of ions back into the tissue, thus altering the isotonic or slightly hypertonic sweat into a hypotonic fluid. The morphologic features of the cells that form the duct are modified for this function. Two to three layers of cells, depending upon the level in the skin, form the wall of the duct. The cells of all layers join by interlocking lateral margins and desmosomes. Luminal cells are joined by tight junctions and are modified by microvilli as they face the cavity. Microfilaments within the microvilli insert into a periluminal filamentous zone that includes microfilaments, intermediate filaments, and vesicles. This structure is visible by light microscopy and has been described as the cuticular border. Cells of the duct are rich in mitochondria, particularly the abluminal basal cells, and contain intermediate filaments and glycogen in the cytoplasm.

The lumen of the duct widens as it approaches and enters the epidermis. Within the epidermis, both luminal and basal cells of the duct synthesize

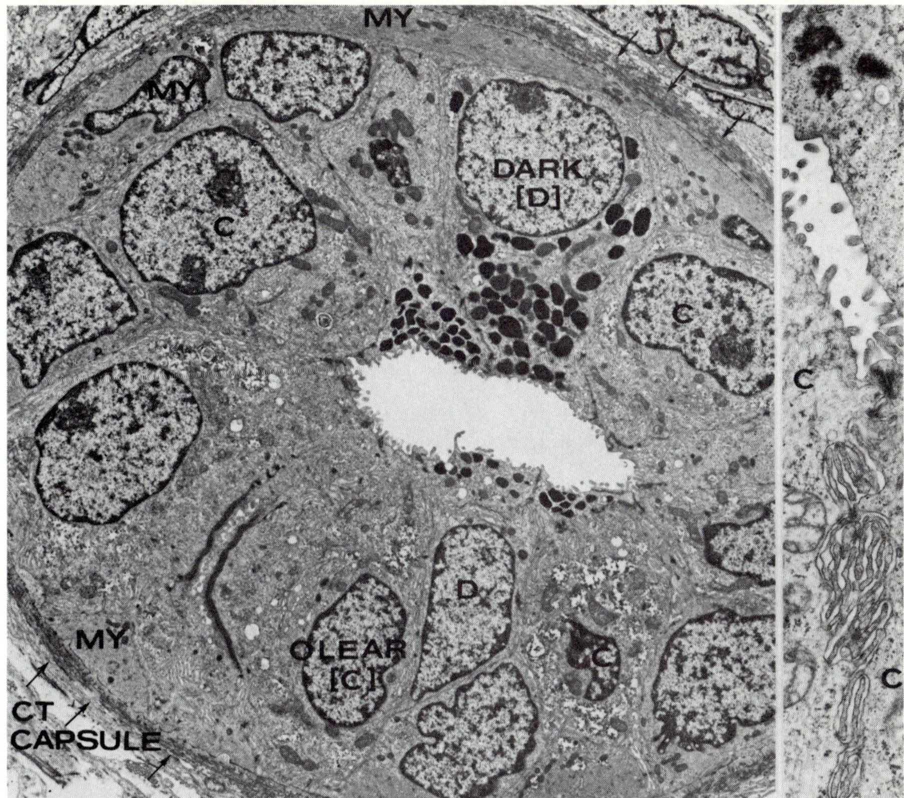

Figure 1-16 Section through one secretory coil of an eccrine sweat gland. The clear (C) and dark (D) secretory cells and the myoepithelial (MY) cells are evident. A connective tissue capsule (CT) surrounds the coil. ×4300 in the original magnification. An intercellular canaliculus between two clear cells is shown in the narrow right-hand segment. ×15,400 in the original magnification.

a globular form of keratohyalin and develop large numbers of multivesicular bodies (containing lysosomal enzymes) in the cytoplasm. The cells keratinize near the epidermal surface to form several layers of squamae that reinforce (and occasionally plug) the opening of the sweat pore.

The Apocrine Sweat Gland

Apocrine sweat glands[38] and eccrine sweat glands have a number of common structural characteristics, as well as features that are unique to each. Both have secretory cells that contain granules, myoepithelial cells, modifications of the cells lining the glandular and ductal segments, and a thick connective tissue capsule. Apocrine glands, however, are fewer in number, more restricted in distribution, generally larger in size, and located deeper in the dermis.

Apocrine sweat glands are found in the axillae, anogenital regions, abdomen, face, and scalp. Specialized apocrine glands include the ceruminous glands of the external auditory meatus and the areola of the breast. Only in the axilla are the numbers of apocrine glands high enough to form a 1:1 ratio with the eccrine sweat glands.

The Secretory Segment

Apocrine glands, like eccrine sweat glands, are also simple, blind tubes with the secreting endpiece highly coiled and embedded in subcutaneous fat. Only one type of secretory cell composes the single-layered cuboidal or columnar glandular epithelium. Cuboidal cells tend to have more microvilli at the luminal border. Columnar cells tend to bulge into the lumen beyond the junctions at their apical-lateral margins. Both cuboidal and columnar cells seal the lumen from the glandular tissue by junctional complexes at the apical borders.

The secretory cells have rough endoplasmic reticulum, mitochondria, multiple Golgi zones, and cytoplasmic granules. They all contain at least one type of secretory granule, and some cells contain several different morphologically distinct granules. A membrane-bound, PAS-positive, electron-dense granule called the true secretory granule is present in all cells. It is believed to arise in the Golgi or from the rough endoplasmic reticulum. It contains small, opaque particles and small lipid droplets organized on a filamentous matrix. A second granule type, found in only certain cells, is believed to form from rodlike structures in the rough endoplasmic reticulum. These granules can become extraordinarily large with the accumulation of ferritin particles, small and large lipid droplets, and lipofuscin material. A small, dense core granule, which may be a precursor to the secretory granule, has been described as a third population of granules.[38,39] A clear, oily secretion containing protein, carbohydrate, ammonia, and lipid is moved from the broad lumen of the gland, where it is retained, into the duct.

Myoepithelial cells in the apocrine gland are arranged in the same manner as in the eccrine sweat gland and also assist in the movement of fluid into the duct, either actively or by providing resistance to changes in luminal volume.[40]

The Apocrine Sweat Duct

The apocrine sweat duct has three layers of cells in the epithelial wall. Luminal cells resemble those of the eccrine sweat duct in having a microvillous border and a periluminal filamentous zone. Basal cells contain multiple mitochondria and glycogen, although resorption of fluid and/or ions is not believed to occur in the ductal segment, as it does in the eccrine gland. The duct of the apocrine gland lacks its own orifice and, instead, merges with the infundibular portion of the hair canal, thus conveying its product to the surface of the skin, mixed with sebaceous secretion. Because of this association with the follicle, apocrine glands are also referred to as epitrichial glands.

The Nail

Nails are hard, keratinized plates that protect the terminal digits and improve the dexterity of the fingers. The nail is the end product of dead, differentiated matrix cells.

Histologic and Fine Structure of the Nail

Four structurally and functionally distinct epithelial zones of the nail are revealed by tracing the epidermal surface from point A to point B in Fig. 1-17. These zones have been described collectively as the nail unit.[41] The first zone is the proximal nail fold or eponychium.[42] This is an upper fold of tissue that lies directly above the most proximal (deepest) portion of the nail plate. It has dorsal and ventral surfaces. The dorsal surface is continuous with the epidermis on the dorsum of the digit. It undergoes typical epidermal keratinization and has conspicuous rete ridges at the dermal-epidermal junction. The underlying dermis is richly vascularized and may contain sweat glands. The cuticle is an extension of the stratum corneum of the dorsal proximal fold.

The organization of the epidermis changes abruptly where the tissue folds inward as the ventral surface of the proximal nail fold (Fig. 1-17). The cellular layers and the dermal-epidermal junction become flattened; a granular layer remains, but the cornified cells merge imperceptibly with

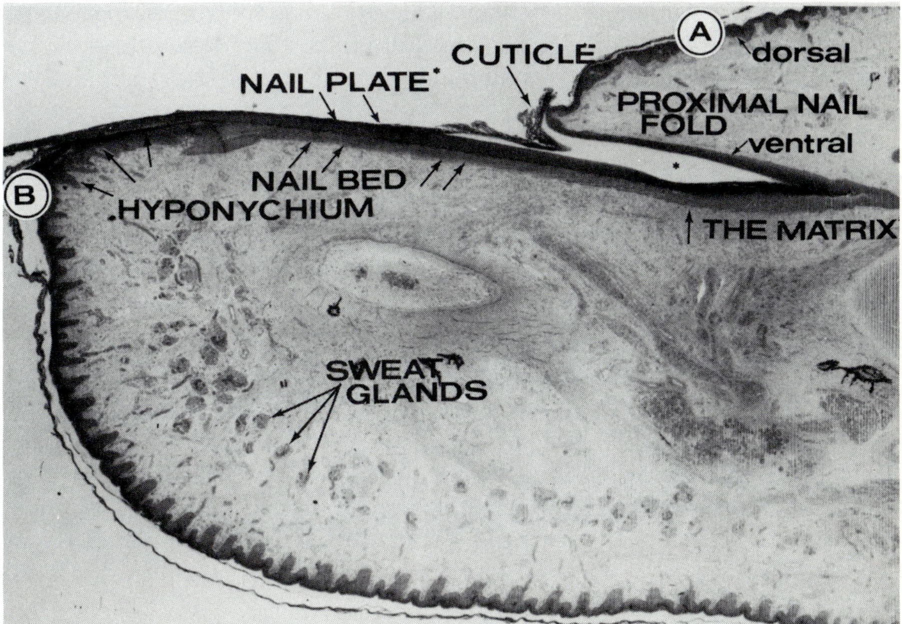

Figure 1-17 Section through a terminal digit of a newborn human infant. The four epithelial regions of the nail unit are traced along the surface from point A to point B. $\times 18$ in the original magnification.

the nail plate or are desquamated from the surface and pushed outward, contributing to the cuticle. There is controversy as to whether the ventral, proximal nail fold epithelium contributes cells to the nail plate. Some believe that it synthesizes a thin dorsal plate of the nail and thus refer to this surface of the proximal fold as the dorsal matrix.[43]

The ventral aspect of the proximal nail fold ends at the terminal portion of the root of the nail. Continuing distally from the root is another epithelial region that is the primary germinative tissue for the nail plate, named the matrix,[41] the ventral matrix,[42] or the intermediate matrix.[43] The matrix extends distal to its junction with the nail bed, the distal border of the lunula.

The matrix epithelium is thick, and the basal layers extend into the dermis in prominent "rootlike" rete ridges (Fig. 1-17). The cells in the upper layers of the matrix lack keratohyalin and keratinize in a manner similar to that of parakeratosis; cornified cells have a thickened envelope and densely packed filaments and often contain remnants of the nucleus. Cell division occurs continuously in all areas of the matrix, pushing cells within the tissue upward and forward diagonally. The direction of growth is a function of the orientation of matrix germinal cells. The size of the matrix determines the thickness of the nail.

The next epithelial region of the nail unit is the nail bed (Fig. 1-17). It is seen externally as the pink portion of the nail. In sections, the tissue is recognized by its longitudinal ridges and grooves. The dermis beneath the ridges includes a dense capillary network, numerous arteriovenous anastomoses, and abundant lymphatics. Like the nail matrix, the nail bed epithelium lacks a granular layer and keratinizes parakeratotically. The cornified cells produced in the nail bed adhere tightly to the undersurface of the nail but do not contribute appreciably to the substance of the nail.

The final epithelial zone of the nail unit is the hyponychium, which lies beneath the free tip of the nail. The tissue is comparable to epidermis and the epithelium of the dorsal proximal nail fold. Keratohyalin granules are present in a granular layer, and differentiation of cells occurs in an outward direction. Cornified squamae shed from the surface collect beneath the unattached extension of the nail in the same manner as with the cuticle.

DERMIS

The regions of the dermis are defined primarily by differences in the size and density of collagen fiber bundles, assembly (maturity) of elastic fibers, types and density of cells, and position of vascular plexuses. The two major zones, the papillary and reticular regions, are involved differently in systemic and genetic diseases and respond dissimilarly to environmental assaults.[44]

Connective Tissue Matrix Molecules of the Dermis

The dermal matrix is composed of fibrous and nonfibrous matrix molecules. The fibrous proteins impart bulk, density, and tensile strength to skin but also allow for compliance and elasticity. Filamentous glycoproteins in the dermis function in cell-matrix attachment. Nonfibrous matrix molecules, such as proteoglycans, form the ground substance that influences the osmotic properties of skin, permits cellular migration in a more fluid milieu, and serves as an integrative, continuous medium for all the other structural elements.

Regions of the Dermis (Table 1-1)

Papillary Dermis

The papillary dermis contains small bundles of small-diameter collagen fibrils. Biochemical and immunohistochemical analyses of this region reveal

Table 1-1

COMPARISON OF THE STRUCTURE AND COMPOSITION OF THE PAPILLARY AND RETICULAR DERMIS

Characteristics	Papillary Dermis	Reticular Dermis
Matrix organization	Loose, fine collagen fibers	Dense; intermediate and coarse collagen fibers
Collagen types	I, III, V, VI; type 1 procollagen	I, III, V, VI
Fibronectin	Present in a linear pattern; may concentrate along the dermal-epidermal junction; intense immunofluorescence staining	Present in reticulate pattern; low-intensity immunofluorescence staining except around vessels and in sheaths of epidermal appendages
Collagenase	Activity can be demonstrated	Activity can be demonstrated
Elastic fibers	Immature oxytalan and elaunin fibers	Elaunin and fully mature elastic fibers
Cellularity	Dense cellularity	Sparse cellularity
Fibroblast morphology	Active by morphologic criteria; basophilic	Less active by morphologic criteria
Fibroblast proliferation	Greater proliferative capacity	Less proliferative capacity
Vascular organization	Microcirculation; capillary loops	Distributing vessels, microcirculation associated with appendages

Source: Modified from LT Smith et al, Structure of the dermal matrix during development and in the adult. *J Invest Dermatol* 79:96s, 1982.

the presence of types I, III, V, and VI collagen and types I and III procollagen.[44] Elastic fibers are present only as bundles of microfibrils coated with soluble elastin (oxytalan fibers) or with small amounts of cross-linked elastin (elaunin fibers).[28] Cells are more abundant in the papillary dermis than in the reticular dermis, the fibroblasts have greater mitotic activity, and the density of blood vessels is greater. The papillary dermis continues around the epidermal appendages as the periadnexal connective tissue and is equivalent to the finely organized matrix surrounding the vessels. A horizontal plexus of blood vessels forms an approximate border between the papillary and reticular regions. Capillary loops project toward the epidermis from the horizontal plexus.

A thin layer of connective tissue immediately underlying the epidermal basal lamina forms a special region of the papillary dermis described as the subepidermal band or reticular lamina. Anchoring fibrils insert directly into the collagen of this tissue. Immunofluorescence staining has localized fibronectin and type I procollagen to this zone.

Reticular Dermis

The bulk of the dermis is the reticular dermis. It includes large bundles of collagen fibrils and mature elastic fibers that have a high proportion of elastin relative to the microfibrillar component. In normal dermis, elastic fibers are located between collagen bundles and are seen in sections as bordering their perimeters. The same collagens present in papillary dermis are also characteristic of the reticular dermis. Types I and III collagen are the primary constituents of the large fiber bundles. Type V collagen surrounds the bundles, and type VI is dispersed throughout the dermal matrix.[44] The epidermal appendages extend deep into the reticular dermis, where they either terminate or penetrate even deeper into the subcutaneous tissue. Vessels pass vertically through the reticular dermis, connecting a horizontal subcutaneous plexus with the subpapillary plexus and giving off microcirculatory networks to the hair follicles and sweat glands. The reticular dermis has fewer cells than the papillary dermis, although fibroblasts, macrophages, and mast cells are found in the interstitium between collagen bundles.

The uppermost portion of the reticular dermis in some individuals forms a distinct region that can be identified as an intermediate dermis. The size of collagen fibrils and fiber bundles in this region is intermediate between those of the papillary dermis and the deep reticular dermis. Elaunin elastic fibers are characteristic of this zone. This level of the dermis appears to be particularly susceptible to trauma and is a plane of low resistance that cleaves with applied shearing forces.

Cells of the Dermis

Fibroblasts, macrophages, and mast cells are regular residents of the dermis (Fig. 1-18). Small numbers of inflammatory cells also may collect around blood vessels.

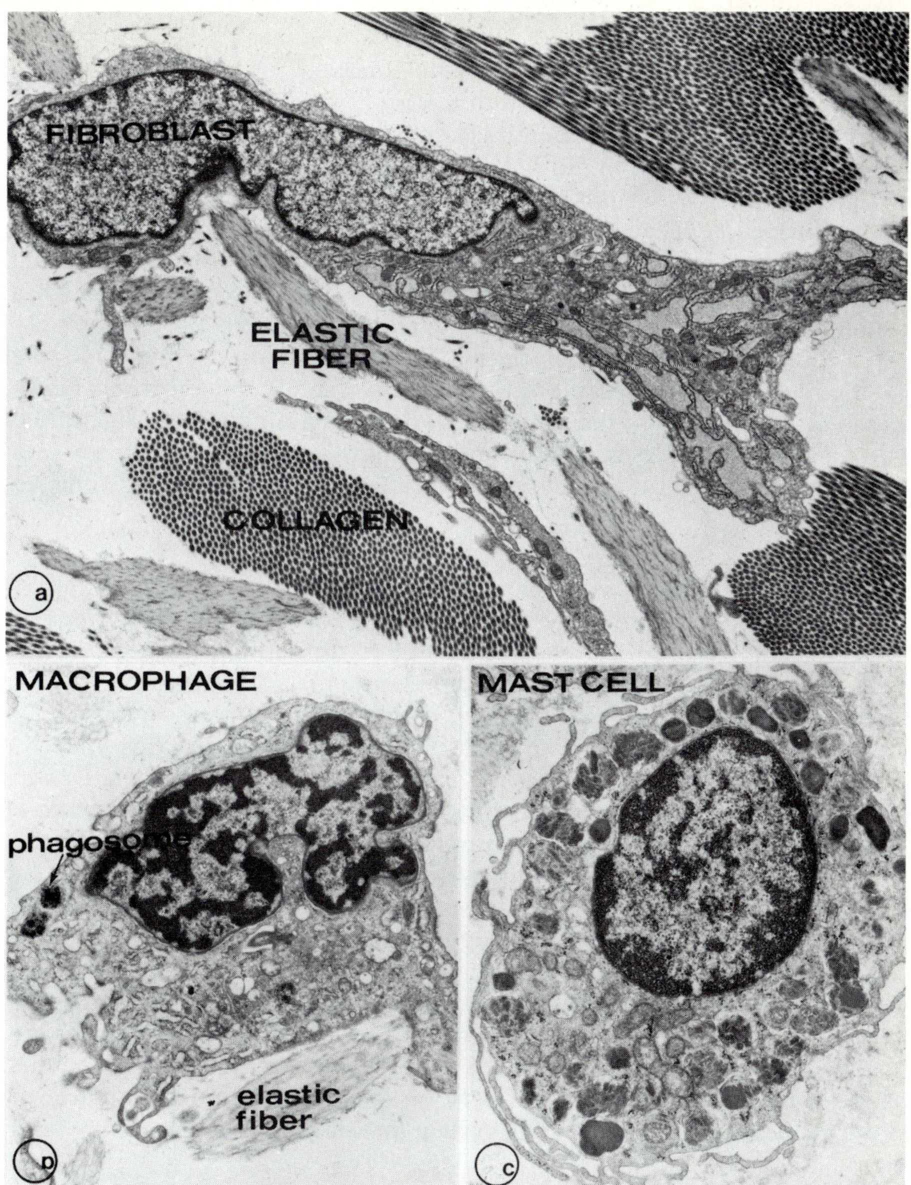

Figure 1-18 Common cells of the dermis. (*a*) Fibroblast surrounded by collagen fiber bundles and elastic fibers. Note the dilatation of the rough endoplasmic reticulum. ×6250 in the original magnification. *(From J Invest Dermatol 79:97s, 1982.)* (*b*) Macrophage. ×7000 in the original magnification. (*c*) Mast cell. Note the difference in morphology of various granules in the cytoplasm and the microvilli of the cell surface. ×13,200 in the original magnification.

The Fibroblast

The dermal fibroblast is a mesenchyme-derived cell that is responsible for the synthesis, destruction, and remodeling of the connective tissue matrix. Its shape depends upon its position relative to the fibrous matrix. Fibroblasts are usually found between bundles of collagen fibrils and in close association with elastic fibers and individual collagen fibrils. They rarely invade a collagen fiber bundle. Fibroblasts can be recognized by their well-developed rough endoplasmic reticulum, one or more regions of Golgi, and few, if any, phagocytic vacuoles (Fig. 1-18*a*). Focal densities evident along the plasma membrane are sites where proteins of the extracellular matrix (e.g., fibronectin) associate with elements of the cytoskeleton through receptors and integral membrane proteins. Fibronectin on the surface of the fibroblast assists in binding it to collagen. The fibroblast also synthesizes and secretes enzymes (e.g., collagenase and gelatinase) responsible for degradation and remodeling of the collagen matrix.

The Macrophage

Macrophages are common in the dermis (Fig. 1-18). They are derived from precursor cells in the bone marrow that differentiate into promonocytes and monocytes in the blood and then into macrophages in the tissue. Differentiation of the macrophage and development of phagocytic activity involve the synthesis and activation of several acid hydrolases and cell surface markers. Like other cells of this lineage, macrophages bear Fc and C3b receptors and possess histocompatibility antigens on the cell surface.[45] Fully differentiated macrophages are no longer capable of division.

Late-stage macrophages are large and have one or more nuclei, intermediate filaments, and an abundance of lysosomes and phagocytic vacuoles that may contain a variety of recognizable or unrecognizable, engulfed cellular debris (Fig. 1-18*b*). Macrophages that do not contain phagosomes are often difficult to distinguish from fibroblasts; both have similar organelles and well-developed rough endoplasmic reticulum. Macrophages are involved in synthesis and secretion of hydrolytic enzymes, components of the complement system, a variety of soluble factors that enhance or suppress T-lymphocyte activity, certain prostaglandins, interferon, and others.

Mast Cells

Mast cells are specialized, bone marrow–derived, secretory cells that are abundant within the connective tissue matrix. They are present in all regions of the dermis, but are most commonly found in the upper dermis around vessels and epidermal appendages and in the subcutaneous fat (Fig. 1-18*c*). Mast cells possess a round or oval nucleus and abundant darkly staining cytoplasmic granules. The cell surface is modified by microvilli and, like fibroblasts, mast cells are surrounded by a coat of fibronectin that helps to position and anchor them to the connective tissue matrix at sites of inflammation or wound repair, where they proliferate. Different populations of granules with varying types of internal structure are recognized (Fig. 1-18*c*).

Vascular Supply of the Skin

The vasculature of the skin is limited to the dermis, where it is composed of distributing and collecting vessels that link plexuses of microcirculatory vessels in the papillary dermis, subcutaneous tissue, and surrounding epidermal appendages.[46,47] Vessels of the dermis have a thicker vascular wall, supported by smooth muscle, pericytes, and collagen and elastic connective tissues, compared with vessels of the subcutaneous tissue or with those of comparable size found in other organs. It has been suggested that the extensive development of the connective tissue and cellular layers around the dermal vessels may add support to a tissue that is constantly subjected to shearing forces.

Small cutaneous branches of musculocutaneous arteries enter the deep reticular dermis from the subcutaneous fat, branch, and then ascend vertically through the dermis toward the epidermis. Branches connect adjacent ascending arterioles and extend to hair follicles and eccrine sweat glands, where they ramify into plexuses that encompass the hair bulb and secretory segments of the glands. The ascending arterioles terminate at the deep border of the papillary dermis, where they branch into a horizontal, subpapillary arteriolar plexus. As mentioned above, this plexus and its related venous channels appear to form a boundary between the papillary dermis and the intermediate level of the reticular dermis. Capillaries project from the plexus toward the epidermis, then drain into the horizontal venous channels organized in parallel layers above and below the arteriolar plexus.[46]

Most of the vessels in the subpapillary plexus are postcapillary venules. They are distinguished ultrastructurally from their arteriolar counterparts by the structure of the basal lamina. Several layers of basal lamina, usually separated by individually spaced collagen fibrils, surround the postcapillary venules, and a single continuous layer envelops the arteriole. The diameters of the arterioles and venules frequently overlap; thus this measurement is useful only if the vessels are side by side, allowing additional morphologic comparisons. The postcapillary venules are prominently involved in inflammatory reactions in the skin. They respond to mediators (e.g., histamine) by developing gaps between endothelial cells that permit extravasation of fluid from the vessel and cell diapedesis. Blood is drained from the subpapillary plexus by descending venules that parallel the ascending arterioles. Valves are present in venules at the dermal-subcutaneous junction.

Direct channels between the arterial and venous circulations also exist in the skin as alternative bypass channels to shunt blood around a congested capillary bed. These structures can have exaggerated development of the smooth muscle coat and are referred to as glomus bodies. They are particularly well developed on the palms and soles.

Lymphatics of the Skin

Lymphatic channels in the skin are important for the clearance of fluid, macromolecules, and cells from the dermis. Deformation of the skin by stretching and pressure guides the substances to the plexus of lymphatic vessels located in the middermis deep to the vessels of the subpapillary vascular plexus. Under normal circumstances, lymph channels are rarely found in the superficial papillary dermis, although a few blind-ending lymphatic loops may project into the dermal papillae. Lymph is drained from the subpapillary plexus to a second plexus positioned at the dermal-subcutaneous junction. It is likely that collection occurs only in the superficial lymphatic capillaries.[48]

The superficial lymphatic vessels are distinguished from blood vessels by a larger luminal diameter, a thin wall consisting largely of an attenuated and occasionally discontinuous endothelium, and the presence of valves. All lymphatic vessels of the skin have a meshwork of elastic fibers as the major supporting tissue of the wall. It has been suggested that the continuity between the mesh of elastic fibers surrounding the vessels and the elastic fiber network in the skin helps direct the movement of substances toward the lymph channels. The vessels of the deeper lymphatic plexus have thicker walls reinforced by smooth muscle.[48]

Cutaneous Innervation

The skin at every point of the body functions as a sensory receptor. Mechanical stimuli and sensations of pain are received by simple (free nerve endings) and complex (corpuscular) receptors. It is quite certain that the various sensory modalities cannot be correlated with a single type of receptor. Motor fibers of the autonomic nervous system supply the eccrine and apocrine sweat glands and smooth muscle of the arrector pili muscle and vessel wall.

Large, myelinated cutaneous branches of musculocutaneous nerves arise segmentally from spinal nerves to innervate the skin. Cutaneous branches of the trigeminal nerve innervate the face. The nerves branch before entering the deep dermis into finer fibers that are still surrounded by a perineurial sheath of collagen and elastic connective tissue and concentrically arranged fibroblasts (Fig. 1-19). Within the trigeminal nerve, epineurial and endoneurial sheaths and Schwann cells envelop fiber bundles and individual fibers. In parallel with the distributing vessels, the nerves form a deep plexus and then ascend to a superficial horizontal subpapillary plexus. Branches from nerves in both plexuses supply various regions and structures of the skin. The extent to which fibers retain their sheaths depends upon their terminal distribution. Although nerves supply the skin segmentally, the boundaries are imprecise and there is overlapping innervation to any given area.

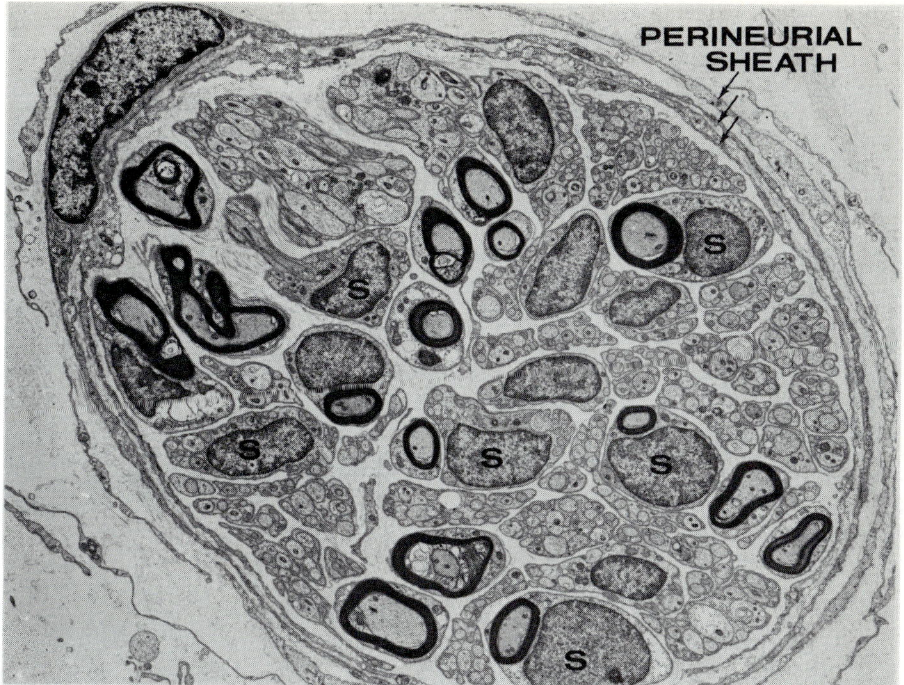

Figure 1-19 Myelinated and unmyelinated nerve fibers of a nerve belonging to the deep plexus in the reticular dermis. S = Schwann cells. ×4550 in the original magnification.

Free Nerve Endings

Free nerve endings are widespread. They are undoubtedly the most important sensory receptors of the body. In humans, they are never totally free of investing layers. Schwann cells and a basal lamina accompany even the finest terminals. Free nerve endings are found most commonly in the papillary dermis just beneath the epidermis (Fig. 1-8). They are branches from the subpapillary plexus or from the network of fibers that surrounds the hair follicle. The latter fibers supply the follicular orifice at the dermal-epidermal junction. Cauna[49] has described penicillate and papillary fibers within the papillary dermis.

The penicillate fibers are separate branches of a nerve that are ensheathed collectively by processes from the same Schwann cell. Their appearance in reconstructed serial sections of hairy skin is responsible for their name. They are suggested to be rapidly adapting receptors that receive external, probably multimodal, nonmechanical stimuli. Papillary fibers branch from the nerves that innervate the follicle and extend to the orifice of the follicle.

Free nerve endings[50] and corpuscular receptors are also present in nonhairy, ridged skin, where they project individually and vertically into about 60 percent of the dermal papilla, without the overlapping distribution characteristic of the penicillate endings. They probably function in fine discrimination.

Other free nerve endings in the skin are associated with specific structures such as hair follicles, individual Merkel cells, and complex Merkel cell receptors in the epidermis that have received various names, depending upon their location and the species (e.g., touch domes, Hederiform endings, Iggo's capsule, Pinkus corpuscles, Haarscheibe, etc.). Motor fibers en route to the eccrine sweat gland, arrector pili muscle, and sebaceous gland are carried along with the sensory fibers in the same distribution.

Corpuscular Receptors

Corpuscular sensory receptors are mechanoreceptors that have a capsular core and an inner core and contain both neural and nonneural components.[51] The capsule is a continuation of the perineurium, and the lamellated portion of the core is formed by wrapping of the Schwann cell about preterminal and terminal regions of the fiber. The size of these receptors depends upon their location within the skin (the deeper structures being larger) and, in some cases, upon the age of the individual. Remodeling of the receptors occurs throughout life.

DEVELOPMENT OF THE SKIN

The coordinated events in epidermal and dermal development, including the development of the vascular and nervous tissues within the skin, begin (visibly) in the second month of embryonic life and are not fully complete until several months after birth. Throughout all stages of development, the differentiation of skin is regulated by a multitude of intrinsic (genetic, metabolic) and extrinsic (microenvironmental) controls.[52,53]

First-Trimester Development

During the first trimester the skin changes from a single-layered ectoderm, basal lamina, and thin layer of mesenchyme to a template of adult skin.

By the end of the third month, the epidermis is stratified to three to four cell layers: basal, intermediate (one or two), and periderm. All cells are joined by desmosomes and contain a large amount of glycogen in their cytoplasm. Basal cells form hemidesmosomes with the basal lamina. Langerhans cells and melanocytes invade the epidermis, Merkel cells either invade the epidermis or differentiate in situ, and the primordia of the epidermal appendages form in at least some regions of the body (Fig. 1-20).

The periderm is the most superficial epidermal layer present only during embryogenesis. It forms at 3 to 4 weeks gestational age, when the epidermis becomes bilayered, and persists as a single blanket of cells covering the developing epidermis proper until keratinization of the interfollicular epidermis is completed in the 24th week. The periderm divides to keep pace with the expanding surface until the second trimester, when it appears to grow only by increasing in diameter. Periderm cells enlarge and undergo

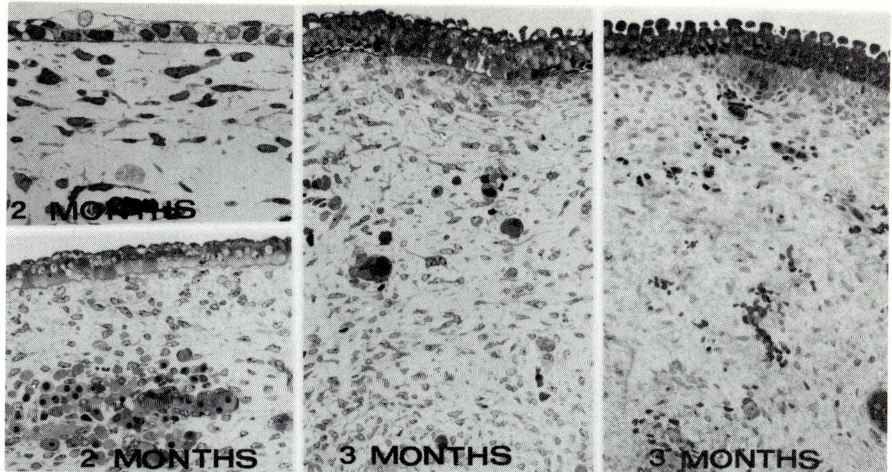

Figure 1-20 Full-thickness skin from embryos and fetuses. Note the stratification of the epidermis and the structure of the periderm cells in each sample. The dermis changes from a watery mesenchyme to a fibrous matrix by the end of the third month. Two months—top ×600, all others ×250 in the original magnification. (*Micrographs courtesy of Lynne T. Smith.*)

a series of morphologic changes that increase the membrane surface area of the cells at the border facing the amniotic cavity, thus suggesting that the periderm may have a role in the exchange of substances between the fetus and amniotic fluid before keratinization[54] (Figs. 1-20 through 1-22).

Development of the epidermal appendages is initiated by localized proliferations of basal cells, which grow into the dermis as cords of cells (eccrine and apocrine sweat glands and pilosebaceous units) or as a fold (nail fold). The process is thought to be induced by interactions between aggregations of certain mesenchymal cells and the epidermis, although the specific molecular interactions are still unclear. Differentiation of each structure occurs primarily in the second trimester, although the nail assumes a more definitive structure by the end of the first trimester. A summary of the development of each of the epidermal appendages has been included in reviews of cutaneous development.[52,53]

Early in the first trimester, the dermis consists of a cellular mesenchyme and an extracellular matrix that is rich in nonfibrous components, especially hyaluronic acid, thus giving the skin a gelatinous texture (Fig. 1-20). Collagen fibers are associated primarily with the cell surface and the basal lamina. Toward the end of the third month, mesenchymal cells become more fibroblastic in appearance and bundles of collagen fibrils are organized in the intercellular space. All of the dermal collagens present in adult dermis are synthesized, although the ratios of at least types I and III collagen are different from those in the adult. The level of type III collagen is elevated, consistent with the presence of a mechanically more compliant tissue. Only the microfibrillar component of the elastic fiber can be recognized at this age.

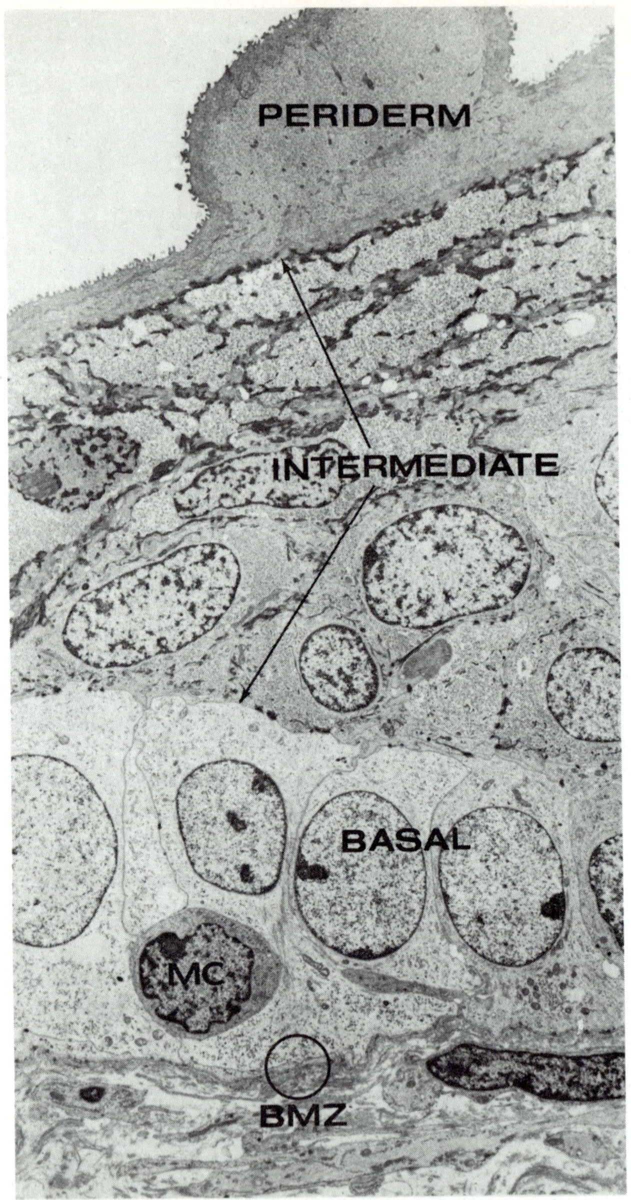

Figure 1-21 Full-thickness epidermis from a fetus of 15 weeks estimated gestational age. Basal cells have less glycogen than intermediate cells. The periderm cells typically have one or more blebs projecting from the surface. All the components of the BMZ are fully formed. A melanocyte (MC) is evident among the basal cells. ×4000 in the original magnification.

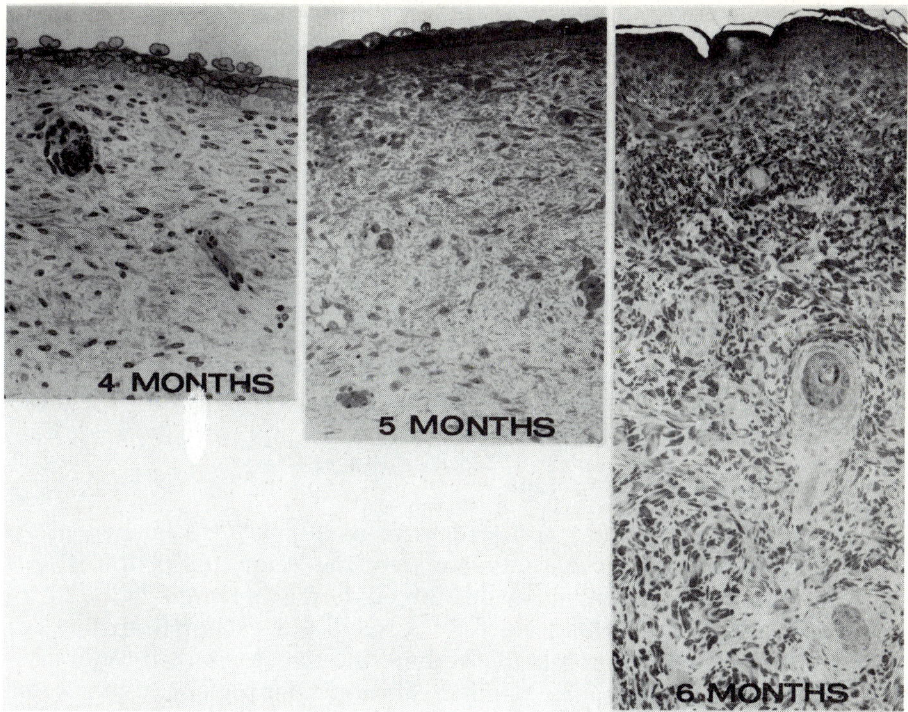

Figure 1-22 Full-thickness skin from second-trimester fetuses. Note the changes in epidermal surface morphology and the progressive increase of connective tissue matrix. ×250 in the original magnification. (*Micrographs courtesy of Lynne T. Smith.*)

Networks of vessels and nerves enter the dermis early in the first trimester (Fig. 1-20). A single horizontal plane of vessels is organized during the second month at the border between the dermis and subcutaneous tissue. Fine capillaries are recognized within the dermis and subcutaneous tissue, presumably as branches from the plexus. In the third month, a second plexus is organized within the tissue of the dermis between the presumptive papillary and reticular dermal regions. Subsequent additions to the vasculature at all levels continue in relation to the increased complexity of the dermal-epidermal junction, development of epidermal appendages, and increased thickness of the dermis. Although the basic pattern of vessels is assembled early, its definitive architecture is not established until after birth, coincident with the function of vessels in thermoregulation and the complete establishment of cutaneous structure (reviewed in Refs. 52 and 53).

Unmyelinated nerve fibers accompany vessels within the dermis. Small fibers grow toward the epidermis and in some instances penetrate it; however, intraepidermal nerves are transient. They withdraw as the epidermis increases in stratification and are rarely found after birth. In contrast to adult fibers, where a Schwann cell usually envelops a single fiber, Schwann cells in fetal nerves can enclose as many as 100 axons within a single "pocket." Segregation of fibers begins in the larger nerves during the first trimester, and with this isolation, myelination proceeds. Pacinian corpuscles are the earliest encapsulated receptors to form. In some regions of the body, they are present by 12 weeks (reviewed in Refs. 52 and 53).

The structure of the skin during the first trimester is simple compared with that of adult skin, but the biochemical properties of the cells and matrix of all regions suggest that many of the adult markers correlated with differentiation (e.g., keratins, antigens of the dermal-epidermal junction, matrix proteins) are expressed. Onset of expression appears to occur at the time of the embryonic-fetal transition, at 8 weeks estimated gestational age. It is not known how these coordinate changes are regulated.

Second-Trimester Development

The primordia of tissues and structures of the skin established in the first trimester undergo differentiation over the 3 months of the second trimester. At the end of this period, the epidermis is keratinized and the periderm is sloughed. Hairs are fully formed and extend from the skin surface, the nail plate is complete, and eccrine sweat glands develop over the general body surface. The papillary and reticular regions of the dermis are clearly delineated. Continued accretion of the matrix occurs throughout the remaining months of development; even at birth, the thickness of the dermis is substantially less than that of the adult.[55] The collagen fibrils and fiber bundles are small in diameter compared with those of the adult, and the elastic fibers are immature in structure and composition. Substantial additions to the dermis occur postnatally (Fig. 1-22).

Continual remodeling of the capillary beds occurs throughout the second and third trimesters, and even after birth, in accord with the continued development of the epidermis and its appendages. Capillary loops are present before birth only in a few regions (e.g., palms, soles, nail fold) where rete ridges and dermal papillae are organized at the dermal-epidermal junction. They are not stabilized or present elsewhere until several weeks after birth.

Third-Trimester Development

The structures and regions of the skin are established well before the third trimester; thus this period is largely one of maturation. The stratum corneum thickens, the dermal-epidermal junction begins to acquire an irregular interface created by alternating ridges and papillae, and the dermis and subcutaneous fat increase in thickness. It is unlikely that the eccrine sweat glands function in utero, but this is a peak period of activity of the sebaceous glands, which become quiescent after birth and remain so until the onset of puberty.

REFERENCES

1. Steinberg MS et al: On the molecular organization, diversity and functions of desmosomal complexes, in *Junctional Complexes of Epithelial Cells.* CIBA Foundation Symposium 125. New York, Wiley, 1987, p 3.
2. Tseng SCG et al: Correlation of specific keratins with different types of epithelial differentiation: monoclonal antibody studies. *Cell* 30:361, 1982.
3. Gelfant S: Cycling-noncycling cell transitions in tissue, aging, immunological surveillance, transformation and tumor growth. *Int Rev Cytol* 70:1, 1981.
4. Lavker RM, Sun T-T: Heterogeneity in basal keratinocytes: morphological and functional correlations. *Science* 215:1239, 1982.
5. Landmann L: Epidermal permeability barrier: transformation of lamellar granule-disks into intercellular sheets by a membrane-fusion process, a freeze-fracture study. *J Invest Dermatol* 87:202, 1986.
6. Lonsdale-Eccles JD et al: A phosphorylated keratohyalin-derived precursor of epidermal stratum corneum basic protein. *J Biol Chem* 255:2235, 1980.
7. Dale BA et al: Assembly of stratum corneum basic protein and keratin filaments in macrofibrils. *Nature* 276:729, 1978.
8. Elias PM: Lipids and epidermal permeability barrier. *Arch Dermatol Res* 270:95, 1981.
9. Elias PM: Epidermal lipids, membranes and keratinization. *Int J Dermatol* 20:2, 1981.
10. Green H: The keratinocyte as a differentiated cell type. *The Harvey Lectures Series* 74:101, 1979.
11. Suzuki H et al: Changes in nuclear DNA and RNA during epidermal keratinization. *Cell Tissue Res* 184:155, 1977.
12. Karasek J: Nuclear morphology of transitional keratinocytes in normal human epidermis. *J Invest Dermatol* 91:243, 1988.
13. Brody I: An ultrastructural study on the role of the keratohyalin granule in the keratinization process. *J Ultrastruct Res* 3:84, 1959.
14. Holbrook KA, Odland GF: Regional differences in the thickness (cell layers) of the human stratum corneum: an ultrastructural analysis. *J Invest Dermatol* 62:415, 1974.
15. Scott IR et al: Histidine-rich protein of the keratohyalin granules: source of the free amino acids, urocanic acid and pyrrolidone carboxylic acid in the stratum corneum. *Biochim Biophys Acta* 719:110, 1982.
16. Menton DN, Eisen AZ: Structure and organization of mammalian stratum corneum. *J Ultrastruct Res* 35:247, 1971.
17. Holbrook KA et al: The appearance, density and distribution of melanocytes in human embryonic and fetal skin revealed by the anti-melanoma monoclonal antibody, HMB-45. *Anat Embryol* 180:443, 1989.
18. Jimbow K et al: Some aspects of melanin biology: 1950–1975. *J Invest Dermatol* 67:72, 1976.
19. Katz SI et al: Epidermal Langerhans cells derived from cells originating in the bone marrow. *Nature* 282:324, 1979.
20. Rodriguez EM, Caorsi I: A second look at the ultrastructure of the Langerhans cell of the human epidermis. *J Ultrastruct Res* 65:297, 1978.
21. Takahashi S, Hashimoto K: Derivation of Langerhans cell granules from cytomembrane. *J Invest Dermatol* 84:469, 1985.
22. Romani N et al: Cultured human Langerhans cells resemble lymphoid dendritic cells in phenotype and function. *J Invest Dermatol* 93:600, 1989.
23. Moll I et al: Intraepidermal formation of Merkel cells in xenografts of human fetal skin. *J Invest Dermatol* 94:359, 1990.
24. Hartschuh W et al: The Merkel cell, in J Bereiter-Han et al (eds), *Biology of the Integument,* vol 2: *Vertebrates.* Berlin, Springer, 1986, p 606.
25. Hartschuh W et al: Chromogranin A in the mammalian Merkel cell: cellular and subcellular distribution. *J Invest Dermatol* 93:614, 1985.
26. Gottschaldt K-M, Vahle-Hinz C: Merkel cell receptors: structure and transducer function. *Science* 214:183, 1981.

27. Westgate G et al: Bullous pemphigoid antigen localization suggests an intracellular association with hemidesmosomes. *J Invest Dermatol* 84:218, 1985.
28. Cotta-Pierera G et al: Oxytalan, elaunin, and elastic fibers in the human skin. *J Invest Dermatol* 66:143, 1976.
29. Sakai L et al: Type VII collagen is a major structural component of anchoring fibrils. *J Cell Biol* 103:1577, 1986.
30. Woodley DT: The molecular organization of the basement membrane, in J Uitto, A Perejda (eds), *Connective Tissue Disease: Molecular Pathology of the Extracellular Matrix*. New York, Marcel Dekker, 1987, p 141.
31. Kazama T et al: Effect of enzyme digestion on anionic sites and charge selective permeability of dermo-epidermal junction. *J Invest Dermatol* 93:814, 1989.
32. Holbrook KA et al: Morphogenesis of hair follicles during the ontogeny of the human skin, in GE Rogers et al (eds), *The Biology of Wool and Hair*. London and New York, Chapman and Hall, 1989, p 15.
33. Spearman RIC: The structure and function of the fully developed follicle, in A Jarrett (ed), *Physiology and Pathophysiology of the Skin*. New York, Academic Press, 1977, vol 4, p 1294.
34. Sengel R: Role of extracellular matrix in the development of skin and cutaneous appendages, in JW Lash, L Saxén (eds), *Developmental Mechanisms: Normal and Abnormal*. In *Progress in Clinical and Biological Research*. New York, Alan R. Liss, 1985, p 123.
35. Nazzaro-Porro M et al: Effects of aging on fatty acids in skin surface lipids. *J Invest Dermatol* 73:112, 1979.
36. Hashimoto K: The eccrine sweat gland, in A Jarrett (ed), *The Physiology and Pathophysiology of the Skin*. New York, Academic Press, 1978, vol 5, p 1544.
37. Sato K et al: Mechanical properties and functions of the myoepithelium in the eccrine sweat gland. *Am J Physiol* 237:C177, 1979.
38. Hashimoto K: The apocrine gland, in A Jarrett (ed), *Physiology and Pathophysiology of the Skin*. New York, Academic Press, 1978, vol 5, p 1575.
39. Bell M: The ultrastructure of the human axillary apocrine glands after epinephrine injection. *J Invest Dermatol* 63:147, 1974.
40. Sato K: Pharmacological responsiveness of the myoepithelium of the isolated human axillary apocrine sweat gland. *Br J Dermatol* 102:235, 1980.
41. Zaias N: *The Nail in Health and Disease*. New York, Spectrum, 1980.
42. Rynne U, Orfanos CE: The human nail: structure, growth and pathological changes. *Curr Probl Dermatol* 9:102, 1981.
43. Spearman, RIC: The physiology of the nail, in A Jarrett (ed), *Physiology and Pathophysiology of the Skin*. New York, Academic Press, 1978, vol 5, p 1812.
44. Holbrook KA, Byers PH: Skin is a window on heritable disorders of connective tissue. *Am J Med Genet* 34:105, 1989.
45. Stingl G et al: Analogous functions of macrophages and Langerhans cells in the initiation of the immune response. *J Invest Dermatol* 71:59, 1978.
46. Braverman IM: Ultrastructure and organization of the cutaneous microvasculature in normal and pathologic states. *J Invest Dermatol* 93:2s, 1989.
47. Ryan TJ: Structure, pattern and shape of the blood vessels of the skin, in A Jarrett (ed), *The Physiology and Pathophysiology of the Skin*. New York, Academic Press, 1973, vol 2, p 577.
48. Ryan TJ: Structure and function of lymphatics. *J Invest Dermatol* 93:18s, 1989.
49. Cauna N: The free penicillate nerve endings of the human hairy skin. *J Anat* 115:277, 1973.
50. Cauna N: Fine morphological characteristics and microtopography of the free nerve endings in human digital skin. *Anat Rec* 198:643, 1980.
51. Halata Z: The mechanoreceptors of the mammalian skin: ultrastructure and morphological classification, in A Brodal et al (eds), *Advances in Anatomy, Embryology and Cell Biology*. New York, Springer-Verlag, 1975, vol 50, p 1.
52. Holbrook KA: Structure and function of the developing human skin, in LA Goldsmith

(ed), *Biochemistry and Physiology of the Skin,* 2d ed. Oxford, Oxford University Press, in press.
53. Holbrook KA: Structural and biochemical organogenesis of skin and cutaneous appendages in the fetus and neonate, in RA Polin, WW Fox (eds), *Neonatal and Fetal Medicine, Physiology and Pathophysiology.* New York, Grune & Stratton, in press.
54. Holbrook KA, Odland GF: The fine structure of developing human epidermis: light, scanning and transmission electron microscopy of the periderm. *J Invest Dermatol* 65:16, 1975.
55. Holbrook KA: A histological comparison of infant and adult skin, in HI Maibach, EK Boisits (eds), *Neonatal Skin Structure and Function.* New York, Marcel Dekker, 1982, p 3.

2

Aging of the Skin

Barbara A. Gilchrest

Reflections on the aging process in skin have been offered from time immemorial by both medical and lay authors. Early histological, physiological, and biochemical studies of aging human skin are well summarized in the 1964 and 1978 *Symposia on the Biology of Skin*,[1,2] which clearly portray the organ's gradual physiological decline and increasing individual variability with age.

More recent studies (reviewed in Refs. 3 and 4) avoid earlier confusion between aging changes and age-related environmental insults such as chronic sun exposure; between developmental changes (conception to maturity) and aging changes (maturity to senescence); and between aging changes and manifestations of age-associated diseases or age-associated hormonal changes such as menopause. Of these, the first is by far the most important, as sun-induced "premature aging" or photoaging of the skin has been widely confused with the true aging process. In most individuals, sun damage is indeed responsible for the majority of clinically evident age-associated cutaneous changes, but unlike intrinsic aging, it is readily preventable.

MORPHOLOGICAL CHANGES

The major clinically apparent aging changes in sun-protected skin include *dryness* (by which is meant roughness), fine wrinkling, laxity, and a variety of proliferative lesions. Sun-exposed skin has, in addition to these changes, elastosis (a pebbly, yellowed quality due to alteration of elastic fibers), irregular hyperpigmentation and depigmentation, telangiectases, coarse wrinkling, and actinic keratoses (rough, red, precancerous patches of atypical epidermal cells).

The histological features associated with aged human skin are well described.[3,4] The major changes are listed in Table 2-1 and shown schematically in Fig. 2-1. The most striking and consistent change is flattening of the dermal-epidermal junction, with effacement of both the dermal papillae and the epidermal rete pegs. This results in a considerably smaller contiguous surface between the two compartments, and presumably less "communication" and nutrient transfer and less resistance to shearing forces. The average epidermal thickness in sun-protected skin probably remains constant with advancing age, but variability in thickness and in the size of individual keratinocytes increases. At the electron-microscopic level, sun-protected old skin is characterized by some widening of the interkeratinocyte spaces; by reduplication of the lamina densa and the anchoring fibril complex in the basement membrane zone; and by loss of the numerous microvillous projections of basal cells into the dermis, which greatly increase the dermal-epidermal interface in young adult skin. Dermal microfibril bundles, the terminal arborizations of elastic fibers believed to assist in anchorage of the basement membrane, are also reduced with age, although the number of hemidesmosomes and anchoring fibrils per unit length of dermal-epidermal junction appears to be unchanged.[5] The average thickness and degree of compaction of the stratum corneum appear to be constant with age. *Skin surface patterns,* a patchwork of fine lines that may be determined by the papillary dermal architecture, reveal a slight age-

Table 2-1

HISTOLOGICAL FEATURES OF AGING HUMAN SKIN

Epidermis	Dermis	Appendages
Flat dermal-epidermal junction	Atrophy (loss of dermal volume)	Graying of hair
Variable thickness	Fewer fibroblasts	Loss of hair
Variable cell size and shape	Fewer mast cells	Conversion of terminal to vellus hair
Occasional nuclear atypia	Fewer blood vessels	Abnormal nail plates
Loss of melanocytes	Shortened capillary loops	Fewer glands
Fewer Langerhans cells	Abnormal nerve endings	

Source: Modified from BA Gilchrest.[3]

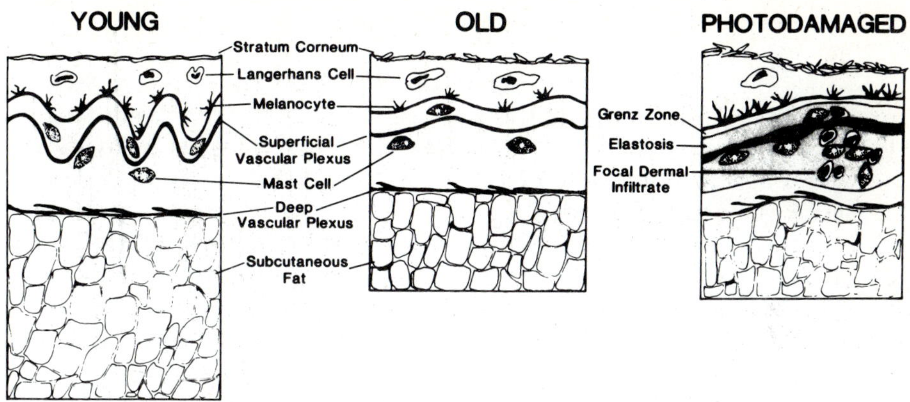

Figure 2-1 Histological features of young, old, and photodamaged skin. Schematic drawings contrast the age-associated changes in normal (sun-protected) young skin, chronologically old skin, and photoaged (photodamaged middle-aged to old) skin. With age alone, there is a marked flattening of the dermal-epidermal junction; loss of dermal and subcutaneous mass; shortened capillary loops, with a corresponding reduction in the area of the superficial vascular plexus; and reduced numbers of Langerhans cells, melanocytes, and mast cells. Photodamaged old skin differs from sun-protected old skin in that it is often hyperkeratotic and has an alternating, variably atrophic and hyperplastic epidermis with nuclear atypia; a prominent band of tinctorially altered collagen and elastic fibers termed *elastosis;* focal perivascular infiltrates composed of lymphocytes, macrophages, and mast cells; a severely attenuated superficial vascular plexus with focal marked dilatation; and a narrow band of apparent sparing, a Grenz zone, that is in fact a subtle scar below the epidermis. Compared to old sun-protected skin, photodamaged skin has a further reduction in Langerhans cell number but an increase in melanocyte number, with marked variation in the size and number of dendrites. [*From BA Gilchrest: Physiology and pathophysiology of aging skin, in LA Goldsmith (ed), Biochemistry and Pathophysiology of the Skin, 2d ed, Oxford, Oxford University Press, in press.*]

associated loss of regularity in sun-protected areas, that is much more pronounced in exposed areas.

A decrease in the number of enzymatically active melanocytes per unit surface area of the skin, approximately 10 to 20 percent of the remaining cell population in each decade, has been repeatedly documented. It is not known whether the cells truly disappear or simply become undetectable by ceasing to produce pigment, but in either case, the body's protective barrier against ultraviolet (UV) light is reduced. Melanocyte number in habitually sun-exposed skin is approximately twice that in comparable sun-protected sites but, again, declines with advancing age. The number of melanocytic nevi (moles) also progressively decreases with age from a peak of 15 to 40 in the third or fourth decade to an average of approximately 4 by the eighth decade, with further subsequent decline.[6,7]

Langerhans cells, approximately 25 to 50 percent as numerous as melanocytes, are an epidermal cell population believed to be responsible for recognition of foreign antigens. A 20 to 50 percent reduction in the number of morphologically identifiable epidermal Langerhans cells occurs between early and late adulthood[8–10] and may account in part for the age-associated decrease in immune responsiveness observed in old skin. A further 50 percent reduction occurs in chronically sun-exposed old skin.[11,12]

Dermal thickness has been reported to decrease gradually by approximately 20 percent during adulthood,[13] although a more recent study using very sensitive instrumentation found a decrease in total dermal thickness only after age 70 years.[14] The remaining dermis is relatively acellular and avascular. In one study, an approximately 50 percent reduction in mast cells and a 30 percent reduction in venular cross-sections were noted in the papillary dermis of buttock skin from old adults compared with young adult controls, and these histological changes were associated with a corresponding response following a standardized UV exposure.[15] The striking age-associated loss of the vascular bed, and especially of the vertical capillary loops that occupy dermal papillae in young skin, is believed to underlie many of the physiological alterations in old skin. The marked reduction in the vascular network surrounding hair bulbs and eccrine, apocrine, and sebaceous glands may be responsible for their gradual atrophy with age.

Precise histological concomitants of fine wrinkling, if any, are unknown, although age-related loss of elastin fibers may contribute. Elastosis, the characteristic tinctorial changes and ultrastructural disorganization of elastic fibers in sun-damaged dermis, is similarly believed to cause the more pronounced wrinkling observed in photoaged skin. Contractions of connective tissue septae within the subcutaneous fat appear to be responsible for deep age-associated expression lines.[16]

Age-related changes in hair color, density, and distribution are widely recognized. Graying is due to progressive and eventually total loss of melanocytes from the hair bulb. The melanocytes remaining in gray hairs may be vacuolated, and the hair matrix and shaft contain fewer melanin granules than those of normally pigmented hair. Loss of melanocytes is believed to occur more rapidly in hair than in skin because the cells are called upon to proliferate and manufacture melanin at maximal rates during the anagen phase of the hair cycle, while epidermal melanocytes are comparatively inactive throughout their life span. Scalp hair is believed to gray more rapidly than other body hair because its anagen (growth phase) to telogen (resting phase) ratio is considerably greater than that of other body hair. Advancing age is also accompanied by a gradual decrease in the number of hairs. Those that remain may be smaller in diameter and grow more slowly.

Eccrine glands decrease approximately 15 percent in average number during adulthood in most body sites, although gland density on the scalp appears to be constant. Similar quantification has not been performed for apocrine glands. Lipofuscin ("age pigment") gradually accumulates with age in the secretory cells of both eccrine and apocrine glands.[17] Sebaceous gland size and number appear not to change with age despite evidence of decreased function.[18]

Pacinian and Meissner's corpuscles, the cutaneous end organs responsible for pressure perception and light touch, progressively decrease to approximately one-third their initial average density between the second and ninth decades of life, as determined histochemically in two body sites. Further, with advancing age, individual end organs display greater variation in size and irregularities in structure. There are very few histologically demonstrable aging changes in Merkel's corpuscles or in free nerve endings.

PHYSIOLOGICAL CHANGES

Table 2-2 lists the major functions of the skin that decline with age. Many of the entries are necessarily interrelated or overlapping.

An age-associated decrease in epidermal turnover rate of approximately 50 percent between the third and seventh decades has been determined by a study of desquamation rates for cells of the stratum corneum at selected body sites.[19] Other investigators have reported a corresponding 100 percent prolongation in the stratum corneum replacement rate in old versus young men.[20] The thymidine labeling index of the epidermis has been reported to decline nearly 50 percent with age,[21] but other investigators find no difference in this parameter and instead implicate apoptosis (cell death and disappearance during transit from the basal layer to the stratum corneum) in the age-associated decrease in desquamation rate.[22] The linear growth rate for nails also decreases by approximately 30 to 50 percent between early and late adulthood.[23]

Repair rates in the skin likewise decline with age, whether measured in terms of wound closure, regeneration of blister roofs (epidermal cell migration and mitosis), collagen deposition, or development of wound tensile strength.

Neoplasia is associated with aging in virtually all organ systems but is especially characteristic of skin. One or more benign proliferative growths are present in nearly every adult beyond age 65 years,[24,25] and most individuals have dozens of lesions. In the United States, basal cell and squamous cell carcinomas outnumber all other human malignancies combined and are strongly related to both increasing age and sun exposure. Melanoma, a less common but more often fatal malignancy, is also statistically related to age and sun exposure. Well-documented increases in the incidence of these malignancies of approximately three- to four-fold

Table 2-2

FUNCTIONS OF HUMAN SKIN THAT DECLINE WITH AGE

Cell replacement	Immune recognition
Injury response	Vascular responsiveness
Barrier function	Thermoregulation
Chemical clearance	Sweat production
Sensory perception	Sebum production
Vitamin D production	Mechanical protection

Source: Modified from BA Gilchrest.[3]

over the past 25 years[26] have justifiably heightened interest in the relationship between aging or photoaging and skin cancer. Increasing cumulative exposure to UV light (sunlight) and increasing induction times from early exposures surely accompany aging, but other factors may include the above-mentioned losses of Langerhans cells and melanocytes and a possibly reduced repair capacity for UV-altered cellular DNA, although the latter finding is controversial.[27]

An age-related decrease in the barrier function of intact stratum corneum, as well as decreased clearance of absorbed materials from the dermis, has been reported for several substances. More recent work suggests that age effects on percutaneous drug absorption depend in part on drug structure being significantly reduced in old skin for hydrophilic substances but unchanged for hydrophobic substances.[28]

Decreased sensory perception was documented in old skin more than three decades ago, using several techniques: threshold stimulus for light touch, vibratory sensation, and corneal sensation. Spontaneous sweating in response to dry heat, measured on digit pads, was reduced more than 70 percent in healthy old subjects compared with young control subjects. This finding was attributable primarily to decreased sweat output per gland.

Highly accurate techniques for measurement of sebum secretion rates have documented an exponential decline of approximately 23 percent per decade throughout adulthood, beginning in the second decade.[29] This age-associated decline in sebum secretion closely parallels the decline in serum androgen levels, to which sebaceous glands are exquisitely sensitive. The clinical effects of decreased sebum production, if any, are unknown. There is no direct relationship to xerosis.[18]

Decreased vascular responsiveness in the skin of older individuals has been documented by measuring vasodilation and transudation after application of standardized irritants to young and old subjects. Intensity of erythema following a standardized UV exposure is also decreased with age in normal skin,[15] although factors other than decreased vascular responsiveness may also contribute. Compromised thermoregulation, which predisposes the elderly to hypothermia and heat stroke, may be due in part to reduced vasodilation or vasoconstriction of dermal arterioles, in part to decreased eccrine sweat production, and in part to loss of subcutaneous fat, all of which occur with advancing age.

Dermal-epidermal separation occurs more readily in the elderly under experimental conditions, as might be anticipated from the histological finding of reduced interdigitation between the dermis and epidermis. The poor adhesion between these two cutaneous compartments in the elderly undoubtedly explains their propensity to "torn" skin and superficial abrasions following minor trauma such as bandage removal and to bulla formation in edematous sites. It may also contribute to the increased prevalence of certain blistering diseases in the elderly.

An age-associated decrease in immune function is well documented both systemically and in the skin,[3] where it is manifested by a relative inability of older subjects to become sensitized to neoantigens and to react to recall antigens.[30,31]

It is widely presumed but not rigorously established that age-associated changes in cellular immunity contribute to the markedly increased incidence in the elderly of such disorders as skin cancer and herpes zoster. Humoral immunity is also measurably impaired in otherwise healthy old adults.[32] One study suggests an age-associated decrease in the human antibody response to neoantigens, particularly for antibodies of the thymus-dependent IgG class,[33] and another documents a marked reduction with age in the percentage of subjects aged 20 to 75 years with positive wheal-and-flare reactions to a standard battery of potential allergens.[34]

An endocrine function of human skin suspected to decline with age is vitamin D production. With age, there is a striking reduction in the epidermal content of 7-dehydrocholesterol,[35] the compound converted to previtamin D by sun exposure, a change that may limit vitamin D production in old skin.

BIOCHEMICAL AND BIOPHYSICAL CHANGES

The water content of the stratum corneum decreases with age,[36] although there appears to be no change in the water content of the total skin.[21]

The proportion of recently synthesized human dermal collagen is small and does not vary with age in adults.[36,37] However, there is a significant decrease with age in the percentage of total collagen that is incompletely cross-linked, from approximately 25 percent at age 30 years to approximately 10 percent at age 75 years, with a proportionate increase in the percentage of insoluble collagen from approximately 70 to 88 percent.[38] Ketoamine-linked glycosylation of insoluble dermal collagen also increases with age,[37] possibly related to slower collagen turnover or higher average glucose levels in the tissue. The recently characterized nonreducible collagen cross-link histidinohydroxylysinonorleucine also increases throughout adulthood in human skin.[39] The total collagen content of skin and the ratio of collagen types I and III are relatively constant, with type III constituting approximately 20 percent of the total, increasing slightly after age 60 years.[40]

Prolyl and lysyl hydroxylase, enzymes necessary for intercellular stabilization of the collagen triple helix and for its intermolecular cross-linking, show an age-associated decline in activity in human skin, primarily during the fetal and postnatal development periods, although cultured dermal fibroblasts from donors ranging in age from a few months to 94 years do not.[41]

Dermal elastin is less well studied than collagen. However, elastin fibers have been reported to show progressive cross-linkage and calcification with age in sun-protected adult skin,[42] and cultured dermal fibroblasts derived from old adults have markedly decreased levels of mRNA for elastin compared to fibroblasts from fetuses or even middle-aged adults,[37] consistent with the decreased elastin biosynthetic capacity of old skin.

Mechanical properties of the skin are also reported to change with age during adulthood. There is progressive loss of elastic recovery, consistent with gradual destruction of the dermal elastin network, decreased extensibility,[43] and marked prolongation of the time required for excised skin of elderly versus young adults to return to its original thickness after compression.[44]

REFERENCES

1. Montagna W (ed): *Advances in the Biology of Skin,* vol 6: *Aging.* Oxford, Pergamon, 1965.
2. Montagna W et al (eds): Special issue on aging. Proceedings of the 28th Symposium on the Biology of Skin. *J Invest Dermatol* 73:1, 1979.
3. Gilchrest BA: *Skin and Aging Processes.* Boca Raton, FL, CRC Press, 1984.
4. Kligman AM, Takase Y: *Cutaneous Aging.* Tokyo, University of Tokyo Press, 1988.
5. Tidman MJ, Eady RAJ: Ultrastructural morphometry of normal skin dermal-epidermal junction: the influence of age, sex and body region on laminar and nonlaminar components. *J Invest Dermatol* 83:448, 1984.
6. Maize JC, Foster G: Age-related changes in melanocytic nevi. *Clin Exp Dermatol* 4:49, 1979.
7. MacKie RM et al: The number and distribution of benign pigmented moles (melanocytic naevi) in a healthy British population. *Br J Dermatol* 113:167, 1985.
8. Gilchrest BA et al: Effects of chronologic aging and ultraviolet irradiation on Langerhans cells in human epidermis. *J Invest Dermatol* 79:85, 1982.
9. Thiers BH et al: The effect of aging and chronic sun exposure on human Langerhans cell populations. *J Invest Dermatol* 82:223, 1984.
10. Scheibner A et al: Langerhans cell and melanocyte distribution in "normal" human epidermis: preliminary report. *Australas J Dermatol* 24:9, 1983.
11. Delo VA et al: Density of Langerhans cells (LC) in normal vs. chronic actinically damaged skin (CADS) of humans. *J Invest Dermatol* 76:330, 1981.
12. Gilchrest BA et al: Chronologic and actinically-induced aging in human facial skin. *J Invest Dermatol* 80:81S, 1983.
13. Black MM: A modified radiographic method for measuring skin thickness. *Br J Dermatol* 81:661, 1969.
14. de Rigal J et al: Assessment of aging of the human skin by in vivo ultrasonic imaging. *J Invest Dermatol* 93:621, 1989.
15. Gilchrest BA et al: Chronologic aging alters the response to ultraviolet-induced inflammation in human skin. *J Invest Dermatol* 79:11, 1982.
16. Pierard GE, Lapiere CM: The microanatomical basis of facial frown lines. *Arch Dermatol* 125:1090, 1989.
17. Cawley EP et al: Lipofuscin ("wear and tear" pigment) in human sweat glands. *J Invest Dermatol* 61:105, 1973.
18. Downing DT et al: Changes in sebum secretion and the sebaceous gland. *Dermatol Clin* 4:419, 1986.
19. Leyden JJ et al: Age-related differences in the rate of desquamation of skin surface cells, in RD Adelman et al (eds), *Pharmacological Intervention in the Aging Process.* New York, Plenum, 1978, p 297.
20. Baker H, Blair CP: Cell replacement in the human stratum corneum in old age. *Br J Dermatol* 80:367, 1967.
21. Kligman AM: Perspectives and problems in cutaneous gerontology. *J Invest Dermatol* 73:39, 1979.
22. Marks R: Measurement of biological aging in human epidermis. *Br J Dermatol* 104:627, 1981.
23. Orentreich N et al: The effect of aging on the rate of linear nail growth. *J Invest Dermatol* 73:126, 1979.

24. Tindall JP, Smith JG: Skin lesions of the aged. *JAMA* 186:1039, 1963.
25. Beauregard SB, Gilchrest BA: A survey of skin problems and skin care regimens in the elderly. *Arch Dermatol* 123:1638, 1987.
26. Glass AG, Hoover RN: The emerging epidemic of melanoma and squamous cell skin cancer. *JAMA* 262:2097, 1989.
27. Hanawalt PC: On the role of DNA damage and repair processes in aging: evidence for and against, in HR Warner et al (eds), *Modern Biological Theories of Aging,* New York, Raven Press, 1987, vol 31, p 183.
28. Roskos KV et al: The effect of aging on percutaneous absorption in man. *J Pharmacol Biophys* (in press).
29. Jacobsen E et al: Age-related changes in sebaceous wax ester secretion rates in men and women. *J Invest Dermatol* 85:483, 1985.
30. Waldorf DS et al: Impaired delayed hypersensitivity in an aging population: association with antinuclear reactivity and rheumatoid factor. *JAMA* 203:831, 1968.
31. Roberts-Thomson JC et al: Aging, immune response and mortality. *Lancet* 2:368, 1974.
32. Pahwa SG et al: Decreased in vitro humoral response in aged humans. *J Clin Invest* 67:1094, 1981.
33. Ammann AJ et al: The antibody responses to pneumococcal capsular polysaccharides in aged individuals. *Proc Soc Exp Biol Med* 164:312, 1980.
34. Barbee RA et al: Immediate skin-test reactivity in a general population sample. *Ann Intern Med* 84:129, 1976.
35. MacLaughlin J, Holick MF: Aging decreases the capacity of human skin to produce vitamin D_3. *J Clin Invest* 76:1536, 1985.
36. Potts RO et al: Changes with age in the moisture content of human skin. *J Invest Dermatol* 82:97, 1984.
37. Uitto J et al: Cutaneous aging: molecular alterations in elastic fibers. *J Cutan Aging Cosmet Dermatol* 1:13, 1988.
38. Schnider SL, Kohn RR: Effects of age and diabetes mellitus on the solubility and nonenzymatic glycosylation of human skin collagen. *J Clin Invest* 67:1630, 1981.
39. Yamauchi M et al: Aging and cross-linking of skin collagen. *Bichem Biophys Res Commun* 152:898, 1988.
40. Lovell CR et al: Type I and III collagen content and fibre distribution in normal human skin during ageing. *Br J Dermatol* 117:419, 1987.
41. Musad S et al: Prolyl and lysyl hydroylase activities of human skin fibroblasts: effect of donor age and ascorbate. *J Invest Dermatol* 75:404, 1980.
42. Partridge SM: Biological role of cutaneous elastin, in W Montagna et al (eds), *Advances in the Biology of Skin.* New York, Meredith, 1970, vol 10, p 69.
43. Leveque JL et al: Influence of aging on the in vivo extensibility of human skin at a low stress. *Arch Dermatol Res* 269:127, 1980.
44. Daly CH, Odland GF: Age-related changes in the mechanical properties of human skin. *J Invest Dermatol* 73:84, 1979.

3

The Skin as an Organ of Protection

Ronald Marks

Human skin acts as a vital defensive structure, separating the delicate inner organs and tissues from the potentially hostile external environment. Its protective roles are necessary for our well-being. When it is remembered that the skin over the limbs and trunk is, for the most part, only 1 to 2 mm thick, it seems astonishing that it is able to offer such a range of protective capacities.

MECHANICAL PROTECTION

Human skin does not provide quite the same mechanical protection as the integument of an alligator or rhinoceros, but nonetheless it affords an essential defensive covering. The stratum corneum and dermis each play a role in this protective function.

Stratum Corneum

The stratum corneum is only 15 to 20 μm thick (Fig. 3-1) over most of the body, but it is still tough enough to resist penetration by the great majority of objects with which we come into daily contact. It may not resist penetration by the attacking mouthparts and stings of insects, by thorns and claws, and by other hard, sharp objects, but we would be much worse off with a softer structure. Over the palms and soles, the horny layer is much thicker than elsewhere; it may be 500 μm thick or

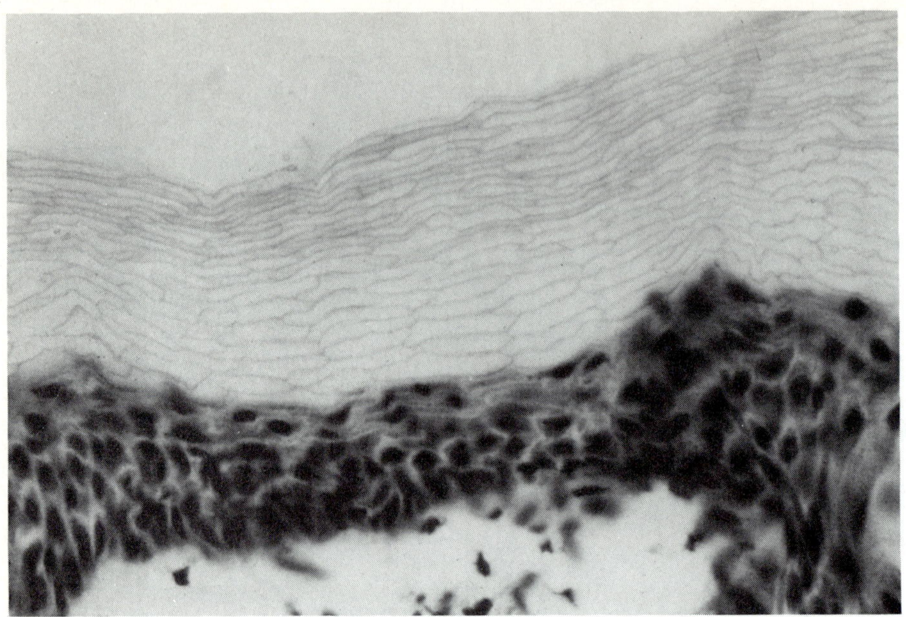

Figure 3-1 Photomicrograph of cryostat-sectioned tissue treated with an alkaline solution to make the structure more easily visible. Note the delicate arrangement of the thin corneocytes (horn cells). ×40 in the original magnification.

more. Clearly, this thickened layer offers increased protection, which is in keeping with the needs of these anatomical regions.

The mechanical properties of the stratum corneum are difficult to study in vivo because of its intimate attachment to other underlying structures. It is possible to test the stratum corneum in vitro, although the act of removing this structure from the rest of the skin may influence its properties. Furthermore, the stratum corneum is an extremely deliquescent membrane, and in vitro it rapidly takes up water, so that during a test cycle the ambient environment has to be controlled. Like all tissues it has viscoelastic properties, although its elastic properties are predominant. In other words, the structure tends to return to its original shape after a deforming force has been removed.

Much of the strength of the horny layer in resisting deforming forces stems from the toughness of the bonds between adjacent corneocytes. This binding force or cohesive quality is also important in modulating desquamation. During desquamation, single corneocytes fall off the skin surface, while new cells become differentiated and are added to the deeper portion of the stratum corneum, keeping the structure of constant thickness. To permit corneocytes to become free at the surface, the binding forces between the cells gradually decrease through a still uncharacterized mechanism. The binding forces within the stratum corneum can be measured with a device known as a cohesograph.

When adequately hydrated, the stratum corneum is flexible and resilient, permitting an astonishing range of movement of limbs and digits. Abnormal stratum corneum (as in the ichthyotic disorders—see Chap. 9) cannot retain adequate amounts of water and is brittle and inflexible. For this reason, fissures are common accompaniments of conditions in which there is an abnormal stratum corneum for any reason (Fig. 3-2).

Dermis

The bulk of the mechanical strength of the skin resides in the fibrous connective tissue elements of the dermis. It is the collagen fibers in particular that give the characteristic toughness to skin. The elastic fibers probably have the task of binding the collagenous fibers together and to the epidermis to make the skin structure behave as a single unit. Between the fibers of the dermis is a viscous, hygroscopic ground substance composed of proteoglycans (chondroitin sulfate, hyaluronic acid, and keratan sulfate). This material is also important to the physical functioning of skin both in supplying a permissive medium for the dermal connective tissue fibers and in imparting resilience at low stress levels.

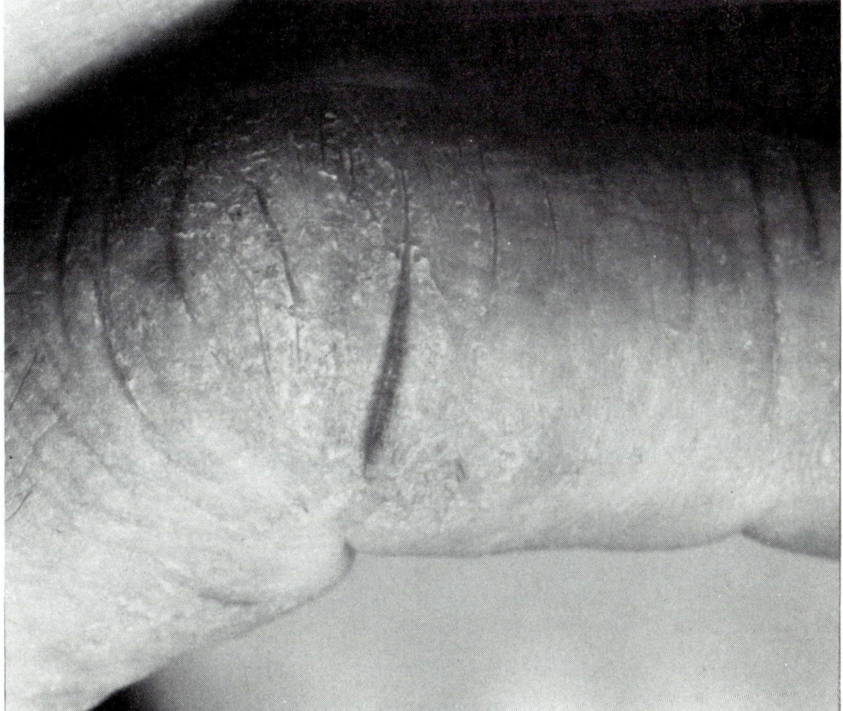

Figure 3-2 Patch of eczema on a finger with a painful, large fissure resulting from inflexible stratum corneum.

When the mechanical properties of skin are tested in vivo, it becomes apparent that they are anisotropic; that is, they differ according to the orientation of the test stimulus. This finding is due to specific orientations of the collagen fiber network, so that there is an in vivo resting tension. This is why a round hole made in the skin rapidly assumes an oval shape. Lines drawn to represent the direction of maximum resting tension in vivo are known as Langer's lines. Traditionally, surgical incisions are made along these lines to minimize the tendency of wounds to gape and to reduce scars.

A variety of techniques has been used to test the mechanical properties of skin in vivo, including methods that record the forces generated after extending, elevating, indenting, or twisting the skin. All of these tests reveal the anisotropy mentioned above, as well as time dependence. The latter feature signifies that the mechanical properties of skin depend on the rate of delivery of the mechanical stimulus and on the recent stress history of the part being tested.

Characteristically, skin behaves as a viscoelastic structure when a strain is applied (Fig. 3-3). The first part of the stress-strain curve is the result of the viscous property of skin. The second, straighter part of the curve is the elastic region in which the skin returns to its original length after the stimulus has been withdrawn.

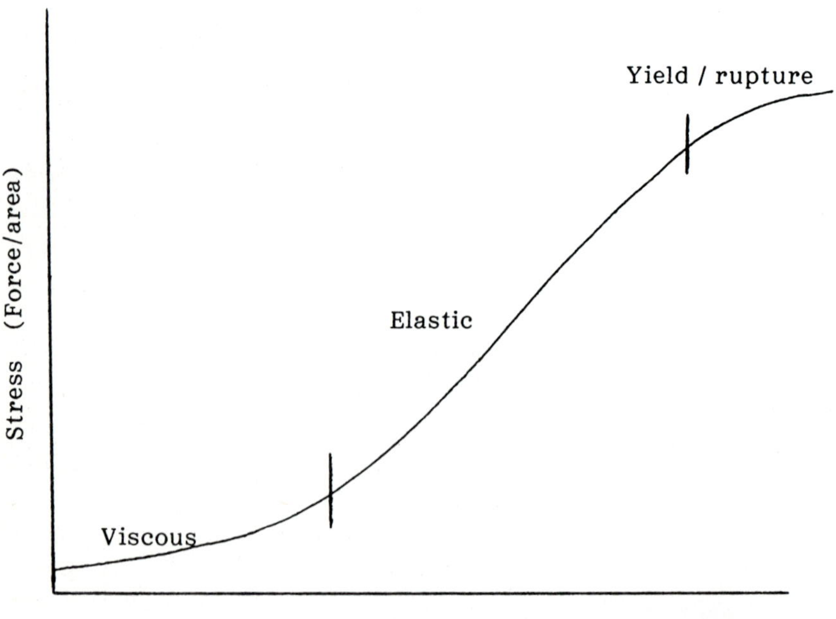

Figure 3-3 Idealized typical stress-strain curve for skin showing various regions.

Exposed skin becomes damaged by solar ultraviolet radiation. The damaged skin becomes "old-looking" and wrinkled and takes on a yellowish discoloration due to an altered staining and morphology of the collagen known as dermal elastotic degenerative change. This damaged skin loses its resilience, firmness, and elasticity. Covered skin also alters with age, but less dramatically, and shows a characteristically increased stiffness.

TRANSEPIDERMAL WATER LOSS

Water tends to evaporate from body tissues, which are 70 to 75 percent water, to the somewhat drier ambient atmosphere. This potentially hazardous process is hindered by the stratum corneum, which, when optimally hydrated, contains only 35 percent water. Nonetheless, the stratum corneum does permit the diffusion of some water vapor across its structure. In healthy persons and without obvious sweating, about 0.5 liter of water is lost per day by this process of transepidermal diffusion. The rate of water loss can be measured by a device known as an evaporimeter, which contains two water sensors mounted one above the other. The normal water loss is 0.5 to 1.0 $mg/cm^2/h$. In certain skin diseases such as psoriasis and eczema there is faulty epidermal differentiation, so that an abnormal and inefficient stratum corneum is formed. This abnormal horny layer may allow through 10 to 12 times more water than normal, which can result in serious dehydration. The same problem arises in burn patients.

It is thought that the main passage of water through the stratum corneum is around the individual cornified cells. When the stratum corneum is progressively removed by adhesive tape, the water loss gradually increases at the site of stripping. The intercellular space in the stratum corneum contains sheets of a glycolipid (a ceramide) that unfurl from extruded minute, membrane-bound lamellar bodies present in the granular cell layer of the epidermis. It is this substance that may well be responsible for the "waterproofing" role of the stratum corneum.

PENETRATION OF DRUGS AND TOXIC SUBSTANCES

The stratum corneum acts as the rate-limiting membrane preventing permeation into the skin of substances encountered in the environment. This function is essential, protecting against intoxication after contact with a wide variety of potentially hazardous natural materials and artificial products. In fact, all molecules are capable of diffusing into the skin, but some do so much more readily than others. The stratum corneum is a lipid-rich structure. In general terms, the more lipophilic a substance, the more readily it will diffuse across into the skin.

It is not certain which specific components of the stratum corneum's structure are responsible for the diffusion barrier quality of the membrane, but the intercellular lipids must be considered as playing a major role. Research findings indicate that as with transepidermal water loss, molecules diffuse inward around cornified cells rather than through them. It is theoretically possible for substances to diffuse through adnexal orifices, i.e., sweat gland and hair follicle openings. The exact role that these structures play in permitting permeation of materials through the stratum corneum is not known. This pathway of penetration has come to be known as shunt diffusion, though whether these pathways reach their potential as shunts is not entirely clear.

There is considerable variation in the rate of penetration of substances at different body sites. This variation is due in part to variation in stratum corneum thickness and may be due in part to the size of corneocytes, which varies from site to site. The humidity of different body sites also affects the rate of penetration; a moist stratum corneum is a less efficient barrier. There may also be inherent site differences relating to the biochemical composition of the intercellular cement material. The groin and genital areas and the retroauricular sites are more easily penetrated than other body sites; by contrast, truncal skin away from the flexures is probably penetrated with the greatest difficulty.

Molecules diffuse through the stratum corneum passively; there is no active transport through the skin. The passive diffusion process is governed by Fick's law, in which

$$\text{Flux} = \frac{KD}{\delta}\Delta C$$

where K = the partition coefficient (describing the ease with which a substance enters the stratum corneum, i.e., its solubility in this tissue relative to its solubility in the solvent in which it is presented to the skin), D = the diffusion constant, δ = the thickness of the stratum corneum, and ΔC = the difference in concentration on either side of the stratum corneum of the molecule in question. In general, molecules with a molecular weight of over 500 find it difficult to diffuse through the stratum corneum, but size is by no means the only consideration.

Any breach of the stratum corneum or any skin disorder that results in faulty keratinization and an abnormal stratum corneum will increase the rate of diffusion of substances through it. In general terms, occlusion of the skin surface enhances the rate of diffusion. There are also substances that, by virtue of their effect on the cornified layer, enhance the penetration of other materials applied to the skin. These penetration-enhancing substances include urea, salicylic acid, and organic solvents such as dimethyl sulfoxide.

The diffusing potential of a substance and the barrier qualities of the stratum corneum can be investigated in vitro using diffusion chambers (Fig. 3-4). In vivo, it is difficult to determine the rate of diffusion of substances, but either the appearance of the material to be tested in the urine or blood is measured or the amount of material that diffuses into the stratum corneum and skin at various time points is assessed.

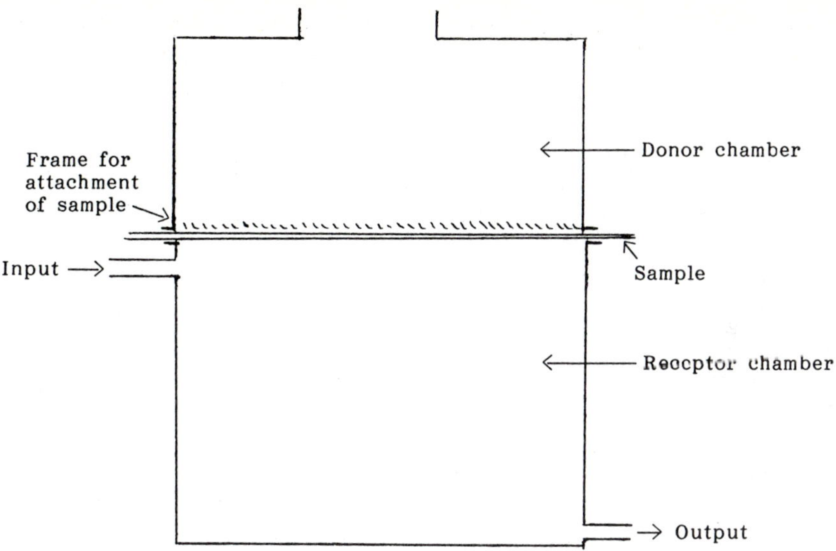

Figure 3-4 Diagram of a diffusion chamber to study percutaneous penetration in vitro.

PROTECTION AGAINST MICROBIAL INVASION

Skin is colonized by various commensal microorganisms, predominantly gram-positive bacteria (*Propionibacterium acnes*) and gram-positive cocci (*Staphylococcus epidermidis*), as well as yeast-like *Pityrosporum* species (*Pityrosporum ovale*). In addition, a mite known as *Demodex folliculorum* is found in the larger hair follicles of many normal individuals. For the most part, these commensal organisms do not invade and do not cause any serious disease. Skin comes in contact with a variety of potentially more harmful viruses, bacteria, and fungi, and one important aspect of the skin's barrier properties is the protection it provides against infection.

For the most part, the intact skin surface is inimical to microbes, and they gain a foothold only when the surface is breached or fissured due to injury or disease. The secretion of sebum from sebaceous glands in the hair follicles can provide the right microenvironment in which parasitic microorganisms can proliferate and invade. This observation explains why these adnexal structures are the most often infected part of the skin. However, it is also true that normal sebum and sweat contain substances that inhibit the growth of certain microorganisms. Damp, sodden skin is more easily injured, and microbes grow more prolifically in this environment. Hence, wet skin is more easily infected than dry skin.

The usual pH of the skin surface is approximately 5.6—the so-called acid mantle of the skin. It has been supposed that this pH aids in reducing the transient population of potentially harmful bacteria, but this hypothesis has not been well received in recent years.

PROTECTION AGAINST THERMAL STIMULI AND HEAT REGULATION

Heat regulation is vital to the maintenance of a constant internal body temperature. Metabolic processes provide the source of body heat. Heat conservation is assisted by fat, vasoconstriction, hair, and muscular activity. Its loss, when necessary, is engineered by sweating and vasodilatation. These subjects are covered in Chap. 4.

The skin provides poor protection against thermal damage both to itself and deeper tissues. However, the stratum corneum does have some insulating properties—particularly at sites at which it is normally quite thick, such as on the palms and soles.

PROTECTION AGAINST SOLAR ULTRAVIOLET RADIATION

Exposed skin is constantly threatened by damage from solar ultraviolet radiation. The damage sustained may be acute, causing erythema, inflammation, and even blistering (i.e., "sunburn"), or it may result in a more serious chronic change such as neoplastic skin disease or a group of degenerative changes in the skin known as photoaging. These latter conditions are due to changes in the dermal connective tissue known as solar elastotic degeneration, and cause functional and cosmetic disabilities.

The major mechanism by which skin protection is obtained is the production of the brown/black pigment known as melanin. This pigment is synthesized from phenylalanine on cytoplasmic organelles (melanosomes) in cells known as melanocytes that reside in the basal layer of the epidermis. They inject the melanin that they synthesize into surrounding keratinocytes, where it provides protection by absorbing the harmful ultraviolet radiation.

After exposure to ultraviolet radiation, melanin synthesis is enhanced (sun tanning). The melanin pigment is carried upward with the keratinocytes to the stratum corneum (Fig. 3-5), but the stratum corneum itself appears to provide some protective quality against ultraviolet radiation.

NOCIOCEPTION, LOCOMOTORY FUNCTION, AND AGGRESSIVE FUNCTION

The inability to feel pain often results in serious damage to the skin. In some instances, extensive and persistent ulcers result from repetitive, inadvertent minor traumas. Clearly, an intact cutaneous afferent peripheral nervous system is a major component of the protective function of the skin.

The ridging of the palms and soles and the prolific sweating capacity of these sites promote a firm grip on contact surfaces, facilitating locomotion. The extensibility of the skin is also vital to all limb movement.

Finally, and for completeness, one must add the old adage that "the best form of protection is attack." The human species is poorly equipped

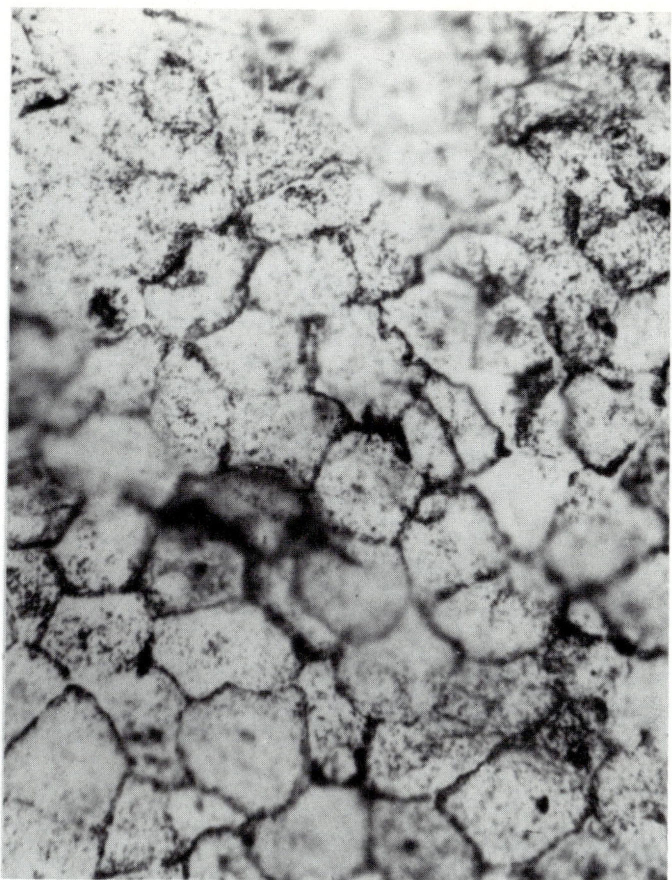

Figure 3-5 Photomicrograph of a sample of stratum corneum removed by the technique of skin surface biopsy and stained with a silver stain to show melanin granules. ×40 in the original magnification.

for aggression, but the analogs of claws—the nails—should be seen as adnexal structures and do have this potential.

SELECTED READINGS

Marks R: Mechanical properties of skin. In: L. Goldsmith (ed), *Biochemistry and Physiology of the Skin*, 2d ed. Oxford, Oxford University Press, in press.

Marks R et al (eds): *The Physical Nature of Skin*. Lancaster, United Kingdom, MTP Press, 1988.

Marks R, Plewig G (eds): *The Stratum Corneum*. Heidelberg, Springer-Verlag, 1983.

Millington PF, Wilkinson R (eds): *Skin*. Cambridge, Cambridge University Press, 1983.

Scott RC et al (eds): *Prediction of Percutaneous Penetration—Methods, Measurements, Modelling*. London, IBC Technical Services, 1990.

4

Temperature Regulation in the Skin

Robert J. Scheuplein

NORMAL BODY TEMPERATURE

Most tissues and organs of the human body function best when they are maintained at a relatively constant temperature near 37°C. The usual range of rectal temperature is 37 ± 1°C, but it is often a degree or two less in the morning and can increase several degrees after heavy exercise. Between environmental extremes of 15°C (60°F) and 54°C (130°F), the nude body is capable of maintaining indefinitely a normal body "core" temperature very close to 37°C (98.6°F)[1] (Fig. 4-1). This is the temperature of the central organs of the body such as the heart, lungs, abdominal viscera, and brain. These may be regarded as contained in a shell of peripheral tissues about 1 inch thick that includes principally the skin and subcutaneous fat. Approximately one-half of the human body lies in this peripheral zone, which is subject to wide variations in temperature in response to environmental extremes. It is only the deep body temperature, or core temperature, that is held sensibly constant—and even this definition depends upon allowing the core region to shrink a little in response to cold environments (Fig. 4-2).

SKIN TEMPERATURE

The temperatures of the peripheral tissues (e.g., skin, muscles, and subcutaneous tissues) are generally lower than the visceral temperatures

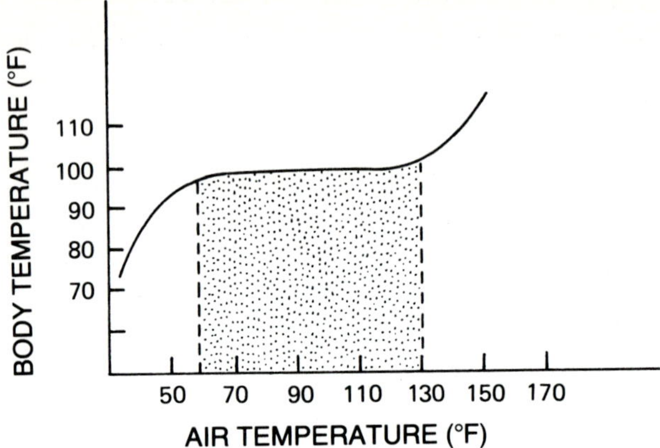

Figure 4-1 Physiological temperature regulatory mechanisms are capable of maintaining body temperature within a narrow range, roughly 98.6±3.6°F over wide extremes of environmental temperature. [*From TB Fitzpatrick et al (eds), Dermatology in General Medicine, 3d ed, New York, McGraw-Hill, 1987, p 348.*]

and are subject to much wider fluctuations. The body surface temperature varies over different parts of the skin but normally lies between that of the body core and that of the surrounding tissues, although rapid evaporation of sweat can lower it below both. Skin temperature T_s may fluctuate between 20 and 40°C without damage. However, prolonged exposures to cold or hot environments, causing local skin temperature as

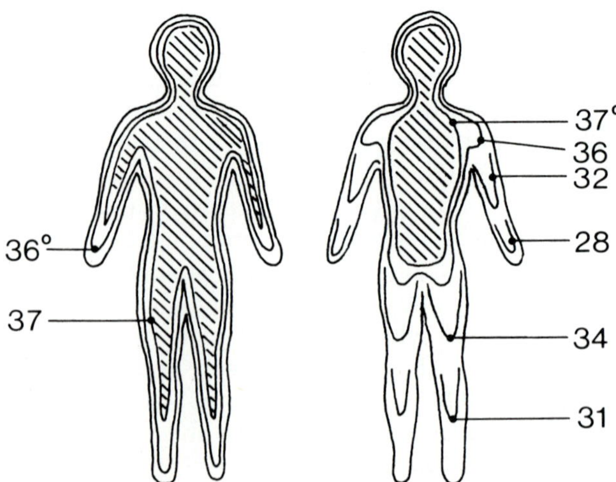

Figure 4-2 The dimensions of the "peripheral tissue" and those of the body core must expand or contract in response to thermoregulatory requirements and the temperature of the surroundings. (*Left*) the temperature isotherms in a warm environment; (*right*) a cold environment. [*From TB Fitzpatrick et al (eds), Dermatology in General Medicine, 3d ed, New York, McGraw-Hill, 1987, p 348.*]

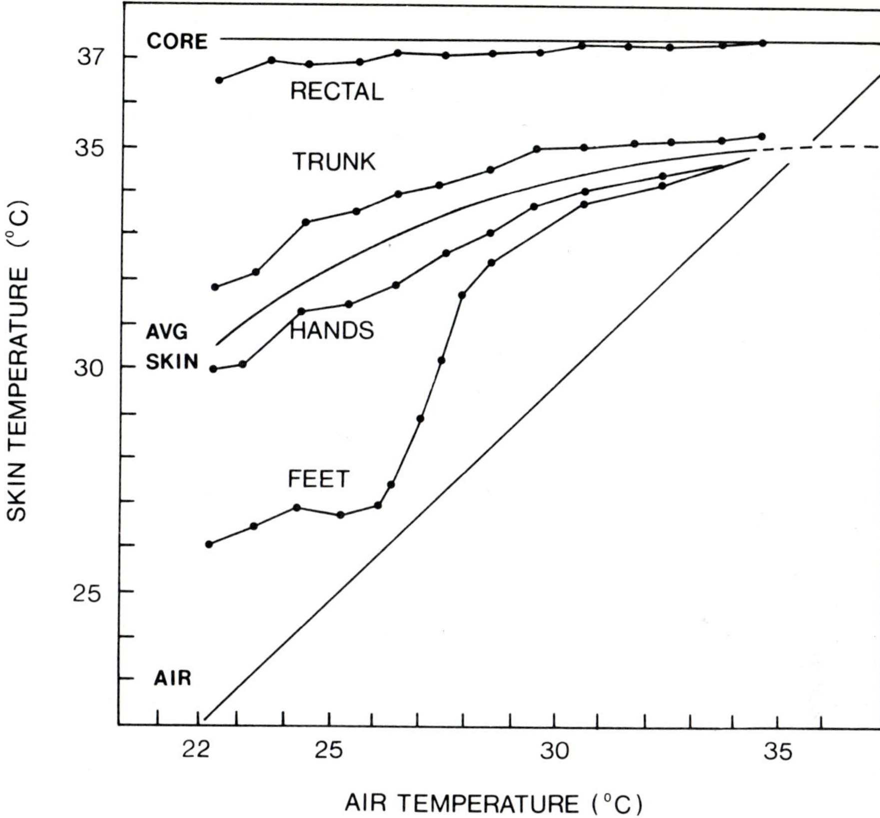

Figure 4-3 Temperatures over the body surface range widely without danger of impairment of function. In cold air the feet have a temperature close to that of the environment. An average skin temperature can be calculated by weighting local skin temperatures by the fraction of body area that each region represents. (*Redrawn from EF Dubois, Heat loss from the human body, Bull NY Acad Med 15:143, 1939.*)

low as 18°C or as high as 45°C, are usually associated with body pain and injury. Under heat stress, skin temperature rises and approaches 35°C over the whole body. Despite increasing environmental temperature, the evaporation of sweat can maintain a relatively cool skin between 30 and 35°C and a stable core temperature of 37°C (Fig. 4-3). When considering hypothalamic temperature regulation, one normally refers to core temperature T_c; when considering the exchange of thermal energy between the skin and the environment, the skin temperature T_s is the appropriate quantity.

BEHAVIORAL AND PHYSIOLOGICAL TEMPERATURE REGULATION: ROLE OF THE SKIN

To accomplish the regulation of body temperature, two different systems are employed: behavioral regulation, involving conscious use of intelligence to promote thermal comfort, and physiological regulation, employing the involuntary responses of the body's temperature-sensing, heat production, and control mechanisms. The skin plays an important role in both types of temperature regulation. Human behavioral regulation against the cold operates in a manner entirely different from the behavioral defense against overheating.[2] The sensation of coldness on the skin is distinctly unpleasant. It is an effective deterrent against exposure to cold stress, and the mechanisms of peripheral cold reception, i.e., at the skin, provide the principal driving impulses for the behavioral defense against cold stress. In contrast, the sensation of warmth on the skin is pleasant under a variety of conditions.

The role of skin in the autonomic regulation of temperature can be understood by remembering that core temperature is controlled by balancing heat production and heat loss, the latter occurring mostly through the skin. The role of the skin in conserving and eliminating heat may be considered in terms of its own heat conductivity, the convection in cutaneous blood vessels, and the excretion of sweat. These internal processes, in turn, influence the heat exchange with the environment by radiation, conduction, convection, and sweat evaporation.

HYPOTHALAMIC REGULATION OF TEMPERATURE

The core temperature of the body is regulated primarily by negative feedback mechanisms operating mainly through a temperature-sensitive area in the anterior hypothalamus. Heat-sensitive neurons located in the preoptic area increase their output as the temperature of the blood perfusing them increases. When the temperature decreases, the rates of discharge decrease. From the preoptic area, signals radiate to various other portions of the hypothalamus to control either heat production or heat loss. The human thermostat is set to a precise reference temperature, usually very close to 37°C, and responses to temperature changes are exquisitely sensitive. The reference temperature represents that control temperature at which the transition is made between the activation of heat production and heat dissipation mechanisms. A mere 0.01°C rise in hypothalamic temperature is sufficient to increase the dissipation of heat through sweating by 6 ml sweat per hour and to raise the blood flow through the skin by 1.5 ml sweat per minute.

This is not the whole story because thermoregulatory mechanisms are directly responsive to skin temperature apart from any change in blood temperature. For example, shivering may occur immediately upon exposure to cold well before the cooling has had time to decrease the temperature of the circulating blood. Recent studies suggest that in addition to temperature receptors located in the skin and temperature-sensitive neurons in the hypothalamus, there are core receptors located deep within the body.[3] Apparently the hypothalamus integrates the sensory information from all these sources and is also influenced by circulatory pyrogens and monoamines. The manner in which this integration is accomplished is unknown.

EFFECT OF SKIN TEMPERATURE

All biologic tissues have a sensitivity to temperature, usually an increase in activity of two- to three-fold for a 10°C change in temperature. But certain cells in the skin have an unusually high temperature sensitivity; it is these cells that are suspected of serving as temperature detectors or *thermoreceptors*. These thermoreceptors are distributed unevenly over the skin in a punctate or spotty fashion, and they are functionally of two kinds: those that increase their firing rate in response to increasing temperature (warm spots) and those activated by decreasing temperature (cold spots). Changes in environmental temperature can be sensed first by the skin's thermoreceptors, and it has been shown that these signals can inhibit sweating and excite shivering. But their influence is modifying rather than determinative, and whether in response to heat or cold stress, the hypothalamic (core) temperature must first attain the critical level or set point. For example, the metabolic rate remains at the basal level regardless of the skin temperature until the hypothalamic temperature drops below the critical level of 37.1°C (Fig. 4-4*a*). At lower central temperatures the metabolic rate is excited by cold thermoreceptors. However, the influence of skin temperature is relatively weak. A drop of only 0.3°C in central temperature has the same effect on metabolic rate as a drop of 10°C in skin temperature. As the skin temperature drops below 20°C, firing rates of cold receptors decline and there is diminished influence on the metabolic rate.[2,4]

Similarly, sweating does not occur unless the central temperature exceeds 37°C regardless of skin temperature (Fig. 4-4*b*). Once this hypothalamic temperature is attained, lowering skin temperature and activating cold thermoreceptors inhibit sweating. The sweat rate appears to be independent of warm receptors; there is no augmentation of sweating above 33°C. As indicated in Fig. 4-4, a skin temperature in excess of 31°C effectively prevents increased heat production and a skin temperature less than 29°C effectively inhibits sweating. These temperature thresholds vary slightly for different individuals.

THERMAL BALANCE

The core temperature is maintained by the balance between heat production and heat loss:

$$H_{\text{produced}} - H_{\text{lost}} = \frac{dQ}{dt} = \frac{CMdT}{dt}$$

The change in heat content with time (dQ/dt) is more usefully expressed in terms of body's specific heat C = 0.83 kcal °C^{-1} kg^{-1}, mass M, and temperature T. When environmental thermal stress changes, heat production and heat loss are transiently out of balance and heat is added or lost to the body. Because of its high heat capacity, the body is able to accept substantial changes in heat content with only slight changes in

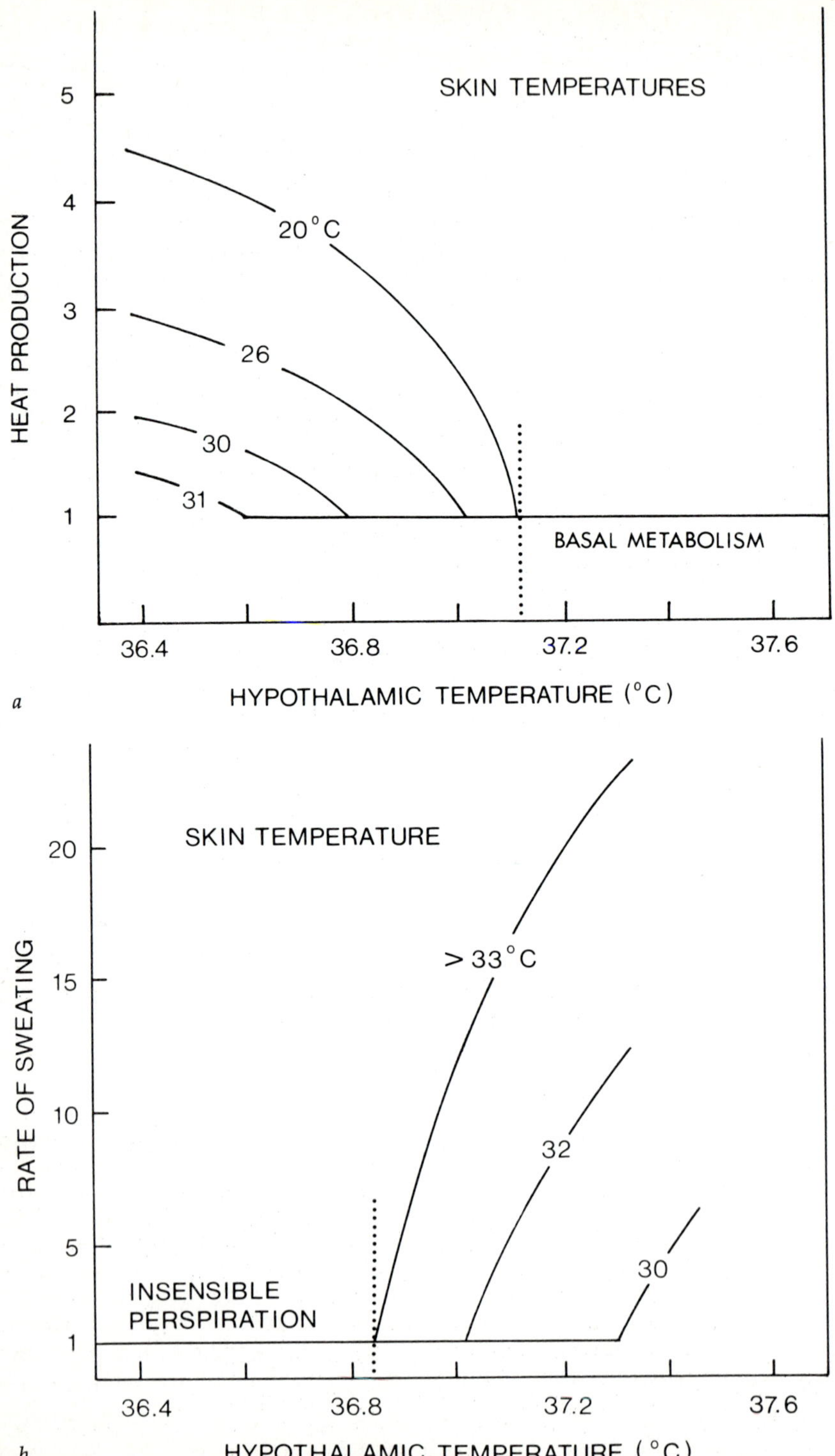

SKIN TEMPERATURES
HEAT PRODUCTION
5
4
3
2
1
20°C
26
30
31
BASAL METABOLISM
36.4
36.8
37.2
37.6
HYPOTHALAMIC TEMPERATURE (°C)
a
SKIN TEMPERATURE
RATE OF SWEATING
20
15
10
5
1
> 33°C
32
30
INSENSIBLE
PERSPIRATION
36.4
36.8
37.2
37.6
HYPOTHALAMIC TEMPERATURE (°C)
b

temperature. Approximately 58 kcal is required to raise the temperature of a 70-kg adult by 1°C, that is,

$$Q = CM\,\Delta T = 0.83 \times 70 \times 1 = 58 \text{ kcal}$$

Normally, the human body generates this much heat in about 30 to 40 min. As the body approaches a state of thermal equilibrium, dQ/dt decreases to zero, and heat production and heat lost are again equal. When thermal balance is maintained in a long-term steady state, body temperature stabilizes at constant values, and the conditions for balance can be summarized by the relationship

$$M = E + R = C_d + C_v$$

where M = total heat produced by body metabolism
E = heat transferred by evaporation of water from cutaneous surface and from lungs
R = heat transferred by radiation
C_d = heat transferred by conduction
C_v = heat transferred by convection

The last three quantities in the equation above can be either positive or negative, depending on whether the surface of the skin is cooler or hotter than the environment. Metabolic heat reaching the skin surface is transferred to the environment by radiation, conduction, convection, and/or evaporation. Exchange by these processes depends not only on the physical conditions of the environment, temperature, and humidity but also on two physical conditions of the skin, its temperature and its wetness due to sweating.[5]

HEAT PRODUCTION

As the energy foods are oxidized in metabolizing tissues, large amounts of energy are released. This is not thermal energy originally, i.e., long-wavelength heat energy, but chemical energy of higher quanta.

◀ **Figure 4-4** (*a*) Effect of skin and core temperatures on heat production. Until the hypothalamic (core) temperature falls below a critical level (37.1°C in the given example), the metabolic rate remains at the basal level. As the core temperature decreases below 37.1°C, the metabolic rate increases rapidly at a rate that depends on skin temperature. High skin temperatures reduce metabolic heat production and lower the critical level or set point. Above a skin temperature of 31°C, little elevation of metabolic rate occurs. (*b*) Effect of skin and core temperatures on sweating rate. Sweating does not occur unless the hypothalamic (core) temperature exceeds a critical level [36.8°C, a different subject than in (*a*)]. Above this temperature, sweating increases very rapidly with slight increases in core temperature. Sweat rate is independent of skin temperatures above 33°C; otherwise, low skin temperatures depress sweating and raise the critical level or set point. [*Drawn from TH Benzinger, C Kitzinger, Microcolorimetry: New methods and objectives, in JD Hardy (ed), Temperature—Its Measurement and Control in Science and Industry, New York, Reinhold, 1963, vol 3, p 43.*]

HEAT DISTRIBUTION

Heat is distributed from the sites of production to the skin and the epithelial linings by combined conduction and vascular convection. The tissue compartments that exhibit the greatest variability in blood flow are the skin, muscles, and splanchnic area; of these, the flow through the skin and muscle is of special importance.

SKIN BLOOD FLOW

Heat regulation is the primary function of the skin's circulation; its flow is 10 to 20 times that required to supply metabolites and oxygen. Under basal conditions roughly 8.5 percent or 450 ml/min of the total blood flow passes through the skin,[6] and it may be greatly increased or decreased with thermal stress.

Since the heat conductivity and specific heat of blood are high, large amounts of heat can be transported to the skin and dissipated with only small changes in the temperature of the blood. The blood flowing through the hands and feet is particularly significant, since this blood flow is extremely high and is under efficient vasoconstrictor control. In contrast, blood flow to the arms and legs is mainly under vasodilator control and seemingly is more closely related to the metabolic requirements of these more muscular regions.[6] It is important to realize that the skin is not a uniform structure; the primary regulative blood vessels engaged in radiative and convective heat loss are limited to the distal extremities and the ears and lips. The rest of the skin, although able to transfer heat passively or through vasodilator mechanisms, is not under sympathetic control.

SPECIALIZED ARCHITECTURE OF BLOOD VESSELS IN SKIN

The circulatory apparatus in the skin consists of the usual nutritive arteries, capillaries, and veins, along with vascular structures concerned primarily with heat transfer.

An extensive subcutaneous venous plexus can hold large quantities of blood, whose rate of flow can be markedly altered.

Arteriovenous (AV) anastomoses are plentiful in the feet, hands, lips, nose, and ears, and they may be used to regulate temperature by opening and closing. Part of the heat produced by exercising muscles can be lost from overlying skin in a similar manner. Superficial veins transport blood from working muscles to the skin without passing into the central circulation.

Blood supplied to the arms and legs by large arteries can return by either of two routes: by superficial veins near the skin surface or by deep venae comitantes (companion veins adjacent and parallel to the main arteries). The apportionment of blood between these two avenues of venous return is under sympathetic control and is extremely important to heat conservation under cold conditions and heat dissipation under warm conditions.

TISSUE INSULATION

The difference in the core and skin temperature ($T_c - T_s$) leads to a natural definition of tissue insulation. The total steady-state heat flux through the skin can be expressed by

$$j_H = \frac{T_c - T_s}{I_t} = \frac{\Delta T}{R}$$

where I_t = the total insulation or thermal resistance

Body insulation is conceptualized as the resistance to heat flow offered by the peripheral tissue layers across which the temperature changes from T_c to T_s. The total insulation includes both tissue and clothing components; in a normally dressed individual in a neutral temperature environment this is 0.1°C $\text{kcal}^{-1}\ \text{h}^{-1}\ \text{m}^{-2}$. Heat-induced vasodilation may reduce this to 0.02 and vasoconstriction can increase it to 0.3°C $\text{kcal}^{-1}\ \text{h}^{-1}\ \text{m}^{-2}$. The insulating layer affects heat transfer in three different ways: by direct changes in insulation I_t through alterations in the quantity of blood flow, by varying its thickness and the amount of tissue available for cooling, and by permitting skin temperature to drop, thus lowering T and reducing heat flow.

RESPONSE TO COLD

When blood colder than normal passes into the preoptic region of the hypothalamus, various heat conservation and production mechanisms become stimulated (Fig. 4-4*a*). The sympathetics are excited, and this causes the blood vessels in the skin to constrict powerfully. The flow of warm blood from the core to the skin is decreased, thereby decreasing the transfer of heat to the body surface. The temperature of the skin drops to approach the air temperature, and this lowers the temperature gradient and further decreases heat loss. Stimulation of the sympathetic nerves also causes the secretion of epinephrine and norepinephrine by the adrenal medulla. These hormones increase the metabolic rates of all cells, thereby increasing heat production. Impulses from the preoptic hypothalamus also activate the primary motor center for shivering, which, in turn, increases the tone of all the muscles. The resulting increase in muscle metabolism can increase heat production by as much as 50 percent. When muscle tone increases beyond a critical level, the stretch reflex begins to oscillate, shivering occurs, and body heat production can increase as much as two to four times normal.

RESPONSE TO HEAT

When blood warmer than normal passes into the preoptic hypothalamus, the heat production center becomes inhibited and heat production mechanisms become inoperative. Any increased metabolism caused by prior sympathetic stimulation ceases and muscular tone diminishes. The blood vessels in the skin dilate, allowing blood to accumulate and heat to be lost rapidly. Vasodilatation also occurs reflexly through direct warming of the skin surface. In addition to reversing the heat-promotion mechanisms, stimulation of the heat center produces sweating and panting.

PHYSICAL MECHANISMS OF HEAT TRANSFER TO THE ENVIRONMENT

All matter radiates and absorbs electromagnetic energy. The amount of energy gained or lost by an object through radiation depends on its surface area, its emissive power (i.e., its radiating power relative to an ideal radiator—a black body), and the difference in temperature between it and other objects in the environment. Human skin, regardless of color, is nearly a perfect black body.[7] Because of our relatively low absolute temperature (T_s = 32 to 33°C = 350K), the skin's black-body emission curve is in the infrared range (0.7 to 20 μm) and has only a barely perceptible maximum at about 9.5 μm. This means that we radiate and absorb heat by infrared radiation in this range with almost perfect efficiency. Were the environment at thermal equilibrium with us, we would all be at this same temperature, radiating and absorbing these same wavelengths. But far more intense sources of radiation such as the sun or manufactured objects, a hot stove, for example, upset this idealized thermal equilibrium. Since skin temperature is ordinarily limited to less than 35°C, an environmental radiant temperature T_R higher than this normally means heat gain, while a T_R less than 32°C usually results in heat loss. The heat flux from the skin to the environment under a 4°C temperature differential is about 36 kcal/h, or about 40 percent of the total heat exchange. (This assumes a total metabolic rate of 85 kcal/h appropriate to a resting adult of average size.)

Conduction and Convection

Conduction is the direct transfer of thermal energy by atomic or molecular collisions without their actual interchange. Conduction ordinarily does not play a predominant role in thermoregulation. However, under cold stress and strong vasoconstriction, the insulating tissue shell surrounding the body core loses heat, principally by conduction. The fact that heat is lost more slowly by this process than when the blood is flowing is vital to heat conservation.

Thermal convection is the transfer of molecules moving in groups carrying their thermal energy with them. Pumping of blood by the heart is an example of forced convection. Natural convection occurs when warm air rises from the body surface. The skin exerts a frictional drag in the air surrounding it, so that a layer of air whose thickness depends upon the air velocity adheres to it. Figure 4-5 shows the considerable effect that even a small ambient wind of only 8 mi/h has on reducing the thickness of the insulating air layer. The heat that is convected from the skin must first be conducted through this air layer before it passes to the environment.

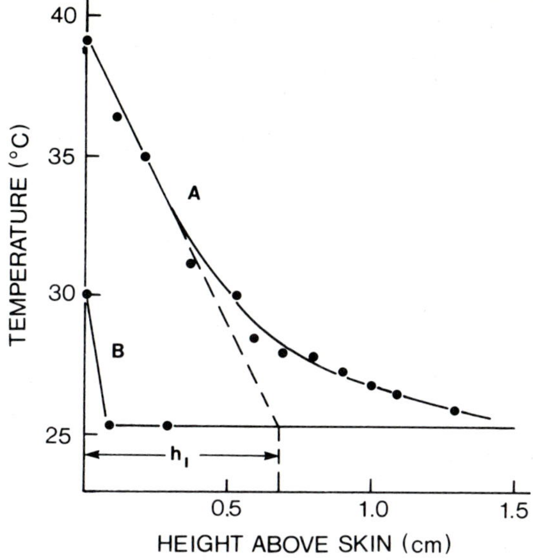

Figure 4-5 The temperature profile shows the thickness of the boundary layer next to the skin in the absence of wind (A) and in a wind of 8 mi/h (B). The "effective" or truly still air thickness in the absence of wind has been constructed (h_1). (*Drawn from RT Tregear, Physical Functions of Skin, London, Academic, 1966.*)

EVAPORATIVE HEAT LOSS AND THE SWEATING MECHANISM

Figure 4.4 illustrates the rapid increase in sweat rate that occurs once the critical hypothalamic temperature (set point) is exceeded. For every gram of water evaporated from the skin or from the membranes of the respiratory tract, 580 cal heat is lost. Only about 7 percent of the total metabolic heat is lost by respiration; more than 100 percent can be lost through the evaporation of sweat. Sweat rates in unacclimatized individuals can reach 3 to 4 liters per hour for short periods, but over a 24-h period the rate of sweating rarely exceeds 0.6 liter per hour. This value, 600 ml/h, is an estimate of the sweat rate that can be maintained indefinitely. In the absence of active sweating, approximately 10 ml/h water is lost through the skin by passive diffusion—sometimes called insensible perspiration.

Sweating is at least a two-step process: (1) precursor fluid formation and (2) the resorption and exchange of many of the components of this fluid by the sweat duct. The precursor fluid is very close to the plasma concentration in sodium and chloride, i.e., 140 mg per liter. Lactate, urea, and potassium are the other major chemical components. As the fluid passes through the duct, resorption of sodium and exchange of some of the other components occur. In a manner similar to its effect on the renal tubule, aldosterone increases the resorption and retention of sodium and excretion of potassium. Because of these active resorption and exchange processes, normal sweat on the skin surface is always hypotonic to plasma.

ACCLIMATIZATION

Repeated exposure of active individuals to either hot or cold environments produces physiological changes that lead to a greater degree of "thermoregulatory fitness." The process is called artificial acclimatization and is similar but inferior to the natural acclimatization acquired by long-term residence or that exhibited by persons indigenous to a given environment.[8]

Hot Environments

When individuals who have not recently been exposed to severe heat have to work hard under hot-wet conditions, their endurance is low. They rapidly become flushed, their respiration rate increases, they may hyperventilate, they suffer from postural hypotension, and they soon may undergo a hypotensive collapse. Both skin and body temperatures rise significantly. In the unacclimatized person, the circulatory collapse is brought about by a rapid peripheral vasodilation that is triggered locally by a hot skin and centrally by a slight overall rise in body temperature. Anastomoses are opened, and in combination with cutaneous vasodilation a considerable increase in the volume of the peripheral vascular bed occurs. As a result of a now inadequate blood volume, there is a partial failure of the venous return and acute circulatory collapse. The onset of sweating is delayed, and cardiovascular collapse may occur before any significant sweating is established. During the acclimatization process, plasma volume increases; in addition, there is increased salt retention by both sweat and urine as a consequence of increased secretion of aldosterone. Finally, the rate of sweating increases and commences at progressively lower rectal temperatures.[9] Vasomotor responses also improve; vasoconstriction increases, and there is a progressive decline in the peripheral blood flow. Skin temperature may be 2 to 3°C lower when an individual is fully acclimatized.

Cold Environments

The human is a tropical animal whose "critical" temperature in still, dry air is about 28°C.[10] Below this temperature, clothes or muscular activity are required to maintain a normal body temperature. Humans rarely become completely acclimatized to cold environments. Physiological temperature regulation in cold climates depends upon vasoconstriction to conserve heat and/or chemical thermogenesis, shivering, or exercise to produce it. These are mostly refractory to acclimatization, however, so humans generally rely on behavioral temperature regulation. They select insulative clothing and adopt appropriate behavior to ensure that they remain warm and comfortable. Some degree of acclimatization apparently does occur; for example, individuals in the Arctic develop basal metabolic rates 20 percent above normal.

DISTURBANCES IN THERMOREGULATION

Heat Cramps and Heat Exhaustion

Cramping pains in the muscles, low blood pressure, pallor, vertigo and nausea, vomiting, and fainting can occur in individuals engaged in prolonged, very active, heat-producing work. The symptoms are caused by sodium chloride depletion that accompanies profuse sweating. They are rapidly relieved by taking salt and can be prevented by taking extra salt beforehand. These symptoms can occur because temperature regulation has priority over the maintenance of salt and water balance despite their severe depletion.[11]

In cystic fibrosis there is a defect in the ability of eccrine sweat ducts to resorb and hence conserve sodium. Consequently, patients with this disorder produce abnormally salty perspiration, and under severe heat stress they can suffer massive salt depletion and extreme symptoms of heat exhaustion. Oral administration of physiological saline during periods of hot weather easily prevents heat casualties in these patients.

Heat Stroke or Hyperpyrexia

Sometimes after exposure to extreme temperatures people may collapse, become unconscious, and die within a short time with temperatures of over 41°C. The symptoms are due to a rapid decline and finally a cessation of sweating. There is some evidence that this may be related to what is commonly called "sweat gland fatigue," the decline in sweating seen during exposure to severe heat.[12] But the physiological pathology of heat stroke is not well understood. Hot, dry skin and a rising internal temperature accompanied by periods of delirium and unconsciousness are signs of this dangerous syndrome.[11,13]

Fever

Fever, which commonly means a body temperature above the usual normal range, is often used to designate the high temperatures associated with infections and other febrile diseases. Such fevers are thought to be the result of an increased hypothalamic "set point" caused by the direct action of a circulating pyrogen. Endogenous pyrogens are produced in the bloodstream 30 to 60 min after the intravenous infection of extracts of infectious bacteria, pathogenic fungi, or viruses.[14] It has been suggested that aspirin and other antipyretics act by inhibiting cyclooxygenase, thereby blocking the production of prostaglandin E_1, a potent fever inducer and perhaps the ultimate pyrogen.[15]

Accidental Hypothermia

Accidental hypothermia is a fall in body core temperature to below 35°C by exposure to a low ambient temperature. The victims are most often healthy youngsters or adults who run into difficulties in cold climatic conditions. Physical and mental exhaustion, combined with inexperience of the circumstances, are contributing factors. Hypothermic incidents of this kind have occurred during mountain hiking, navigation competitions, skiing, white-water excursions, and swimming. When a person exercises in a wet-cold environment, oxygen intake can be 50 percent higher than it is when exercising in a dry-cold environment. This obligatory drain is exhausting in unfit people and accounts for the premature fatigue commonly associated with cold exposure accidents. The combination of wind and wetting reduces the effective thermal insulation of a typical clothing ensemble to one-tenth of its normal value.[16] This makes the insulation of subcutaneous fat as important in wet-cold conditions as it is in immersion in cold water. Exercising in wet-cold conditions causes general discomfort, and the rectal temperature tends to decrease unless the workload is heavy—in which case it cannot be sustained for long. Another contributing factor may be the dysfunction of motor nerves in the cold, leading to clumsiness in walking and in manual dexterity.[17]

REFERENCES

1. Hammel HT: Regulation of internal body temperature. *Annu Rev Physiol* 30:641, 1968.
2. Benzinger TH: Peripheral cold reception and central warm reception, sensory mechanisms of behavior and autonomic thermostasis, in JD Hardy et al (eds), *Physiological and Behavioral Temperature Regulation*. Springfield, Ill, Charles C Thomas, 1968, p 831.
3. Hardy JD: Peripheral inputs to the central regulation for the body temperature, in S Itoh et al (eds), *Advances in Climatic Physiology*. Tokyo, Igaku-Shoin, 1972, p 417.
4. Benzinger TH: Heat regulation: homeostasis of central temperature in man. *Physiol Rev* 49:672, 1969.
5. Gagge AP, Nishi Y: Heat exchange between human skin surface and thermal environment, in DHK Lee et al (eds), *Handbook of Physiology*, sec 9: *Reactions to Environmental Agents*. Bethesda, American Physiological Society, 1977.
6. Hertzmann AB, Randall WC: Regional differences in the basal and maximal rates of blood flow in the skin. *J Appl Physiol* 1:234, 1948.
7. Hardy JD, DuBois EF: The technique of measuring radiation and convection. *J Nutr* 15:461, 1937.
8. Ladell WSS: Terrestrial animals in humid heat: Man, in DB Dill et al (eds), *Handbook of Physiology*, sec 4: *Adaptation to the Environment*. Washington, American Physiological Society, 1964, p 625.
9. Morimoto T: Acclimatization of sweating mechanism to hot environments, in A Jarrett (ed), *The Physiology and Pathophysiology of the Skin*. London, Academic, 1978, vol 5, p 1645.
10. Wilkerson JR et al: Critical temperature of unacclimatized male caucasians. *J Appl Physiol* 33:451, 1972.
11. Leithead CS, Lind AR: *Heat Stress and Head Disorders*. Philadelphia, Davis, 1964.
12. Sargent F: Depression of sweating in man: so-called "sweat gland fatigue," in W Montagna et al (eds), *Advances in Biology of Skin*. New York, Pergamon, 1962, vol 3, p 163.
13. Lind AR: Pathophysiology of heat exhaustion and heat stroke, in M Khogali, JRS Hales (eds), *Heat Stroke and Temperature Regulation*. Sydney, Academic Press, 1983, p 312.
14. Wood WB Jr: The pathogenesis of fever, in S Mudd (ed), *Infectious Agents and Host Reactions*, Philadelphia, Saunders, 1970, p 146.

15. Stitt JT et al: PGE_1 fever: its effect on thermoregulation at different low ambient temperatures. *Am J Physiol* 227:622, 1974.
16. Pugh LGCE: Cold stress and muscular exercise, with special reference to accidental hypothermia. *Br Med J* 2:333, 1967.
17. Hirvonen J: Accidental hypothermia, in P Lomax, E Schonbaum (eds), *Body Temperature Regulation, Drug Effects and Therapeutic Implications.* New York, Marcel Dekker, 1979, p 664.

5

Percutaneous Absorption

Peter Buchan and Jean-Claude Jamoulle

Percutaneous absorption may be defined as the passage of substances from the surface through the skin, where they may enter the systemic circulation via the capillary network and lymphatics or remain located subcutaneously. This subject is of interest not only in the field of dermatology but also in the fields of cosmetics, environmental toxicology, and transdermal drug delivery. Only in the case of transdermal drug delivery is percutaneous absorption a deliberate aim, presenting simply a potential for systemic side effects in the other cases. The development of new dermatological products presents the challenge of increasing local activity without causing a concomitant rise in systemic activity.

This chapter briefly reviews the main features of percutaneous absorption and the barrier function of the skin in its healthy, damaged, and diseased states. Some excellent books are available to the reader seeking more detailed information.[1–6]

BARRIER, RESERVOIR, AND METABOLIC FUNCTIONS OF SKIN

The skin plays an important role as a protective organ, controlling the penetration of xenobiotics into the viable tissues and the systemic circulation and the excretion of other substances such as water. The various events following the application of a drug to the skin are shown schematically in Fig. 5-1. On liberation from its vehicle, a drug may penetrate the skin via either the stratum corneum or skin appendages such as the hair follicle

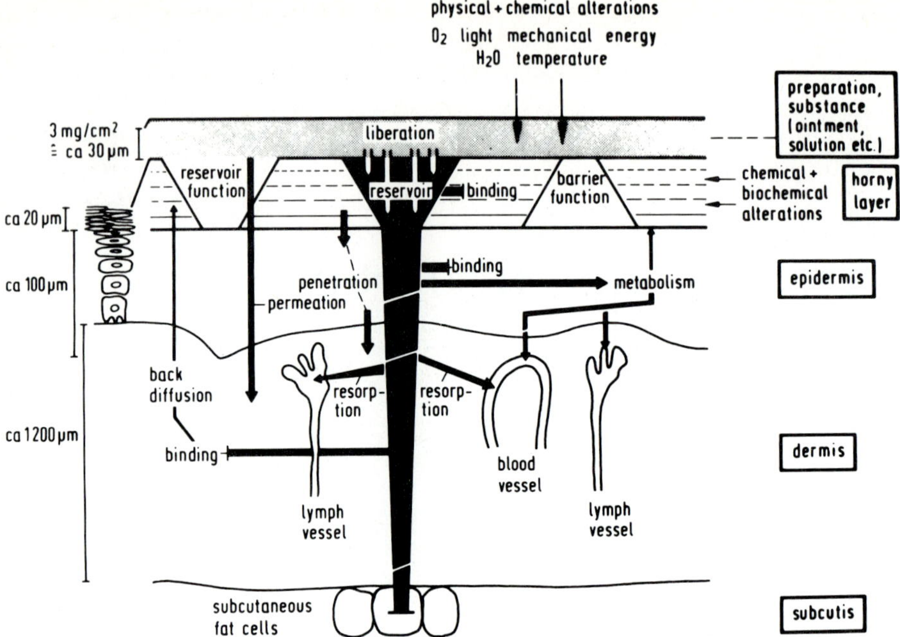

Figure 5-1 Local events subsequent to the application of a drug or substance to the skin surface.

(so-called shunt pathways), then traverse through the epidermis to the dermis for removal by the microcirculation. During diffusion the drug may be bound to macromolecules and undergo metabolism. Although it has been clearly demonstrated that certain substances accumulate in appendages such as the hair follicle that may be important for targeted delivery,[7] the contribution of these pathways to overall absorption has yet to be quantified, and there is little doubt that, in general, the stratum corneum represents the major barrier to penetration in the skin.

As epidermal cells progress outward to form the stratum corneum, membrane-coating granules or Odland bodies are exocytosed, forming a multilamellar structure of lipid bilayers containing molecules of cholesterol, fatty acids, acylglucosylceramide, and acylceramides. It is currently believed that the arrangement of this multilamellar structure constitutes a selective barrier to penetration.

When the distribution of penetrating substances in various skin layers is examined during percutaneous absorption experiments, the highest concentrations are usually found in the stratum corneum. While this is compatible with the passage through the stratum corneum forming the rate-limiting step in percutaneous absorption, it has been shown that the stratum corneum also acts as a reservoir after removal of excess material remaining on the surface of the skin following topical application. This observation was originally made with corticosteroids[8] but has since been found to apply to many other substances, such as antifungals and retinoids.

The ability of the skin to metabolize hydrocarbons and steroids has been known for some time and has been studied in detail. When the total field of cutaneous metabolism is reviewed, it becomes apparent that skin can perform most of the phase one and phase two transformations associated with hepatic enzyme activity.[9–11] This xenobiotic metabolizing activity is performed largely by the viable epidermis, which can be regarded as the counterpart to the liver in terms of first-pass metabolism of drugs administered by the topical and oral routes, respectively.

Metabolites formed on the passage of xenobiotics through the epidermis may be biologically inactive or may express activities not possessed by the parent substance. Thus, polycyclic aromatic hydrocarbons are activated in skin by oxidative metabolism, a step necessary for expression of their carcinogenic potential, whereas other topically applied substances may be subject to a first-pass metabolic step that reduces their pharmacological activity.

METHODS FOR STUDYING PERCUTANEOUS ABSORPTION

To obtain the most meaningful results, percutaneous absorption should be studied under the most relevant conditions, namely, after appropriate topical exposure in humans. However, this is often impossible due to ethical problems with potentially toxic substances and to analytical limitations when the rate and extent of absorption are low. When possible, such studies are of much value.[12,13] As a result, a variety of alternative techniques have been developed.

A widely used in vitro technique involves applying a test substance to the surface of excised skin or an artificial membrane suspended across a diffusion cell and measuring the appearance of the test substance in the fluid bathing the underside of the skin in a receptor chamber.[14] Human skin maintained in a viable state most closely resembles the in vivo situation, although artifacts can occur particularly due to the loss of a functional capillary network and metabolic function.

Due to their indirect nature, noninvasive in vivo techniques must be verified as suitable for estimating percutaneous absorption. Techniques of particular utility are the measurement of transepidermal water loss, which indicates the general state of the skin barrier and has been shown to correlate well with the absorption of certain substances applied to different areas of the body,[15] and measurement of the quantity of drug in the upper layers of the stratum corneum removed by serial tape stripping, which predicts very accurately the amount of substance absorbed after a single administration and a relatively short exposure period.[16]

PHARMACOKINETIC ASPECTS

A pharmacokinetic approach to percutaneous absorption is essential for analyzing the physiological mechanisms involved and their interaction with the penetrant and vehicle, and for predicting the outcome of percutaneous absorption under diverse circumstances.

Substances traverse the skin barrier by passive diffusion, the driving force being the higher concentration at the outer surface. In its simplest form the diffusional flux, $J = A \cdot Kp \cdot \Delta C$, where J is quantity per unit time, A is area of skin, Kp is the permeability coefficient, and ΔC is the difference in concentration across the skin. The permeability coefficient reflects the overall contribution of the different layers to barrier function and can be further defined by $Kp = D \cdot Km \cdot 1^{-1}$, where D is the diffusion coefficient, Km is the skin:vehicle partition coefficient, and 1 is the distance traversed by the diffusing substance. The pharmacokinetic parameter to be studied depends on the situation in question. Obviously, in the case of a transdermal administration of a drug such as scopolamine, where an optimum blood level is to be maintained, the rate of absorption is important. On the other hand, when chronic topical exposure can give rise to a chronic systemic effect, the total amount absorbed daily may be more important than the rate of absorption. The total pharmacokinetic behavior with regard to systemic activity will, of course, depend also on the further distribution, metabolism, and excretion of the substance concerned. The topical route often involves repeated administration. Estimation of percutaneous absorption should take into account not only the frequency and duration of exposure but also the possibility of nonlinear pharmacokinetics through drug- or vehicle-induced changes in barrier function by damage or healing processes or through induction or inhibition of skin-metabolizing enzymes.

INTERACTIONS INVOLVING SKIN, PENETRANT, AND VEHICLE

Because percutaneous absorption is a passive diffusion phenomenon, it depends on the physicochemical interaction involving the test substance, its vehicle, and the barrier presented by the skin under the influence of any relevant external factors (Fig. 5-2).

Occlusion is an external influence that can affect the vehicle and the stratum corneum; the latter becomes hydrated, selectively facilitating the penetration of certain substances. Iontophoresis also falls into the category

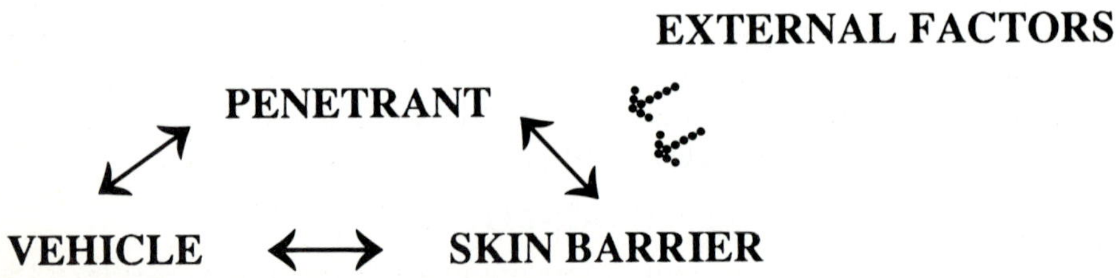

EXTERNAL FACTORS

PENETRANT

VEHICLE ⟷ SKIN BARRIER

Figure 5-2 Interactions in percutaneous absorption.

of external influences and is being intensively studied as a means to increase the penetration of otherwise poorly penetrating substances.[17]

Since the semipermeable nature of the cutaneous barrier depends on the anatomical and biochemical composition of skin, changes in these aspects due to variations within the normal physiological state or external factors may result in altered percutaneous absorption.

Under normal physiological conditions, important intraindividual differences have been observed with respect to the site of application in humans. In addition, clear regional variations in percutaneous absorption exist. In general, absorption is high in the scrotum, jaw angle, forehead, axilla, and scalp and low in the forearm, palm, and foot arch.[18]

The results using ^{14}C-labeled substances indicated that percutaneous absorption may be decreased in elderly people, particularly for less lipid-soluble compounds.[19] The in vitro penetration of tritiated water, alcohols, and fatty acids through human skin samples is similar in full-term infants and adults but greatly elevated in preterm infants, demonstrating incomplete barrier function.[20] Therefore, the newborn must nevertheless be considered at higher risk for the systemic effects of topical administration due to immature metabolism, both cutaneous and systemic, a greater surface-to-volume ratio, and other conditions such as occlusive dressings or clothing.

Studies on homologous series of molecules have illustrated the importance of physicochemical properties such as the octanol:water partition coefficient in percutaneous absorption. With moderately nonpolar substances, increasing lipophilicity results in increasing permeability, supporting the idea of a lipoidal pathway for passage through the skin.[21] However, this does not hold for extremely nonpolar molecules, whose passage from the stratum corneum appears to be impeded by the more aqueous environment of the lower layers of the epidermis, suggesting in their case a rate-controlling step beyond the stratum corneum. At the other end of the scale, the permeation of more polar molecules does not seem to depend on the octanol:water partition coefficient. Water channels in the stratum corneum or passage via shunt routes provided by skin appendages may be the explanation for this behavior.

The vehicle can exert an influence at two levels: first, by liberating the penetrant from the vehicle into the stratum corneum and, second, by influencing the barrier properties of the stratum corneum directly or indirectly. The liberation of a penetrant from the vehicle into the stratum corneum depends on its "readiness" to leave the vehicle—expressed as thermodynamic activity—and the partition coefficient created between the vehicle and the stratum corneum.[2] Since the thermodynamic activity is highest at saturation of the penetrant in the vehicle, it is argued that a true comparison of the potential ability of different vehicles to augment the penetration of a given test substance should be made not at equal concentrations but at saturation of the test substance in the vehicles.

In fact, it is likely that most formulations will have some effect on the stratum corneum. Indirectly, an ointment-type formulation may form an occlusive layer, increasing the water content of the stratum corneum. A wide range of organic solvents and surfactants such as propylene glycol, dimethylsulfoxide, oleic acid, and pyrrolidine derivatives have been shown to enhance penetration through the stratum corneum, an effect attributed to different interactions with the lipid bilayers of the intercellular spaces. The penetration enhancers appear to possess different mechanisms of action, varying in efficacy depending on the penetrant in question and exhibiting synergism with certain combinations of enhancers. Much of the current interest in penetration enhancers is related to transdermal delivery systems that are often limited by low percutaneous absorption.

DAMAGED SKIN

Removal of the stratum corneum by stripping represents the extreme case and has been used by several workers as a reference for assessing the degree of diminution in barrier function. The permeability of rat skin to water increases in relation to the degree of physical damage inflicted and returns to normal levels during the repair process.[22] Although damage induced by chemicals such as sodium laurylsulfate has been shown to increase percutaneous absorption, chemical insults seem to have less effect than physical injury. Ultraviolet irradiation can also lead to increased absorption, depending on the duration of exposure.[23]

In rats suffering from essential fatty acid deficiency, transepidermal water loss and percutaneous absorption of hydrocortisone increase in relation to the disease state.[24] These changes probably result from a disruption in the balance of stratum corneum lipids essential to barrier function.[25]

DISEASED SKIN

Human dermatological disease represents a category of abnormal or damaged skin conditions in which changes in skin permeability are of particular practical relevance. Although it can be reasoned that diseases characterized by deviations in the anatomical and biochemical features related to barrier functions should result in altered skin permeability, definitive studies are far more difficult to conceive than in the cases of deliberately damaged skin discussed above. Despite problems such as the number of and uniformity of sample sites, adequate controls (uninvolved contralateral sites or matched normal subjects), concomitant treatment, exacerbation or remission of disease, and analytical limitations, certain studies have yielded useful information.

After topical application of triamcinolone acetonide or desoxymethasone to psoriatic patients, higher concentrations were found in involved compared to non-involved skin.[1] On the other hand, when estimated by urinary elimination in normal and psoriatic subjects, the percutaneous absorption of hydrocortisone and anthralin did not differ between the two groups of subjects.[26,27] These apparently contradictory findings may be explained by the differential influence of diseased skin on local and systemic bioavailability.

By measuring serum cortisol levels during dexamethasone-induced adrenocortical suppression, Turpeinen[28] recently demonstrated a positive correlation between the percutaneous absorption of hydrocortisone and the severity of the disease in children suffering from atopic dermatitis. In adults suffering from chronic atopic dermatitis, the percutaneous absorption of hydrocortisone increased during exacerbation and decreased during remission of the disease.[29]

It should be borne in mind that possible changes in percutaneous absorption depend not only on the nature and severity of the disease, but also on the drug in question and on drug-induced changes in barrier function such as irritation or healing of the disease. When considering both the therapeutic efficacy and the possible local and systemic side effects of a topical therapy, an understanding of percutaneous absorption is crucial. Factors such as age, site of application, occlusion, vehicle, and disease state should be taken into account in order to relate the quantity and frequency of applied drug to its potential pharmacological activities.

REFERENCES

1. Schaefer H et al; *Skin Permeability*. Berlin, Springer-Verlag, 1982.
2. Barry BW: *Dermatological Formulations: Percutaneous Absorption*. New York, Marcel Dekker, 1983.
3. Skerrow D, Skerrow CJ: *Methods in Skin Research*. New York, Wiley, 1985.
4. Shroot B, Schaefer H: *Pharmacology and the Skin*, vol 1: *Skin Pharmacokinetics*. Basel, Karger, 1987.
5. Bronaugh RL, Maibach HI: *Percutaneous Absorption*, 2d ed. New York, Marcel Dekker, 1989.
6. Scott RC et al: *Prediction of Percutaneous Penetration*. London, IBC Technical Services, 1990.
7. Schaefer H et al: Follicular penetration, in RC Scott et al (eds), *Prediction of Percutaneous Penetration*. London, IBC Technical Services, 1990, p 163.
8. Vickers CFH: Existence of reservoir in the stratum corneum. *Arch Dermatol* 88:20, 1963.
9. Pannatier A et al: The skin as a drug-metabolizing organ. *Drug Metab Rev* 8:319, 1978.
10. Kappus H: Drug metabolism in the skin. *Handls Exp Pharm* 87:123, 1989.
11. Noonan PK, Wester RC: Cutaneous metabolism of xenobiotics, in RL Bronaugh, HI Maibach (eds), *Percutaneous Absorption*, 2d ed. New York, Marcel Dekker, 1989, p 53.
12. Feldmann RJ, Maibach HI: Percutaneous penetration of steroids in man. *J Invest Dermatol* 52:89, 1969.
13. Chandrasekaran SK et al: Pharmacokinetics of drug permeation through human skin. *J. Pharm Sci* 67:1370, 1978.
14. Franz TJ: The finite dose technique as a valid in vitro model for the study of percutaneous absorption. *Curr Probl Dermatol* 7:58, 1978.
15. Lotte C et al: In vivo relationship between transepidermal water loss and percutaneous penetration of some organic compounds in man: effect of anatomic site. *Arch Dermatol Res* 279:351, 1987.
16. Rougier A et al: In vivo correlation between stratum corneum reservoir function and percutaneous absorption. *J Invest Dermatol* 81:275, 1983.
17. Sloan JB, Soltani K: Iontophoresis in dermatology. *J Am Acad Dermatol* 15:671, 1986.
18. Feldmann RJ, Maibach HI: Regional variation in percutaneous penetration of ^{14}C cortisol in man. *J Invest Dermatol* 48:181, 1967.

19. Roskos KV et al: The effect of aging on percutaneous absorption in man. *J Pharmacokinet Biopharm* 17:617, 1989.
20. Fisher LB: Studies on the permeability of infant skin, in RL Bronaugh, HI Maibach (eds), *Percutaneous Absorption,* 2nd ed. New York, Marcel Dekker, 1989, p 135.
21. Roberts M et al: Permeability of human epidermis to phenolic compounds. *J Pharm Pharmacol* 29:677, 1977.
22. Scott RC et al: Permeability of abnormal rat skin. *J Invest Dermatol* 86:201, 1986.
23. Lamaud E, Schalla W: Influence of UV irradiation on penetration of hydrocortisone: in vivo study in hairless rat skin. *Br J Dermatol* 111:152, 1984.
24. Schalla W et al: Therapeutic variables and pharmacokinetics in topical therapy, in B Shroot, H Schaefer (eds), *Pharmacology and the Skin,* vol 1: *Skin Pharmacokinetics.* Basel, Karger, 1987, p 199.
25. Elias PM: Membranes, lipids and the epidermal permeability barrier, in R. Marks, EL Christophers (eds), *The Epidermis in Disease,* Lancaster, England, MTP Press, 1981, p 1.
26. Wester RC et al: In vivo percutaneous absorption of hydrocortisone in psoriatic patients and normal volunteers. *J Am Acad Dermatol* 8:645, 1983.
27. Wester RC et al: In vivo percutaneous absorption of drugs in psoriatic patients and normal volunteers. *Clin Pharmacol Ther* 41:175, 1987.
28. Turpeinen M: Influence of age and severity of dermatitis on the percutaneous absorption of hydrocortisone in children. *Br J Dermatol* 118:517, 1988.
29. Turpeinen M et al: Percutaneous absorption of hydrocortisone during exacerbation and remission of atopic dermatitis in adults. *Acta Derm Venereol (Stockh)* 68:331, 1988.

6

Cutaneous Sensation and the Pathophysiology of Pruritus

Jeffrey D. Bernhard

The skin and brain derive from the same embryonic layer and, in many respects, the skin functions as an "external nervous system" that provides continuous information to the central nervous system. The tactile functions of the skin are critical to human growth, development, and behavior.[1] The sense of touch is the first to develop in the human embryo, when it is less than 6 weeks old. Young animals deprived of maternal touching do not develop normally.[1] Touching is one of most people's favorite ways to demonstrate affection.

The eyes, ears, mouth, nose, and skin utilize a remarkable variety of sensory receptors to receive stimuli from the environment.[2] Chemoreceptors detect taste, smell, blood oxygen level, and other factors that affect the chemistry of the body. Electromagnetic receptors detect light on the retina. Thermoreceptors detect changes in temperature. Mechanoreceptors detect touch, pressure, vibration, tickle, and position. Nociceptors in the skin and internal organs detect pain and damage to tissues. The term *nociceptor* comes from the Latin *nocere,* "to hurt or injure," which also appears in the clinical dictum *primum non nocere* ("first, do not harm").

CUTANEOUS RECEPTORS, NERVES, AND NEURAL PATHWAYS

The nerves that supply the skin begin as large, myelinated branches of musculocutaneous nerves that arise from spinal nerves.[3] In general, sensory nerves supply the skin in geometric segments known as *dermatomes*. These nerves terminate in a rich supply of free nerve endings and specialized corpuscular receptors. Most corpuscular or mechanoreceptors have onion-like structures composed of a capsule and an inner core (Fig. 6-1). Compression of a corpuscle indents or changes its shape in such a way that ion channels are opened and an action potential is generated in the nerve to which it is connected. Pacinian corpuscles (after F. Pacini, Italian anatomist, 1812–1883) lie in the deep dermis and subcutaneous tissue and respond to vibrational stimuli. Meissner's corpuscles (after G. Meissner, German anatomist and physiologist, 1829–1905) are located in the dermal papillae of the fingers and toes and are involved in the sensation of touch. Other specialized sensory structures, such as "touch domes" in hairy skin, Ruffini's end organs (after A. Ruffini, Italian anatomist, 1864–1929), and Merkel's discs (after F.S. Merkel, German anatomist, 1845–1919) are involved in cutaneous sensation as well.[4,5] In contrast to corpuscular receptors, in which the nerve terminal functions as a signal transducer, it appears that the Merkel cell (see Chap. 1) acts as the transducer in Merkel receptors.[5]

The most numerous and important sensory receptors in the skin are free nerve endings that form a finely arborizing network just beneath the epidermis near the dermal-epidermal interface (Fig. 6-1).[6] Also known as *penicillate* (L. *penicillus*, "brush" + *-ate*) nerve endings, these receptors are

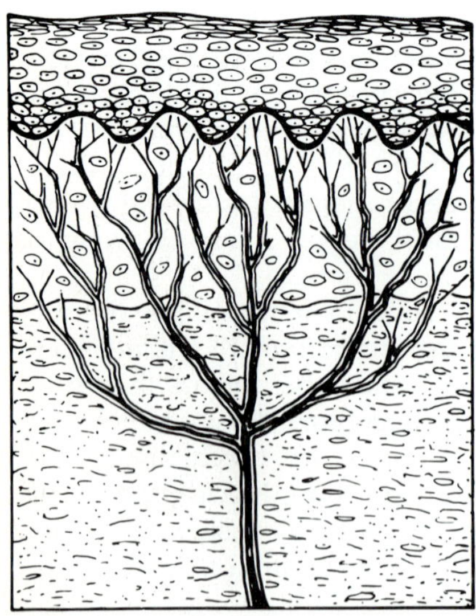

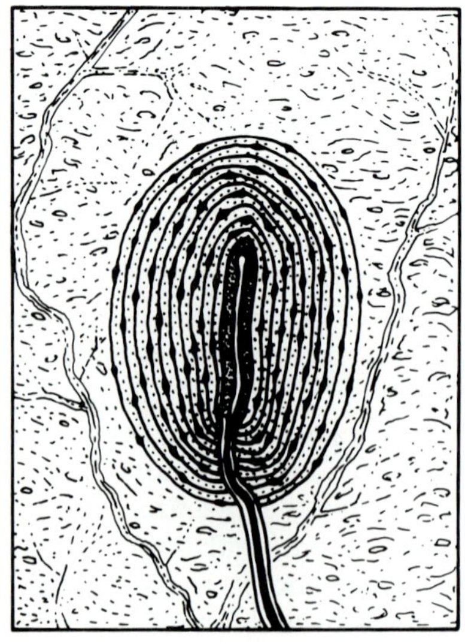

Figure 6-1 On the left, finely arborizing free nerve endings that serve the sensations of itch and pain terminate near the dermal-epidermal junction. A typical corpuscular receptor is shown on the right.

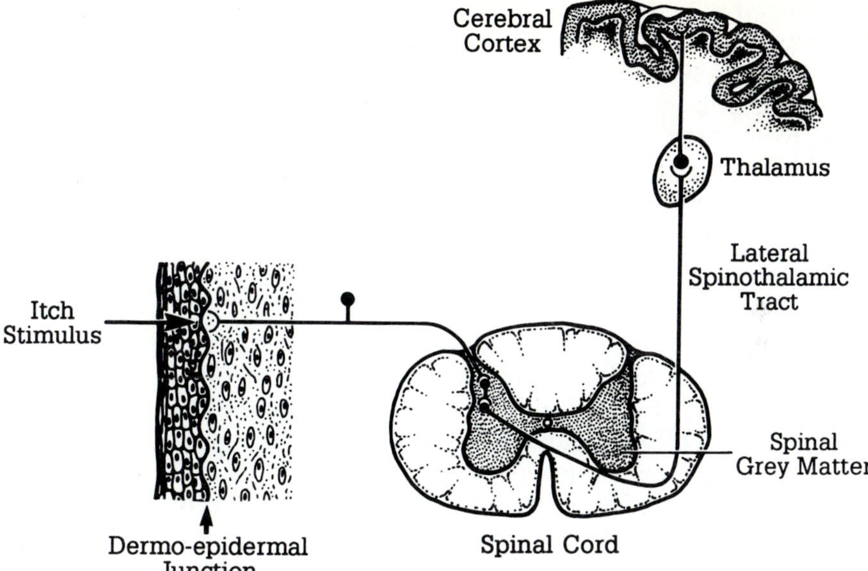

Figure 6-2 A simplified diagram of the neuroanatomical pathway for itching. Crossing takes place above the level of entry to the spinal cord, not at the same level, as the diagram suggests. Interneurons in addition to those shown may be present. Some neurons of the spinothalamic tract terminate at lower levels than are shown. Pain is also transmitted in the spinothalamic tract. (*Modified from Greaves.*[7])

involved in the perception of touch, temperature, pain, and itching. Small, myelinated ganglion cell axons carrying itch information terminate on neurons in the posterior horn of the spinal cord. Second-order cells then send their axons across the midline into the spinothalamic tract, where they ascend to the thalamus. Thalamic neurons then project to the sensory cortex (Fig. 6-2). At different levels along this pathway, competing sensations, psychological factors, and pharmacological agents may reduce or magnify the perceived itch. Portions of the trigeminal system are presumably responsible for processing itch information from the face. However, clinical details of the pathway are scant.

Many textbooks suggest that itch is a variety of pain, since both sensations are served by similar receptors and nerves. However, although itch and pain may travel through shared neural pathways (e.g., the spinothalamic tract in the spinal cord), most authorities now agree that they are separate, unique sensations.[7–9] Several observations lead to this conclusion. Itching elicits the reflex or desire to scratch; pain provokes a withdrawal response. Itching and pain can both be felt on the same area of skin at the same time, and their intensity may vary independently. Morphine, which relieves pain, often causes itching. Pruritic stimuli exert their action at or near the dermal-epidermal junction; pain is elicited from deeper nerve endings in the skin. Recent electrical stimulation studies also support the proposition that itch and pain are carried by different populations of primary sensory neurons.[8] This conclusion is consistent with the "labeled line" principle, according to which different sensory modalities (such as sight, sound, touch, and pain) travel along specific nerves and terminate at specific points in the central nervous system.[2] Precisely how the free, unmyelinated, penicillate nerve endings that function as itch receptors work is not known, but it is reasonable to suspect that they contain receptors for certain chemicals known to evoke itching, such as histamine and kallikrein.[10]

CHEMICAL MEDIATORS OF PRURITUS

Histamine is the most well-known chemical mediator of itching, but it is not the only one and in many instances may not be the most important. This is evident from the observation that antihistamines are not helpful in many patients with generalized or other types of pruritus. Furthermore, experimental histamine injections sufficient to elicit itching always produce a visible wheal and flare, while many patients with generalized itching have no visible skin changes. Endopeptidases, substance P, certain opioid peptides, prostaglandins, and related substances may affect itching in various ways (Fig. 6-3).[7] A number of endogenous proteases, including trypsin, chymotrypsin, and fibrinolysin, cause itching when injected into human skin. Although some proteases are potent histamine releasers, certain others must act independently of histamine, because antihistamines have no effect on their action.[11] On the other hand, substance P, a vasoactive peptide present in the central nervous system and in peripheral nerves, probably acts by releasing histamine.[12] Opioid peptides may affect the perception of itch in both the peripheral and central nervous systems.[13]

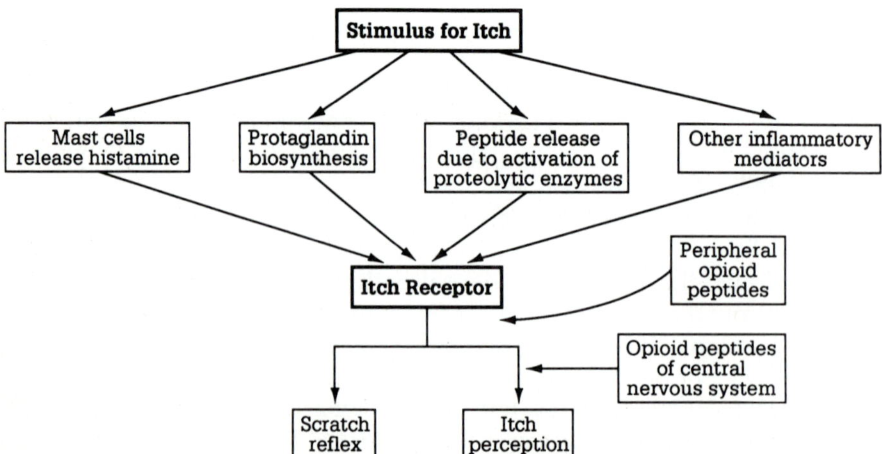

Figure 6-3 Chemical mediators of pruritus. Some molecules may act directly on the itch receptor. Others may enhance or inhibit itching by acting at the level of the itch receptor, peripheral nervous system, or central nervous system. (*Modified from Greaves.*[7])

Prostaglandins also seem to play an indirect role in pruritus, probably by sensitizing free nerve ending receptors to histamine or other pruritogens.[14,15] The amount of histamine required to elicit itching in skin that has been pretreated with prostaglandin E_1 is reduced by one-half. Some chemicals, such as the prostaglandins and other arachidonic acid metabolites derived from cell membranes, are released when the skin is damaged or inflamed by disease; these may contribute to itching in many inflammatory skin diseases, such as psoriasis. Mechanical, electrical, and thermal stimuli can also provoke itching when applied to the skin.[7] One practical implication of the variety of chemicals and physical factors that stimulate itching is that no single pharmacological intervention, such as the use of antihistamine drugs, is effective in treating all patients with different types of pruritus. It is ironic that we have no single medication for the treatment of itching as good as aspirin is for pain.

SKIN DISORDERS ASSOCIATED WITH PRURITUS

Itching is an important and distressing feature of many skin disorders, especially certain inflammatory diseases such as atopic dermatitis and psoriasis. Why some diseases cause itching and others do not is not entirely clear. Why some conditions lead to pruritus in some patients but not in others is even more mysterious. In urticaria (hives), immediate hypersensitivity leads to histamine release from mast cells and causes itching in most patients. Urticaria is the prototypical histamine-mediated disorder, and usually responds well to treatment with antihistamines and elimination of the underlying cause. In scabies and allergic contact dermatitis, delayed immunologic hypersensitivity reactions to an exogenous agent lead to an inflammatory reaction and the release of a variety of mediators that may be pruritogenic. In fiberglass dermatitis, mechanical irritation of the skin leads to itching. In others, such as lichen planus, the mechanism is not apparent, but the accumulation of inflammatory cells near the dermal-epidermal junction, where free nerve endings are profuse, suggests a possible link. Molecules such as peptides and prostaglandins, which either cause or enhance pruritus, are released during inflammatory reactions. Pruritus may be especially intense in scabies, dermatitis herpetiformis, atopic dermatitis, and some cases of hives. The term *psoriasis*, which comes from the Latin *iasis*, "a condition," and *psor-*, "of itching," can be intensely pruritic. Some of the most important pruritic skin diseases are listed in Table 6-1.[16]

SYSTEMIC DISORDERS ASSOCIATED WITH PRURITUS

A variety of serious medical problems, such as Hodgkin's disease, liver disease, and renal disease, can cause generalized itching, occasionally as the first indication of illness. Generalized pruritus is therefore a symptom of cardinal medical significance.[16] A patient with generalized pruritus may have secondary skin lesions caused by rubbing or scratching, but these

Table 6-1

SOME DERMATOLOGIC DISORDERS ASSOCIATED WITH PRURITUS

Infestation
Scabies
Pediculosis
Inflammatory
Dermatitis herpetiformis
Bullous pemphigoid
Atopic dermatitis
Allergic contact dermatitis
Psoriasis
Lichen planus
Urticaria
Drug hypersensitivity
Infections
Varicella
Dermatophytosis
Folliculitis
External causes
Fiberglass dermatitis
Irritant dermatitis
Insect bites (e.g., fleas)
Miscellaneous
Xerosis (dry skin—common)
Anogenital pruritus
Sunburn
Mastocytosis

Source: Modified from Bernhard.[16]

are not specific and are not helpful in arriving at a diagnosis of the underlying cause. Sometimes, however, subtle but specific primary lesions of a recognizable skin disorder are present; for this reason, the patient who presents with pruritus of undetermined origin should undergo repeated careful examination for a primary skin disease such as those listed in Table 6-1. Drugs, external factors such as fiberglass exposure, and infested pets are also important causes of generalized itching, with or without specific skin lesions. Once the presence of a primary skin disease and external factors have been excluded, it is necessary to consider the possibility of a systemic, or internal, cause of generalized itching. A partial list of systemic disorders associated with generalized pruritus is given in Table 6-2. The evaluation of a patient with pruritus of undetermined origin is an important and difficult task for the physician, especially when one considers the wide range of possibilities and the expense and discomfort

Table 6-2

SOME SYSTEMIC DISORDERS ASSOCIATED WITH GENERALIZED PRURITUS

Hepatic
- Obstructive biliary disease
- Intrahepatic cholestasis of pregnancy
- Drug-induced cholestasis

Renal disease—chronic renal failure

Metabolic and endocrine disorders
- Hyperthyroidism
- Hypothyroidism
- Carcinoid syndrome
- Systemic mastocytosis

Hematologic disorders
- Polycythemia vera
- Paraproteinemia
- Iron deficiency

Malignant diseases
- Hodgkin's disease
- Visceral malignancy (rare)
- Cutaneous T-cell lymphoma (mycosis fungoides)

Drug hypersensitivity

Parasitic infestations

Psychiatric disorders (uncommon)

Source: Modified from Bernhard.[16]

that may be involved in testing for them. Such an evaluation should be carefully guided by the results of a thorough history, review of systems, and general physical examination, not by the uncritical use of laboratory tests and procedures designed to exclude every possibility.[16]

Chronic Renal Disease[17]

Uremic pruritus is probably the most common variety of generalized itching with an internal cause encountered in clinical medicine today. Prior to the advent of hemodialysis, itching was a recognized feature of chronic renal failure. The fact that itching is still a significant problem for many patients who undergo chronic hemodialysis suggests that at least one chemical not adequately removed by the procedure is responsible. Surprisingly, the severity of itching is not directly related to the severity of the underlying renal disease, as measured by individual parameters of renal function, such as the serum creatinine or blood urea nitrogen level. Pruritus in hemodialysis patients responds to ultraviolet B phototherapy, oral activated charcoal ingestion, and oral administration of the ion exchange resin cholestyramine. The first presumably inactivates one or more unidentified circulating pruritogens; the second and third presumably bind them. In some hemodialysis patients, itching seems to be related to secondary hyperparathyroidism and responds to subtotal parathyroidectomy.

Hepatobiliary Disease

Obstructive biliary disease frequently causes itching. Although some evidence suggests that bile acids and salts are responsible, it has not been possible to establish a direct relationship between skin or blood levels of these compounds and the presence or degree of pruritus. According to one hypothesis, bile salts cause itching not because of a direct effect on the skin but because of a toxic effect on hepatocyte cell membranes, leading to the release of still unidentified pruritogenic substances, some of which may be novel metabolites of cholesterol.[18] Pregnancy and a number of drugs, such as phenothiazines, estrogens, and anabolic steroids, can also produce itching because they cause cholestasis. Extrahepatic biliary obstruction caused by a tumor can also lead to cholestatic pruritus. Itching is the most frequent symptom of primary biliary cirrhosis and may be the presenting complaint in more than one-half of the patients who develop it.[19]

Hematologic and Lymphoproliferative Disorders

Thirty percent or more of patients with Hodgkin's disease are afflicted by severe pruritus, which, moreover, may be the earliest symptom and presenting complaint. Cutaneous T-cell lymphoma (mycosis fungoides) is often intensely pruritic. Itching after a hot shower is said to be characteristic of polycythemia vera, but it also occurs after contact with water in a number of other disorders, such as aquagenic pruritus, aquagenic urticaria, heat urticaria, and preexisting dermatoses.[20] Iron deficiency, even in the absence of overt anemia, may lead to itching in some cases, but the true frequency and significance of this association remain to be established. In systemic mastocytosis, which may cause generalized pruritus in the absence of skin lesions, histamine release from an excessive number of mast cells is presumably responsible. Pruritus in other hematologic and lymphoproliferative disorders may be attributed in some instances to histamine release from abnormal cells or increased numbers of basophils, but otherwise they remain unknown.

Endocrine Disorders

Ten percent or more of patients with hyperthyroidism complain of itching, and in a number of cases it is this problem that first leads them to seek medical attention. Hypothyroidism also causes itching, perhaps because of dry skin. Diabetes mellitus is often mentioned as a cause of itching. Although localized pruritus of the anogenital area occurs in diabetes, generalized pruritus without a rash is not common.[21] In some cases, anogenital pruritus in diabetes is caused by *Candida* or dermatophyte fungus infection.

SCRATCHING

Although it may be "better than riches to scratch where it itches," scratching has undesirable effects of its own and can contribute to the appearance of secondary infection. Repeated rubbing and scratching of a small area leads to a change known as *lichenification,* in which the skin thickens and develops accentuated skin markings. How scratching relieves itching is not known. According to one theory, the neural stimulus from scratching breaks up reverberating circuits in the segment of the spinal cord into which impulses from a pruritic site pass.[22] According to the "gate theory," various factors may diminish itching through modulation of afferent stimuli at the level of the spinal cord or above. Sufficiently hard scratching simply substitutes pain for itch.

TREATMENT[16]

The most basic and important objective is to determine whether an underlying skin disease, systemic disease, or external factor is present and then to treat or eliminate it. Symptomatic treatment of itching falls into four main categories. First, the patient must be educated to eliminate or reduce provocative factors, such as excessive bathing and woolen fabrics. Second, soothing topical preparations, such as menthol lotions, help some people. Third, systemic chemical treatment may be helpful. In urticaria or other conditions in which histamine may be involved, antihistamines are helpful. In other cases, antihistamines may help because of their sedative effect. Opiate antagonists, such as naloxone, may turn out to be helpful in the treatment of certain cases of itching.[23] Fourth, physical modalities such as ultraviolet B phototherapy are helpful in certain types of pruritus, such as that associated with chronic hemodialysis.[24]

REFERENCES

1. Montagu A: *Touching. The Human Significance of the Skin,* 3d ed. New York, Harper & Row, 1986.
2. Guyton AC: Sensory receptors and their basic mechanisms of action, in AC Guyton, *Textbook of Medical Physiology,* 7th ed. Philadelphia, Saunders, 1986, p 572.
3. Holbrook KA, Wolff K: The structure and development of skin, in TB Fitzpatrick et al (eds), *Dermatology in General Medicine,* 3d ed. New York, McGraw-Hill, 1987, p 93.
4. Guyton AC: Somatic sensations. I. The mechanoreceptive sensations, in AC Guyton, *Textbook of Medical Physiology,* 7th ed. Philadelphia, Saunders, 1986, p 580.
5. Iggo A, Andres KH: Morphology of cutaneous receptors. *Annu Rev Neurosci* 5:1, 1982.
6. Shelley WB, Arthur RP: The neurohistology and neurophysiology of the itch sensation in man. *Arch Dermatol* 76:296, 1957.

7. Greaves MW: Pathophysiology of pruritus, in TB Fitzpatrick et al (eds), *Dermatology in General Medicine*, 3d ed. New York, McGraw-Hill, 1987, p 74.
8. Tuckett RP: Itch evoked by electrical stimulation of the skin. *J Invest Dermatol* 79:368, 1982.
9. Denman ST: A review of pruritus. *J Am Acad Dermatol* 14:375, 1986.
10. Fjellner B: Experimental and clinical pruritus. *Acta Derm Venereol (Stockh)* Suppl 97:1, 1981.
11. Hägermark Ö: Studies on experimental itch induced by kallikrein and bradykinin. *Acta Derm Venereol (Stockh)* 54:397, 1974.
12. Hägermark Ö et al: Flare and itch induced by substance P in human skin. *J Invest Dermatol* 71:233, 1978.
13. Bernstein JE et al: Antipruritic effect of an opiate antagonist, naloxone hydrochloride. *J Invest Dermatol* 78:82, 1982.
14. Greaves MW, McDonald-Gibson W: Itch: the role of prostaglandins. *Br Med J* 3:608, 1973.
15. Hägermark Ö et al: Potentiation of itch and flare responses in human skin by prostaglandins E_2, H_2 and a prostaglandin endoperoxide analogue. *J Invest Dermatol* 69:527, 1977.
16. Bernhard JD: Clinical aspects of pruritus, in TB Fitzpatrick et al (eds), *Dermatology in General Medicine*, 3d ed. New York, McGraw-Hill, 1987, p 78.
17. Gilchrest BA et al: Clinical features of pruritus among patients undergoing maintenance hemodialysis. *Arch Dermatol* 118:154, 1982.
18. Ghent CN: Pruritus of cholestasis is related to effects of bile salts on the liver, not the skin. *Am J Gastroenterol* 82:117, 1987.
19. Roll J et al: The prognostic importance of clinical and histologic features in asymptomatic and symptomatic primary biliary cirrhosis. *N Engl J Med* 308:1, 1983.
20. Steinman HK, Greaves MW: Aquagenic pruritus. *J Am Acad Dermatol* 13:91, 1985.
21. Neilly JB et al: Pruritus in diabetes mellitus: investigation of prevalence and correlation with diabetes control. *Diabetes Care* 9:273, 1986.
22. Ayres S: The fine art of scratching. *JAMA* 189:1003, 1964.
23. Bernstein JE: Neuropeptides and the skin, in LA Goldsmith, (ed), *Biochemistry and Physiology of the Skin*. New York, Oxford University Press, 1983, p 1217.
24. Gilchrest BA et al: Ultraviolet phototherapy of uremic pruritus: long-term results and possible mechanisms. *Ann Intern Med* 91:17, 1979.

7

The Skin as an Immunologic Organ

Daniel N. Sauder

For many years, it was believed that the skin could be a target for immune-mediated damage but had no direct role in immune function. However, the passive role of skin in immune events is no longer a tenable theory. Over the last 15 years, it has become clear that the skin represents the peripheral arm of the immune system and, as such, is composed of at least three components: the epidermal Langerhans cells, the epidermal T cells, and the hormone-like immunoregulatory and pro-inflammatory glycoproteins termed cytokines. Together these components play a major role in epidermal immunity and function. Streilein used the designation skin-associated lymphoid tissue (SALT) to describe this immune function of the skin.[1] This chapter summarizes the functions of major components of SALT.

LANGERHANS CELLS

The epidermal Langerhans cell, with its antigen-presenting ability, was one of the first members of SALT to be actively studied. Langerhans cells represent only a small subpopulation (3 to 4 percent) of epidermal cells. They are recognized under the light microscope following staining for membrane ATPase. Langerhans cells are highly dendritic and reside in a suprabasal level of the epidermis. Ultrastructurally, they have a distinctive intracytoplasmic granule termed a Langerhans cell granule or Birbeck granule.[2]

The potential immunologic role of Langerhans cells was suggested by Silberberg et al. in the 1960s, although proof was provided only in the late 1970s with the studies of Stingl, Katz, and co-workers.[2–4] Langerhans cells were found to bear Fc-IgG and C3 receptors. Langerhans cells are derived from bone marrow precursors and bear Ly-5/T200/CD45[5] antigens that are present on virtually all hematopoietic cells (Table 7-1). Langerhans cells from atopic dermatitis patients bear small amounts of surface IgE.[6] Langerhans cells express class I and class II major histocompatibility complex (MHC) antigens on their surface, as well as CD1 and CD4 antigens.[2]

Functional Properties of Langerhans Cells

Langerhans cells are potent stimulators of antigen-specific T-cell activation. Antigen presentation is thought to involve two signals that are presented to T cells. The first signal involves uptake, processing, and presentation of the antigen in association with class II molecules on the T cell and the T-cell receptor. A second antigen is also thought to be required. This antigen is a nonspecific signal that appears to be mediated by interleukin-1 (see the following section). Langerhans cells are believed to play a critical role in generating T-cell-dependent immune responses in the skin. Langerhans cells are extremely potent in their ability to activate T cells, more potent than macrophages and peripheral blood mononuclear cells.

Antigen Presentation by Langerhans Cells

$CD4^+$ (helper) T cells do not recognize free antigen but rather antigen on the surface of other cells termed antigen-presenting cells. Early studies of antigen presentation by antigen-presenting cells suggested that direct contact between the antigen-presenting cell and the T cell was required

Table 7-1

PHENOTYPIC AND FUNCTIONAL PROPERTIES OF LANGERHANS CELLS

Phagocytosis	±
Nonspecific esterase	+
Adenosine triphosphatase	+ +
Class I MHC antigens	+
Class II MHC antigens	+ +
Fc-IgG receptors	+
C3 receptors	+
IL-2 receptors	±

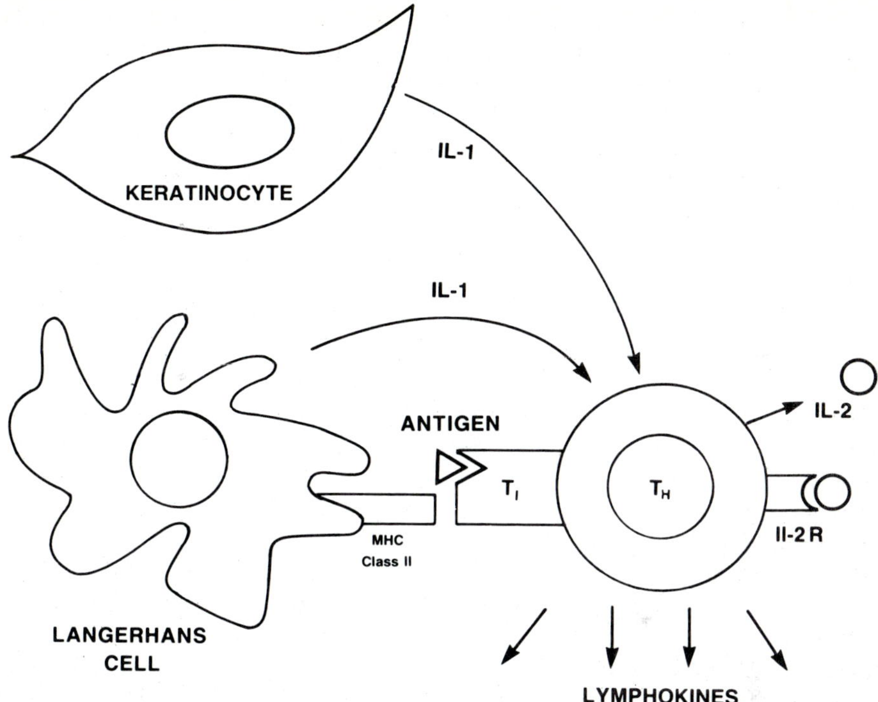

Figure 7-1 Antigen presentation by epidermal cells. The first signal is provided by Langerhans cells in association with class II MHC molecules to the CD4$^+$ (helper) T cell (T_H) via the T-cell antigen receptor (T_i). The second signal is provided by the release of IL-1 by Langerhans cells or the keratinocyte. This leads to expression of IL-2 receptors on the T cell and secretion of IL-2, leading to clonal expression of the T cell in response to the initial antigen.

for T-cell activation. Current understanding of T-cell activation suggests that a CD4$^+$ T cell receives two signals for optimal antigen presentation. The first signal involves uptake and processing in which large antigens are degraded to fragments that are more recognizable by the T cells. These fragments are associated with class II MHC molecules as the antigen-presenting cells.

The second signal, a nonspecific amplification signal, provided by the antigen-presenting cell, is mediated by interleukin-1 (IL-1). Following activation, CD4$^+$ T cells express a receptor for another soluble helper factor termed interleukin-2 (IL-2), and a subpopulation of CD4$^+$ T cells also secrete IL-1 (Fig. 7-1).

Since IL-1 was believed to be necessary for optimal antigen presentation, studies were undertaken to determine if Langerhans cells could produce it. Unexpectedly, these studies led to the finding that the main cellular source for IL-1 in the skin was the keratinocytes, not the Langerhans cells.[7]

Thus, IL-1, which provides the second amplification signal to the T cell, can also be provided by the keratinocyte, and since keratinocytes outnumber Langerhans cells by more than 20:1, keratinocytes may be the major source of this second amplification.

In Vivo Functions of Langerhans Cells

The in vitro functions of Langerhans cells have been well established by direct experimentation. In vivo functions have been extrapolated from in vitro data and supported by studies of conditions that alter Langerhans cell function. Ultraviolet (UV) light results in morphologic changes to Langerhans cells both in vitro and in vivo.[8] Application in vivo of contact allergens to UV-irradiated epidermis does not lead to sensitization but rather to specific immunologic unresponsiveness mediated by $CD8^+$ (suppressor) T cells.[9]

Langerhans cells from patients infected with human immunodeficiency virus-1 (HIV-1) also appear to be impaired. In 1984, Belsito et al. reported a decrease in Langerhans cells in patients with acquired immunodeficiency syndrome (AIDS) or AIDS-related complex (ARC.)[10] Tschachler et al. have shown that HIV-1 proteins can be detected in Langerhans cells from AIDS and ARC patients.[11] HIV-1-like virions have been shown to bud from Langerhans cell membranes, and Langerhans cells appear to be profoundly damaged by HIV-1. These changes may lead to a decrease in skin immune surveillance mechanisms, which may contribute to infectious and neoplastic complications of AIDS. In addition, since Langerhans cells have evidence of intact virion, these cells in the skin could be a vehicle for transmission of the virus.

Role of Langerhans Cells in Allergic Contact Dermatitis

In 1980, Toews et al.[12] found that Langerhans cells were required for the induction of allergic contact dermatitis. Mouse skin that had a decreased density of Langerhans cells, such as that of the tail, failed to induce contact dermatitis but led to specific immunologic tolerance. Similarly, if the allergen was applied to UV-irradiated skin (which caused a decrease in Langerhans cell density), tolerance was induced. It was primarily the results of these and similar studies that led to understanding of the role of Langerhans cells in allergic contact dermatitis.

Mechanisms of Allergic Contact Dermatitis

Allergic contact dermatitis represents a prototype of delayed-type hypersensitivity reactions. It can be divided into two phases: the induction phase, in which immunity to the allergen occurs, and the elicitation phase, in which the inflammatory response occurs upon reexposure to the allergen.

Induction Phase

Most chemicals capable of inducing allergic contact dermatitis require binding to carrier proteins before they can be recognized by the immune system. This carrier protein may be provided by either keratinocytes or Langerhans cells. Chemicals that require a carrier protein to be recognized by the immune system are termed haptens.

When skin comes in contact with these haptens, a cascade of events occurs. First, the hapten penetrates the stratum corneum and enters the epidermis. This process is probably assisted by keratinocytes, either through direct phagocytosis or through the release of keratinocyte-derived cytokines. These cells then internalize the antigen, process it, then externalize it on its cell surface in association with class II MHC molecules. The antigen-bearing Langerhans cells then present the antigen to the T cell. Whether this occurs in the epidermis or dermis or at the regional lymph node is unknown. However, the regional lymph node is not required for this process, and sensitization can occur in the skin. Langerhans cells and sensitized T lymphocytes then migrate from the skin to the draining lymph node, where they enter the paracortical areas. In these areas they proliferate and differentiate. Some of these lymphocytes migrate back to skin sites where the initial allergen was located. Other lymphocytes remain in the regional lymph node as long-lived memory cells.

Elicitation Phase

The elicitation phase occurs after sensitization has taken place when the skin is reexposed to the initial allergen. Elicitation can also occur if the initial allergen persists at the site of induction.

During the elicitation phase, lymphocytes migrate to the skin, although only a small proportion of infiltrating lymphocytes are sensitized. The unsensitized lymphocytes respond to cytokines released by the sensitized lymphocytes, by Langerhans cells, and by keratinocytes. During the elicitation phase, keratinocytes express class II MHC molecules on their surface; this is thought to enhance migration of lymphoid cells. Not only are effector T lymphocytes generated during induction and elicitation of allergic contact dermatitis, but $CD8^+$ T lymphocytes as well. Under normal circumstances, the effector signal is too strong to be inhibited by the suppressor signal. However, in certain circumstances, such as when an allergen is applied to areas of decreased Langerhans cell density, suppression overcomes sensitization. This process may be mediated by Thy-1^+ dendritic epidermal cells.

IMMUNE FUNCTION OF KERATINOCYTES

Keratinocytes have recently been shown to synthesize and secrete hormone-like polypeptide molecules collectively called cytokines. The term cytokine is a generalization of the term lymphokine, which refers to polypeptide products of activated lymphocytes involved in cellular immunity.[13] Initially, cytokines were named according to their biologic activity in a particular assay rather than on the basis of their biologic properties. To free the nomenclature of definitions based on bioassays, the term interleukin (between leukocytes) was introduced. There are currently eight interleukins (Table 7-2).

The interleukins represent only one subgroup of cytokines. Cytokines also include the hemopoietic colony-stimulating factors (CSFs), cytolysins, interferons, growth factors, and suppressor or inhibitory factors.

Under appropriate stimulation, keratinocytes can synthesize and secrete a surprisingly large array of cytokines,[7,14–20] including IL-1, IL-3 (murine), IL-6, IL-8, and the hematopoietic colony-stimulating factors (CSFs), including granulocyte colony-stimulating factor (GM-GSF), and transforming growth factors α and β (Table 7-3, Fig. 7-2).

Keratinocytes can be induced to synthesize these cytokines in response to a variety of stimuli, including UV light, bacterial infections, and trauma. Cytokines released from keratinocytes can then influence a variety of lymphoid functions (Table 7-3).

In addition to secreting cytokines, keratinocytes respond to a variety of cytokines. For example, keratinocytes can migrate and proliferate in response to IL-1.[21,22]

In the normal epidermis, Langerhans cells are the only cells that express class II MHC antigens. However, under certain circumstances, keratinocytes can express these antigens. For example, interferon γ released by lymphocytes can induce expression of class II MHC molecules on

Table 7-2

BIOLOGIC ACTIVITY OF THE INTERLEUKINS

IL-1	Multiple pro-inflammatory and immunoregulatory activities, including: Neutrophilia Chemotaxis for T cells and keratinocytes Mitogen for thymocytes and fibroblasts
IL-2	T-cell growth factor Activates natural killer cells Induces lymphokine-activated killer cells
IL-3	Pluripotent hematopoietic growth factor
IL-4	Growth factor for B cells and resting T cells
IL-5	Increases proliferation of activated B cells Stimulates eosinophil colony function
IL-6	Induces growth of pre-B cells Induces production of acute phase proteins by hepatocytes
IL-7	Stimulates proliferation of lymphoid progenitor cells (T- and B-cell precursors)
IL-8	Neutrophil chemoattractant T-cell chemoattractant

Table 7-3

KERATINOCYTE-DERIVED CYTOKINES

Cytokine	Messenger RNA	Bioactivity
Interleukins		
IL-1α	+	+
IL-1β	+	+
IL-2	−	−
IL-3	+ (murine)	+ (murine)
IL-4	−	−
IL-5	−	−
IL-6	+	+
IL-7	−	−
IL-8	+	+
CSFs		
Macrophage CSF	+ (murine)	+ (murine)
Granulocyte-macrophage CSF	+	+
Granulocyte CSF	+ (murine)	+ (murine)
Transforming growth factors (α, β)	+	+
Fibroblast growth factor	+	+
Interferons		
Interferon α	+	+

keratinocytes[23,24] and increase the expression of these molecules, which in turn may lead to enhanced antigen presentation to T cells.

In addition to inducing class II MHC molecules on keratinocytes, interferon γ can induce an adhesion molecule on keratinocytes termed intercellular adhesion molecule-1 (ICAM-1).[25] The ICAM-1 molecule is part of a class of adhesion molecules that are important in cell-cell interaction. These molecules play an important role in promoting interaction between T cells and epidermal cells.

T CELLS IN THE SKIN

Lymphocytes are normally present in the skin. Some of them represent a recirculating pool of T cells. A subset of recirculating T cells displays special affinity for skin. This is seen in diseases such as cutaneous T-cell lymphoma, but it has also been demonstrated that lymphocytes from lymph nodes draining cutaneous sites of induction of contact dermatitis selectively migrate back to the skin.

THY-1 AND DENDRITIC EPIDERMAL CELLS

Murine skin also contains a unique lymphoid cell expressing Thy-1 antigen on its surface.[26,27] These cells also express T3, a unique marker for

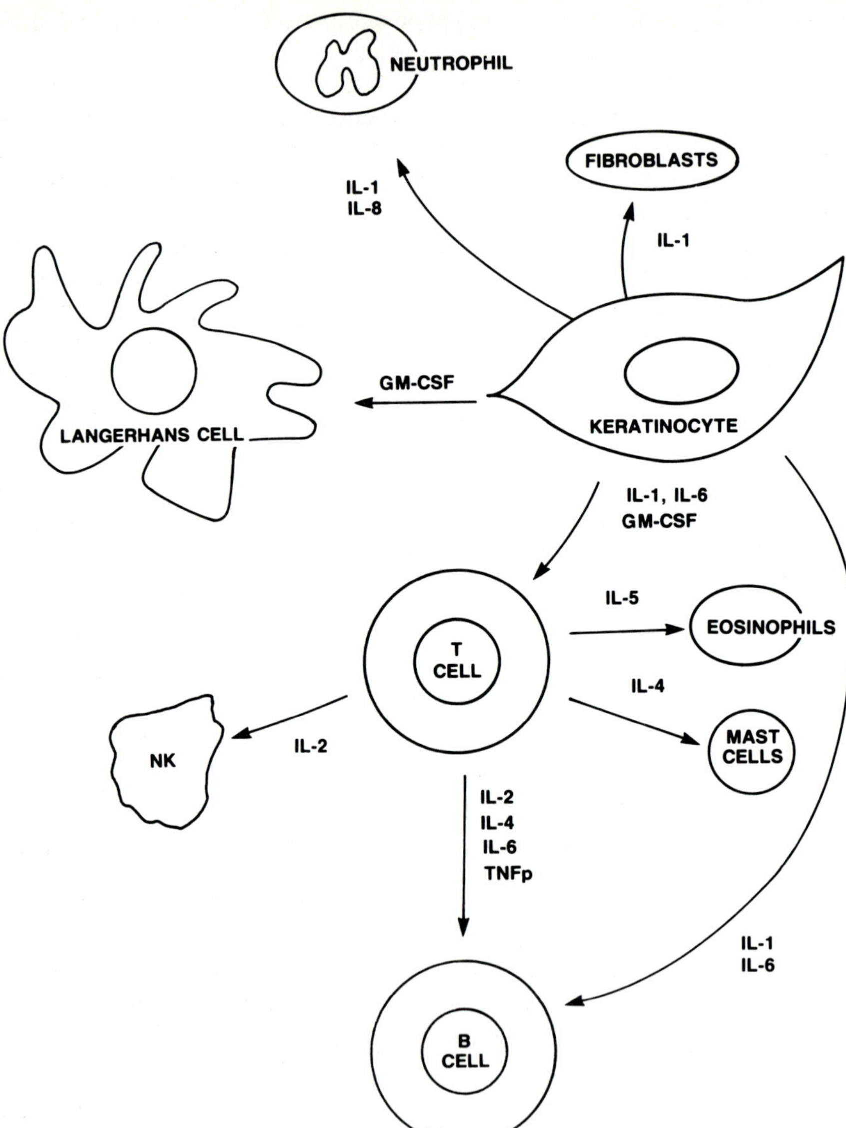

Figure 7-2 The cytokine cascade. Keratinocytes synthesize and secrete a wide array of cytokines, including IL-1, IL-6, IL-8, and GM-GSF, which in turn influence a host of inflammatory and immunoregulatory cell types.

thymus-derived cells, and a T-cell receptor composed of the products of the γ and δ genes but not of the α and β genes.[28]

This novel cell type of T-cell lineage is termed the Thy-1^+ dendritic epidermal cell. These cells may function as alternative antigen-presenting cells that appear to act primarily by down-regulating the immune response.[29] Thy-1^+ dendritic epidermal cells have also been shown to possess some natural killer activity in vitro[30] and thus may function as killer cells in immune surveillance in the epidermis.

Thy-1$^+$ dendritic epidermal cells express Thy-1, CD3, and Asialo GM-1 molecules on their surface but do not express CD4, CD8, or MHC class II molecules. These cells proliferate in vitro in response to IL-2. The human equivalent of murine Thy-1$^+$ dendritic epidermal cells has not yet been conclusively identified.

Thus, the peripheral arm of the immune system designated by Streilein as skin-associated lymphoid tissue is composed of Langerhans cells, keratinocytes, and epidermotropic T cells. This system is probably intimately involved in normal homeostasis and in host defense mechanisms against foreign invaders. Functional impairment of this system by UV light or by certain pathogens, such as HIV-1, may result in cutaneous neoplasms or infections.

REFERENCES

1. Streilein JW: Skin-associated lymphoid tissues (SALT): origins and functions. *J Invest Dermatol* 80:12S, 1983.
2. Stingl G et al: The immune function of epidermal cells, in DA Norris (ed), *Immune Mechanisms in Cutaneous Disease.* New York, Marcel Dekker, 1989, p 3.
3. Stingl G et al: Epidermal Langerhans cells bear Fc and C3 receptors. *Nature* 268:245, 1977.
4. Tamaki, K et al: Ia antigens in mouse skin are predominantly expressed on Langerhans cells. *J Immunol* 123:784, 1979.
5. Flotte TJ et al: Demonstration of T200 in human Langerhans cell surface membranes. *J Invest Dermatol* 82:535, 1984.
6. Barker JN et al: Surface-bound immunoglobulin E on antigen-presenting cells in cutaneous tissue of atopic dermatitis. *J Invest Dermatol* 90:117, 1988.
7. Sauder DN et al: Biology and molecular biology of epidermal thymocyte activating factor. *Ann NY Acad Sci* 548:241, 1988.
8. Aberer W et al: Ultraviolet light depletes surface markers of Langerhans cells. *J Invest Dermatol* 76:202, 1981.
9. Elmets CA et al: Analysis of the mechanism of unresponsiveness produced by haptens painted on skin exposed to low dose ultraviolet radiation. *J Exp Med* 158:781, 1983.
10. Belsito DV et al: Reduced Langerhans cell Ia antigen and ATPase activity in patients with the acquired immunodeficiency syndrome. *N Engl J Med* 310:1279, 1984.
11. Tschachler E et al: Epidermal Langerhans cells—a target for HTLV-III/LAV infection. *J Invest Dermatol* 88:233, 1987.
12. Toews GB et al: Epidermal Langerhans cell density determines whether contact sensitivity or unresponsiveness follows skin painting with DNFB. *J Immunol* 124:445, 1980.
13. Balkwill FR, Burke F: The cytokine network. *Immunol Today* 11:229, 1989.
14. Bell TV et al: Expression of mRNA homologous to interleukin-1 in human epidermal cells *J Invest Dermatol* 88:375, 1987.
15. Kupper TS et al: Human keratinocytes contain mRNA indistinguishable from monocyte interleukin-1. *J Exp Med* 64:2095, 1986.
16. Danner M, Luger TA: Human keratinocytes and epidermoid carcinoma cell lines produce a cytokine with interleukin-3-like activity. *J Invest Dermatol* 88:353, 1987.
17. Kupper TS et al: Keratinocyte derived T-cell growth factor (KTGF) is identical to granulocyte macrophage colony-stimulating factor (GM-CSF). *J Invest Dermatol* 91:185, 1988.
18. Sauder DN et al: Molecular and functional characterization of keratinocyte cytokines that induce B cell growth. *Clin Res* 37:695A, 1989.

19. Coffey RJ et al: Production and auto-induction of transforming growth factor—α in human keratinocytes. *Nature* 328:817, 1987.
20. Akhurst RJ et al: Localized production of TGF-β mRNA in tumor promoter-stimulated mouse epidermis. *Nature* 331:363, 1988.
21. Sauder DN et al: Autocrine growth stimulation of human keratinocytes by epidermal cell derived thymocyte activating factor. *Arch Dermatol Res* 280:71, 1988.
22. Martinet N et al: Identification and characterization of chemoattractants for epidermal cells. *J Invest Dermatol* 90:122, 1988.
23. Gaspar AA, Katz SI: Induction and functional characterization of class II MCH (Ia) antigens on murine keratinocytes. *J Immunol* 140:2956, 1988.
24. Niederwieser D et al: IFN-mediated induction of MHC antigen expression on human keratinocytes and its influence on in vitro alloimmune responses. *J Immunol* 140:2556, 1988.
25. Dustin ML et al: Adhesion of T lymphoblasts to epidermal keratinocytes is regulated by interferon γ and is mediated by intercellular adhesion molecule 1 (ICAM-1). *J Exp Med* 167:1323, 1988.
26. Tschachler E et al: Expression of Thy-1 antigen by murine epidermal cells. *J Invest Dermatol* 81:282, 1983.
27. Bergstresser PR et al: Thy-1 antigen-bearing dendritic cells populate murine epidermis. *J Invest Dermatol* 81:286, 1983.
28. Stingl G et al: Thy-1 dendritic epidermal cells express T3 antigen and the T cell receptor gamma chain. *Proc Natl Acad Sci USA* 84:4586, 1987.
29. Cruz PD et al: UV-irradiated Ia^+ and Thy-1+ epidermal cells induce down regulation of contact hypersensitivity. *J Invest Dermatol* 90:552, 1988.
30. Caughman SW et al: Culture and characterization of murine dendritic Thy-1^+ epidermal cells. *J Invest Dermatol* 86:615, 1986.

SECTION TWO

MORPHOLOGY OF CUTANEOUS LESIONS

8

The Structure of Skin Lesions

Jeffrey D. Bernhard and Thomas B. Fitzpatrick

The skin is unique among the organ systems because of its direct and immediate accessibility to visual inspection, physical examination, and histopathologic analysis. This provides an unparalleled opportunity for clinicopathologic correlation. Furthermore, diseases of many other organ systems may be associated with, and often recognized by, specific cutaneous signs.

The accurate recognition and description of cutaneous lesions has been referred to as "the living gross pathology of the skin."[1] Darier, a French dermatologist, referred to the basic lesions as the "alphabet" for reading the language of the skin. The physician must not only look at but *read* the skin for what it may reveal about the patient and the pathophysiology of disease. The following description of the basic lesions is thus provided as an introduction to the basic clinical nomenclature of dermatology.[2–4]

Table 8-1 lists the basic lesions with regard to the component and level of the skin affected, along with some examples of diseases from the text.

MACULE

A *macule* (Fig. 8-1) is a circumscribed, flat lesion that differs from the surrounding skin because of its color. It may result from alterations in any layer or component of the skin. Macules may be of any size or shape. They may result from hyperpigmentation, hypopigmentation, vascular

Table 8-1

CLINICAL CLASSIFICATION OF SKIN LESIONS ACCORDING TO THE COMPONENT OF THE SKIN PRIMARILY INVOLVED*

Skin Compartment/Lesion	Disease Example
1. Epidermis	
a. Keratinocytes	
(1) Scaling macules, papules, or plaques	Psoriasis, eczema
(2) Vesicles and bullae	Pemphigus
(3) Pustules	Acne, pustular psoriasis
(4) Exudative lesions	Impetigo
(5) Atrophy (diffuse or circumscribed)	Lupus erythematosus
b. Melanocytes	
(1) Localized and diffuse hypomelanosis	Vitiligo
(2) Localized and diffuse hypermelanosis	Neurofibromatosis
2. Dermal-epidermal interface	
a. Vesicles	Pemphigoid
b. Bullae	Pemphigoid
c. Scaling macules	Lupus erythematosus
d. Papules	Lichen planus
e. Plaques	Lichen planus
3. Dermis	
a. Connective tissue	
(1) Papules and nodules	Dermatofibroma
(2) Ulcers	Venous stasis
(3) Sclerosis (diffuse or circumscribed)	Scleroderma
(4) Edema	Urticaria
(5) Atrophy (diffuse or circumscribed)	Necrobiosis lipoidica
b. Blood vessels	
(1) Erythematous macules, papules, plaques	Erythema multiforme
(2) Edema (wheal)	Urticaria
(3) Purpura	Vasculitis
(4) Infarcts	Thromboembolism
(5) Telangiectasia	Sun-damaged skin
4. Panniculus adiposus	
a. Connective tissue	
(1) Nodules	Erythema nodosum
(2) Atrophy	Trauma
b. Blood vessels	
(1) Nodules	Polyarteritis nodosa
c. Lipocytes	
(1) Nodules	Lipoma
(2) Atrophy	Liquefying panniculitis

* Some lesions may involve more than one component of the skin in combination. For example, cutaneous T-cell lymphoma involves both dermis and epidermis.

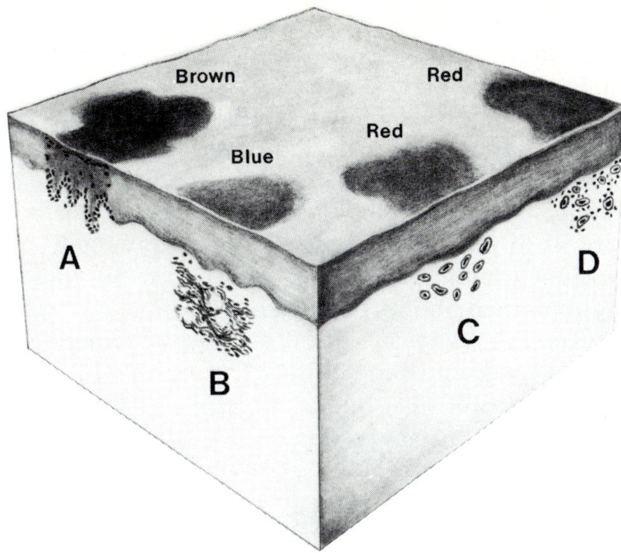

Figure 8-1 Macule. (A) Epidermal hyperpigmentation. (B) Dermal pigmentation. (C) Erythema. (D) Purpura. [*From TB Fitzpatrick et al (eds), Dermatology in General Medicine, 3d ed, New York, McGraw-Hill, 1987, p 26.*]

abnormalities such as capillary hemangioma and capillary dilation (erythema), or purpura (extravasated red blood cells). In some conditions, such as tinea versicolor, macules may be associated with very fine scale.

Telangiectasias are permanent dilations of capillaries that may or may not disappear with application of pressure. They form nonpulsatile, fine, bright-red lines or net-like patterns on the skin. They are usually macular and are normal findings on the face (malar areas, nose) in persons chronically exposed to wind and sun. They are a prominent feature of the erythematous color noted in cutaneous lupus erythematosus. In addition, they may occur in the skin around the nail bed in certain collagen-vascular disorders, such as lupus erythematosus and dermatomyositis, on the face and trunk in scleroderma, and in areas of radiodermatitis. Generalized forms of telangiectasia occur infrequently and are inherited rarely.

Lesions caused by extravasated red blood cells are included under the term *purpura*. *Petechiae* are small, pinpoint, purpuric spots that are often seen in thrombocytopenic states. *Ecchymoses* are larger, bruise-like, purpuric lesions. Pressing a glass slide (diascopy test) on the border of a red lesion is a simple and reliable method for differentiating redness caused by vascular dilation (erythema) from redness caused by extravasated erythrocytes or erythrocyte products (purpura). If the redness remains under the pressure of the slide, the lesion is purpuric.

An *infarct* is an area of cutaneous necrosis resulting from occlusion of blood vessels, as in vasculitis and bacterial emboli. Cutaneous infarcts have a variegated, dusky red to grayish hue. They start as irregularly shaped macules, sometimes depressed slightly below the plane of the skin and often surrounded by a pink zone of hyperemia. Infarcts may be tender and may ulcerate.

Macules may occur as disseminated, small, erythematous lesions, as in drug eruptions, or may be confluent and cover a whole extremity or one-half of the face, as in capillary hemangioma (nevus flammeus). Macules may be pigmented—for example, a café-au-lait color, as in neurofibromatosis; brown, as in melanocytic nevi (moles); gray, as in collections of dermal melanocytes (mongolian spots); or white, as in vitiligo or postinflammation hypopigmentation. The blue color of some clinical lesions results in part from the scatter of light (Tyndall phenomenon) as it passes through the turbid medium of the dermis.

PAPULE

A *papule* (Fig. 8-2) is a small, solid, elevated lesion. Most papules are smaller than 0.5 cm in diameter, and the major portion projects above the plane of the surrounding skin. Oblique lighting with a flashlight in a darkened room is often necessary to detect the slight elevation. The lesion can be the result of metabolic deposits, localized hyperplasia of cellular components of the epidermis or dermis, or localized cellular infiltrates in the dermis. Superficial papules with sharp borders are seen when the lesion is the result of an increase in the number of epidermal cells or melanocytes, as in verruca vulgaris or melanocytic nevi.

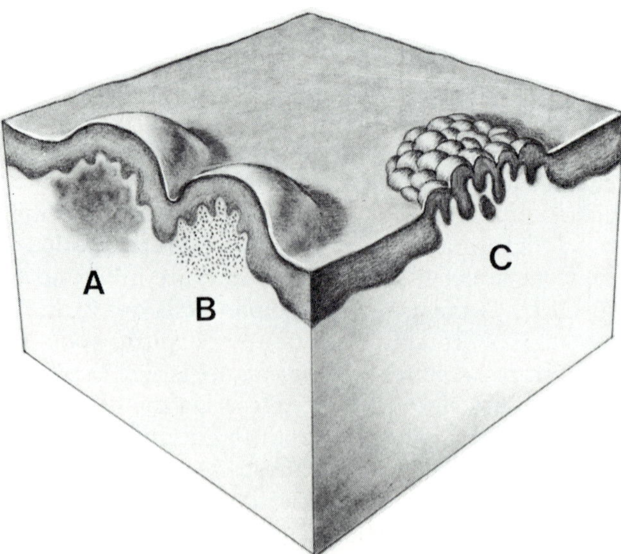

Figure 8-2 Papule. (A) Metabolic deposit in dermis. (B) Cellular infiltrate in dermis. (C) Localized hyperplasia of cellular elements. [*From TB Fitzpatrick et al (eds), Dermatology in General Medicine, 3d ed, New York, McGraw-Hill, 1987, p 28.*]

Papules may have a variety of shapes. They may be acuminate (pointed), as in miliaria rubra (prickly heat rash); dome-shaped, as in molluscum contagiosum; or flat-topped, as in lichen planus.

Other features, such as color, are also important in the identification of papular lesions. Red papules are seen in psoriasis, with a superimposed scale that produces bleeding when removed. A copper color is noted in the lesions of secondary syphilis. In flat-topped papules, a violaceous hue and fine, net-like, white markings on the surface suggest the diagnosis of lichen planus. Purpuric, hemorrhagic, or necrotic papules are noted in cutaneous necrotizing vasculitis and meningococcemia. Melanocytic nevi and early malignant melanoma often occur as rounded, brown or black papules. Skin tags (acrochordons) are pedunculated or filiform lesions with normal skin color.

A papule may consist of multiple small, closely packed, projecting elevations known as a vegetation. Vegetations may be covered with a thick, dry scale and called *keratotic* (as in common warts) or may be soft and smooth (as in condyloma acuminatum). Seborrheic keratoses are common vegetative lesions, especially in older persons. The term *maculopapular* is frequently used in a variety of ways. Because macules are flat and papules are raised, we consider it imprecise and prefer to use more explicit terms in describing a rash.

PLAQUE

A *plaque* (Fig. 8-3) is an elevation above the skin surface that occupies a relatively large area in comparison with its height above the skin. Plaques

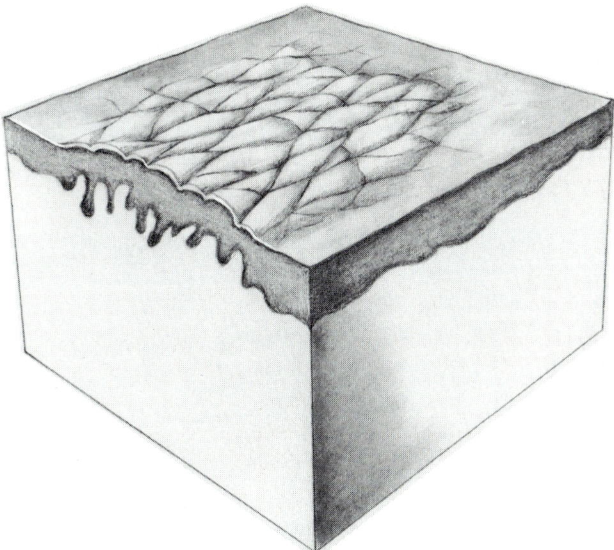

Figure 8-3 Plaque. [*From TB Fitzpatrick et al (eds), Dermatology in General Medicine, 3d ed, New York, McGraw-Hill, 1987, p 29.*]

are often formed by a confluence of papules, as in psoriasis. The typical lesion of psoriasis is an erythematous plaque with silvery layers of scale.

Repeated rubbing, especially in people with chronic eczema, leads to areas of *lichenification*. Proliferation of keratinocytes and stratum corneum, in combination with changes in the collagen of the underlying dermis, causes lichenified areas of skin to appear as thickened plaques with accentuated skin markings.

NODULE

A *nodule* (Fig. 8-4) is a palpable, solid, round or ellipsoidal lesion of varying size; it can be located in the epidermis or extend into the dermis or subcutaneous tissue. Nodules can develop as a result of benign or malignant proliferation of any component of the skin or subcutaneous tissue. For example, keratinocyte proliferation occurs in verruca vulgaris and basal cell carcinoma. Melanocyte proliferation occurs in melanocytic nevi and malignant melanoma. Proliferation of connective tissue elements occurs in dermatofibroma.

Nodules in the dermis and subcutis may indicate systemic disease and result from inflammation, neoplasms, or metabolic deposits. For example, tuberculosis, the deep mycoses, xanthomatosis, lymphoma, and metastatic neoplasms all can present as cutaneous nodules. Kaposi's sarcoma in the acquired immunodeficiency syndrome may appear as purple nodules, papules, and plaques. Erythema nodosum presents as tender subcutaneous nodules on the legs. Foreign-body reactions, insect bites, and bacteria are

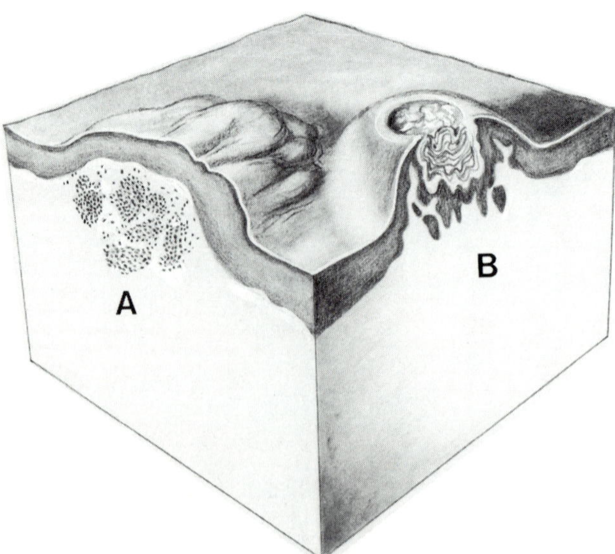

Figure 8-4 Nodule. (A) Dermal nodule. (B) Epidermal nodule. [*From TB Fitzpatrick et al (eds), Dermatology in General Medicine, 3d ed, New York, McGraw-Hill, 1987, p 30.*]

among other causes of nodular lesions. Since nodules may indicate serious systemic disease, biopsy and culture of unidentified persistent nodules should always be performed.

Tumor is a general term for any mass, benign or malignant, and is sometimes used to indicate a large nodule.

It is often helpful to describe a nodule with measurements and with modifying adjectives such as *hard, firm, soft, fleshy, cystic, warm, movable, fixed,,painful,* or *painless*. The surface of a nodule should also be described—for example, as smooth, keratotic, or ulcerated. There is some semantic confusion in distinguishing nodules, tumors, and large papules. In most cases, it is simpy best to include measurements and descriptive terms that convey the important characteristics of the lesion in question.

WHEAL

A *wheal* (hive) (Fig. 8-5) is a rounded or flat-topped, elevated lesion that is characteristically evanescent. Its borders are often sharp and move over hours. These lesions are the result of edema in the upper layer of the dermis. Hives are red, but if the amount of edema is sufficient to compress superficial vessels, they may be white, particularly in the center. Wheals may be 3 to 4 mm in diameter, as in cholinergic urticaria, or 10 to 12 cm, as in urticaria caused by penicillin. In wheals that persist for more than 24 h, a biopsy specimen should be obtained to rule out necrotizing vasculitis.

Angioedema is a deep, edematous reaction that leads to tissue swelling

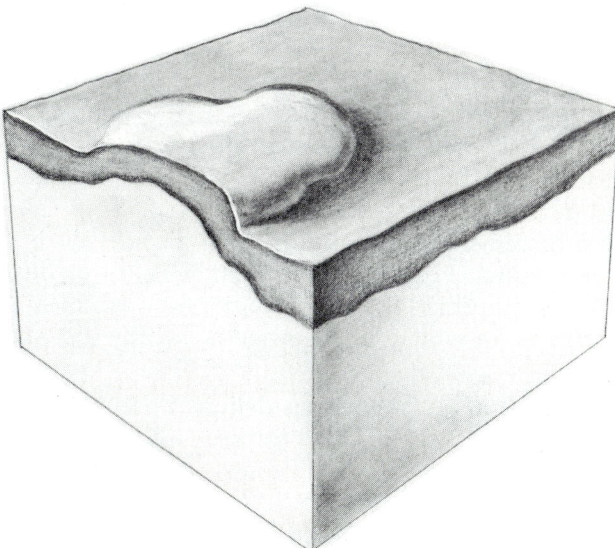

Figure 8-5 Wheal. [*From TB Fitzpatrick et al (eds), Dermatology in General Medicine, 3d ed, New York, McGraw-Hill, 1987, p 31.*]

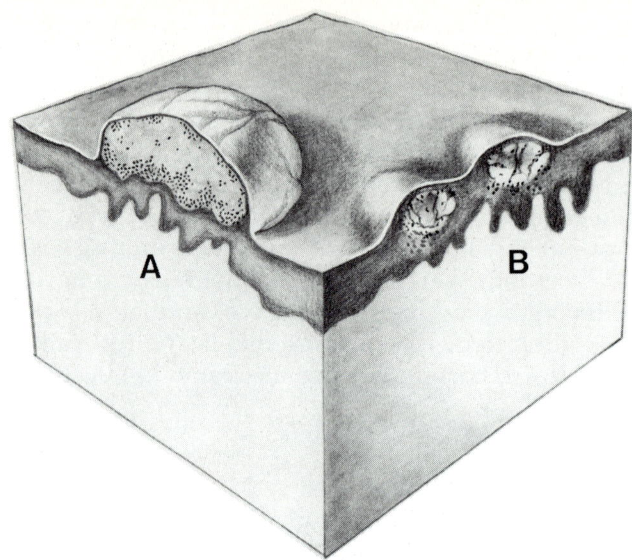

Figure 8-6 Vesicle. (A) Subcorneal. (B) Spongiotic. [*From TB Fitzpatrick et al (eds), Dermatology in General Medicine, 3d ed, New York, McGraw-Hill, 1987, p 32.*]

and that often occurs in areas with very loose dermis and subcutaneous tissue, such as the lip. It may also occur on the hands and feet.

VESICLE AND BULLA

A *vesicle* (Figs. 8-6 to 8-8) is a circumscribed, elevated lesion that contains fluid. Often its walls are so thin that they are translucent, and the serum, lymph, blood, or extracellular fluid is visible. A vesicle with a diameter greater than 0.5 cm is a *bulla*.

Vesicles and bullae arise from cleavage at various levels of the skin; the cleavage may be within the epidermis or in the region of the dermal-epidermal interface. Cleavage just beneath the stratum corneum produces a subcorneal vesicle or bulla, as in impetigo. Intraepidermal vesiculation may result from intercellular edema (spongiosis), as is characteristically seen in delayed hypersensitivity reactions of the epidermis (e.g., in contact eczematous dermatitis). Loss of intercellular bridges, or desmosomes, is known as *acantholysis*. This type of intraepidermal vesiculation is seen in pemphigus vulgaris, in which the cleavage is usually just above the basal layer.

Viruses cause a curious "ballooning degeneration" of epidermal cells, as in herpes zoster, herpes simplex, variola, and varicella. Viral bullae often have a depressed (umbilicated) center.

Pathological changes at the dermal-epidermal interface may cause sub-epidermal vesicles and bullae, as in bullous pemphigoid and erythema multiforme. The amount of pressure required to collapse the lesion may help predict whether a bulla is intraepidermal or subepidermal, as the former tend to be more fragile.

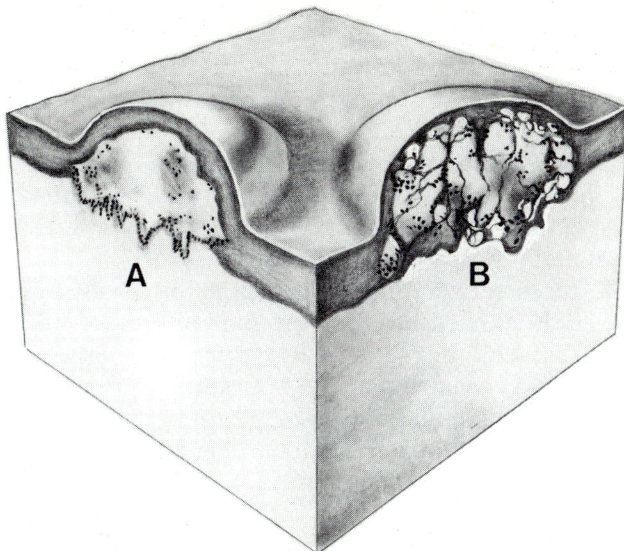

Figure 8-7 Vesicle. (A) Acantholytic. (B) Balloon degeneration. [*From TB Fitzpatrick et al (eds), Dermatology in General Medicine, 3d ed, New York, McGraw-Hill, 1987, p 32.*]

When the epidermis is lost, usually as a result of vesiculation, the circumscribed denudation is known as an *erosion* and appears as a moist, slightly depressed lesion. An erosion does not scar because it involves only the epidermis. If the inflammation and loss of tissue extends into the papillary dermis, an *ulcer* occurs and scarring results.

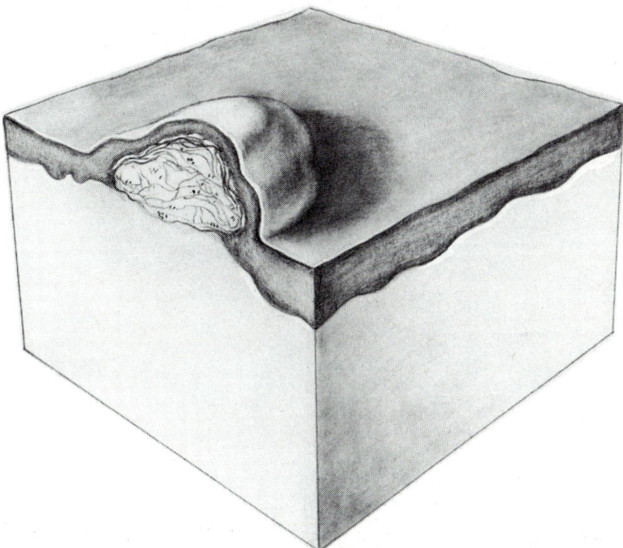

Figure 8-8 Vesicle. Subepidermal. [*From TB Fitzpatrick et al (eds), Dermatology in General Medicine, 3d ed, New York, McGraw-Hill, 1987, p 33.*]

PUSTULE

A *pustule* (Fig. 8-9) is a circumscribed lesion that contains pus. Pus is a white to yellow-green fluid that contains neutrophils and cellular debris. Infectious pathogens may be present or the lesion may be sterile, as in the lesion of pustular psoriasis. Depending on the nature of the exudate, pustules may appear white, yellow, or green-yellow and may vary in size and shape. Follicular pustules are conical, usually contain a hair in the center, and generally heal without scarring.

Pustules are characteristic of acne, pustular psoriasis, and some drug eruptions, especially those caused by bromide or iodide. Vesicular lesions of some viral diseases (varicella, variola, vaccinia, herpes simplex, and herpes zoster) may become pustular. A Gram's stain and culture of the exudate from pustules should always be performed.

A *furuncle* is a deep, necrotizing form of folliculitis with an accumulation of pus. It feels warm and is red and tender. Several furuncles may coalesce to form a *carbuncle.*

A *sinus* is a connecting tract or fistula between the surface of the skin and an underlying structure such as an abscess, which is a collection of pus formed by the disintegration of tissue. A sinus near the rectum may be seen in rectal abscess, carcinoma of the bowel, or granulomatous colitis (Crohn's disease).

CYST

A *cyst* is a sac or closed cavity that contains liquid or semisolid material (fluid, cells, and cell products). Cysts may have an epithelial, endothelial,

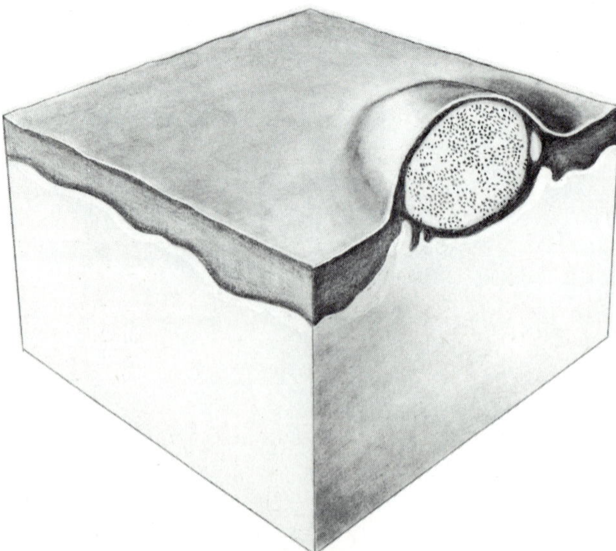

Figure 8-9 Pustule. [*From TB Fitzpatrick et al (eds), Dermatology in General Medicine, 3d ed, New York, McGraw-Hill, 1987, p 34.*]

or membranous lining. A spherical or oval nodule or papule may be suspected of being a cyst if, on palpation, it is resilient. The most common cysts are epidermal (keratinous) cysts, which are lined with squamous epithelium and produce keratinous material. Cysts of pilar (hair follicle) origin are lined with multilayered epithelium that will not mature through a granular layer and are called *pilar cysts.*

ATROPHY

Epidermal atrophy results from a decrease in the number of epidermal cell layers. Atrophic epidermis may or may not retain the normal skin lines and is often associated with some alteration in the dermis. A common change of this sort is seen on sun-exposed surfaces of elderly individuals, where the skin may be finely wrinkled and more transparent than normal.

Dermal atrophy results from a decrease in the papillary or reticular dermal connective tissue and usually appears as a depression in the skin. It occurs in the striae of pregnancy and in Cushing's disease. Dermal atrophy may follow inflammation or trauma, with or without ulceration. An example is necrobiosis lipoidica diabeticorum, in which loss of skin markings, increased translucence, and localized depression of the skin result in a distinctive clinical picture seen on the skin of some patients with diabetes mellitus. Atrophy in the panniculus also causes depressions of the skin, as in progressive lipodystrophy.

ULCER

An *ulcer* (Fig. 8-10) is a lesion in which there has been destruction of the epidermis and dermis. Certain features that are helpful in determining the cause of ulcers include location, borders, base, discharge, and any associated features of the lesion or surrounding skin, such as nodules, excoriations, varicosities, hair distribution, presence or absence of sweating, and adjacent pulses. Venous stasis ulcers are accompanied by pigmentation and, occasionally, by edema or sclerosis. They begin most commonly on the medial aspect of the ankle or lower leg. Hypertensive or ischemic ulcers tend to start on the lateral aspect of the ankle or foot. Factitial lesions often have artificial shapes including straight, angular borders. Excoriations that have enlarged into ulcers have a similar appearance but may be accompanied by the residua of an underlying dermatosis (e.g., eczematous dermatitis associated with chronic venous insufficiency). Decubitus ulcers occur at pressure points.

Ulceration can occur as a result of tissue infarction in areas of large-vessel or small-vessel occlusion or constriction caused by various factors: embolus, thrombosis, cryoprecipitates, and necrotizing vasculitis of various sorts. Ulceration occurs in tumors, such as basal cell carcinoma, and in granulomatous nodules caused by a variety of infectious agents such as fungi, parasites, and bacteria.

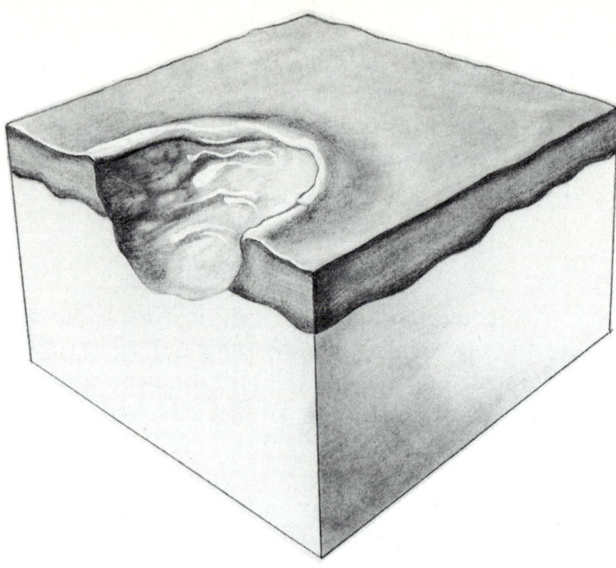

Figure 8-10 Ulcer. [*From TB Fitzpatrick et al (eds), Dermatology in General Medicine, 3d ed, New York, McGraw-Hill, 1987, p 35.*]

SCAR

A *scar* occurs wherever ulceration or sufficient damage to the dermis has taken place, and its appearance reflects the pattern of healing. Scars may be hypertrophic or atrophic and may be sclerotic, or hard, as the result of collagen proliferation. Scarred skin often loses the normal skin lines and appendages. Scars may occur in the course of acne and in varicella-zoster virus infection. Raynaud's disease, syphilis, tuberculosis (especially on the face), and leprosy (on the digits) may produce loss of tissue, or *mutilations,* that alter major anatomic structures.

SCALE

The end product of keratinization is the cornified cell of the outermost layer of the skin, the stratum corneum. When keratinocyte production occurs at an increased rate, as in psoriasis, immature cells that retain nuclei reach the skin surface; this condition is called *parakeratosis.* Parakeratotic cells may pile up and contribute to the formation of *scales* (Fig. 8-11). A scale is thus a flake or flat plate of stratum corneum that may be one or many cell layers thick. Scales are seen in a variety of other conditions (e.g., dermatophyte infections, pityriasis rosea, and secondary syphilis). Densely adherent scales that have a gritty feel (like sandpaper) are typically seen in solar keratosis. Fish-like scales occur in a group of disorders known as the *ichthyoses* and result from prolonged retention of stratum corneum cells.

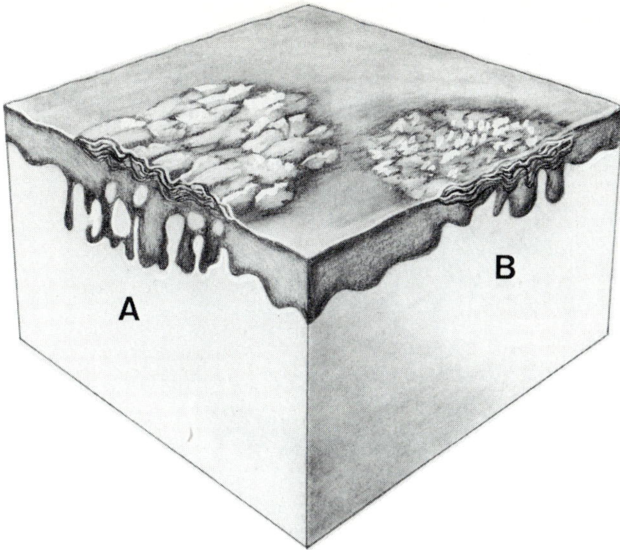

Figure 8-11 Scale. (A) Parakeratotic scale surmounting psoriasiform epidermal hyperplasia. (B) Densely adherent scale from localized increase in the stratum corneum. [*From TB Fitzpatrick et al (eds), Dermatology in General Medicine, 3d ed, New York, McGraw-Hill, 1987, p 37.*]

CRUST

A *crust* (Fig. 8-12) results when serum, blood, or purulent exudate dries on the skin surface; it is characteristic of pyogenic infections. Crusts may be thin, delicate, and friable or thick and adherent. They are yellow when formed from dried serum, green or yellow-green when formed from purulent exudate, or brown or dark red when formed from blood. Crusts may be present in acute eczematous dermatitis and impetigo (honey-colored crusts).

GANGRENE AND SPHACELUS

Gangrene refers to a severe necrotizing and sloughing process. Gangrene that results from arterial occlusion is characterized by a sharply demarcated blue-black color. Gangrene from streptococcal or clostridial infection may begin with vesicles that become purplish black and are followed by rapid necrosis of whole segments of skin.

A *sphacelus* is a densely adherent, dry, necrotic membrane occurring in the floor of an ulcer. It is seen in decubitus ulcers, ulcers due to x-ray damage, diphtheritic ulcers, or any ischemic ulcer or factitial dermatosis.

EXCORIATION

Excoriations are superficial excavations of epidermis that result from scratching. They may be linear or punctate. They are frequently found in

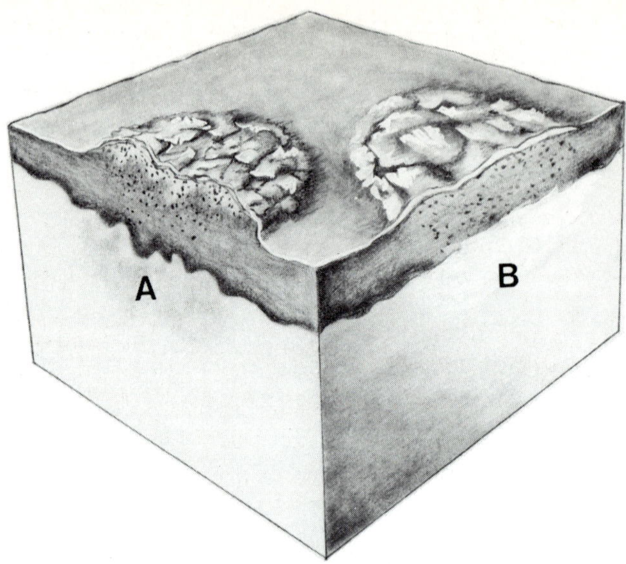

Figure 8-12 Crust. (A) Thin, friable, superficial crust. (B) Thick, adherent exudate and crust. [*From TB Fitzpatrick et al (eds), Dermatology in General Medicine, 3d ed, New York, McGraw-Hill, 1987, p 38.*]

many types of pruritus and are concomitants of pruritic skin disease, such as atopic eczema.

FISSURE

Fissures are linear cleavages or cracks in the skin and may be painful. They occur particularly in dermatitis of the hands and feet, especially with excessive drying of the skin. Fissures are frequently noted in perianal psoriasis, at the angles of the mouth (perlèche), in chronic eczematous dermatitis, and in psoriasis of the palms and soles.

SCLEROSIS

Sclerosis is caused by an accumulation of collagen in the dermis. It is manifested by circumscribed or diffuse hardening or induration and is often detected more easily by palpation than by inspection. Sclerosis is a component of morphea, linear scleroderma, systemic scleroderma, and porphyria cutanea tarda. Sclerosis occurs in chronic stasis dermatitis and chronic lymphedema.

GENERAL CONSIDERATIONS IN DERMATOLOGIC DIAGNOSIS

In making a dermatologic diagnosis, several features other than the nature of the primary lesion are important. These include the distribution, shape, and arrangement of lesions on the body. For example, psoriasis often involves the scalp, elbows, and knees. Atopic dermatitis frequently involves the flexural aspects of the elbows and knees. The most characteristic lesions of erythema multiforme are shaped like rings, targets, or bull's-eyes, and they are usually distributed on the extremities. An annular (ring-like) shape is often seen in immunologically mediated disorders and suggests that immunoreactants or inflammatory mediators are involved in a process of diffusion from a central point. Some infections, such as impetigo, dermatophytosis (ringworm), and the skin lesion of Lyme disease (erythema chronicum migrans) also give rise to annular lesions that enlarge from a central point of inoculation. *Arrangement* refers to the way lesions are grouped: for example, the bullae of herpes zoster are characteristically grouped closely together in the distribution of a single dermatome.

Except in certain instances, the pathophysiologic factors that determine the shape, arrangement, and distribution of lesions remain largely a matter of conjecture. Jagged, irregular infarcts correspond to the distribution of underlying blood vessels affected by occlusive processes such as thromboembolism. Trauma plays a role in the localization of psoriasis to sites such as the knees. Ultraviolet radiation–induced damage to nucleic acids appears to be important in determining the photodistribution of lesions in systemic lupus erythematosus. The astute clinician combines a knowledge of the structure of skin lesions and the pathophysiology to arrive at diagnoses that can be made in no way other than by careful physical examination of the skin.

REFERENCES

1. Jackson R: *Morphological Dermatology. A Study of the Living Gross Pathology of the Skin.* Springfield, Ill, Charles C Thomas, 1979.
2. Fitzpatrick TB, Bernhard JD: The structure of skin lesions and fundamentals of diagnosis, in TB Fitzpatrick et al (eds), *Dermatology in General Medicine,* 3d ed. New York, McGraw-Hill, 1987, p 20.
3. Fitzpatrick TB, Bernhard JD: Skin lesions of general medical significance, in E Braunwald et al (eds), *Harrison's Principles of Internal Medicine,* 11th ed. New York, McGraw-Hill, 1987, p 232.
4. Winkelmann RK (chairman): Glossary of basic dermatology lesions. *Acta Derm Venereol (Stockh)* Suppl 130, 1987.

SECTION THREE

DISORDERS OF THE EPIDERMIS

9

Biology of the Epidermis and Pathophysiology of Psoriasis and Certain Ichthyosiform Dermatoses

Howard P. Baden

The epidermis is an organized, stratified epithelium. Its major cellular component is the keratinocyte, but it also contains melanocytes, Langerhans cells, and Merkel cells. The epidermis consists of three compartments designated germinative, differentiated, and cornified (Fig. 9-1). It is the last that forms the barrier layer of the skin, which prevents the entrance of toxic substances and microorganisms and the loss of water and electrolytes.

NORMAL EPIDERMIS

Kinetics

The epidermis constantly renews itself, with stratum corneum cells shed at the surface and replaced by new cells constantly formed by mitosis in the basal layer. Although the basal cell layer makes up the predominant portion of the germinative cell compartment in the normal epidermis, at least a portion of the second row is also capable of cell division. Above the germinative compartment are the viable differentiated cells that form the spinous layer and the more superficial granular layer. The size of these compartments varies in different areas of the skin and with the state of tissue normalcy. Spinous cells are larger than basal cells because of an increase in the cytoplasmic volume of the differentiated cells. The granular layer contains one or two rows of oval, horizontally oriented cells containing

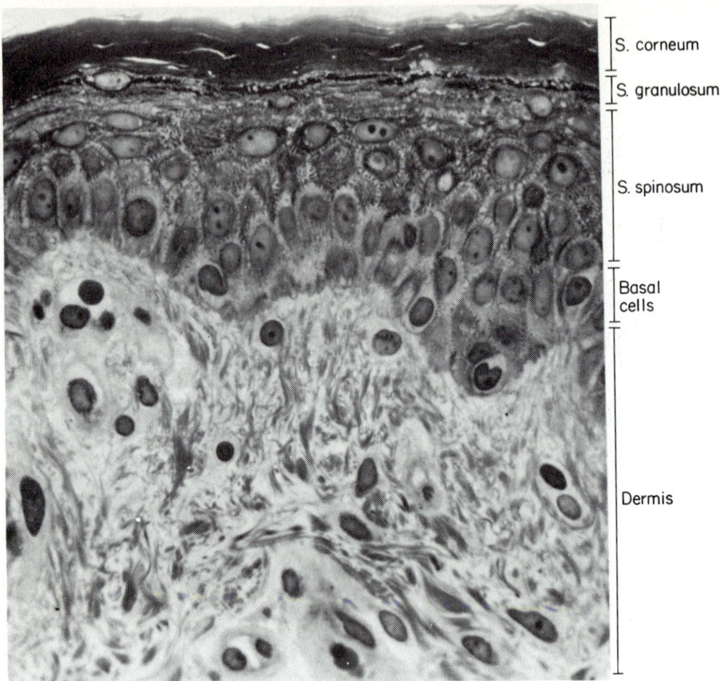

Figure 9-1 Histological section of the skin showing the various layers of the epidermis. ×400 in the original magnification. [*From TB Fitzpatrick et al (eds), Dermatology in General Medicine, 2d ed, New York, McGraw-Hill, 1979, p 44.*]

cytoplasmic (keratohyalin) granules. The third compartment of epidermal cells is the stratum corneum overlying the stratum granulosum. It is distinguished by a loss of cellular detail, the absence of nuclei, and flattened cells. It is considered a nonviable end product of epidermal cell differentiation.

The epidermal cells appear to be organized into units in which a number of germinative and differentiated cells are surmounted by a single flattened stratum corneum cell. Since the cells increase in size as they ascend, there is a greater number of cells in the lower layers. In most areas of the body the stratum corneum cells are carefully stacked, with their edges overlapping in a very precise manner[1] (Fig. 9-2). When the epidermal turnover rate is increased, this orderly stacking is lost; this process is associated with a loss of barrier function. Normally, the epidermis of the palms and soles turns over faster than that of the rest of the body, and the stratum corneum shows a haphazard arrangement of cells.

Replacement of the epidermis takes about one month and has been determined by pulse labeling of the epidermis with ^{14}C-glycine and determining when the radioactivity is lost from the surface. As cells pass

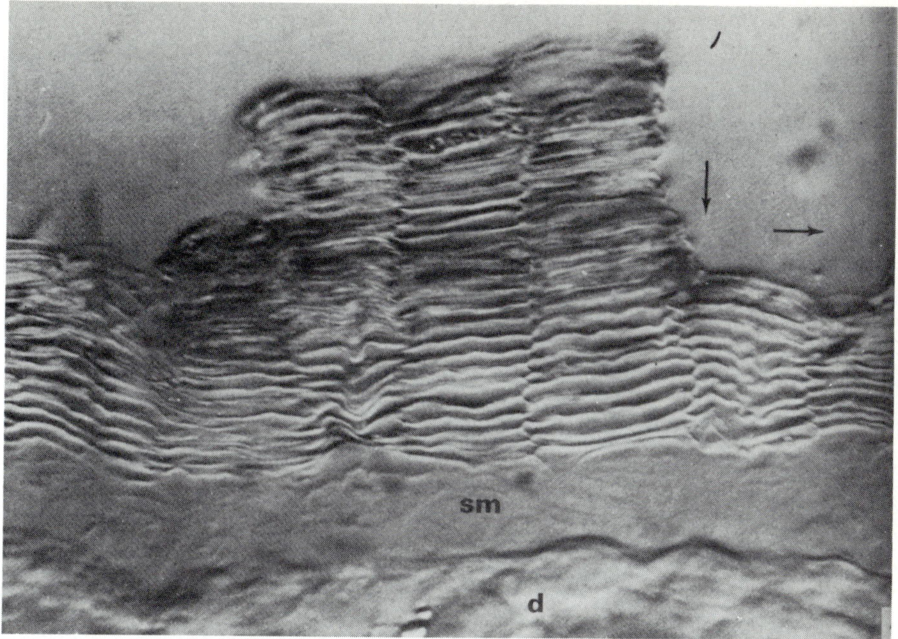

Figure 9-2 Scanning electron micrograph of skin. The stratum corneum has been swollen to show layering. d = dermis; sm = stratum malpighium. [*From DN Menton, AZ Eisen.*[1]]

through the epidermis, they spend about half their time in the viable layers and the remainder in the stratum corneum.

The cycle of an epidermal basal cell, like that of other dividing cells, has been divided into different periods (Fig. 9-3). Following mitosis, a cell enters the G_1 interphase period, in which it carries on most of its metabolic activities. In response to a specific stimulus the cell begins the DNA synthesis (S) period, during which DNA is doubled in preparation for mitosis. A relatively short postsynthetic (G_2) phase then occurs followed by an equally brief mitotic period (M). The G_1 period repeats, during which time the two daughter cells separate but both remain in the basal layer. The mechanism responsible for the movement of cells into the differentiating spinous layer has not been determined, but it is not simply a response to cell division and "pressure" to move up. It has been suggested that some cells in the basal layer are blocked in G_1 and do not cycle (G_0) unless the epidermis is stimulated to undergo hyperplasia.

Internal and external factors influence epidermal cell proliferation. Diurnal variations in mitotic activity have been reported in human skin, with an increase in the number of epidermal cells synthesizing DNA during the night.[2] A tissue-specific epidermal mitotic inhibiting substance called chalone has been described, which is a glycoprotein with a molecular

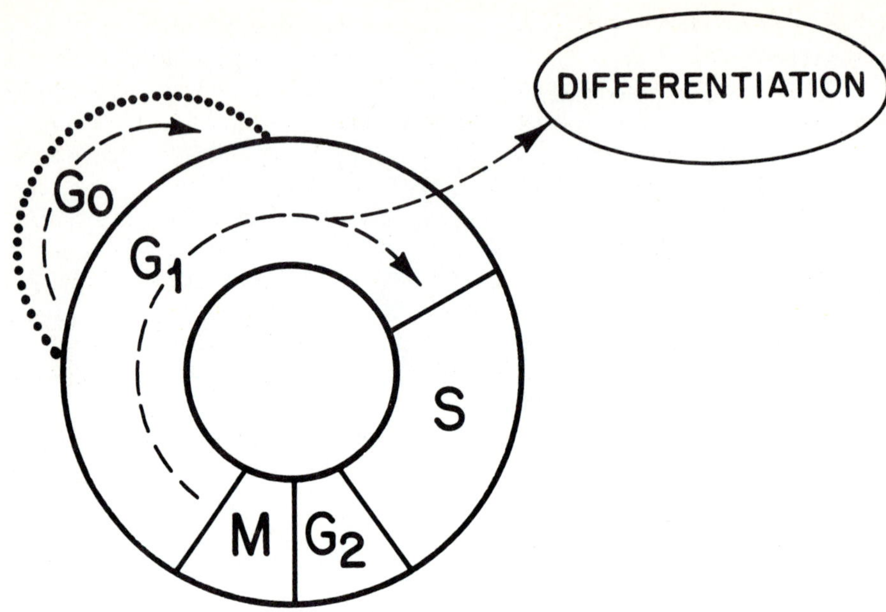

Figure 9-3 Cell cycle.

weight of 35,000.[3] An epidermal growth factor, a polypeptide with a molecular weight of 6000, has been shown to stimulate epidermal proliferation in vivo and in vitro.[4] A large number of reports have appeared describing the effect of a variety of other growth factors and cytokines on cultured keratinocytes, but their effect on intact tissue remains to be determined. At the molecular level, cyclic nucleotides and prostaglandins have also been suggested as regulators of epidermal proliferation, especially as revealed by studies in psoriatic epidermis.[5] External factors that affect epidermal proliferation are those that injure the skin, such as wounding and ultraviolet radiation.

Subcellular Structures

Differentiation of the epidermis is a complex process involving a number of metabolic pathways that must proceed in an orderly manner in order to achieve normal cornification. A summary of these processes is shown in Fig. 9-4, which indicates the locations where they occur.

Fibrous Proteins

The major structural protein of the epidermis is fibrous keratin. It has a helical configuration, as demonstrated by x-ray diffraction analysis, and is organized into intracellular tonofilaments, as seen by electron microscopy

(Fig. 9-5). Keratin is a double-stranded α-helical molecule consisting of polypeptide chains of molecular weights between 40,000 and 70,000.[6] As revealed by sodium dodecylsulfate (SDS) polyacrylamide gel electrophoresis (PAGE) analysis, normal epidermal keratins consist of four major proteins of molecular weights 50, 56.5, 58, and 65 to 67 kd. In other human epithelial tissues that also contain fibrous proteins, a different composition is observed (Fig. 9-6), pointing to the heterogeneity of the keratin molecules.[7] This is further complicated by the findings that keratins can be grouped into two families, acidic and basic, and that members from each family form a pair that leads to the formation of the fibrous proteins. In epidermis, for example, the acidic 50-kd component pairs with the basic 58-kd one, and the acidic 56.5-kd component pairs with the basic 67-kd one.

Studies of cloned keratin genes have shown that the keratin molecule consists of a central helical core of 300 to 350 amino acids and flanking

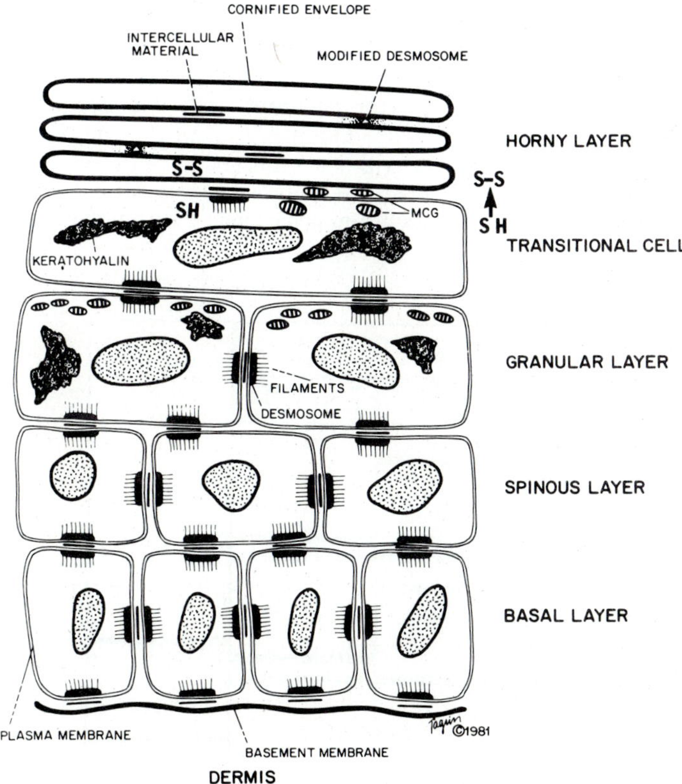

Figure 9-4 Schematic representation of the epidermis showing various structural components. The keratins are in the reduced form (SH) in the viable layer and oxidized (S-S) in the stratum corneum.

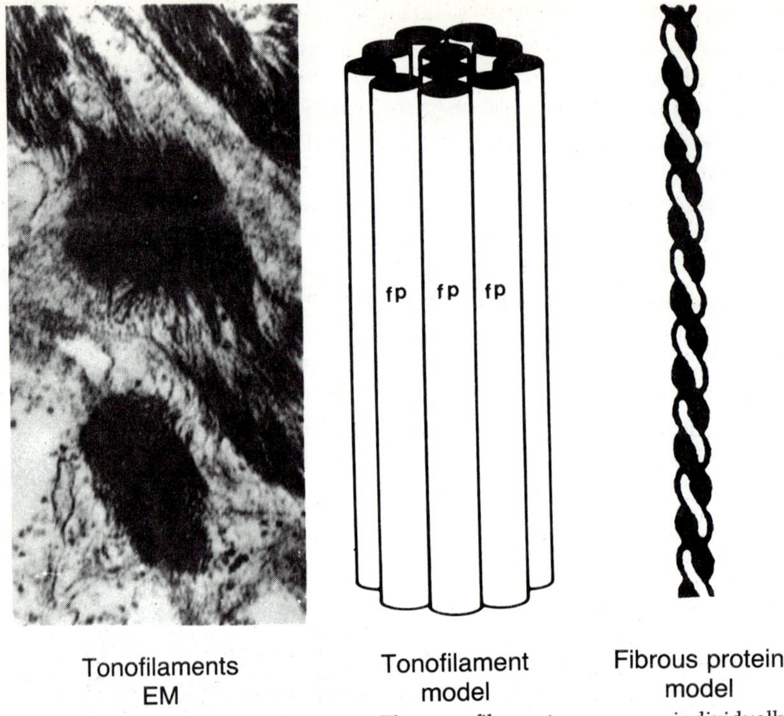

Figure 9-5 Structure of tonofilaments. The tonofilaments are seen individually and in bundles streaming out of the desmosome. The tonofilament consists of groups of fibrous protein molecules (fp) that contain two different polypeptide chains in the basic subunit.

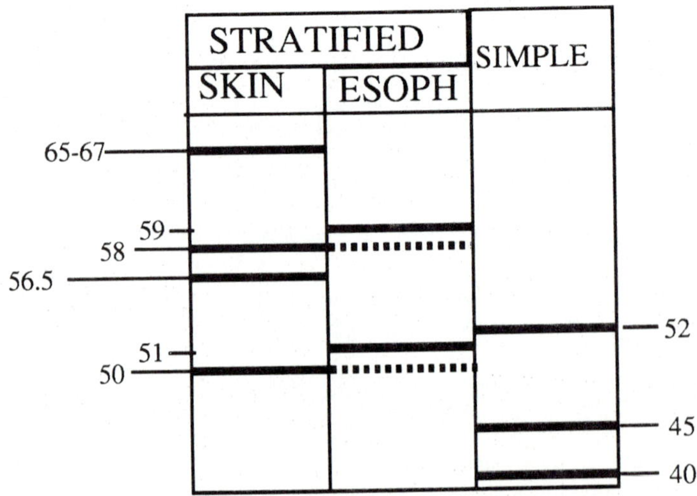

Figure 9-6 Keratin polypeptides of epidermis and epithelial tissues. Molecular weights are $\times 10^{-3}$.

nonhelical regions at the N-terminal and C-terminal ends. The helical cores are remarkably conserved in the various keratin molecules, and differences in the proteins are primarily related to the size and sequence of the terminal ends. The initial step in forming the fibrous proteins is the assembly of individual peptides into a double-stranded, coiled molecule. The exact mechanism by which the 80-Å filament is formed is not precisely known but must involve side-to-side as well as end-to-end interactions. The filaments become organized, so that they attach to a perinuclear ring and extend through the cytoplasm to the attachment plaques of the desmosome on the plasma membrane (Fig. 9-7). This plasma membrane–nuclear link probably plays an important role in coordination of cellular activities.

Synthesis of keratin starts in the basal layer and continues throughout the living epidermis. In the basal layer only the 50-kd and 58-kd proteins

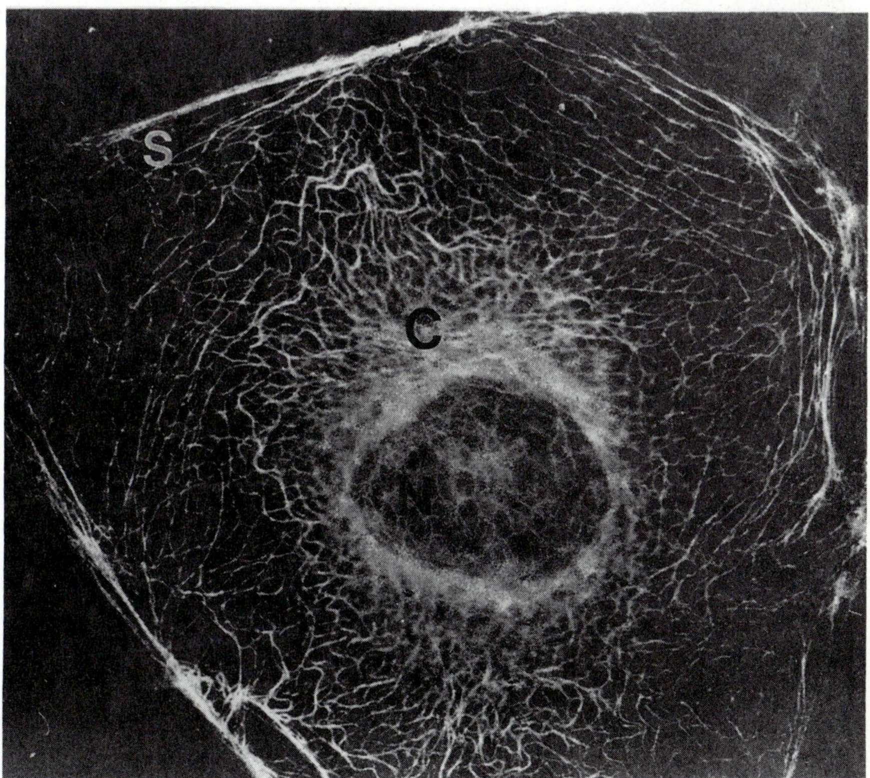

Figure 9-7 Pattern of intermediate filament network in an epithelial cell. N = nucleus; C = cytoplasm; S = cell surface. [*From RD Goldman, GN Dessev, Intermediate filaments: problems and perspectives, in GE Rogers et al* (eds), *The Biology of Wool and Hair, London and New York, Chapman and Hall, 1989, p 89.*]

are made, whereas the 56.5-kd and 65- to 67-kd ones are synthesized in increasing amounts in the suprabasal cells.[7] In the viable epidermis the keratins contain cysteine residues, while in the stratum corneum they are oxidized to cystine, enhancing the insolubility of the proteins. Other posttranslational modifications of the keratins have been reported. Phosphorylation has been documented and explains in part the charge heterogeneity that has been observed in two-dimensional electrophoresis.[8] The ε-(γ-glutamyl) lysine cross-link (Fig. 9-8) has also been observed in the fibrous proteins extracted from the epidermis, although the cornified envelope is thought to the major site at which cross-linking occurs.[9] Conversion of peptide-bound citrulline has been reported, although filaggrin appears to be the major protein that is modified this way.[10] Finally, proteolytic degradation occurs continuosly throughout the stratum corneum so that the keratins become reduced in size and are more difficult to separate by electrophoresis.

Desmosomes

An important structural component of the epidermis is the desmosome,[11] which anchors cells to one another and to which the filamentous proteins attach (Fig. 9-9). A number of components have been identified but there is not uniform agreement on their exact location in the desmosome (Fig. 9-10). DP III is now called plakoglobin and is found entirely within the plaque. DG I a,b,c (desmoglein) and DG II a,b run from the plaque into the intercellular space and are glycoproteins. In addition to the need to define the location of the structural proteins more precisely, there remains

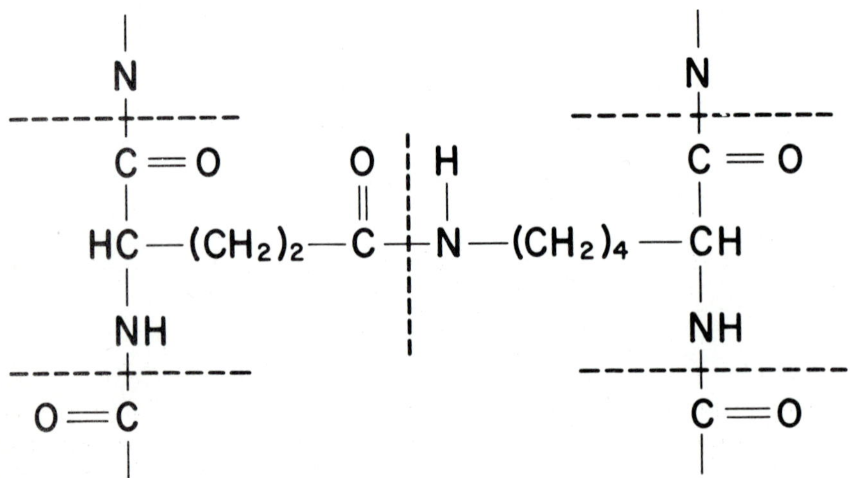

Figure 9-8 The ε-(γ-glutamyl) lysine cross-link connecting amino acids in peptide linkage. (From HP Baden, Keratinization in the epidermis, Pharmacol Ther 7:393, 1979.)

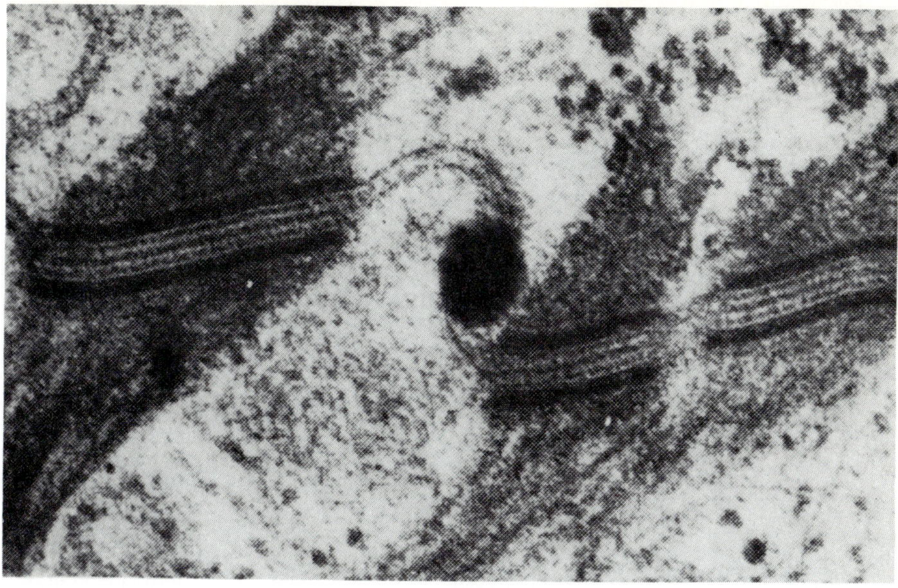

a

T
AP
IL
OL
DL
IC
DL

b

Figure 9-9 (*a*) Electron micrograph of a desmosome showing the various layers. ×64 in the original magnification. (*b*) Schematic representation of a desmosome. IC = intercellular contact layer; DL = distal light layer; OL and IL = outer and inner leaflets of the plasma membrane; AP = attachment plaque; T = tonofilaments. (*Part a from AS Zelickson, Ultrastructure of Normal and Abnormal Skin, Philadelphia, Lea & Febiger, 1967, p 62.*)

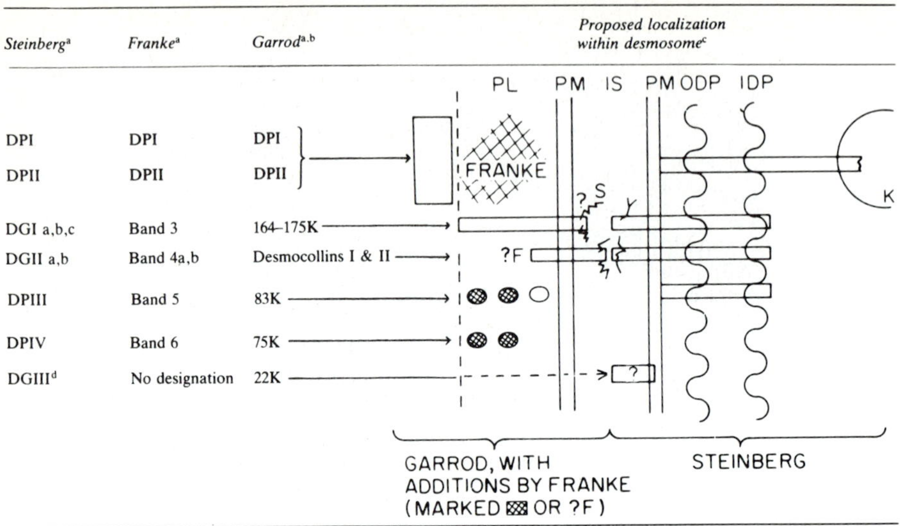

Steinberg[a]	Franke[a]	Garrod[a,b]	Proposed localization within desmosome[c]
DPI	DPI	DPI	
DPII	DPII	DPII	
DGI a,b,c	Band 3	164–175K	
DGII a,b	Band 4a,b	Desmocollins I & II	
DPIII	Band 5	83K	
DPIV	Band 6	75K	
DGIII[d]	No designation	22K	

Figure 9-10 Designation and localization of desmosomal proteins. ([a]) DP = desmoplakin; DG = desmoglein. ([b]) Mr is given in thousands. ([c]) PL = plaques; PM = plasma membrane; IS = intercellular space; S = sugar; ODP = outer dense plaque; IDP = inner dense plaque; K = keratin. Franke has desmoplakin entirely within the plaque. (*From Junctional Complexes of Epithelial Cells, New York, Wiley, 1987, p 67.*)

the question of how the filaments attach to the plaque and specifically how the cells are held together. The latter issue is important in order to understand how cells move through the epidermis and still maintain their attachment to one another. In addition, there are a number of diseases in which the cells separate from one another (acantholysis) as a result of disruption of the desmosome; we would like to understand the mechanism.

Keratohyalin

Another important structure in the epidermis is the keratohyalin granule (Fig. 9-11), which is seen in the uppermost viable layer as a large, darkly staining particle. By electron microscopy this material, at least in the rat, has been shown to consist of two components, one of which is rich in cystine polypeptides and appears to give rise to the cornified envelope of the cell.[12] The other identified component is a basic protein rich in histidine and arginine that is thought to act as a matrix material surrounding filaments in the stratum corneum. Labeled amino acid incorporation studies have shown that keratohyalin proteins are synthesized in the granular layer and are not accumulated cellular debris, as originally suggested.

The basic keratohyalin protein has been purified from human epidermis and found to have a molecular weight of 37 kd.[13] A precursor of this protein with a molecular weight of about 300,000 has been identified. It is

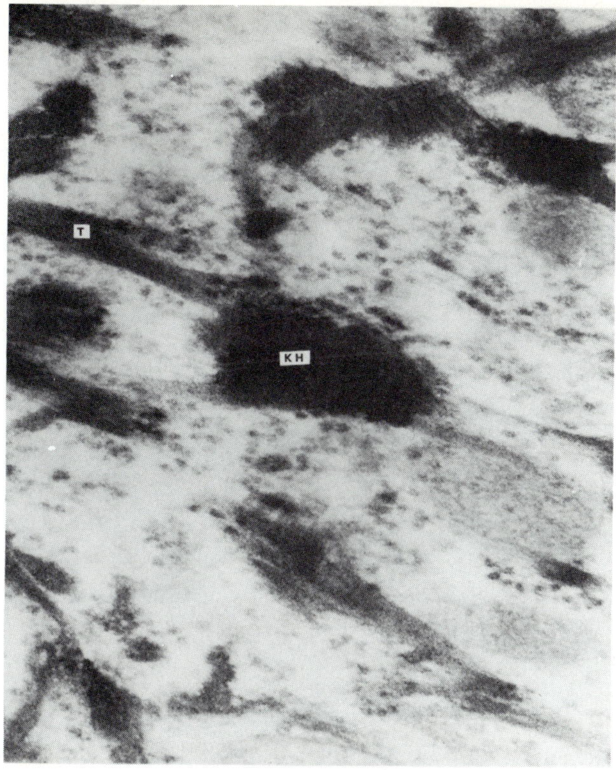

Figure 9-11 Electron micrograph of keratohyalin granules (KH). T = tonofilaments. ×38 in the original magnification. (*From HP Baden, Keratinization in the epidermis, Pharmacol Res 7:393, 1977. Micrograph courtesy of R. Lavker.*)

phosphorylated and then broken down by proteolytic enzymes into the basic protein, now called filaggrin. The addition of filaggrin to a suspension of filamentous protein induces the formation of rope-like structures that by electron microscopy resemble the keratin pattern of matrix and fibrous proteins seen in normal stratum corneum.[14] Thus, filaggrin acts as a matrix protein in which the fibrous protein is embedded. In the stratum corneum, filaggrin is altered by the enzymatic conversion of peptide-bound arginine to citrulline, which reduces its positive charge and allows it to detach from the fibrous protein. Filaggrin then undergoes further hydrolysis to free amino acids and their derivatives, which act as water-binding substances and are important in maintaining the water content of the stratum corneum.

Cornified Envelope

A thick envelope is formed beneath the plasma membrane of granular cells that cannot be solubilized by denaturing solvents even when a

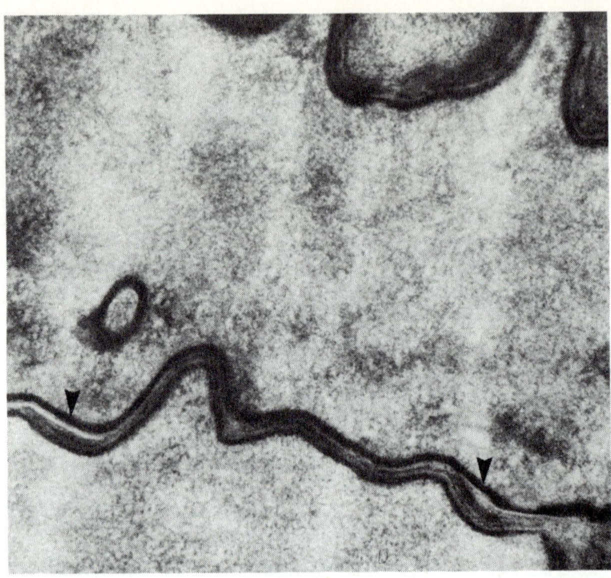

Figure 9-12 Electron micrograph of stratum corneum showing the thickened cell envelope (arrowheads). ×66 in the original magnification. (*From AS Zelickson: Ultrastructure of Normal and Abnormal Skin, Philadelphia, Lea & Febiger, 1967, p 97.*)

reducing agent is present[15] (Fig. 9-12). This structure, the cornified envelope, is rendered insoluble by the formation of ϵ-(γ-glutamyl) lysine cross-links. Cytoplasmic and membrane-associated precursors have been identified in whole epidermis and cultured epidermal cells.[16–18] The most thoroughly studied of these is involucrin, an acidic protein in which 50 percent of the amino acidues are glutamine, which has been shown to be a substrate for transglutaminase. Although originally reported to be present only in primates, involucrin-like proteins have been recognized in other mammals. The other precursors have been shown to be more widely distributed in mammals, and vary in composition and size in the different animals that have been studied. The transglutaminase responsible for the cross-linking is membrane associated and keratinocyte specific.[19]

Membrane-Coating Granules

Specialized 0.1- to 0.5-μm ovoid bodies, membrane-coating granules, are observed in the upper spinous and granular layers. They are surrounded by a 30-Å-thick membrane and have an internal structure of lamellae with alternating density (Fig. 9-13). They are extruded into the intercellular space at the base of the stratum corneum and partially disintegrate to give rise to lamellar sheets. These sheets are a mixture of lipid and protein and are likely the principal diffusion barrier in the stratum corneum. Phos-

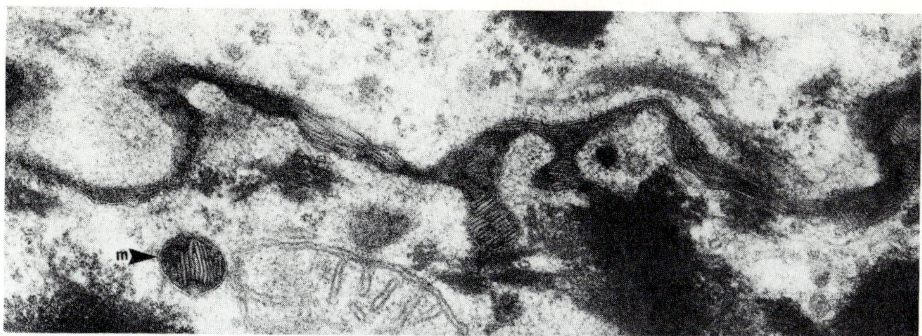

Figure 9-13 Electron micrograph of epidermis showing membrane-coating granules (m) within a cell and in the intercellular space. *(From PM Elias et al, Mammalian epidermal barrier layer lipids: composition and influence on structure, J Invest Dermatol 69:531, 1977.)*

pholipids are present in the granular layer but are replaced by neutral lipids in the stratum corneum.[20] This change in lipid distribution is critical to the function of the stratum corneum as a barrier to the diffusion of water. In addition to its role as a diffusion barrier, intercellular material is thought to be important for the cohesion and eventual separation of stratum corneum cells. The details of this process have not been delineated.

Cornification

The conversion of the viable granular cells to dead horny cells is associated with a number of other changes. There is breakdown and reabsorption of many subcellular organelles, including nuclei, mitochondria, Golgi, and others. Most of the proteins and nucleic acid that are not incorporated into the keratinized products are also broken down and reabsorbed. Although some enzymes may remain in the stratum corneum, the metabolic pathways for energy production and synthesis of macromolecules no longer operate. Finally, the water content drops from 70 percent in the granular layer to 30 percent in the stratum corneum.

New Concepts of the Keratinocyte

In the past several years, it has become apparent that the keratinocyte may carry out functions other than synthesizing the stratum corneum barrier. The first clue to this hypothesis was the demonstration that keratinocytes may produce interleukin-1 (IL-1). It has now been shown that the cells can synthesize IL-6, IL-8, granulocyte-macrophage colony-stimulating factor, and macrophage colony-stimulating factor.[21] In addition, the keratinocyte may develop receptors for IL-1, IL-4, tumor necrosis factor, and α and γ interferons. Thus, the epidermis may excrete cytokines that initiate or modify the inflammatory process in the skin and, at the same time, can be affected by factors that in turn modify their response.

Keratinocytes have also been shown to respond to growth factors; the most well-described ones are epidermal growth factor and transforming growth factors α and β.[22] The former two are thought to be stimulatory and the latter inhibitory. It has also been shown that keratinocytes can synthesize the transforming growth factors, and with the α factor, there may be autoinduction.

At present there is little direct evidence linking the cytokines and growth factors to disease, but it seems likely that such evidence will be found. Our understanding of dermatologic diseases will be enhanced as our knowledge about the action of these factors increases.

PSORIASIS

Psoriasis is a common cutaneous disease affecting about one percent of the population, with the onset in 70 percent of patients by age 20. Although it is generally agreed that there is a genetic component to the disease, there is disagreement as to whether the mode of inheritance is polygenic or dominant.

Studies of histocompatibility antigens have been done in psoriasis. Some reports have shown increased frequencies of HLA-A1, -B13, and -B17,[23,24] while in other studies HLA-B37 was significantly elevated. These diverse findings may reflect differences in the racial and ethnic origins of the various populations that have been studied. As pointed out by Murray et al.,[23] the increased frequency of a number of HLA alloantigens and the changed association of these alloantigens in patients with psoriasis compared with the control population suggest a multifactorial genetic influence. Henseler and Christophers[25] studied a large population of patients with psoriasis in Germany and reported that patients with early-onset disease (less than 20 years) have an inheritable form that is more severe than the form occurring in patients over 40.

The earliest psoriatic lesion is an erythematous papule 2 to 5 mm in diameter surmounted by a fine scale. The lesion then enlarges to a more typical thick plaque with a silvery, micaceous scale (Fig. 9-14). Characteristically, the lesions of psoriasis remain sharply demarcated from the surrounding normal skin. As smaller lesions enlarge, they coalesce to form large plaques that may continue to grow in a centrifugal manner or form large geographic or gyrate configurations.

Although the disease may occur explosively, the onset is usually insidious, with the first lesions commonly localized to the scalp, elbows, and knees or at sites of trauma. There is no clear explanation why certain body areas are more prone to develop lesions, except that trauma may be a factor. The usual course is a series of exacerbations and remissions, with lesions varying in size and configuration from patient to patient and in the same patient from time to time.

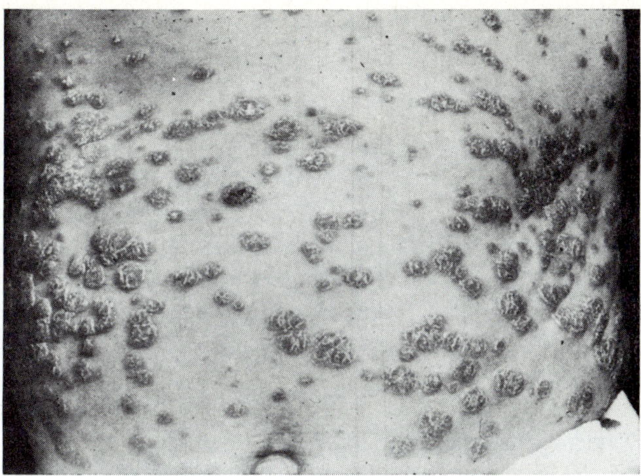

Figure 9-14 Photograph of psoriasis showing raised lesions of varying size covered with a white scale.

Epidermis and dermis both appear to be abnormal in psoriasis. Histologically there is thickening of the stratum corneum, with retention of nuclei (parakeratosis) and long, club-shaped rete (epidermal) ridges, which results in marked thickening (acanthosis) of the epidermis[26] (Fig. 9-15). The granular layer is decreased or absent, and collections of neutrophils are seen under the stratum corneum. The dermal papillae are elongated

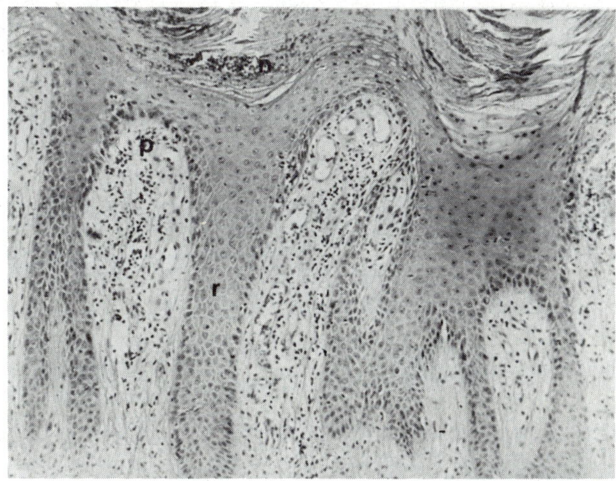

Figure 9-15 Histological section of a psoriatic plaque showing elongation of the epidermal ridges (r) and dermal papillae (p). There is parakeratosis and an accumulation of neutrophils (n) under the stratum corneum. ×60 in the original magnification.

and club-shaped distally. There is dilatation and tortuosity of the capillary loops. Although these changes are highly characteristic of psoriasis, they are not specific.

There is increased turnover of the epidermis, which results in the shedding of large amounts of scale[27]; studies have been performed in an attempt to quantitate these abnormalities. Experimental methods involved the use of ^{14}C-glycine as a protein label and tritiated thymidine as a DNA label for autoradiographic analysis. Serial biopsy specimens then display the outward progression of labeled cells in vivo. In normal skin initial labeling is confined to the basal cell layer and some suprabasal cells, whereas in psoriatic skin the lower three layers of cells are involved in active mitosis. The transit time through the viable layer in the hyperplastic, psoriatic epidermis is only 48 h compared with about 13 days in normal skin. Since psoriatic cells retain their nuclei in the horny layer (parakeratosis), the transit time can be followed through this cellular compartment as well. This too has been shown to be 48 h. Studies of transit time in normal stratum corneum indicate that it is 13 to 14 days. In summary, the turnover for the entire normal epidermis is 26 to 27 days, whereas in psoriatic epidermis it is 4 days.[28] Not only is the turnover time markedly shortened but the population of germinative cells is expanded.

A similar technique using tritiated thymidine has been employed to determine whether the cell cycle of individual germinative cells is faster in psoriatic than in normal epidermis. The duration of the germinative cell cycle in normal skin was calculated to be about 300 h and in psoriasis to be 37.5 h. Therefore, not only is the germinative cell population in psoriasis enlarged but the germinative cell cycle of the individual cell is about one-fourth as long as that of the normal epidermal cell.

Several investigators have challenged this evidence of shortening of the cell cycle.[29] They offer the alternative explanation that many epidermal cells in G_1 are inhibited and that in psoriatic lesions these resting cells are released and begin to divide, thus increasing the proliferative cell pool. Current evidence supports the shortened cell cycle in psoriasis but also invokes recruitment of normally resting cells into the actively dividing pool.

Biochemical studies that have tried to identify a chemical defect have shown that there is increased consumption of oxygen and glucose in psoriatic epidermis and that the oxidative pathways are increased to a greater extent than the anaerobic ones.[30] The enzymes of the glycolytic pathway, the hexose monophosphate shunt, and the Krebs cycle have all been shown to be markedly increased in activity, a fact that correlates with the overall increase in metabolic activity in the epidermal cell. Studies on lipid metabolism have shown that there is an increase in the total lipid and phospholipid content and in the ratio of free cholesterol to esterified cholesterol.

There is, in addition, an increase in DNA and RNA in the stratum corneum, which is probably a reflection of the retention of subcellular particles in the stratum corneum. The amount of breakdown products of nucleic acid is increased, as well as the amount of neutral soluble proteins, which also reflects retention of macromolecules.[31]

In psoriasis, variation in the expression of keratin polypeptides occurs in the epidermis. The most constant finding is a reduction in the 67- to 65-kd and 56.5-kd components and the appearance of the 48- and 56-kd ones. The latter two represent a pair of keratins associated with hyperproliferative keratinocytes. They are not specific for psoriasis but can also be observed in other diseases, including skin cancers.[32] The pattern of uninvolved psoriatic epidermis is normal, and the pattern of treated lesions also returns to normal. These findings are most consistent with an abnormality in the regulation of keratin gene expression.

Keratohyalin granules are generally reduced or absent histologically in psoriatic epidermis and reappear as the lesion goes into remission. Little or no staining was observed when psoriatic epidermis was studied by indirect immunofluorescence using an antibody to filaggrin. Histochemical staining for protein-bound histidine, in which keratohyalin is enriched, shows decreased amounts of the amino acid, and incorporation of labeled histidine is markedly reduced in psoriatic epidermis. These data suggest that the absence of granules reflects a decreased amount of the protein that is its major constituent. Electron-microscopic studies have shown that the morphology of the epidermis is disturbed. In particular, the normal keratin pattern (e.g., filaments embedded in a matrix) is not seen. An additional histological feature is a reduction in the thickness of the membrane that surrounds stratum corneum cells to half of its normal value of about 160 Å.

Cyclic nucleotides have been studied in the epidermis because they are known to be associated with regulation of cell turnover. Levels of cyclic AMP have been found to be normal, but cyclic GMP and the cyclic GMP/cyclic AMP ratio are elevated.[5] No specific abnormality has been demonstrated in the synthetic or degradative enzymes. Since similar changes in cyclic nucleotides have been associated with hyperplasia in other tissue, this may also be important in the epidermis. It has not been established whether this change is specific for psoriasis or occurs in other disorders that show epidermal hyperplasia.

Studies of arachidonic acid metabolism have found that levels of arachidonic acid, 12-L-hydroxy-5,8,10,14-eicosatetraenoic acid (HETE), and prostaglandin E_2 (PGE_2) are elevated in lesions of psoriasis compared with normal skin. Glucocorticoids, which are known to produce regression of psoriatic lesions, normalize the level of arachidonic acid and reduce the HETE concentration.[33] This appears to be the result of inhibition of phospholipase A, which converts phospholipids to arachidonic acid.

Levels of the polyamines putrescine, spermine, and spermidine are elevated in lesional epidermal tissue; these increases are associated with activation of ornithine decarboxylase activity. Elevated levels of polyamines in tissue have been associated with hyperplasia and with elevated levels of cyclic AMP. Although cyclic AMP is not elevated in whole epidermis, there may be areas in the epidermis (e.g., basal layer) where this elevation occurs. Studies on cultured epidermal cells suggest that elevated levels of cyclic AMP are associated with an increased rate of cell turnover.

A relationship exists in many tissues between the cyclic nucleotide, prostaglandin, and polyamine pathways. PGE_2 is known to activate adenyl cyclase and raise cyclic AMP, and this may also be true for HETE in the epidermis. Increased levels of cyclic AMP result in increased synthesis of polyamines, which leads to cellular hyperplasia. Whether this general scheme applies to psoriatic epidermis and what starts this cascade remain speculative for the present.

It is apparent that the pathogenesis of psoriasis is not entirely understood, but evidence points most strongly to a defect in regulation of epidermal turnover and differentiation. The multiple metabolic pathways in the epidermis must be highly coordinated so that the final product, the stratum corneum barrier, is precisely formed. It is not surprising that a perturbation in regulation could result in the disturbance of a number of macromolecular pathways, resulting in the multiple abnormalities that have been observed.

In this discussion the epidermis has been considered as an isolated tissue. However, this is clearly not the case, since dermal-epidermal interaction is critical to normal functioning of both tissues. It is conceivable that the primary defect lies in the dermis or even in the immune system of the body and that the epidermis is reacting to this defect. Indeed, fibroblasts from psoriatic skin have been shown to induce hyperplasia in normal epidermis using a synthetic dermis model.[34] Furthermore, abnormalities have been described in the blood vessels of psoriasis at both the structural and functional levels.[35] Abnormalities of the immune system are less well understood but may prove to be very important.[36] Recently it has been shown that cyclosporin given systematically can significantly ameliorate the disease.[37] One aspect of the disorder that appears to be explained in immunologic terms is the accumulation of neutrophilic polymorphonuclear leukocytes. It has been found that psoriatic plaques contain increased amounts of a serine proteinase that cleaves the fifth complement protein, yielding the chemotactic peptide C5a, which attracts neutrophils.[38] However, HETE and leukotriene B_4 may also play a role, since they are known to regulate neutrophil function.[39]

Finally, a list of potential components of the pathogenesis in some of which an abnormality has been described is given in Table 9-1. Many if not all of these represent secondary events, with the primary disturbance remaining unknown. There is a growing belief that this may be a defect in the signal-transduction system of the keratinocyte and that this defect is related in some way to the immune system.

Table 9-1

POSSIBLE COMPONENTS OF THE PATHOMECHANISM OF PSORIASIS

Cellular	Intercellular	Intracellular
Fibroblasts	Epidermal growth factor (EGF)	Phospholipase A_2
Keratinocytes	12-HETE, LTB_4	Guanylate cyclase-cGMP
Endothelial cells	Prostaglandins: PGE_2, $PGF_2\alpha$	Adenylate cyclase-cAMP
Granulocytes	Platelet activating factor (PAF)	Phospholipase C-DG/IP_3
Monocytes	Interleukins: IL-1	Tyrosine kinase
Dendritic cells	Interferons: IFN-α, IFN-γ	Calmodulin
T lymphocytes	Complement $C5_a$ des arg	Ornithine decarboxylase

Source: Modified from JD Bos.[36]

ICHTHYOSIS

There are several disorders associated with rather thick accumulation of stratum corneum. Ichthyosis vulgaris (dominant) and sex-linked ichthyosis are two disorders with fairly constant clinical features of this type.[40] The fish-like scales seen on the extensor surfaces of the extremities and trunk are responsible for the name (Fig. 9-16). These disorders start early in life and change very little with age. They usually improve in very warm, humid climates, apparently from loosening of the scales.

Histological examination of the skin in both disorders shows a stratum corneum that is thicker than normal but of normal structure. In ichthyosis vulgaris the granular layer is absent or markedly diminished (Fig. 9-17), while in sex-linked ichthyosis it is present in normal amounts.[41]

The fibrous proteins appear to be normal in both diseases, as are the results of cell kinetic studies. This fits with the fact that the patients do not shed excessive amounts of scale in spite of their thickened stratum corneum. No consistent abnormalities have been reported in the other subcellular organelles, such as membrane-coating granules and desmosomes.

The skin may return to a normal appearance following treatment with topical agents such as propylene glycol, α-hydroxy acids, and salicylic acid (called keratolytics) that cause separation of cells at the surface of the skin. A similar result occurs when patients are kept in a warm, humid environment for prolonged periods. These treatments cause a decrease in the

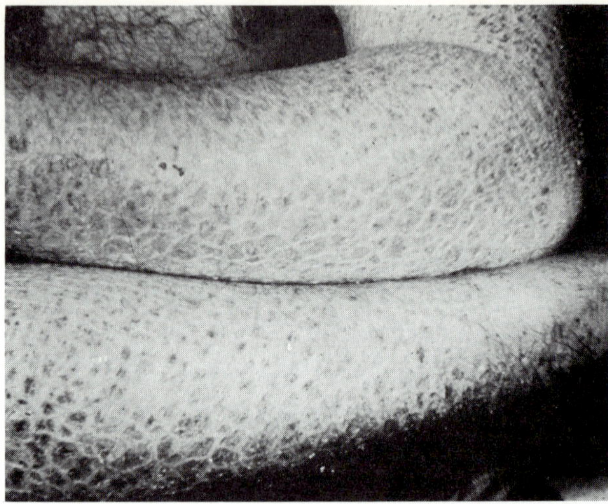

Figure 9-16 X-linked ichthyosis showing dark scales. [*From AEH Emory, DL Rimion (eds)*], *Principles and Practice of Medical Genetics, Edinburgh, Churchill Livingstone,* 1983, p 656.)

cohesive bonds between cells and allow separation of cells. The former method is more efficient because it may remove material from between cells, while hydration causes swelling of the tissue and makes mechanical separation easier. These findings have led to the hypothesis that the abnormality in these two types of ichthyosis is retention of stratum corneum

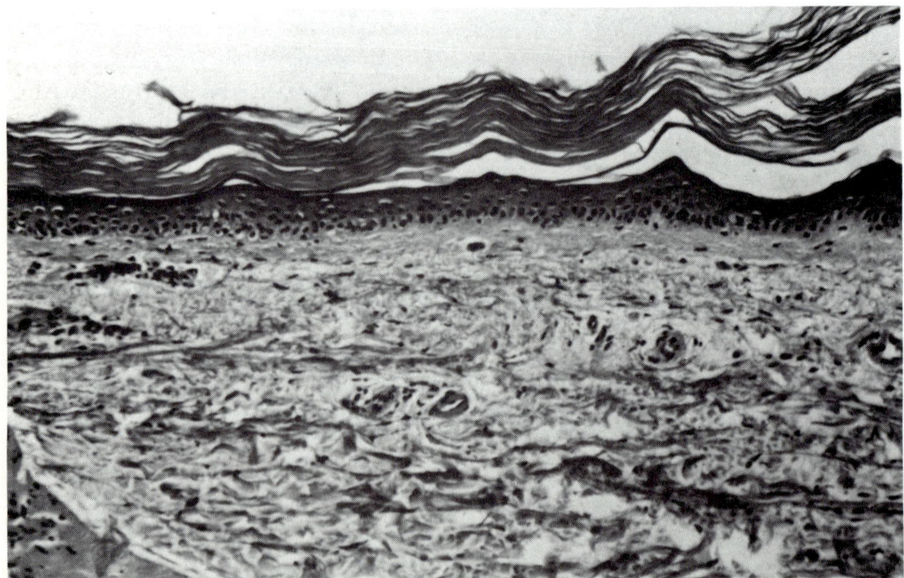

Figure 9-17 Photomicrograph of skin with ichthyosis vulgaris. There is no granular layer. ×100 in the original magnification.

as a result of a failure in the normal mechanism of cell separation. It is not known whether there is an accumulation of an excessive amount of an abnormal type of cementing substance or whether some specific enzyme-mediated lysis mechanism is malfunctioning. Since these two disorders have different modes of inheritance, different genes are involved and the abnormality may not be the same for both.

Recently a specific microsomal enzyme defect, steroid sulfatase (arylsulfatase C) deficiency, has been found in sex-linked ichthyosis[42–44] but not in other types of ichthyosis. This deficiency has been noted in cultured fibroblasts and epidermal cells of individuals with sex-linked ichthyosis. It has also been shown that cholesterol sulfate is present in increased amounts in the stratum corneum of patients with X-linked ichthyosis, presumably as a result of a sulfatase deficiency.[45] Ichthyosis-like changes have been observed with other abnormalities of lipid metabolism such as Refsum's disease, in which phytanic acid accumulates as a result of an absence of the enzyme α-phytanic acid α-hydroxylase involved in its catabolism.[46] In patients given large amounts of nicotinic acid or triparanol, chemicals that inhibit lipid synthesis, dryness and scaling similar to the appearance of ichthyosis develop.

It is not clear how different disorders of lipid metabolism could give rise to thickening of the stratum corneum, but it is known that lipids are deposited in the intercellular space as the stratum corneum develops. This material appears to function as a barrier as well as a cementing substance. It is not unreasonable to speculate that disturbances in the composition of this material might give rise to the abnormal adherence of stratum corneum cells.[47]

Numerous other hereditary and acquired disorders are associated with accumulation of stratum corneum, including another form of ichthyosis known as lamellar ichthyosis.[48] The response to various therapeutic modalities has been poor in many of these conditions, but the development of synthetic analogues of vitamin A, known as retinoids, appears to be an important therapeutic breakthrough.

Vitamin A is a fat-soluble isoprenoid with a six-membered cyclohexane ring and an 11-carbon side chain. The most common form of vitamin A in mammalian tissues and marine fish is an ester of *trans*-retinol. Carotenoids are precursors of vitamin A present in plants that are converted enzymatically to the vitamin in the intestinal wall. Retinyl esters are hydrolyzed in the intestinal lumen to retinol. This is reconverted in the mucosal cells to retinyl esters, which are transported via chylomicrons to the liver. The esters are hydrolyzed to retinol palmitate and stored in cellular membranes. When vitamin A is needed by peripheral tissue, the retinyl palmitate is hydrolyzed to retinol, bound to a specific carrier protein[49] (retinol-binding protein) in a 1:1 ratio, and secreted into the circulation, where this complex is bound to one molecule of prealbumin. This complex attaches to a specific surface receptor on a peripheral cell that releases retinol into the cell. The retinol then combines with another carrier protein, cytosol-retinol-binding protein (CRBP),[50] and then is transported to the cell nucleus.

Retinoic acid is absorbed into the portal circulation and carried by serum albumin and is not stored. There is a specific cytoplasmic-retinoic acid-binding protein that functions similarly to CRBP.[51]

The minimal daily requirement of vitamin A for adults is about 1000 units, and for children it is about 500 units (1 IU = 0.3 μg retinol).

Vitamin A deficiency is seen most commonly in chronic diseases affecting fat absorption but can also occur with chronic dietary inadequacy. About 15 percent of the U.S. population has concentrations in plasma below the accepted limits; most of these are black or Mexican-American infants and children.[52] The skin changes consist of dryness and follicular keratotic papules. Other changes include night blindness, xerosis of the eyes and bronchorespiratory tract leading to infection, and retarded growth and development. Hypervitaminosis A can result from chronic ingestion of excess retinol or acute ingestion of very high doses (in excess of 1 million units per day). Typical symptoms and signs are irritability, headache, desquamation of the skin, bone pain, hair loss, and hepatomegaly.

The biochemical basis for the actions of vitamin A has been under intensive investigation, especially with renewed interest in vitamin A analogues as therapeutic agents. The finding of cytosol-binding proteins suggests an effect similar to that of the hormones; that is, vitamin A may act at the transcription level to control synthesis of specific proteins. Vitamin A has also been shown to influence translation through an effect on tRNA. It has been shown that vitamin A is involved in the glycosylation of proteins, and a mannosyl retinyl phosphate intermediate has been identified that can donate mannose groups to protein.[53] Furthermore, the vitamin can control the biosynthesis of glycosaminoglycans. Labilization of lysosomes is readily demonstrated in cultured chick tissue, particularly in bone.

Retinol and retinal can be interconverted in the body, and both can be converted to retinoic acid, but the latter pathway is irreversible. Retinol, retinal, and retinoic acid can correct abnormalities of growth and development in deficient animals, but only the former two can correct the visual and fertility problems. The action of vitamin A in the visual cycle has been well described and will not be reviewed.

Vitamin A supplementation had been used to treat a variety of cutaneous diseases but fell into disuse because of lack of rigorous proof of efficacy and concern about toxicity. Two analogues have become available for clinical use that appear to be efficacious without producing serious toxicity, particularly with respect to the liver and central nervous system (Fig. 9-18). The *cis* isomer has been used primarily in this country for diseases characterized by hyperkeratoses and has resulted in marked shedding of thickened stratum corneum.[54] Inflammatory components of the diseases are only modestly improved. The drug appears to act by reducing the

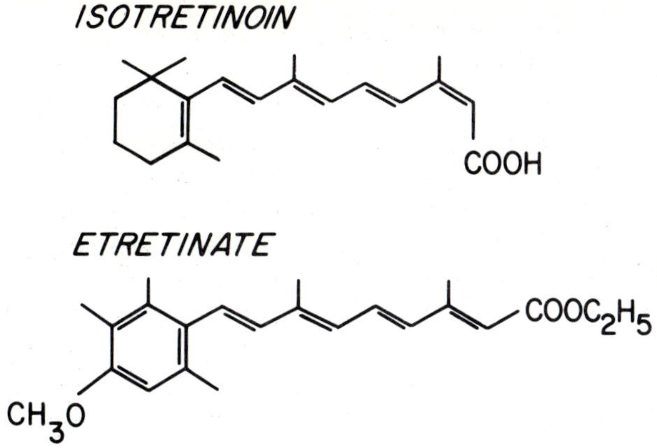

ISOTRETINOIN

COOH

ETRETINATE

$COOC_2H_5$

CH_3O

Figure 9-18 Structure of retinoids.

cohesiveness of stratum corneum cells. Levels of lysosomal enzymes in lesions of treated patients have not been elevated, indicating that the vitamin does not work by a hydrolytic mechanism. It has been suggested that the vitamin might work by modification of glycoproteins that are known to be present on cell surfaces, but this has not yet been studied in depth.

The loss of cohesion of epidermal cells also has been reproduced in vitro by exposing epidermal cell cultures to retinoids during the growth phase.[55] The dose used was 1 μg/ml of *trans*-retinoic acid, which is not toxic to the cells but results in increased shedding of cells. Electron micrographs of cultures show fewer cell layers and wider spaces between cells, with many microvilli on the surface of the cell. Although increased numbers of lysosomes are observed, the amount of lysosomal enzymes is not increased. These effects are also observed with retinol and *cis*-retinoic acid.

Another change observed in cultured cells is an increase in the amount of neutral soluble protein and a decrease in the amount of cross-linked fibrous keratins. A decreased number of desmosomes was not appreciated in culture but has been reported in vivo.

It thus appears that a major effect of retinoids is to decrease the attachment of cornified cells. It should be kept in mind that this is found with pharmacologic doses of retinoids and may be an exaggeration of a normal action of the vitamin or an entirely different toxic action, for example, on the cell membranes.

Etretinate, a new synthetic retinoid, appears to have an additional effect when used in psoriasis. Some patients have complete clearing of the lesions, with disappearance of redness as well as loss of scales. Histological examination of lesions during treatment shows toxic effects on the epidermal cells initially, and there may be a greater inhibition of cell turnover than is observed with the other retinoids.

EPIDERMOLYSIS BULLOSA

Epidermolysis bullosa simplex (Fig. 9-19) is a dominantly inherited disorder associated with blistering of the skin in areas of mechanical trauma.[56] There are several genetic variants. The generalized type appears at birth or shortly afterward, while the local type appears later. Blistering is usually worse in the summer months. The condition improves, at least in the generalized type, with age. Scarring ordinarily is not a feature of the disease, and nails, hair, mucous membranes, and teeth are usually unaffected. Secondary infection with bacterial pathogens is common, particularly in childhood.

Histological examination of the skin shows cytolysis of basal or suprabasal cells (Fig. 9-20). By electron microscopy this change first appears in the perinuclear region and proceeds to the periphery of the cell. Clumping of the tonofilaments has been observed, but lysis of desmosomes with associated rounding up of cells and separation from one another (acantholysis) has not.

The pathogenesis of the disorder has not been elucidated, but several mechanisms have been considered. The stability of the helical structure of the fibrous protein has been investigated by doing isometric contraction studies of blister tops while heating the tissue in water. This technique determines the temperature at which the α helix unfolds and a cross-β-folded structure forms. This was found to be between 82 and 85°C, the same as for normal tissue.

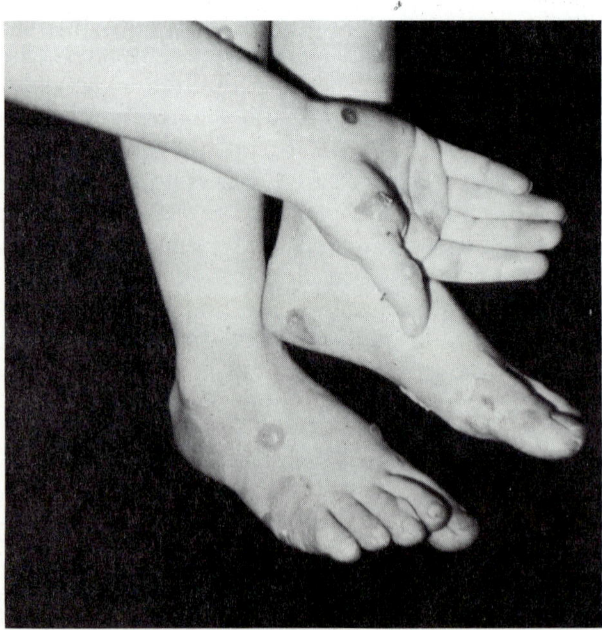

Figure 9-19 Dominant epidermolysis bullosa simplex.

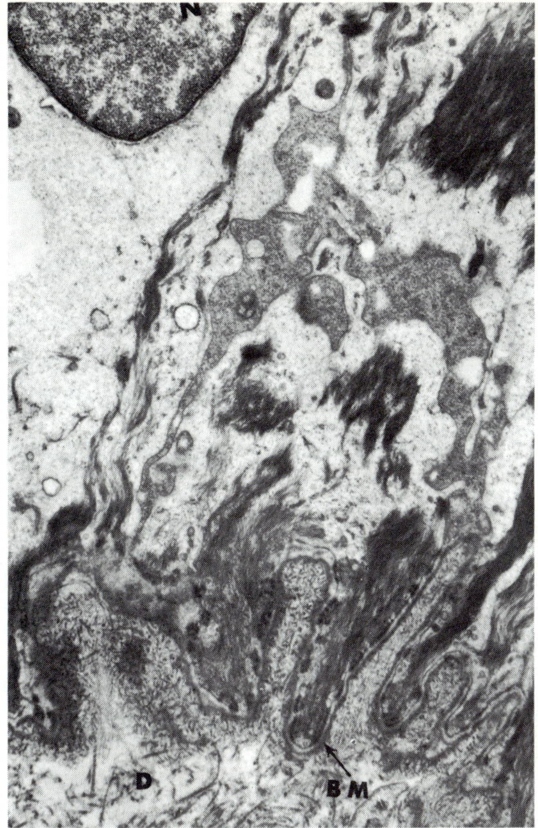

Figure 9-20 Histological section of an early blister from dominant epidermolysis bullosa simplex. Cytolysis of the cells is present. The basement membrane (BM) and dermis (D) are intact. [*From TB Fitzpatrick et al (eds), Dermatology in General Medicine, 3d ed, New York, McGraw-Hill, 1987, p 614.*]

It has been postulated that there is release of lysosomal enzymes into the cytoplasm of the epidermal cell in response to trauma and that this explains the cytolysis that is observed. It should be possible to test this hypothesis for the disease by injuring cultured epidermal cells and testing the effect of specific inhibitors of lysosomal enzymes on subsequent damage to the cells.

The increased severity of the disease in warm weather has several possible explanations. There may be a temperature-sensitive subcellular component in the cell that starts a cascade of events that, again, could be lysosomal in origin. A more likely explanation is that the surface of the skin is more moist in warm weather, which causes swelling of the stratum corneum. This swelling exaggerates irregularities on the skin surface, increasing its frictional properties. This is particularly noticeable on the acral regions of the extremities.

REFERENCES

1. Menton DN, Eisen AZ: Structure and organization of mammalian stratum corneum. *Ultrastruct Res* 35:247, 1981.
2. Schering LE: Mitotic activity in human epidermis. *Anat Res* 135:7, 1959.
3. Bullough WS, Rytomaa T: Mitotic hemostasis. *Nature* 205:573, 1965.
4. Cohen S, Elliot GA: The stimulation of epidermal keratinization by a protein isolated from the submaxillary gland of the mouse. *J Invest Dermatol* 40:1, 1963.
5. Marcelo CL, Voorhees JJ: Cyclic nucleotides, prostaglandins and polyamines in psoriasis. *Pharmacol Ther* 9:297, 1980.
6. Steinert PM, Roop DR: Molecular and cellular biology of intermediate filaments. *Annu Rev Biochem* 57:593, 1988.
7. Sun T-T et al: Monoclonal antibody studies of mammalian epithelial keratins: a review. *Ann NY Acad Sci* 455:307, 1985.
8. Gilmartin ME et al: Phosphorylation of epidermal keratins. *J Invest Dermatol* 75:211, 1980.
9. Abernathy JL et al: The ϵ-(γ-glutamyl) lysine cross-links in human stratum corneum. *J Biol Chem* 252:1837, 1977.
10. Kubilus J et al: The presence of citrulline in epidermal proteins. *Biochim Biophys Acta* 581:114, 1979.
11. Steinberg MS et al: On the molecular organization, diversity and functions of desmosomal proteins, in G Bock, S Clark (eds), *Junctional Complexes of Epithelial Cells.* New York, Wiley, 1987, p 3.
12. Fukuyama K et al: Dense homogeneous deposits of keratohyalin granules in newborn rat epidermis. *J Ultrastruct Res* 38:16, 1972
13. Sybert VP et al: Ichthyosis vulgaris: identification of a defect in synthesis of filaggrin correlated with an absence of keratohyalin granules. *J Invest Dermatol* 84:191, 1985.
14. Dale BA et al: Assembly of stratum corneum basic protein and keratin filaments in macrofibrils. *Nature* 276:729, 1978.
15. Matoltsy AG, Matoltsy MN: The membrane protein of horny cells. *J Invest Dermatol* 46:127, 1966.
16. Baden HP et al: Characterization of monoclonal antibodies generated to the cornified envelope of human cultured keratinocytes. *J Invest Dermatol* 89:454, 1987.
17. Rice RH, Green H: Presence in human epidermal cells of a soluble protein precursor of the cross-linked envelope: activation of the cross-linking by calcium ions. *Cell* 18:681, 1979.
18. Ma AS-P, Sun T-T: Differentiation-dependent changes in the solubility of a 195 kD protein in human epidermal keratinocytes. *J Cell Biol* 103:41, 1986.
19. Thacher SM, Rice RH: Keratinocyte-specific transglutaminase of cultured human epidermal cells: relation of cross-linked envelope formation and terminal differentiation. *Cell* 40:685, 1985.
20. Elias PM: Epidermal lipids, membranes and keratinization. *Int J Dermatol* 20:1, 1981.
21. Kupper TS: Production of cytokines by epithelial tissues. *Am J Dermatopathol* 111:69, 1989.
22. Watt FM: Keratinocyte cultures: an experimental model for studying how proliferation and terminal differentiation are co-ordinated in the epidermis. *J Cell Sci* 90:525, 1988.
23. Murray C et al: Histocompatibility alloantigens in psoriasis and psoriatic arthritis. *J Clin Invest* 66:670, 1980.
24. Russel JT et al: Histocompatibility (HL-A) antigens associated with psoriasis. *N Engl J Med* 287:738, 1972.
25. Henseler T, Christophers E: Psoriasis of early and late onset: characterization of two types of psoriasis vulgaris. *J Am Acad Dermatol* 13:450, 1985.
26. Lever WF, Schaumburg-Lever G: Psoriasis, in *Histopathology of the Skin,* 7th ed. Philadelphia, Lippincott, 1990, p 156.
27. Weinstein GD, Frost P: Abnormal cell proliferation in psoriasis. *J Invest Dermatol* 50:254, 1968.
28. Weinstein GD et al: Cell proliferation in normal epidermis. *J Invest Dermatol* 82:623, 1984.

29. Gelfant S: The cell cycle in psoriasis: a reappraisal. *Br J Dermatol* 95:577, 1970.
30. Halprin KM, Ohkawara A: Carbohydrate metabolism in psoriasis: an enzymatic study. *J Invest Dermatol* 46:51, 1966.
31. Flesch P et al: Water-soluble organic components of psoriatic scales. *Arch Dermatol* 86:476, 1962.
32. Weiss RA et al: Monoclonal antibody analysis of keratin expression in epidermal diseases: a 48- and 56-kdalton keratin as molecular markers for hyperproliferative keratinocytes. *J Cell Biol* 98:1397, 1984.
33. Hammarstrom S et al: Glucocorticoids in inflammatory proliferative skin disease reduces arachidonic and hydroxyeicosatetraenoic acids. *Science* 197:994, 1977.
34. Saiag P et al: Psoriatic fibroblasts induce hyperproliferation of normal keratinocytes in a skin equivalent model in vitro. *Science* 230:669, 1985.
35. Ryan TJ: Microcirculation in psoriasis: blood vessels, lymphatics and tissue fluid. *Pharmacol Ther* 10:27, 1980.
36. Bos JD: The pathomechanisms of psoriasis; the skin immune system and cyclosporin. *Br J Dermatol* 118:141, 1988.
37. Ellis CN et al: Cyclosporine improves psoriasis in a double-blind study. *JAMA* 256:3110, 1986.
38. Lazarus G et al: Polymorphonuclear leukocytes: possible mechanism of accumulation in psoriasis. *Science* 198:1162, 1987.
39. Goetzl EJ: Mediators of immediate hypersensitivity derived from arachidonic acid. *N Engl J Med* 303:822, 1980.
40. Wells RS, Kerr CB: Clinical features of autosomal dominant and sex linked ichthyosis in an English population. *Br Med J* 1:947, 1966.
41. Feinstein A et al: Histology of autosomal dominant ichthyosis vulgaris and x-linked ichthyosis. *Arch Dermatol* 101:524, 1970.
42. Shapiro LJ et al: X-linked ichthyosis due to steroid-sulphatase deficiency. *Lancet* 1:70, 1978.
43. Shapiro LF et al: Enzymatic basis of typical x-linked ichthyosis. *Lancet* 2:756, 1978.
44. Kubilus J et al: Steroid-sulfatase deficiency in sex linked ichthyosis. *Am J Hum Genet* 31:50, 1979.
45. Williams ML, Elias PM: Stratum corneum lipids in disorders of cornification. I. Increased sulfate cholesterol content of stratum corneum in recessive x-linked ichthyosis. *J Clin Invest* 68:1404, 1981.
46. Klenk E, Kahlke W: Uber das Vorkommen der 3,7,11,15-Tetramethyl-hexadecansaure (Phytansaure) in den Cholesterinestern und anderen Lipoidfraktionen der Organe bei einem Krankheitsfall unbekannter genese (Verdacht auf Heredopathia atactica polyneuritiformis [Refsum-syndrom]). *Hoppe-Seyler's Z Physiol Chem* 333:133, 1963.
47. Rehfeld SJ et al: Calorimetric and electron skin resonance examination of lipid phase transitions in human stratum corneum: molecular basis for normal cohesion and abnormal desquamation in recessive x-linked ichthyosis. *J Invest Dermatol* 91:499, 1988.
48. Bernhardt MC, Baden HP: Report of a family with an unusual expression of recessive ichthyosis and review of 42 cases. *Arch Dermatol* 122:428, 1986.
49. Goodman DE: Vitamin A transport and delivery and the mechanism of vitamin A toxicity, in CE Orfanos et al (eds), *Retinoids. Advances in Basic Research and Therapy*. Berlin, Springer-Verlag, 1981, p 31.
50. Sani BP: Localization of retinoic acid-binding protein in nuclei. *Biochem Biophys Res Commun* 75:7, 1977.
51. Ong, DE, Chytil F: Presence of cellular retinol and retinoic acid binding proteins in experimental tumors. *Cancer Lett* 2:25, 1976.
52. Roels OA: Vitamin A physiology. *JAMA* 214:1097, 1970.
53. Quill H, Wolf G: Formation of α-1,2- and α-1,3-linked mannose disaccharides from mannosy retinyl phosphate by rat liver membrane enzymes, in *Modulation of Cellular Interactions by Vitamin A and Derivatives (Retinoids). Ann NY Acad Sci* 359:331, 1981.

54. Elias PM: Epidermal effects of retinoids: supramolecular observations and clinical implications. *J Am Acad Dermatol* 15:797, 1986.
55. Kubilus J et al: Effects of retinoic acid and other retinoids on the growth and differentiation of 3T3 supported human keratinocytes. *In Vitro* 17:786, 1981.
56. Cooper TW et al: The mechanobullous diseases (epidermolysis bullosa), in TB Fitzpatrick et al (eds), *Dermatology in General Medicine*, 3d ed. New York, McGraw-Hill, 1987, p 610.

10

Pathophysiology of Allergic Contact Dermatitis

Donald V. Belsito

Allergic reactions can be broadly divided into B-cell (antibody)- and T-cell (cell)-mediated types. As classified by Coombs and Gell, allergic contact dermatitis represents a type IV cell-mediated reaction, as do delayed-type hypersensitivity to microbial antigens, certain homograft reactions, and some autoimmune diseases. Clinically, allergic contact dermatitis has a variety of appearances, depending upon its duration. Acutely, the eruption is characterized by macular erythema and papules or vesicles, depending on the intensity of the allergic response. Chronically, the condition presents as a lichenified, scaling, occasionally fissured dermatitis, with or without accompanying vesicles. Although the geographic distribution of an eruption might suggest that it is due to a contactant (Fig. 10-1), neither the morphology nor the histopathology (Fig. 10-2) is distinctive. The clinicopathologic differential diagnosis of allergic contact dermatitis includes irritant contact, atopic, nummular, seborrheic, and dyshidrotic dermatitides, among others. In cases of widespread exposure (e.g., from clothing or from airborne or ingested allergens), the disease can present as an erythroderma. Certain features, such as sparing of the axillary vault in textile dermatitis or relative sparing of clothed areas in airborne dermatitis, can give clues to the nature of the disorder. However, only a strong clinical suspicion and judicious use of patch tests will result in appropriate diagnosis and treatment of allergic contact dermatitis.

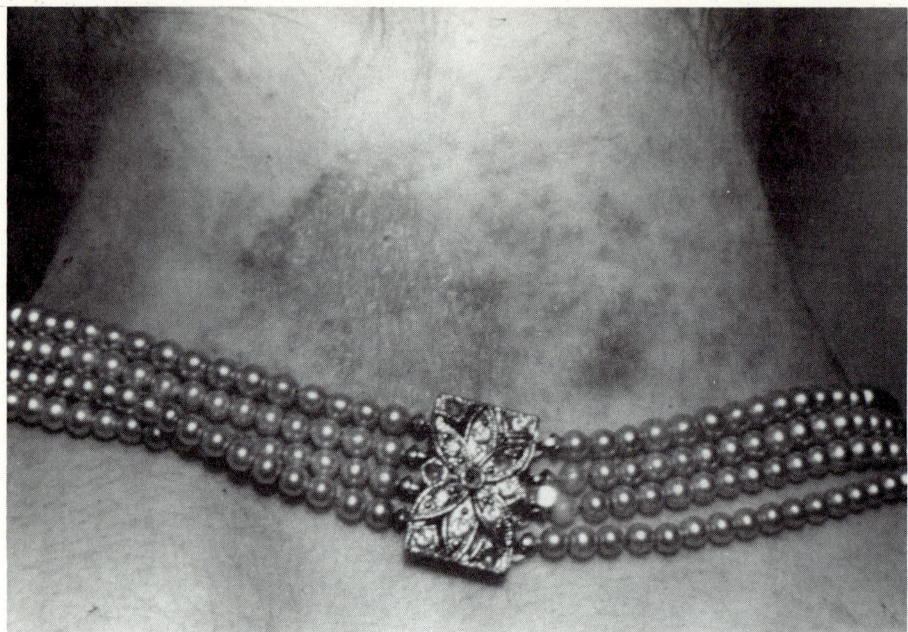

Figure 10-1 Subacute to chronic allergic contact dermatitis to nickel. For several months, the patient had this pruritic, erythematous, papulovesicular eruption, which soon coalesced into plaques over the posterior neck, as well as the earlobes. Patch tests revealed a strong positive reaction to nickel sulfate (2.5% in petrolatum). Nickel is ubiquitous in the environment and is a common sensitizer. This patient was exposed to the allergen present in her jewelry.

THE ALLERGENS

Most environmental contact allergens, which number more than 2800, are haptens, i.e., simple chemicals that must link to proteins to form a complete antigen before they can sensitize.[1] Most haptens are low molecular weight (less than 500 kd), electrophilic molecules that bind to carrier proteins via covalent bonding.[2] The major exception to such covalent bonding occurs among the metallic salts (nickel, cobalt, etc.). Although linkage to protein is critical in transforming a hapten to an allergen, it is not the only requirement for allergenicity, since not all electrophilic, protein-binding substances are haptens.[3] The nature of the antigenic determinants, the type of binding that the hapten forms with the carrier, the final three-dimensional configuration of the conjugate, and a host of unknown factors contribute to the allergenicity of a given chemical.[4] As of 1984–1985, the most frequent contact allergens in the United States included nickel, *p*-phenylenediamine, quaternium-15, neomycin, thimerosal, formaldehyde, cinnamic aldehyde, ethylenediamine, potassium dichromate, and thiurams.[5]

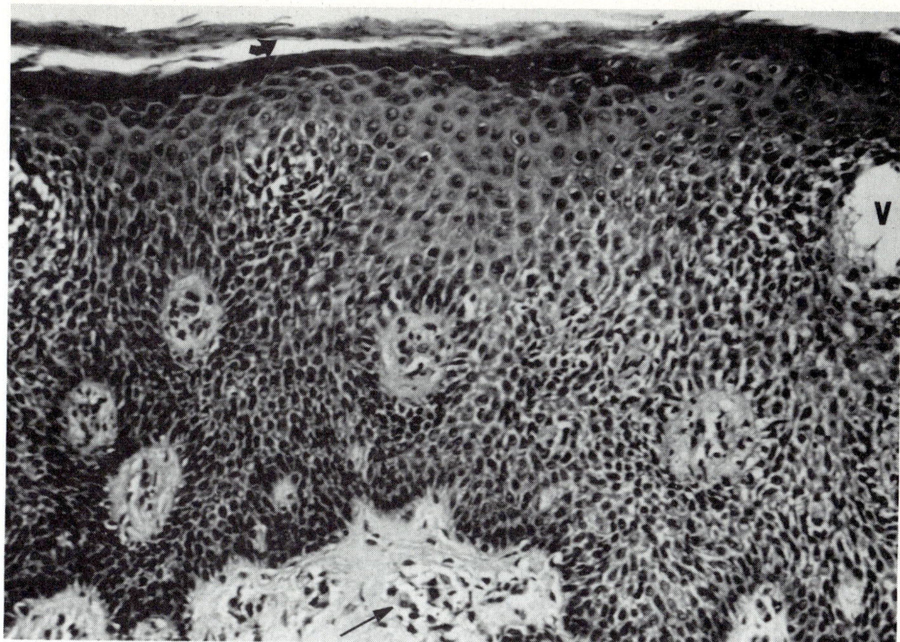

Figure 10-2 Histopathology of subacute allergic contact dermatitis. A biopsy specimen of the rash pictured in Fig. 10-1 shows epidermal intercellular edema and microvesiculation (v), which are characteristic of an allergic response, as well as other eczematous dermatitides. The superficial perivascular infiltrate (→) consists of lymphocytes, macrophages, and, occasionally, eosinophils. The parakeratotic stratum corneum (➔) is indicative of the subacute to chronic nature of this eruption. (Hematoxylin-eosin; ×330 in the original magnification.)

PATHOPHYSIOLOGY

Type IV reactions are marked by an afferent (antigen recognition) and an efferent (response) phase. During the afferent phase, the allergen is "processed" and presented to T cells by the Langerhans cell, the antigen-presenting cell of the skin. Whether this occurs in the skin (peripheral presentation) or in the paracortical (thymus-dependent) areas of the draining lymph nodes (central presentation) is a matter of continued controversy (reviewed in Ref. 6).

Langerhans cells are bone marrow–derived dendritic cells situated within the suprabasilar layer of the epidermis. Under resting conditions, they are the only epidermal cells that express class II (HLA-DR) antigens on their surface.[7] Once it has contacted the antigen, the Langerhans cell must process it. Because of its limited ability to phagocytose, antigen processing by the Langerhans cell is thought to involve ingestion by endocytosis and nonlysosomal degradation of the antigen followed by recycling of antigenic peptides bound to HLA-DR onto the cell surface.[8] Whether keratinocytes cooperate in antigen processing is unknown.

Within 2 to 4 h after stimulation by antigen, migration of Langerhans cells into lymphatic vessels is evident[9]; by 18 to 24 h, antigen-bearing Langerhans cells, capable of transferring sensitization, are found in large numbers in the lymph node.[10] In order for an allergic response to occur, Langerhans cells must process the antigen and present it to CD4+ T cells (T helper cells) with receptors specific for class II antigen and the contact allergen (Fig. 10-3). The antigen-specific receptor on T cells consists of CD3, a transducing protein found on all T cells, coupled with Ti, a heterodimeric protein whose variable regions act as the specific antigen binding site.[11] The reaction of allergic contact dermatitis is also "restricted" by the major histocompatibility complex in that the contact allergen must be presented in the presence of HLA-DR molecules on the antigen-presenting cell.[12] In addition to the CD3–Ti complex, CD4 antigen on T cells acts as an additional recognition site for HLA-DR on antigen-presenting cells.

As Langerhans cells interact with CD3–Ti+, CD4+ lymphocytes, interleukin-1 (IL-1) is synthesized and released by Langerhans cells.[13] IL-1 enhances the immunologic function of the antigen-presenting cell in part by up-regulating class II (HLA-DR) antigen expression on Langerhans cells.[14] Its

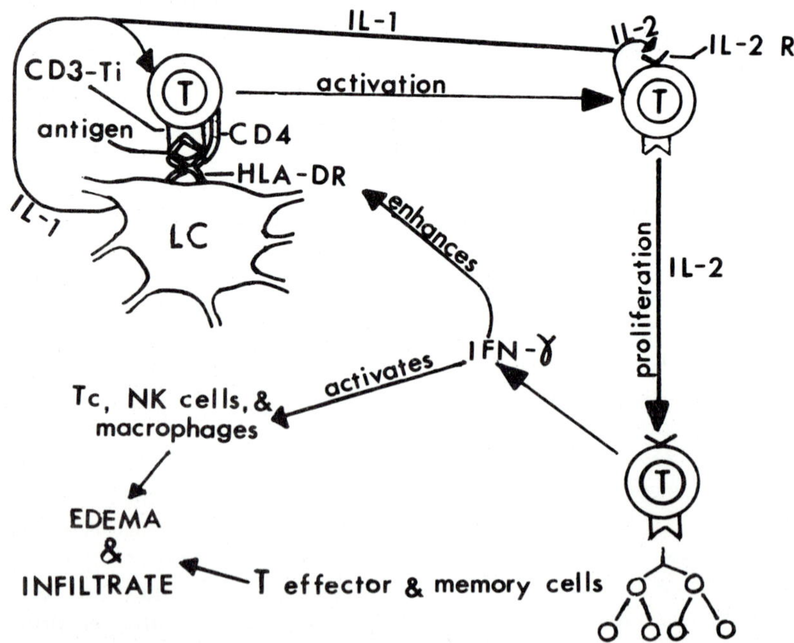

Figure 10-3 An overview of the mechanism of allergic contact dermatitis. See text for details. Antigen (△); CD3-Ti (⌴) = antigen recognition site; CD4 (⅃) = a recognition site for HLA-DR; HLA-DR (⋈) = class II antigen; IFN-γ = interferon-γ; IL-1 = interleukin 1; IL-2 = interleukin-2; IL-2R = IL-2 receptor; LC = Langerhans cells; NK = natural killer cells; T = T cells; Tc = cytotoxic T cells. (*From Belsito DV[6] with permission.*)

primary function, however, is to activate T cells to produce and secrete interleukin-2 (IL-2) and interferon-γ (IFN-γ). Together with IL-1, IL-2 induces its own receptor (IL-2 R) on T cells. Although IL-2 is a product of specifically sensitized $CD4^+$ T cells, it acts nonspecifically to stimulate $CD4^+$ and $CD8^+$ T cells (T suppressor/cytotoxic cells) with and without specific antigen receptors, causing them to proliferate and to secrete IFN-γ.[15] Thus, the final response to a contact allergen is polyclonal and nonspecific; however, the $CD3–Ti^+$, $CD4^+$ T cells do serve to localize the response to the site of challenge via their production of IL-2 and IFN-γ. It is IFN-γ, in conjunction with IL-2, that activates cytotoxic T cells, natural killer (NK) cells, and macrophages.[16] These cells, along with their soluble mediators, eventuate in the epidermal edema (spongiosis) and dermal infiltrate that, although not diagnostic, are characteristic of allergic contact dermatitis. Like IL-1, IFN-γ augments expression of HLA-DR on the antigen-presenting cell,[14] which, at least in vitro, improves its antigen-presenting function.[17]

In addition to its known role in allergic contact dermatitis, IFN-γ induces the production of tumor necrosis factor (TNF) by monocytes.[18] TNF is a cytokine that produces necrosis of selected tumor lines and prevents uptake and storage of triglyceride; therefore, it is also called *cachectin*. What role it might play in allergic contact dermatitis is presently unknown. However, given TNF's known tropism for the skin[19] and its ability to enhance antigen-induced T-cell proliferation,[20] it will likely be shown to contribute, along with other cellular mediators, to the final pathological changes seen. Keratinocyte-derived cytokines may also participate in the immune response. Epidermal thymocyte-activating factor (ETAF) and IL-1 appear to be identical molecules. Although ETAF can induce T cells to produce IL-2 in vitro,[21] it is unclear whether it does so during the in vivo immune response. Keratinocyte-derived T-cell growth factor (KTGF) has some in vitro properties similar to those of IL-2[22]; whether in vivo it stimulates the $CD3–Ti^+$, $CD4^+$ T cell to secrete IFN-γ and whether it has any role in T cell–mediated immunity is not known. Finally, IL-6 may play a role in the immunologic response. Both IL-1 and TNF induce IL-6,[23] a product of a variety of cell types including keratinocytes. IL-6 is known to up-regulate class II antigen on Langerhans cells[14] and to function as a second signal for IL-2 production by mature T cells.[24]

Several studies have indicated that mast cells are activated during allergic contact dermatitis, most likely by a T cell–derived antigen-binding factor.[25] In mice, this factor has been shown to cause mast cell release of serotonin within 2 h after antigenic challenge and to result in antigen-specific swelling of challenged ears at 2 h.[25] Pharmacologic blockade of serotonin prevents not only this early phase of the response but also the delayed (24 to 48 h) reaction.[26] In addition, other investigators have noted a triphasic cutaneous allergic response in mice with peaks at 1.5, 8, and 24 h following antigenic challenge, which was associated with elevation of serum histamine levels at 1 to 4, 12, and 48 h.[27] If, as suggested,[25–27] vasoactive amines are important regulators of allergic contact dermatitis via their induction of endothelial gaps that permit the ingress or egress of effector cells, the first two peaks at 1 to 4 and 12 h would be most relevant, since they correspond more closely to the appearance of the cellular infiltrate, which begins as early as 2 to 4 h and peaks at 24 h.[27] The presence of a third peak of histamine at 48 h,[27] a time of decreased responsiveness, suggests that histamine, which is known to exert a stimulatory effect on $CD8^+$ T lymphocytes,[28] may be involved in down-regulating the reaction in the later stages.

Basophils may play a similar role in down-regulating sensitivity. In humans, 5 to 15 percent of the infiltrating cells in certain contact allergic reactions are basophils, which constitute such a large proportion of the infiltrate only as the reaction is waning.[29] Additional work is needed to clarify the role, if any, of the basophil in regulating allergic contact dermatitis, since a phenomenon termed *cutaneous basophil hypersensitivity* or the *Jones-Mote reaction* occurs concomitantly with allergic contact dermatitis and has thus far confused the matter.[30]

Macrophages may also play a role in turning off the immune response. In response to stimulation by IFN-γ, macrophages produce prostaglandins, especially of the E series.[31] Both prostaglandin E_1 and prostaglandin E_2 inhibit production of IL-2 and expression of the IL-2R.[32] The E series prostaglandins have also been shown to inhibit NK cell activation via their inhibition of IL-2.[33] Thus, soluble mediators such as histamine or prostaglandins, which are responsible for eliciting the reaction, also play an active role in dampening the response. In addition, desquamation of antigen-laden skin, cellular or enzymatic degradation of antigen with destruction of the antigen-presenting cell, and other presently unknown regulatory mechanisms contribute to the resolution of the allergic response.

INFLUENCE OF AGE, GENDER, AND GENETIC INHERITANCE ON ALLERGIC CONTACT DERMATITIS

Clinically, aged individuals have been shown to have various defects in the induction and/or elicitation of allergic contact dermatitis. The precise reason for this decline in contact sensitivity is unknown. Age-related defects involving various participants of the cell-mediated response have been described (reviewed in Ref. 34). Experiments in which contact-sensitized, aged mice injected with naive, young T cells demonstrated normal responses upon antigenic challenge suggest that a failure of T-cell amplification signals and generation of sufficient T effector cells may be the primary deficiencies in aged animals.[35]

The competency of T cell–mediated immune reactions in children is controversial. Patch testing of children with standard concentrations of allergens has reportedly resulted in a high percentage of irritant reactions.[36] Documented allergic reactions are mostly seen in older pediatric patients and are secondary to topical medications or plants. As suggested by Straus, who was able to sensitize 35 of 48 infants (1 to 4 days old) to *Rhus* oleoresin,[37] the apparent hyporesponsiveness of infancy may be due to limited exposure and not to deficient immunity. Similarly, the effects of gender on the incidence of allergic contact hypersensitivity are related to the likelihood of exposure.[38]

Although animal studies have shown strain (presumably genetic) variation in cell-mediated immunity, the evidence of a genetic influence in humans has been slight. Skog found that 5 percent of a defined population could not be sensitized to dinitrochlorobenzene and suggested that this was due to inheritance.[39] In another study, significant genetic association with the capacity to become sensitized to *para*-nitrosodimethylaniline was reported.[40] However, many attempts to correlate human leukocyte antigen haplotype with nickel sensitivity[41] or other allergies[42] have shown no association. Thus, definitive evidence of class II–related influences on allergic contact hypersensitivity in humans is circumstantial at best, perhaps because of our diverse genetic pool.

THERAPEUTIC CONSIDERATIONS

The primary goal in treating allergic contact dermatitis is identification of the offending allergen via patch testing and removal of this substance from the patient's environment. Certain allergens, such as *Rhus* oleoresin and gold, appear to persist locally in the skin for weeks to months following exposure. In these and other similar situations, treatment with physicochemical agents that down-regulate responsiveness may be required. Clinically, glucocorticoids and ultraviolet radiation (ultraviolet B, UVB or psoralens plus ultraviolet A, PUVA) are the agents most widely used.

Glucocorticoids inhibit type IV reactions at multiple points (reviewed in Ref. 6). HLA-DR$^+$ Langerhans cell numbers are decreased, the production and function of IL-1, IL-2, and IFN-γ are inhibited, and T-cell proliferation is decreased. Glucocorticoids are not, however, cytolytic for the T effector cells of allergic contact dermatitis in humans; steroid-induced lymphopenia results primarily from alterations in the trafficking of lymphocytes. Furthermore, under the influence of the products of activated macrophages, CD4$^+$ T cells are resistant to the effects of glucocorticoids. This resistance of CD4$^+$ T cells notwithstanding, corticosteroids effectively inhibit every major aspect of cell-mediated immunity, and they remain a mainstay in the treatment of allergic contact dermatitis.

Like corticosteroids, both UVB and PUVA block induction and elicitation of allergic contact dermatitis in numerous ways (reviewed in Ref. 6). This multifocal blockade of allergic contact dermatitis by phototherapy has been clinically useful in the treatment of occupationally related contact allergy in workers unable or unwilling to change employment.[43,44] Both UVB and PUVA are known to decrease the density of HLA-DR$^+$ epidermal Langerhans cells significantly and to induce epidermal hyperplasia, making it more difficult for the antigen to reach any remaining suprabasilar HLA-DR$^+$ antigen-presenting cells. Furthermore, UVB may alter responsiveness via its induction of keratinocyte-derived prostaglandin E, which has been shown to inhibit the function of IL-2 and NK cells. PUVA blocks lymphocyte proliferation, probably by similar mechanisms. By means of a prostaglandin-induced efferent blockade of the draining lymph node, UVB has also been shown to inhibit lymphocytic trafficking. As a result of this blockade, it is less likely that antigen-bearing Langerhans cells will contact a sensitized lymphocyte in the periphery. Finally, the elevation of prostaglandin E levels may up-regulate suppressor cell function. Curiously, UVB has been shown to enhance levels of soluble IL-1, although this enhancement appears to be counteracted by a UVB-induced epidermal cell-derived inhibitor of IL-1 activity.

In addition to specific immunotherapy, treatment of allergic contact dermatitis should be directed to amelioration of symptoms. Acute, vesicular, weeping eruptions benefit from drying agents such as topical aluminum sulfate/calcium acetate; chronic, lichenfied eruptions are best treated with emollients. Pruritus can be controlled with topical antipruritics or oral antihistamines; topical antihistamines are best avoided given the risk of inducing a secondary allergy in existing dermatitic skin.

REFERENCES

1. Landsteiner K, Chase MW: Studies on the sensitization of animals with simple chemical compounds. IX. Skin sensitization induced by injection of conjugates. *J Exp Med* 73:431, 1941.
2. Dupuis G, Benezra C: *Allergic Contact Dermatitis to Simple Chemicals: A Molecular Approach*. New York, Marcel Dekker, 1982, pp 52–66, 83.
3. Sommer G et al: Epicutaneous induction of hyporeactivity in contact sensitization: demonstration of suppressor cells induced by contact with 2,4-dinitrothiocyanatebenzene. *Immunology* 29:517, 1975.
4. Parker D et al: A comparison of the conjugation of DNTB and other dinitrobenzenes with free protein radicals and their ability to sensitize or tolerize. *J Invest Dermatol* 81:198, 1983.
5. Storrs FJ et al: Prevalence and relevance of allergic reactions in patients patch tested in North America—1984 to 1985. *J Am Acad Dermatol* 20:1038, 1989.
6. Belsito, DV: The pathophysiology of allergic contact hypersensitivity. *Clin Rev Allergy* 7:347, 1989.
7. Rowden G et al: Ia antigen expression on human epidermal Langerhans cells. *Nature* 268:247, 1977.
8. Hanau D et al: Human epidermal Langerhans cells cointernalize by receptor-mediated endocytosis "nonclassical" major histocompatibility complex class I molecules (T6 antigens) and class II molecules (HLA-DR antigens). *Proc Natl Acad Sci USA* 84:2901, 1987.
9. Silberberg-Sinakin I et al: Antigen bearing Langerhans cells in skin, dermal lymphatics and in lymph nodes. *Cell Immunol* 25:137, 1976.
10. Macatonia SE et al: Dendritic cells and the initiation of contact sensitivity to fluorescein isothiocyanate. *Immunology* 59:509, 1986.
11. Reinherz EL et al: The delineation of antigen receptors on human T lymphocytes. *Immunol Today* 4:5, 1983.
12. Schwartz RH: T lymphocyte recognition of antigen in association with gene products of the major histocompatibility complex. *Annu Rev Immunol* 3:237, 1985.
13. Sauder DN et al: Langerhans cell production of interleukin-1. *J Invest Dermatol* 82:605, 1984.
14. Belsito DV et al: Enhancement by various cytokines or 2-beta mercaptoethanol of Ia

antigen expression on Langerhans cells in skin from normal aged and young mice: effect of cyclosporine A. *J Immunol* 143:1530, 1989.
15. Chang TW et al: Cellular origin and interactions involved in gamma-interferon production induced by OKT3 monoclonal antibody. *J Immunol* 128:585, 1982.
16. Vilcek J et al: Interferon-gamma: a lymphokine for all seasons. *Lymphokines* 11:1, 1985.
17. Shimada S et al: Enhanced antigen-presenting capacity of cultured Langerhans cells is associated with markedly increased expression of Ia antigen. *J Immunol* 139:2551, 1987.
18. Beutler B et al: Effect of gamma-interferon on cachectin expression by mononuclear phagocytes: reversal of the lps^d (endotoxin resistance) phenotype. *J Exp Med* 164:1791, 1986.
19. Beutler B et al: Cachectin/tumor necrosis factor: production, distribution, and metabolic fate in vivo. *J Immunol* 135:3972, 1985.
20. Yokota S et al: Enhancement of antigen- and mitogen-induced human T lymphocyte proliferation by tumor necrosis factor-alpha. *J Immunol* 140:531, 1988.
21. Luger TA et al: Murine epidermal cell–derived thymocyte-activating factor resembles murine interleukin 1. *J Immunol* 128:2147, 1982.
22. Kupper TS et al: Keratinocyte-derived T-cell growth factor: a T-cell growth factor functionally distinct from interleukin 2. *Proc Natl Acad Sci USA* 83:4451, 1986.
23. Ray A et al: Activation of the human "$beta_2$-interferon/hepatocyte stimulating factor/ interleukin 6" promoter by cytokines, viruses, and second messenger agonists. *Proc Natl Acad Sci USA* 85:6701, 1988.
24. Garman RD et al: B-cell stimulatory factor 2 ($beta_2$ interferon) functions as a second signal for interleukin 2 production by mature murine T cells. *Proc Natl Acad Sci USA* 84:7629, 1987.
25. Askenase PW et al: T cells produce an antigen-binding factor with in vivo activity analogous to IgE antibody. *J Exp Med* 157:862, 1982.
26. Van Loveren H, Askenase PW: Delayed-type hypersensitivity is mediated by a sequence of two different T-cell activities. *J Immunol* 133:2397, 1984.
27. Kerdel FA et al: Mast cell participation during the elicitation of murine allergic contact hypersensitivity. *J Invest Dermatol* 88:686, 1987.
28. Sahasrabudhe DK et al: Inhibition of suppressor T lymphocytes (Ts) by cimetidine. *J Immunol* 138:2760, 1987.
29. Dvorak HF et al: Morphology of delayed-type hypersensitivity reactions in man. *J Invest Dermatol* 67:391, 1976.
30. Sobel RA et al: Anti–T cell monoclonal antibodies in vivo. I. Inhibition of delayed hypersensitivity but not cutaneous basophil hypersensitivity reactions. *J Immunol* 138:2500, 1987.
31. Gemsa D: Stimulation of prostaglandin E release from macrophages and possible role in the immune response, in E Pick (ed), *Lymphokines.* New York, Academic Press, 1981, p 335.
32. Walker C et al: Lymphokine regulation of activated (G1) lymphocytes: prostaglandin E2–induced inhibition of interleukin 2 production. *J Immunol* 130:1770, 1983.
33. Chun M et al: Enhancement of cytotoxic activity of natural killer cells by interleukin 2 and antagonism between interleukin 2 and adenosine cyclic monophosphate. *Scand J Immunol* 22:375, 1985.
34. Belsito DV et al: Reversal by lymphokines of the age-related hyporesponsiveness to contact sensitization and reduced Ia expression on Langerhans cells. *Arch Dermatol Res* 279:S76, 1987.
35. Belsito DV, Possick LE: Age-related changes in allergic contact hypersensitivity: functional T cell deficiencies are primarily responsible. *J Invest Dermatol* 90:546, 1988.
36. Marcussen PV: Primary irritant patch-test reactions in children. *Arch Dermatol* 87:378, 1963.
37. Straus HW: Artificial sensitization of infants to poison ivy. *J Allergy* 2:137, 1931.
38. Schubert H, Prater E: Sexual differences in contact allergy. *Boll Dermatol Allerg Professionale* 2:35, 1987.

39. Skog E: The influence of preexposure to alkyl benzene sulphonate detergent, soap and acetone on primary irritant and allergic eczematous reactions. *Acta Derm Venereol (Stockh)* 38:1, 1958.
40. Walker FB et al: Genetic factors in human allergic contact dermatitis. *Int Arch Allergy Appl Immunol* 32:453, 1967.
41. Silvennoinen-Kassinen S et al: No significant association between HLA and nickel contact sensitivity. *Tissue Antigens* 14:459, 1979.
42. Valsecchi R et al: HLA antigens and contact sensitivity. *Arch Dermatol* 118:533, 1982.
43. Bruynzeel DP et al: Oral psoralen photo-chemotherapy of allergic contact dermatitis of the hands. *Derm Beruf Umwelt* 30:16, 1982.
44. Mork NJ, Austad J: Short wave ultraviolet light (UVB) treatment of allergic contact dermatitis of the hands. *Acta Derm Venereol (Stockh)* 63:87, 1982.

11

Pathophysiology of Atopic Dermatitis

Jon M. Hanifin

Atopic dermatitis is a chronic inflammatory skin condition characterized by dryness, erythema, and extreme pruritus. The consequent scratching and rubbing lead to lichenification, most typically in the antecubital and popliteal flexures (Fig. 11-1). Usually patients have a personal or family history of atopy (i.e., asthma, allergic rhinitis, food intolerance, atopic dermatitis). The condition is commonly referred to as eczema, neurodermatitis, or, in Europe, prurigo Besnier.

Atopic dermatitis is a very common condition.[1] A survey of dermatologic diseases in the United States showed a prevalence of 2.4 percent in children and 0.7 percent in adults. Because there is no biochemical marker or other diagnostic screening test, subtle clinical features are easily missed and these figures underestimate the true prevalence. A recent study cited an incidence of 10 percent, increased from 3 percent in the past 20 years.[2]

Atopic dermatitis usually begins at an early age, with 60 percent of patients affected in the first year of life and 85 percent within the first 5 years.[3] The dermatitis is typically more constant in the early years; later the tendency is toward symptom-free periods that may last for periods ranging from months to years. However, many patients, especially those with the most severe disease, are extensively affected throughout life. Even with apparently complete remissions, individuals retain a tendency toward dry, sensitive skin and a lifetime risk of renewed disease activity.

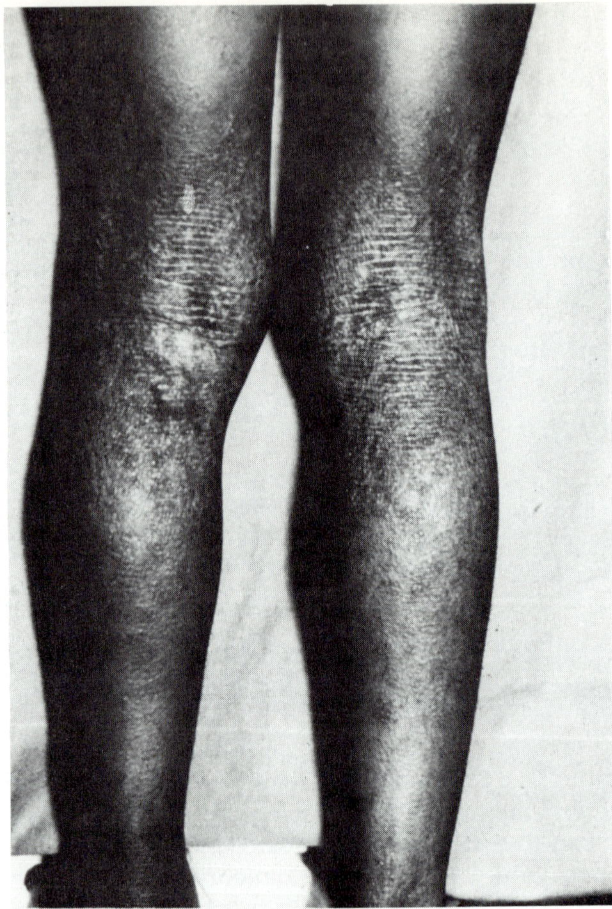

Figure 11-1 Lichenified plaques of atopic dermatitis localized to the popliteal fossae.

HISTOPATHOLOGY

Histological features of atopic dermatitis are the same as those of any of the eczematous diseases. Biopsy specimens from infantile eczema[4] showed intercellular epidermal edema (spongiosis) and a dermal perivascular mononuclear cell infiltrate. Increased numbers of mast cells correlated with the density of the dermal infiltrate.

Studies of Epon-embedded, Giemsa-stained 1-μm specimens from patients with atopic dermatitis showed normal numbers of mast cells with some degranulation in acutely involved areas but significantly increased numbers of mast cells in lichenified skin.[5] Endothelial cell hypertrophy and basement membrane thickening were evident in the superficial venular plexus of acute and chronic lesions, as well as in some areas of uninvolved skin. Both clinically normal skin and the lichenified areas showed demyelination and perineural fibrosis. Acute and chronic lesions showed marked to moderate infiltrates of both lymphocytes and macrophages. Only occasional basophils and eosinophils were evident. Interstitial fibrin deposition was not detected. Increased numbers of Langerhans cells are distributed throughout the epidermis of chronic lesions, though this increase is not evident in uninvolved skin or in areas of acute lesions.[6] Newer immunohistological techniques have shown IgE bound to epidermal Langerhans cells.[7] Other monoclonal antibody studies have revealed the presence of eosinophil cationic proteins in the dermis, indicating that eosinophils infiltrate lesions and then disintegrate, possibly augmenting the inflammatory response.[8] The lymphocytic infiltrate has been characterized as consisting mainly of $CD4^+$ (helper) T cells, most of which also stain with antibody to class II major histocompatibility complex (MHC) antigen, a sign of T-cell activation.

GENETIC ASSOCIATIONS

The familial nature of atopic dermatitis is well established, but the genetic mode of inheritance is unknown. Autosomal dominant, autosomal recessive, and polygenic inheritance all have been suggested. Children of allergic parents show an increased incidence of allergic conditions. In families with one allergic parent, 58 percent of children developed allergic symptoms; if both parents were allergic, 79 percent of offspring were affected.[9] Another study showed that 73 percent of allergic children and only 29 percent of nonallergic children had a family history of allergy.[10]

Studies of twins showed a concordance of 85 percent among monozygotic twins, while concordance in dizygotic twins was no different from that in other siblings.[2] This suggests environmental influences, genetic factors, and multifactorial causation in atopic dermatitis.

IMMUNOLOGIC CONSIDERATIONS

Immunoglobulin E

The clinical association of atopic dermatitis with asthma and allergic rhinitis suggests a possible pathogenic role for IgE antibodies. Eighty percent of patients with atopic dermatitis show immediate skin test reactions to one or more environmental allergens.[3] Serum IgE levels are elevated in approximately the same percentage, and the highest levels tend to occur in patients with extensive skin disease.[11] There is also considerable evidence against a direct pathogenic role for IgE in atopic dermatitis (Table 11-1). Although elevated serum IgE is a prominent feature of atopic dermatitis, it may simply reflect a basic defect of immunoglobulin regulation. Also, because serum IgE is elevated in many other skin conditions, one might surmise that a cutaneous inflammation, like parasitosis, is a stimulus to IgE production. Peripheral blood B lymphocytes from patients with atopic dermatitis, when cultured in the presence of T cells and monocytes, spontaneously produce increased quantities of IgE.

Table 11-1

SERUM IgE AND ATOPIC DERMATITIS

A pathogenic role is suggested by:
- Elevated levels in 80% of patients
- Levels higher than those in asthma or allergic rhinitis
- The fact that more severe disease is generally associated with higher levels

Evidence against a causal relationship includes:
- Typical flexural eczema in patients with agammaglobulinemia
- Normal IgE levels in 20% of patients
- High IgE levels in some conditions (e.g., parasitosis) without dermatitis
- High IgE levels when atopic dermatitis is in remission

This overproduction may also depend upon interleukin-4 (IL-4) and other cytokines.[12]

Cellular Immune Function

Both clinical and immunological observations indicate depressed cell-mediated immunity in atopic dermatitis (Table 11-2). Atopic individuals exhibit unusual susceptibility to cutaneous herpes simplex, vaccinia, molluscum contagiosum, and warts.[11] Delayed-type hypersensitivity is also reduced in atopic dermatitis. Patients are less easily sensitized to *Rhus* (poison ivy) and dinitrochlorobenzene and show decreased delayed skin test reactivity to intradermal tuberculin, candidin, and other microbial

Table 11-2

EVIDENCE OF DEPRESSED CELL-MEDIATED IMMUNITY IN ATOPIC DERMATITIS

Susceptibility to certain cutaneous viral infections
- Herpes simplex
- Vaccinia
- Molluscum contagiosum
- Verruca vulgaris (common warts)

Reduced sensitization to
- *Rhus* oleoresin (poison ivy, etc.)
- Dinitrochlorobenzene
- Miscellaneous environmental contactants

Cutaneous anergy to microbial antigens (e.g., candidin, streptokinase-streptodornase)

Decreased in vitro lymphocyte reactivity to mitogens and antigens

Reduced monocyte and neutrophil chemotaxis

antigens.[13] Although studies have demonstrated depressed in vitro lymphocyte transformation, these responses may be normal during clinical remission and then become abnormal during clinical flares of dermatitis. There does not appear to be a serious central defect of cell-mediated immunity, and patients are not predisposed to systemic infections or internal malignancy.

Studies have indicated reduced circulating T lymphocytes in patients with atopic dermatitis, especially those cells bearing IgG-Fc receptors and expressing CD8, the phenotype of suppressor and cytotoxic T cells.[14] A long-standing hypothesis suggests that absence of a suppressor cell population accounts for elevated IgE production in atopic dermatitis, but this appears to be an oversimplified conceptualization of a much more complex system.

Chemotactic Defects and Staphylococcal Infections

Neutrophil and monocyte chemotaxis is reduced during exacerbations of atopic dermatitis,[15] though these in vitro defects become normal with clinical improvement. In vivo migration of neutrophils to skin windows is reduced in even mildly involved skin. Moreover, serum from patients with severe atopic dermatitis inhibits normal neutrophil and monocyte chemotaxis. Reduced phagocyte migration may predispose to the frequent staphylococcal skin infections that occur in atopic dermatitis. Over 90 percent of persons with atopic dermatitis have coagulase-positive *Staphylococcus aureus* as the predominant organism of their skin flora.[16]

An etiologic role for staphylococci in atopic dermatitis was suggested by studies demonstrating increased serum levels of IgE antibody specific for *S. aureus* in the hyperimmunoglobulinemia E syndrome. However, such increases could not be detected in atopic dermatitis,[17] though colonization with *S. aureus* may trigger release of histamine and other mast cell mediators by nonimmunologic mechanisms, leading to the itching and inflammation of atopic dermatitis.

PHYSIOLOGICAL AND PHARMACOLOGIC ASSOCIATIONS

White Dermographism

Stroking the skin in atopic dermatitis results in a white line known as white dermographism. However, this reaction is not specific and may be seen in other skin conditions, including mycosis fungoides and psoriasis.[18] Photoelectric pulse meter recordings indicate that the blanch is probably due to dermal edema and vasoconstriction.

Responses to Cholinergic Agents and the Delayed Blanch

Intradermal injection of acetylcholine or methacholine initially causes a normal wheal and flare response, but, after a few minutes, the wheal becomes blanched.[19] This delayed blanch reaction may be elicited in 70 percent of patients with atopic dermatitis and is often considered to be a diagnostic sign. However, this reaction also occurs in allergic contact dermatitis.[20] The delayed blanch is blocked by atropine, indicating a muscarinic effect. Whether the blanch is due to edema from increased vascular permeability or to vasoconstriction or both is unresolved. There is some evidence of elevated acetylcholine levels in the skin of patients with atopic dermatitis.[18] This neurotransmitter may be an important link between the central nervous system and the skin and may explain in part the influence of emotional factors in atopic dermatitis.

Nicotinic Acid Response

Topically applied nicotinic acid or esters cause erythema on normal skin. In contrast, application to skin with atopic dermatitis results in either no erythema or a blanch. Again, this effect is not specific and its significance is uncertain.

Catecholamine Studies

Allergic patients show reduced responses to epinephrine in terms of gluconeogenesis and relaxation of bronchial smooth muscle. Observations such as these led Szentivanyi to formulate his theory of β-adrenergic blockade as a basis for atopy.[21] Blockade of β-adrenergic receptors leads to an imbalance in cyclic nucleotide responses, resulting in cholinergic hyperreactivity. Adrenergic receptors are classed as either α or β, based on their relative responses to isoproterenol, epinephrine, and norepinephrine. The increased piloerection in atopic dermatitis may indicate a high level of α-adrenergic tone. Asthmatics have increased α-adrenergic sensitivity, reflected by cutaneous vasoconstriction and pupillary dilatation responses to phenylephrine.[22]

Histamine, Mast Cells, and Basophils

When intramuscular histamine was given to persons with atopic dermatitis, increases in erythema and skin temperature were recorded over the face, neck, and elbow flexures.[23] These findings may reflect increased target tissue reactivity to histamine or may result from increased delivery of histamine to inflamed areas.

Several investigators, using various techniques, have shown increased histamine release by leukocytes from patients with atopic dermatitis.[24,25] While the atopic cells do not apparently bind more IgE, they show a lower threshold for anti-IgE-triggered histamine release. These studies suggest an abnormality of basophil and mast cell regulation by the cyclic nucleotide system or other regulatory pathways.

β-Adrenergic Blockade Theory and Cyclic Nucleotide Abnormalities

Early experimental and clinical observations suggested that atopic tissues might be blocked at the β-adrenergic receptor,[21] permitting the abnormal pharmacologic hyperreactivity characteristic of atopy. Skin from atopic dermatitis patients, when treated with β-adrenergic agonists, failed to inhibit DNA synthesis.[26] Atopic leukocytes showed abnormal functional responses that correlated with subnormal cyclic AMP levels after β-adrenergic stimulation.[27] However, studies also showed reduced leukocyte cyclic AMP levels after histamine and prostaglandin E_1 stimulation, suggesting a defect not limited to the β-adrenergic receptor.[28] Also, direct measurements of β-adrenergic receptor numbers and affinities showed no measurable difference when atopic leukocytes were compared with normal cells.

An alternative mechanism for the reduced cyclic AMP responsiveness in atopy was suggested by the observation of increased cyclic AMP-phosphodiesterase (PDE) activity in untreated, isolated mononuclear leukocytes from patients with atopic dermatitis.[29] This was a consistent finding, and increases were noted even in leukocytes from patients with atopic dermatitis in remission. Thus it appears that the reduced cyclic AMP levels, after stimulation of leukocytes with catecholamines and other agonists, result from rapid breakdown by excess PDE (Fig. 11-2). Using

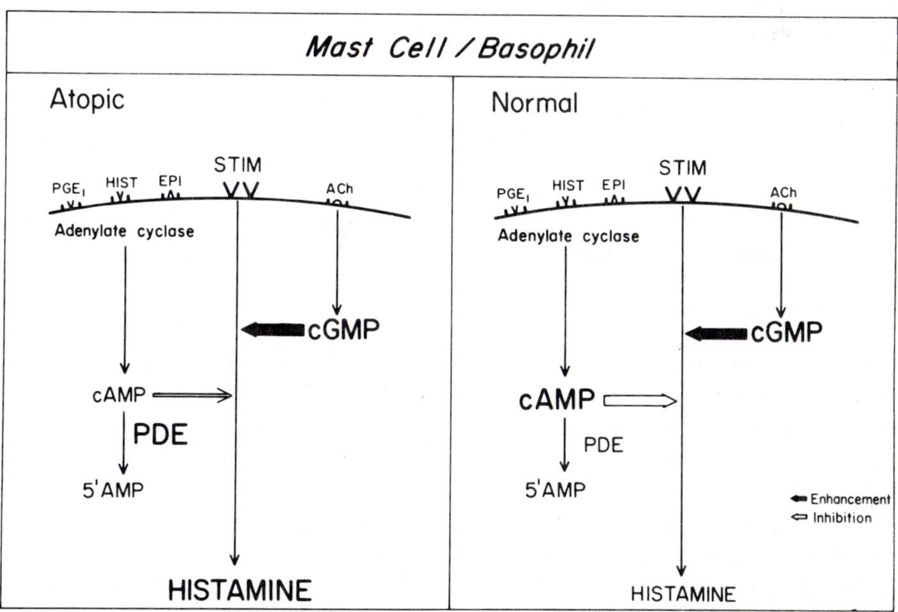

Figure 11-2 Diagrammatic representation of the cyclic AMP (cAMP) regulatory abnormality that may result from increased phosphodiesterase (PDE) activity in atopic cells. Normally the respective enhancing and inhibiting effects of cGMP (cyclic guanosine 3′,5′-monophosphate) and cAMP are balanced in regulating histamine release. Enhancement may be stimulated by acetylcholine (ACh). Activation of adenylate cyclase by prostaglandin E_1 (PGE_1), histamine (HIST), or epinephrine (EPI) would lead to increased cAMP and inhibition of histamine release. In atopic cells, this inhibitory effect is negated by PDE hydrolysis of cAMP to 5′-adenosine monophosphate (5′-AMP), allowing a net enhancement of histamine release.

the mast cell–basophil system as an example, the lack of normal intracellular cyclic AMP responses might allow increased histamine release. In fact, this has been demonstrated in leukocytes from patients with atopic dermatitis.[25] In that study, the abnormal histamine release correlated with increased PDE activity and was normalized when leukocytes were exposed to PDE inhibitors. Additionally, elevated PDE levels in atopic B cells and/or T helper cells might provide a permissive influence accounting for excessive IgE synthesis.[30] Evidence from transplantation studies demonstrates that the atopic trait is transferred with marrow cells.[31] A genetically determined defect resulting in abnormally high PDE activity in various immunocompetent and inflammatory, bone marrow–derived cells might account for the disordered immunologic and pharmacologic abnormalities that characterize atopic dermatitis.

In summary, atopic dermatitis is a condition characterized by chronic or relapsing cutaneous inflammation and pruritus. Patients may show a mild immune deficiency manifested by increased susceptibility to cutaneous viral and staphylococcal infections. Serum IgE levels are generally elevated, but the role of IgE in causing the skin inflammation is uncertain. Increased IgE synthesis with increased releasability of leukocyte histamine appears to reflect a basic regulatory defect. The finding of elevated leukocyte cyclic AMP-PDE in atopy may account for inadequate cyclic nucleotide control of cell functions.

REFERENCES

1. Hanifin JM: Epidemiology of atopic dermatitis, in H Schlumberger (ed), *Monographs in Allergy*. Basel, Karger, 1987, vol 21, p 116.
2. Larsen FS et al: Atopic dermatitis: a genetic-epidemiologic study in a population-based twin sample. *J Am Acad Dermatol* 15:487, 1986.
3. Rajka G: *Essential Aspects of Atopic Dermatitis*. Berlin, Springer-Verlag, 1989.
4. Sedlis E, Prose P: Infantile eczema with special reference to the pathologic lesion. *Pediatrics* 23:802, 1959.
5. Mihm MC Jr et al: The structure of normal skin and the morphology of atopic eczema. *J Invest Dermatol* 67:305, 1976.
6. Uno H, Hanifin JM: Langerhans cells in acute and chronic epidermal lesions of atopic dermatitis, observed by L-dopa histofluorescence, glycolmethacrylate thin section, and electron microscopy. *J Invest Dermatol* 75:52, 1980.
7. Bruynzeel-Koomen C et al: The presence of IgE molecules on epidermal Langerhans cells in patients with atopic dermatitis. *Arch Dermatol Res* 278:199, 1986.
8. Leiferman KM et al: Dermal deposition of eosinophil-granule major basic protein in atopic dermatitis. *N Engl J Med* 313:282, 1985.
9. Kaufman HS, Frick OL: The development of allergy in infants of allergic parents: a prospective study concerning the role of heredity. *Ann Allergy* 37:410, 1976.
10. Freeman GL, Johnson S: Allergic disease in adolescence. I. Description of survey: prevalence of allergy. *Am J Dis Child* 107:549, 1964.
11. Hanifin JM: Atopic dermatitis, in E Middleton, Jr, et al (eds), *Allergy: Principles and Practice*, 3d ed. St Louis, CV Mosby, 1988, vol II, p 1403.
12. Pene J et al: IgE production by normal human lymphocytes is induced by interleukin 4 and suppressed by interferons gamma and alpha and prostaglandin E_2. *Proc Natl Acad Sci USA* 85:6880, 1988.

13. Elliott ST, Hanifin JM: Delayed cutaneous hypersensitivity and lymphocyte transformation: disassociation in atopic dermatitis. *Arch Dermatol* 115:36, 1979.
14. Leung DYM et al: Enumeration of T cell subsets in atopic dermatitis using monoclonal antibodies. *J Allergy Clin Immunol* 67:450, 1981.
15. Hanifin JM et al: Chemotaxis inhibition by plasma from patients with atopic dermatitis. *Acta Derm Venereol (Stockh)* [Suppl] 92:52, 1980.
16. Leyden JJ et al: *Staphylococcus aureus* in the lesions of atopic dermatitis. *Br J Dermatol* 90:525, 1974.
17. Friedman SJ et al: IgE antibodies to *Staphylococcus aureus:* prevalence in patients with atopic dermatitis. *Arch Dermatol* 121:869, 1985.
18. Hanifin JM: Pharmacophysiology of atopic dermatitis. *Clin Rev Allergy* 4:43, 1986.
19. Lobitz WC, Campbell CH: Physiologic studies in atopic dermatitis (disseminated neurodermatitis). I. The local cutaneous response to intradermally injected acetylcholine and epinephrine. *Arch Dermatol Syph* 67:575, 1953.
20. Uehara M, Ofuji S: Abnormal vascular reactions in atopic dermatitis. *Arch Dermatol* 113:627, 1977.
21. Szentivanyi A: The beta-adrenergic theory of the atopic abnormality in bronchial asthma. *J Allergy* 42:203, 1968.
22. Henderson WR et al: Alpha-adrenergic hyper-responsiveness in asthma. *N Engl J Med* 303:263, 1980.
23. Williams DH: Skin temperature reaction to histamine in atopic dermatitis. *J Invest Dermatol* 1:119, 1938.
24. Lebel B et al: Anti-IgE-induced histamine release from basophils in children with atopic dermatitis. *Acta Derm Venereol (Stockh)* [Suppl] 92:57, 1980.
25. Butler JM et al: Increased leukocyte histamine release with elevated cyclic AMP-phosphodiesterase activity in atopic dermatitis. *J Allergy Clin Immunol* 71:490, 1983.
26. Carr RH et al: Failure of catecholamines to inhibit epidermal mitosis in vitro. *J Allergy Clin Immunol* 55:255, 1973.
27. Reed CE et al: Adrenergic mechanisms and the adenyl cyclase system in atopic dermatitis. *J Invest Dermatol* 67:333, 1976.
28. Safko MJ et al: Heterologous desensitization of leukocytes: a possible mechanism of beta adrenergic blockade in atopic dermatitis. *J Allergy Clin Immunol* 68:218, 1981.
29. Grewe SR et al: Elevated leukocyte cyclic AMP-phosphodiesterase in atopic disease: a possible mechanism for cyclic AMP-agonist hyporesponsiveness. *J Allergy Clin Immunol* 70:452, 1982.
30. Cooper KD et al: Phosphodiesterase inhibition by Ro20-1724 reduces hyper-IgE synthesis by atopic dermatitis cells in vitro. *J Invest Dermatol* 84:477, 1985.
31. Agosti J et al: Transfer of allergen-specific IgE-mediated hypersensitivity with allogeneic bone marrow transplantation. *N Engl J Med* 319:1623, 1988.

12

Pathophysiology of Pemphigus

Mary Ann Robledo and Luis A. Diaz

The term *pemphigus* refers to a group of cutaneous diseases that are characterized by the development of intraepidermal blisters and, sometimes, mucosal erosions.[1] These diseases are listed in Table 12-1. All forms of pemphigus are characterized by epidermal cell-cell detachment (acantholysis), which leads to (intraepidermal) vesicle formation, and by IgG autoantibodies directed against antigenic determinants present on the cell surfaces of differentiating keratinocytes.[2]

Both forms of pemphigus foliaceus are easily differentiated from pemphigus vulgaris and its variants such as pemphigus vegetans (Table 12-2). In pemphigus vulgaris the lesions usually appear first on mucosal surfaces, acantholysis is suprabasilar rather than subcorneal, and the autoantibodies recognize a different epidermal glycoprotein.[3]

The most severe form of pemphigus is pemphigus vulgaris, which may occur at any age; its most common onset is in the fourth, fifth, and sixth decades. It is characterized by flaccid, exceedingly fragile, noninflammatory bullae that usually arise on normal-appearing skin. These bullae tend to coalesce and rupture easily, resulting in large, denuded areas that are the predominant clinical feature of this type of pemphigus (Fig. 12-1, top panel). Pemphigus vulgaris involves both the skin and the mucous membranes, and in virtually all cases the initial lesion affects the oral mucosa. Prior to the introduction of corticosteroids in the 1950s, pemphigus vulgaris was considered almost uniformly fatal, due mainly to protein,

Table 12-1

CLINICAL VARIANTS OF PEMPHIGUS

Pemphigus vulgaris
Pemphigus vegetans
Cazenave's pemphigus foliaceus (nonendemic)
Endemic pemphigus foliaceus (fogo selvagem)
Pemphigus erythematosus (Senear-Usher syndrome)
Drug-induced pemphigus

fluid, and electrolyte losses and/or uncontrollable sepsis. Acantholysis is the histological hallmark of all forms of pemphigus.[1] In pemphigus vulgaris, it starts with the development of epidermal intercellular edema, leading to dissolution of intercellular "bridges" and widening of intercellular spaces, and ending finally in cell-cell detachment. These microscopic changes occur in the suprabasilar area, i.e., between the basal and spinous cell layers (Fig. 12-1, middle panel). Basal cells remain attached to the dermis but are laterally detached, adopting the form of a "row of tombstones."[1]

Endemic pemphigus foliaceus or fogo selvagem is similar to the nonendemic form seen in North America and Europe, originally described by Cazenave.[4] It is characterized clinically by superficial blistering and erosive lesions that affect the skin and rarely involve the mucosal surfaces (Fig. 12-2, left panel)[5–8] and histologically by acantholysis involving the subcorneal layers of the epidermis (Fig. 12-2, right top panel). In both forms, circulating autoantibodies in the patients' sera recognize desmoglein I.[9] The major features that distinguish nonendemic pemphigus foliaceus from fogo selvagem are listed in Table 12-2.

Although fogo selvagem occurs mainly in Brazil, where there are approximately 15,000 registered cases,[10] clusters of cases of an endemic fogo selvagem–like disease have been reported in Colombia,[11] El Salvador, Paraguay, and Peru.[12] The disease frequently affects children and young adults; the peak incidence is in the second and third decades of life. This age distribution is quite different from that observed in nonendemic pemphigus foliaceus.

The precise cause of all forms of pemphigus and the mechanisms that initiate the antibody formation are essentially unknown. However, in fogo selvagem, there is strong epidemiological evidence suggesting that an environmental agent is responsible for initiating the disease.[10–12] Drugs such as penicillamine,[13,14] rifampin,[15] and captopril[16] are known to precipitate a pemphigus-like disease with features of pemphigus foliaceus or pemphigus vulgaris.

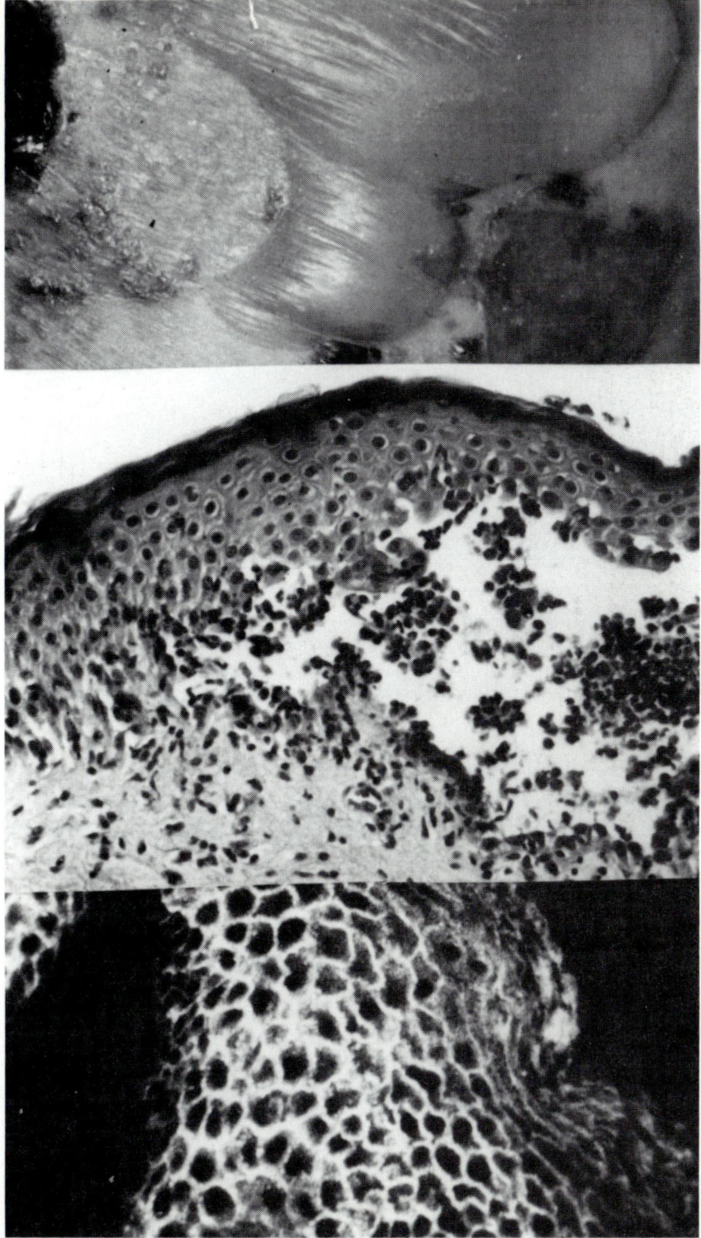

Figure 12-1 *Top panel:* flaccid blisters and erosions in a patient with pemphigus vulgaris. *Middle panel:* histological section of a skin lesion from a pemphigus vulgaris patient demonstrating suprabasilar acantholysis. Hemaloxylin-eosin; × 200 in the original magnification. *Bottom panel:* pemphigus vulgaris autoantibodies shown by indirect immunofluorescence techniques using human skin substrate. The immunofluorescence staining of the epidermal intercellular spaces is indistinguishable among all forms of pemphigus.

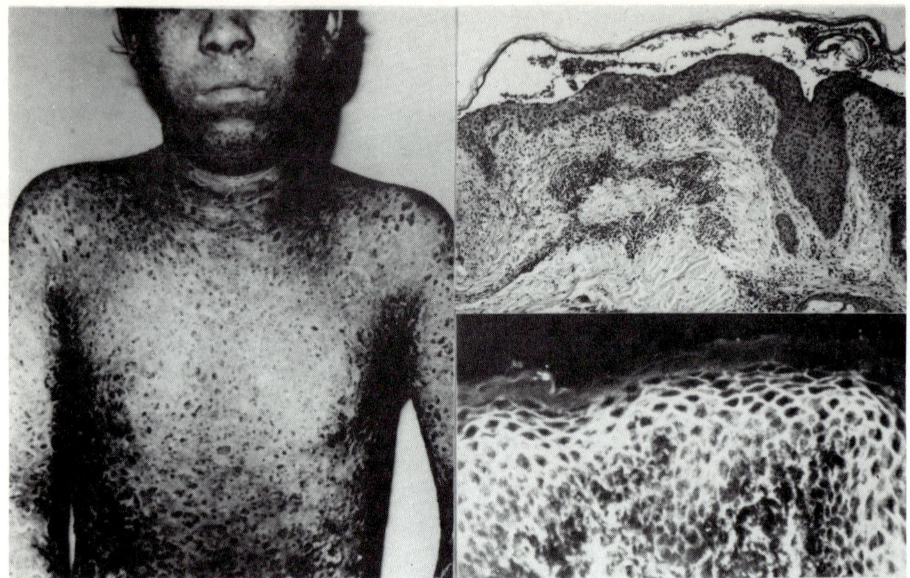

Figure 12-2 *Left panel:* young man with a generalized form of endemic pemphigus foliaceus showing an exfoliative dermatitis. *Right top panel:* histological examination of a vesicular lesion from a patients with pemphigus foliaceus showing a subcorneal vesicle. Hematolylin-eosin; × 200 in the original magnification. *Right bottom panel:* pemphigus foliaceus autoantibodies demonstrated by indirect immunofluorescence.

There is also some evidence that genetic factors may play a role in the development of pemphigus. For example, pemphigus vulgaris occurs in all ethnic and racial groups, but there is a higher incidence in Jews, in whom there is an increased prevalence of the HLA DRw4 phenotype.[17,18] Recently, a study of the genetics of pemphigus vulgaris by restriction fragment length polymorphism analysis reported striking results.[19–22] The authors confirmed that almost all affected individuals have the HLA phenotype DR4 or DRw6. In addition, using cDNA probes for the DQ α and β genes of the major histocompatibility complex, they found a unique and specific DQ β restriction fragment in almost all patients with pemphigus vulgaris that was not detected in the control groups. Preliminary human leukocyte antigen (HLA) studies in fogo selvagem patients have been recently reported[23] in which 58 percent of a group of fogo selvagem patients ($n = 24$) were DR1 positive, while only 20 percent of the control group expressed this marker, indicating a relative risk of 5.5. Additionally, HLA DR4 was found in 42 percent of the patients versus 17 percent of the control group. HLA DR1 and DR4 antigens were found in 83 percent of the fogo selvagem patients. Interestingly, HLA DR7, which was present in 17 percent of the controls, was absent in all fogo selvagem patients studied, suggesting that this antigen may confer resistance to the development of fogo selvagem.

Table 12-2

PEMPHIGUS VULGARIS AND PEMPHIGUS FOLIACEUS

Differential Features	Pemphigus Vulgaris	Endemic Pemphigus Foliaceus (Fogo Selvagem)	Nonendemic Pemphigus Foliaceus (Cazenave)
Distribution	Sporadic	Endemic, Brazil	Sporadic
Cause	Unknown	Environmental?	Unknown
Age	Adults	Children and young adults	Elderly
Familial cases	Rare	Frequently observed	None
Skin Lesions	Deeper, suprabasilar	Superficial, subcorneal	Superficial, subcorneal
Mucosal Lesions	Common	Rare	Rare
Passive Transfer	Suprabasilar disease in mice	Subcorneal disease in mice	?
Antigens	135-kd glycoprotein	Desmoglein I	Desmoglein I
Pregnancy	Neonatal pemphigus	Normal newborns	Normal newborns
Prognosis	Guarded	Variable	Variable

Pemphigus has rarely been associated with other autoimmune disorders such as lupus erythematosus (Senear-Usher syndrome), rheumatoid arthritis, myasthenia gravis, pernicious anemia, Hashimoto's thyroiditis, and tumors such as benign thymomas.[24,25] When this association occurs, the course of pemphigus usually is not affected by the presence of these disorders. Pemphigus has also been associated with various malignancies; however, the incidence of malignancy is not high, and temporal relationships are rare.

Although several important papers have implicated in situ activation of complement[26] or proteases[27] in the production of acantholysis, this chapter covers studies that convincingly demonstrate the pathogenicity of pemphigus autoantibodies. Additionally, we emphasize certain recent studies that explore new hypotheses on the autoantibody-induced acantholysis seen in pemphigus vulgaris and fogo selvagem, respectively.

THE PATHOGENIC ROLE OF PEMPHIGUS AUTOANTIBODIES: CLINICAL OBSERVATIONS

The clinical observations that support a pathogenic role for pemphigus autoantibodies in patients include the following:

Virtually 100 percent of patients with pemphigus have IgG autoantibodies bound to the surface of the epidermal cells both in and around lesions, as shown by direct immunofluorescence techniques (Fig. 12-1, bottom panel; Fig. 12-2, right bottom panel).[28] Complement proteins are also detected in lesional epidermis.[26]

In addition, the serum of virtually all patients with active disease contains antiepithelial cell surface autoantibodies, which can be demonstrated by indirect immunofluorescence procedures using frozen sections of stratified squamous epithelium as tissue substrate.[2,28] The titer of pemphigus autoantibodies detected in the patient's serum correlates well with the clinical activity and extent of disease.[2,28,29] The antigen(s) to which these autoantibodies bind is (are) not restricted to human skin, for these autoantibodies will bind to the cell surface of stratified squamous epithelium from all mammals and birds.[30] Recent studies[10,31–33] found these antigens to be desmosome-associated glycoproteins, suggesting that pemphigus autoantibodies may impair the assembly of desmosomes and induce cell detachment. Further studies are needed to clarify this issue.

There are several reported cases in which mothers with pemphigus vulgaris have given birth to children during a period when their disease was active, and the neonates were born with lesions typical of pemphigus vulgaris.[34,35] These infants were shown to have antiepidermal autoantibodies bound to the cell surface of lesional epidermis and circulating in their serum. In the months following birth, the antiepidermal autoantibodies disappeared and the cutaneous disease improved correspondingly, suggesting that the transplacental transfer of the pathogenic maternal autoantibodies was responsible for the neonatal cutaneous disease. In contrast, newborns from mothers with active nonendemic pemphigus foliaceus[36] and active fogo selvagem[37] showed normal skin and negative serology. Moreover, pemphigus autoantibodies were detected in the baby's epidermis by direct immunofluorescence and were absent in cord blood despite positive serology in the mother.[36] We have tested by indirect immunofluorescence the sera of eight mother-newborn pairs where the mothers had documented fogo selvagem and the babies were born completely normal. Interestingly, the mothers had high titers of IgG4 pemphigus autoantibodies in their sera ($>$1:160), and the cord blood of all newborns showed negative or low titer of antibodies ($<$1:10).

It is possible, therefore, that pemphigus foliaceus autoantibodies do not pass the placenta and that the babies are born with normal skin. It is known that IgG crosses the placenta through an active transport process mediated by Fc receptors and that this transport is IgG subclass restricted (IgG1 = IgG3 $>$ IgG4 $>$ IgG2).[38] It is also possible that IgG4 autoantibodies in fogo selvagem may have a unique restriction by isoelectric point that may also regulate their passage through the placenta, as is the case for other molecules.[39]

Plasmapheresis has been employed for the treatment of patients with pemphigus.[40–42] The rationale for this treatment was that removal of circulating autoantibodies, with a subsequent decrease in their immunofluorescence titer, may lead to clinical improvement of the disease. In fact, with intensive plasmapheresis, it is possible to produce a decrease in circulating autoantibody titers as well as an improvement in the patient. The major drawback of this technique is that the improvement is very brief. With the cessation of plasmapheresis the autoantibody titers quickly rebound, sometimes to a higher level, and the disease flares once again.[42]

DEFINING THE NEONATAL MOUSE MODEL OF PEMPHIGUS VULGARIS

Our laboratory has demonstrated that IgG purified from the serum of patients with pemphigus vulgaris,[43] when given in sufficient doses, induced a blistering disease in neonatal BALB/c mice. The animals were injected intraperitoneally with two divided doses daily. Within 18 to 72 h of the first injection, the animals developed cutaneous blisters and erosions. These lesions had the same clinical, histological, ultrastructural, and immunologic features as those seen in the human disease. These pathological changes were not observed in animals that received comparable doses of pooled normal human IgG. The severity of the disease produced in these animals was dependent on both the total dose of IgG administered and the titer of human pemphigus autoantibody detected in the mouse serum by indirect immunofluorescence. In addition, lesions occurred only as long as the injections were continued. Once the injections were discontinued, new lesions ceased to appear and previous lesions began to resolve.

In summary, the animal model of pemphigus vulgaris confirmed earlier observations in human pemphigus[44] and experimentally induced acantholysis in skin explants[45,46] that the basal cell–dermal attachment remains unaltered even in a fully developed acantholytic vesicle ("tombstone row"). The basal cell hemidesmosomes are intact, and the dermal-epidermal junction is ultrastructurally well defined. The observation that the basal cell–dermal adhesion remains unaltered suggests that the factor or mediator released by suprabasal keratinocytes does not affect the attachment of basal cells to the dermis. This is surprising, for the dermal-epidermal attachment is known to be extremely labile to proteases.[47,48] Therefore, it is conceivable that the epidermal acantholysis induced by pemphigus vulgaris antibodies may go through an early detachment process that is mediated by proteases, but the fully developed acantholytic vesicle may represent the end result of both intra- and extracellular processes rather than of extracellular events alone.

DEFINING THE NEONATAL MOUSE MODEL OF FOGO SELVAGEM

We have also developed a model of fogo selvagem in neonatal mice by injecting fogo selvagem autoantibodies into these animals.[49] The IgG fraction from the sera of 10 patients was purified and injected intraperitoneally into newborn BALB/c mice. Cutaneous blisters and erosions developed within 18 to 72 h (Fig. 12-3, top panel). There was a good correlation between the extent of disease produced in the mice and the immunofluorescence titer of fogo selvagem autoantibodies in the IgG fractions. By light and electron microscopy, the lesions were typical acantholytic blisters in the granular cell layer (Fig. 12-3, middle panel). Suprabasilar acantholysis (typical of the animal model of pemphigus vulgaris) was not present in any of these animals.

This study showed that fogo selvagem autoantibodies produced epidermal lesions in the animal model that were morphologically distinct from those caused by pemphigus vulgaris autoantibodies in the same animals. Thus, these findings yielded a useful in vivo experimental model for comparing and contrasting mechanisms of tissue injury in both diseases. They also demonstrated convincingly that the lesions of fogo selvagem are indeed caused by the autoantibodies.

THE PATHOGENIC AUTOANTIBODY RESPONSE IN FOGO SELVAGEM IS PREDOMINANTLY IgG4

We have demonstrated[50] that fogo selvagem autoantibodies are also restricted to the IgG4 subclass. The purpose of this investigation was twofold: to determine the IgG subclass profile of fogo selvagem autoantibodies in the serum and skin of patients and to evaluate the pathogenicity of fractionated IgG subclass autoantibodies by passive transfer studies in neonatal BALB/c mice.

The IgG subclasses with fogo selvagem autoantibody activity were evaluated in sera from 29 patients with active disease and in lesional skin of 18 patients by immunofluorescence using IgG subclass specific monoclonal antibodies. The predominant fogo selvagem autoantibodies present in all patients were of the IgG4 subclass and in some patients were exclusively of this subclass. IgG1 was present in 23 of 29 patients, although in markedly lower titers than IgG4. In nine patients, IgG2 was present in very low titers. No IgG3 fogo selvagem autoantibody was detected in any patient's sera. Direct immunofluorescence of lesional skin exhibited a preferential deposition of IgG4 in the epidermal intercellular space. The pathogenic effect of IgG4 was demonstrated in experimental animals. IgG fractions containing IgG4 fogo selvagem autoantibody activity were prepared by ammonium sulfate precipitation and diethylaminoethyl (DEAE) cellulose chromatography and passively transferred to neonatal BALB/c mice. The human disease was reproduced clinically, histologically, and immunologically in these animals. Only IgG4 fogo selvagem autoantibodies

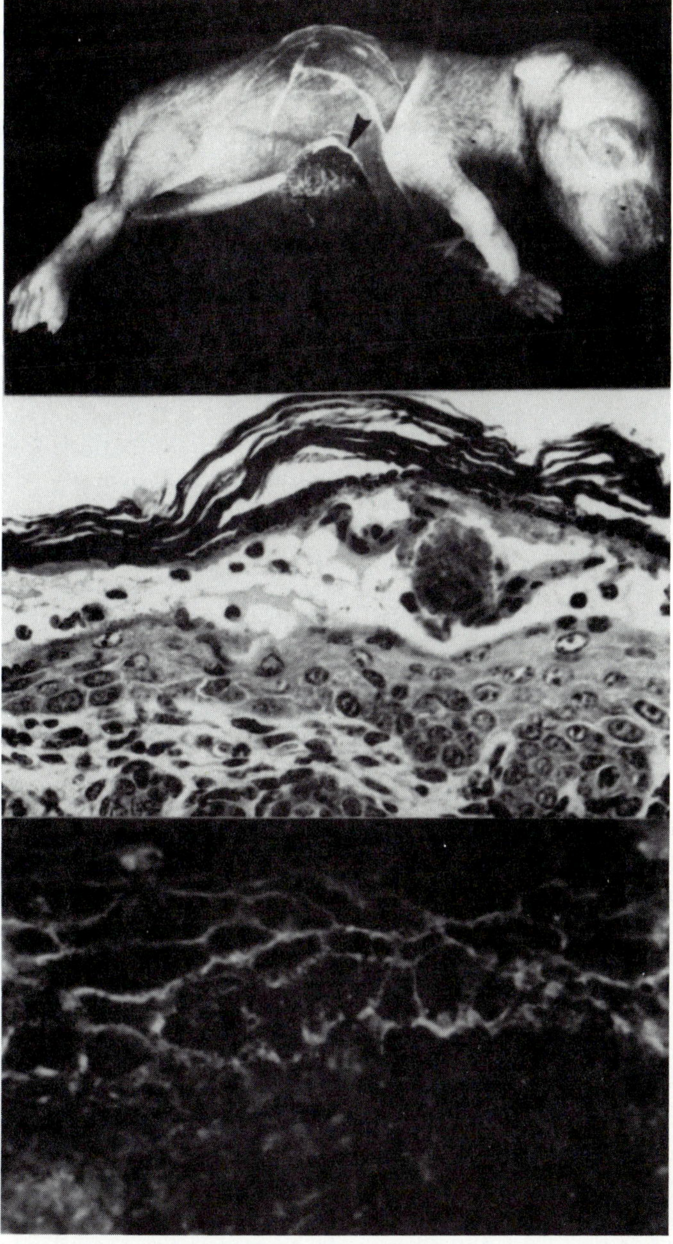

Figure 12-3 *Top panel:* neonatal BALB/c mouse shows a superficial blister (*arrow*) and a positive Nikolsky's sign 16 h after intraperitoneal injection of fogo selvagem IgG (15 mg per gram of body weight per day). *Middle panel:* subcorneal acantholysis in the mouse model of pemphigus foliaceus exhibiting histological features of human pemphigus foliaceus. Hematoxylin-eosin; × 200 in the original magnification. *Bottom panel:* human pemphigus foliaceus autoantibodies bound to the lesional epidermal intercellular space of a mouse injected with the patient's IgG, as shown by direct immunofluorescence.

were bound to lesional mouse epidermis, as determined by direct immunofluorescence, and around the keratinocyte surface, as determined by immunoelectron microscopy. Serum from diseased mice contained high titers of fogo selvagem IgG4 autoantibodies.

Finding IgG4 to be the pathogenic fogo selvagem autoantibody is unexpected because in vitro it has been shown to have poor effector functions compared to the other IgG subclasses. The finding of pathogenic IgG4 autoantibodies in fogo selvagem provides a new model for the study of IgG4-mediated responses, as well as insight into the pathogenesis of a unique autoimmune disease.

Restricted IgG subclass responses may reflect immune stimulation by a certain type of antigen. For example, polysaccharides preferentially stimulate an IgG2 subclass response, whereas certain proteins induce IgG1/IgG3 or IgG1/IgG4 production.[51,52] A restricted IgG4 response has been described in individuals with chronic antigenic stimulation, for example, filariasis[53] and *Hymenoptera* venom exposure.[54] Interestingly, it has been postulated that fogo selvagem may be precipitated by chronic black fly bites.[10]

PEMPHIGUS VULGARIS AND FOGO SELVAGEM AUTOANTIBODIES

Pemphigus vulgaris autoantibodies may cross-link a cell surface antigen and trigger acantholysis, whereas fogo selvagem autoantibodies may impair the function of an epidermal cell adhesion molecule.

The effect of both bivalent $F(ab')_2$ and monovalent Fab′ fragments of pemphigus vulgaris and fogo selvagem IgG on the epidermis of mice was studied in vivo.[55] Purified IgG fractions were obtained from the serum of two patients with active disease and high titers of pemphigus autoantibodies. Bivalent $F(ab')_2$ fragments were prepared by digestion with pepsin, and monovalent Fab′ fragments were prepared from pemphigus vulgaris and fogo selvagem $F(ab')_2$ by reduction/alkylation of these fragments. The purity of these fragments was tested by sodium dodecylsulfate (SDS) polyacrylamide gel electrophoresis and fragment-specific antisera.

When the $F(ab')_2$ fragments of pemphigus vulgaris and fogo selvagem IgG were injected parenterally into neonatal mice, they bound to the epidermal cell surfaces and produced typical acantholytic lesions without detectable C3 deposition. The monovalent Fab′ fragments of pemphigus vulgaris IgG retained the ability to bind to the epidermal cell surface both in vitro and in vivo and had immunofluorescence titers similar to those of the original IgG fraction from which they were obtained. However, although they were administered in the same doses as the bivalent fragments and bound to the epidermal cell surface in vivo, they did not induce acantholysis in the mice. On the contrary, the Fab′ fragments from fogo selvagem IgG continued to bind their epidermal antigens and induced acantholysis in the neonatal mouse model of fogo selvagem.

Since Fab′ fragments are monovalent and cannot cross-link cell surface antigens, one can speculate that cross-linking of the pemphigus vulgaris antigen by intact IgG or $F(ab')_2$ may be the initial signal in the induction of acantholysis in pemphigus vulgaris. Since intact fogo selvagem IgG, its $F(ab')_2$ and its Fab′ fragments are all pathogenic, it is conceivable that binding of these antibody molecules may impair the function of an epidermal cell adhesion antigen. This, in turn, may precipitate acantholysis. These preliminary observations are currently being investigated in more detail. Should they be confirmed, the immunopathological differences between pemphigus vulgaris and pemphigus foliaceus will be further documented. In pemphigus vulgaris the autoantibodies cross-link a surface antigen and are internalized by the keratinocyte. In fogo selvagem the autoantibody may impair the function of a keratinocyte adhesion molecule, as previously postulated.[56,57]

ACKNOWLEDGMENTS

Supported in part by U.S. Public Health Service Grants RO1-AR32599 and RO1-AR32081 from the National Institutes of Health and a research grant awarded by the Dermatology Foundation.

REFERENCES

1. Lever WF: Pemphigus vulgaris, in WF Lever (ed), *Pemphigus and Pemphigoid*. Springfield, IL, Charles C Thomas, 1965, p 116.
2. Beutner EH, Jordon RE: Demonstration of skin antibodies in sera of patients with pemphigus vulgaris by indirect immunofluorescent staining. *Proc Soc Exp Biol Med* 117:505, 1964.
3. Stanley JR et al: Distinction between epidermal antigens binding pemphigus vulgaris and pemphigus foliaceus autoantibodies. *J Clin Invest* 74:313, 1984.
4. Cazenave P: Pemphigus chronique, général forme rare du pemphigus foliace. *Ann Mal Peu* 1:208, 1844.
5. Perry HO: Pemphigus foliaceus. *Arch Dermatol* 83:52, 1961.
6. Brown MV: Fogo selvagem (pemphigus foliaceus). *Arch Dermatol Syphilol* 69:589, 1954.
7. Azulay RD: Brazilian pemphigus foliaceus. *Int J Dermatol* 21:121, 1982.
8. Diaz LA et al: Endemic pemphigus foliaceus—"fogo selvagem". I. Clinical features and immunopathology. *J Am Acad Dermatol* 20:657, 1989.
9. Stanley JR et al: Antigenic specificity of fogo selvagem autoantibodies is similar to North American pemphigus foliaceus and distinct from pemphigus vulgaris. *J Invest Dermatol* 87:197, 1986.
10. Diaz LA et al: Endemic pemphigus foliaceus—"fogo selvagem". II. Current and historic epidemiologic aspects. *J Invest Dermatol* 92:4, 1989.
11. Robledo MA et al: South-American pemphigus foliaceus: study of an epidemic in El Bagre and Nechi, Colombia, 1982 to 1986. *Br J Dermatol* 118:737, 1988.
12. Castro RM et al: Brazilian pemphigus foliaceus. *Clin Dermatol* 1:22, 1983.
13. Degos MMR et al: Pemphigus chez un maladie traité par penicillamine pour maladie de Wilson. *Bull Soc Fran Dermatol Syphilograph* 76:751, 1969.
14. Tan SG, Rowell NR: Pemphigus-like syndrome induced by *d*-penicillamine. *Br J Dermatol* 95:99, 1976.
15. Lee CW et al: Pemphigus foliaceus induced by rifampicin. *Br J Dermatol* 111:619, 1984.
16. Yokel BK et al: Induction of acantholysis in organ explant cultures by *d*-penicillamine and captopril. *Clin Res* 35:726, 1987.

17. Park MS et al: HLA-DRW4 in 91% of pemphigus vulgaris patients. *Lancet* 2:441, 1979.
18. Brautbar C et al: HLA-DRw4 in pemphigus vulgaris patients in Israel. *Tissue Antigens* 16:238, 1980.
19. Szafer F et al: Detection of disease-specific restriction fragment length polymorphisms in pemphigus vulgaris linked to the DQw1 and DQw3 alleles of the HLA-D region. *Proc Natl Acad Sci USA* 84:6542, 1987.
20. Scharf SJ et al: HLA class II allelic variation and susceptibility to pemphigus vulgaris. *Proc Natl Acad Sci USA* 85:3504, 1988.
21. Sinha AA et al: A newly characterized HLA DQb allele associated with pemphigus vulgaris. *Science* 239:1026, 1988.
22. Scharf SJ et al: Sequence analysis of the HLA-DRb and HLA-DQb loci from three pemphigus vulgaris patients. *Hum Immunol* 22:61, 1988.
23. Moraes JR et al: Brazilian pemphigus susceptibility and resistance associated with HLA. *Clin Res* 37:529, 1989.
24. Diaz LA et al: A syndrome of multiple autoimmune reactivity. *Arch Dermatol* 116:77, 1980.
25. Maize JC et al: Pemphigus foliaceous: a case with serological features of Senear-Usher syndrome and other autoimmune abnormalities. *J Am Acad Dermatol* 7:736, 1982.
26. Kawana S et al: Deposition of the membrane attack complex of complement in pemphigus vulgaris and pemphigus foliaceus skin. *J Invest Dermatol* 92:588, 1989.
27. Hashimoto K et al: Anti-cell surface pemphigus autoantibody stimulates plasminogen activator activity of human epidermal cells: a proposed mechanism for the loss of epidermal cohesion and blister formation. *J Exp Med* 157:259, 1983.
28. Beutner EH et al: Autoantibodies in pemphigus vulgaris. *JAMA* 192:682, 1965.
29. Fitzpatrick RE, Newcomer VD: The correlation of disease activity and pemphigus antibody titers in pemphigus. *Arch Dermatol* 116:285, 1980.
30. Diaz LA et al: Phylogenetic studies with pemphigus and pemphigoid antibodies. *Acta Derm Venereol (Stockh)* 58:537, 1979.
31. Eyre RW, Stanley JR: Identification of pemphigus vulgaris antigen extracted from normal human epidermis and comparison with pemphigus foliaceus antigen. *J Clin Invest* 81:807, 1988.
32. Korman NJ et al: Demonstration of an adhering-junctional molecule (plakoglobin) in the autoantigens of pemphigus foliaceus and pemphigus vulgaris. *N Engl J Med* 321:631, 1989.
33. Jones JCR et al: Further analysis of pemphigus autoantibodies and their use in studies on the heterogeneity, structure, and function of desmosomes. *J Cell Biol* 102:1109, 1986.
34. Moncada B et al: Neonatal pemphigus vulgaris: role of passively transferred pemphigus antibodies. *Br J Dermatol* 106:465, 1982.
35. Storer JS et al: Neonatal pemphigus vulgaris. *J Am Acad Dermatol* 6:929, 1982.
36. Eyre WR, Stanley JR: Maternal pemphigus foliaceus with cell surface antibody bound in neonatal epidermis. *Arch Dermatol* 124:25, 1988.
37. Proenca NG et al: Gravidez em doentes com penfigo foliaceo Sul-Americano (fogo selvagem). *An Brasil Dermatol* 54:239, 1979.
38. McNaab T et al: Structure and function of immunoglobulin domains. V. Binding of immunoglobulin G and fragments to placental membrane preparations. *J Immunol* 117:882, 1976.
39. Berlhe A et al: Molecular charge effects on the protein permeability of the guinea pig placenta. *Placenta* 8:365, 1987.
40. Auerbach R, Bystryn J: Plasmapheresis and immunosuppressive therapy. *Arch Dermatol* 115:728, 1979.
41. Swanson DL, Dahl MV: Pemphigus vulgaris and plasma exchange: clinical and serologic studies. *J Am Acad Dermatol* 4:325, 1981.
42. Roujeau JC et al: Plasma exchange in pemphigus. *Arch Dermatol* 119:215, 1983.
43. Anhalt GJ et al: Induction of pemphigus in neonatal mice by passive transfer of IgG from patients with the disease. *N Engl J Med* 306:1189, 1982.

44. Hashimoto K, Lever WF: An ultrastructural study of cell junctions in pemphigus vulgaris. *Arch Dermatol* 101:287, 1970.
45. Hu C-H et al: Epidermal acantholysis induced in vitro by pemphigus autoantibody: an ultrastructural study. *Am J Pathol* 90:345, 1978.
46. Barnett ML: Effect of pemphigus antibodies on desmosomal structure in vitro. *J Invest Dermatol* 70:141, 1978.
47. Medawar PB: Sheets of pure epidermal epithelium from human skin. *Nature* 148:783, 1941.
48. Fukuyama K et al: Ultrastructural studies of newborn rat epidermis after trypsinization. *J Ultrastruct Res* 46:219, 1974.
49. Roscoe JT et al: Brazilian pemphigus foliaceus autoantibodies are pathogenic to BALB/c mice by passive transfer. *J Invest Dermatol* 85:538, 1985.
50. Rock B et al: Restricted heterogeneity of IgG subclass response in endemic pemphigus foliaceus. *N Engl J Med* 320:1463, 1989.
51. Schur PH: IgG subclasses—a review. *Ann Allergy* 58:89, 1987.
52. Persson MAA et al: IgG subclass-associated affinity differences of specific antibodies in humans. *J Immunol* 140:3875, 1988.
53. Ottesen EA et al: Prominence of IgG4 in the IgG antibody response to human filariasis. *J Immunol* 134:2707, 1985.
54. Aalberse RC et al: Serologic aspects of IgG4 antibodies. I. Prolonged immunization results in an IgG4-restricted response. *J Immunol* 130:722, 1983.
55. Rock B et al: Monovalent Fab′ immunoglobulin fragments from endemic pemphigus foliaceus autoantibodies reproduce the human disease in neonatal BALB/c mice. *J Clin Invest,* in press.
56. Diaz LA, Marcelo CL: Pemphigoid and pemphigus antigens in cultured epidermal cells. *Br J Dermatol* 98:631, 1978.
57. Diaz LA: Molecular structure of the epidermal extracellular spaces: a review. *Int J Dermatol* 18:432, 1979.

SECTION FOUR

DISORDERS OF THE EPIDERMAL APPENDAGES

13

Biology of the Sebaceous Gland and the Pathophysiology of Acne Vulgaris

John S. Strauss

BIOLOGY OF SEBACEOUS GLANDS

Sebaceous glands are found everywhere on the human skin except for the palms, soles, and dorsa of the feet. The sebaceous glands are part of the pilosebaceous unit, and their secretion (sebum) flows through the sebaceous duct into the follicular canal. Sebaceous glands also are found on some mucous membranes. Those in the mouth empty directly onto the surface through the gland duct itself. There is great variation in the size and density of the glands; more glands and larger glands are found on the face and scalp compared with other areas of the body. On much of the face in adults, the sebaceous glands are the predominant portion of the follicle. These follicles are called sebaceous follicles (Fig. 13-1) and are the follicles that are involved in acne.

Sebaceous cells enlarge and contain more lipid as they move in a centripetal direction to the center of the sebaceous acini. Mitotic activity is restricted to the peripheral basal cell layer of the gland. Therefore sebaceous gland development involves both mitosis and lipogenesis, and there is evidence that these two processes are independently controlled. Sebaceous gland secretion is a continuous process and is holocrine in nature. However, the capacity of the unprotected skin to hold lipid is limited, and therefore excess lipid is lost. If the skin is protected, the lipid will continue to accumulate.

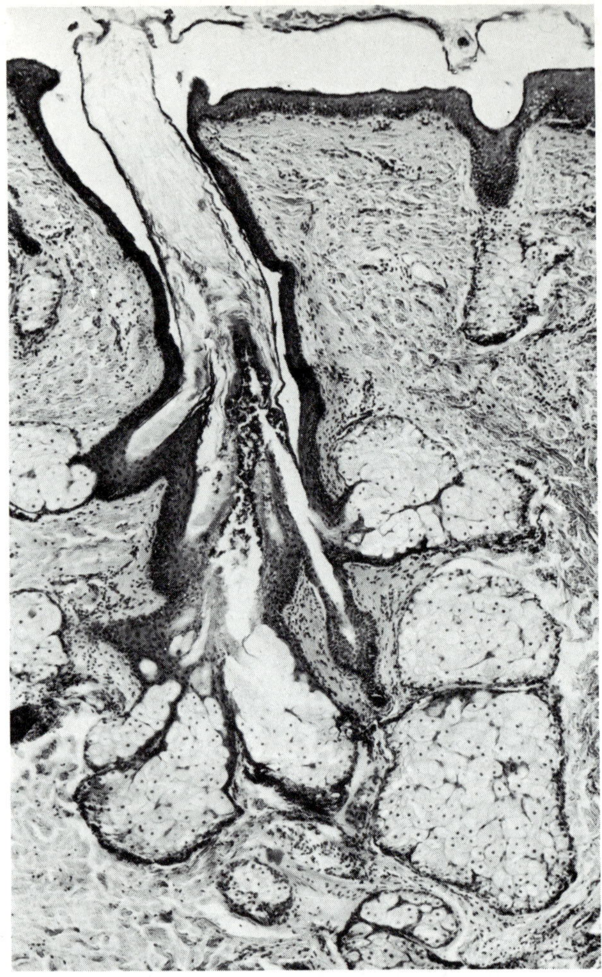

Figure 13-1 Sebaceous follicle from the human cheek. The sebaceous ducts, as well as the widely dilated follicular canal, are filled with keratinous material. A small vellus hair is present. [*From TB Fitzpatrick et al (eds), Dermatology in General Medicine, 3d ed, New York, McGraw-Hill, 1987, p 186.*]

Sebaceous gland growth is under endocrinologic control.[1–3] The prime stimulus for growth in the male is testicular testosterone and its metabolic products such as dihydrotestosterone. In the female, ovarian and adrenal androgens are probably responsible for gland growth. While the glands are large at birth, they undergo atrophy soon afterward and do not enlarge again until the beginning of puberty. Since the sebaceous glands are androgen sensitive, their growth is one of the earliest signs of the pubertal spectrum. After puberty, the glands remain stable in size. In women, they undergo atrophy during menopause, but in men sebaceous gland activity is maintained until approximately 70 years of age. While androgens are of prime importance, there is an important pituitary influence on sebaceous gland activity, and in hypopituitarism, sebaceous gland activity is markedly diminished.

Physiological amounts of estrogens do not influence sebaceous gland development and, therefore, are unimportant in the normal control of the sebaceous gland. However, pharmacologic amounts of estrogen do decrease sebaceous gland activity.[4] This effect is mediated through central inhibition of androgen production. This finding is used in the treatment of severe acne in women.[5]

Because the sebaceous glands are deep in the dermis and do not open directly to the skin surface, it has not been possible to collect sebum, the product of the sebaceous glands, directly. Therefore, skin surface lipids have been used to study sebaceous gland secretion and sebum composition. The skin surface lipids represent a two-compartment system in that they originate from both the epidermis and the sebaceous glands. Since sebaceous and epidermal lipids are distinctly different, the composition of the skin surface lipids will vary depending upon whether the major portion is derived from the epidermis or the sebaceous glands.[6] The approximate composition of sebum and epidermal lipid is given in Table 13-1. Triglycerides and their breakdown products make up approximately two-thirds of both epidermal and sebaceous lipids. Therefore, the concentration of triglycerides and their breakdown products does not vary significantly as the percentage of sebaceous and epidermal lipids changes. On the other hand, since triglycerides are hydrolyzed by bacterial lipases, the concentrations of triglycerides, diglycerides, and free fatty acids may vary greatly in a given individual under various conditions.

Besides triglycerides, the epidermal lipids are cholesterol and cholesterol esters. In contrast, less than 5 percent of sebaceous lipids are cholesterol and cholesterol esters. Wax esters and squalene are uniquely of sebaceous origin and represent the major nontriglyceride fraction of sebum. Therefore,

Table 13-1

APPROXIMATE COMPOSITION OF SEBUM AND EPIDERMAL LIPID

	Sebum, wt (%)	Epidermal Lipid wt (%)
Glycerides and free fatty acids	57.5	65
Wax esters	26.0	—
Squalene	12.0	—
Cholesterol esters	3.0	15
Cholesterol	1.5	20

if most of the skin surface lipids are of epidermal origin, as in childhood, the cholesterol content will be high, whereas the concentration of wax esters and squalene will be low.[7] If, however, most of the skin surface lipid is of sebaceous origin, as in the adult, in whom over 95 percent of facial lipid is from the sebaceous glands,[6] the wax ester and squalene content is high, whereas the cholesterol level is low. Under appropriate conditions, the relative amounts of cholesterol and wax esters or squalene in skin surface lipids can be used as an indication of the relative sebaceous and epidermal contributions to the skin surface lipid.

Since the sebaceous glands are holocrine structures, their secretory activity provides a rough measurement of gland size, and for many years measurements of sebum production have been used to study changes in sebaceous gland activity. It is best to collect the lipids of the forehead by trapping them on absorbing materials such as paper[8] or a dried bentonite slurry.[9] Then the trapped lipid is extracted for quantitative or qualitative analysis. An essential element that must be considered is the contribution of the lipid reservoir of the epidermis. In the most common method, in use for over 20 years, surface lipids are depleted for only 30 minutes.[8] It has now been established that cutaneous reservoir depletion takes as long as 12 to 14 h, and a new collection method takes this fact into consideration.[9] The surface samples are obviously contaminated by epidermal lipids, but less than 5 percent of forehead lipids are of epidermal origin. Therefore, within the limits of the technique, the collected lipids do represent a measure of sebum production and can be used to detect physiological as well as drug-induced changes in sebaceous glands.

ACNE VULGARIS

Acne vulgaris is usually classified as a disease of the sebaceous glands, but it should be classified as a disease of the pilosebaceous unit since the lesions develop in the upper portion of the follicular canal and do not involve the glands primarily. Acne is the most common disease seen by dermatologists, accounting for over 25 percent of all dermatologic office visits. Physicians involved in primary care delivery are also likely to see acne as a presenting complaint quite frequently. Nonetheless, since 80 to 90 percent of all individuals develop some acne in the second and third decades, it is obvious that only a small percentage of those with acne actually consult physicians.

Acne is occasionally present at birth or in the neonatal period. However, it is not until puberty that it becomes a common problem. The disease may be an early manifestation of the pubertal spectrum, and in young females it may precede menarche by more than a year. Acne reaches a peak incidence during the middle to late teenage period, and then the number of cases gradually decreases. In women, acne may persist through the third decade or even later. Acne is slightly more common in males, and severe acne is definitely more common in males.

Etiology and Pathogenesis

While the basic cause of acne is unknown, there is considerable information on its pathogenesis. The disease is multifactorial. Knowledge of the various factors involved in the disease is important, since treatment may be directed at one or more of these causative factors.

Acne develops in sebaceous follicles (Fig. 13-1). These follicles open to the surface by a widely dilated follicular orifice (visible as the so-called pore of the skin of the face) and are wide throughout their entire length. A vellus hair is always present in the follicle, but as it is very small, it may not be apparent from examination of a single microscopic section. Short ducts connect the huge, deeply situated, multiacinar glands to the large follicular duct.

The follicular canal contains keratinous material from the wall of the canal, sebum from the sebaceous glands, and a variable microbial flora. These are all involved in the pathogenesis of the disease.

The primary structural change is an alteration in the pattern of keratinization in the lower portion of the follicular infundibulum (the infrainfundibulum).[10] Normally the keratinous squamae in the follicular canal are loosely organized. In the earliest lesion (the microcomedo), which is not visible clinically, the keratinous material becomes more dense. The cells of the microcomedo are much more coherent and contain amorphous material, which is probably generated by lipid during the process of keratinization. Kinetic studies have demonstrated that there is an increase in cellular turnover, so that more cells are generated per unit period of time.[11]

As a group, patients with acne produce more sebum than do normal persons, and patients with severe acne secrete more sebum than those with mild acne.[12] Nevertheless, there is considerable variation in sebum production within the group of patients with acne, indicating that the disease is not related solely to sebaceous gland activity. Many other facts indicate that sebum plays a role in the overall pathogenesis of the disease. These include the following: sebum is comedogenic[13]; sebum causes inflammation when injected into the skin[14]; acne occurs in the neonatal period when the sebaceous glands are well developed; acne appears as part of the pubertal spectrum at a time when sebaceous gland development occurs; and acne can be controlled by orally administered estrogens, antiandrogens such as cyproterone acetate, and spironolactone and retinoids, all of which inhibit sebaceous gland activity.

Several studies have been done to attempt to demonstrate that sebum from acne patients is different from that in normal individuals. In general, no consistent patterns of change have been observed.[15] However, there is a significant decrease in the level of linoleic acid in sebum,[16] and considerable evidence has been presented to link the low levels of linoleic acid to the pathogenesis of acne.[17] It has been postulated that the low levels of linoleic acid represent the dilution of this essential fatty acid, which is not synthesized in the sebaceous glands, by the newly synthesized sebaceous lipids in the large sebaceous glands characteristically found in patients with acne. In turn, the low concentration of linoleate in sebum induces a localized essential follicular fatty acid deficiency, with the characteristic responses of hyperkeratosis and decreased barrier function within the follicle.[17]

The predominant organism in the follicular flora is an anaerobic pleomorphic diphtheroid, *Propionibacterium acnes.* In the acne age range from 11 to 15 years, practically no *P. acnes* are found in individuals without acne, whereas in patients with acne the geometric mean is 114,800 *P. acnes* per square centimeter.[18] Similar differences are found in 16- to 20-year-old groups, but in older individuals the number of organisms is the same in those with and without acne. While staphylococci, micrococci, and yeasts (*Pityrosporum* species) are also found in the follicle, there is no evidence that they are involved in the acne process.

In spite of the importance of *P. acnes* in the pathogenesis of acne, acne is not a bacterial disease per se, and its response to therapy with antibiotics is not what one would expect from a bacterial disease. Instead, *P. acnes* generates inflammatory agents. Extracellular products of *P. acnes* include enzymes such as lipases, proteases, and hyaluronidases, as well as chemotactic factors. It is these extracellular products and, in turn, their products that cause inflammatory changes.

Indirect evidence that *P. acnes* is responsible for lipolysis and inflammation is supplied by experiments in which suspensions of this organism have been injected into cysts.[19] The injection of viable organisms causes rupture of the cysts and severe inflammation of the surrounding tissues. Very little inflammation is produced by the injection of nonviable organisms into cysts, and injection of living organisms into the dermis induces only a slight to moderate infiltrate of neutrophils.

Clinical Manifestations

The primary site of acne is the face, and to a lesser degree the back, chest, and shoulders. On the trunk, lesions tend to be more numerous near the midline. Acne is a pleomorphic disease consisting of noninflammatory and inflammatory lesions. While one type of lesion may be predominant, close observation usually reveals several types of lesions. Comedones, which are the primary lesions of acne, are noninflammatory (Fig. 13-2). Closed comedones (whiteheads) may be difficult to visualize. They appear as pale, slightly elevated, small papules. They often do not have a clinically visible orifice. Stretching of the skin is an aid in detecting these lesions. Since the closed comedones are the precursors of the large inflammatory lesions, they are of considerable clinical importance. Open comedones (blackheads) develop from closed comedones as the orifice dilates. The open comedo is flat or slightly raised, with a central follicular impaction. While comedones are the primary lesions of acne, they are not

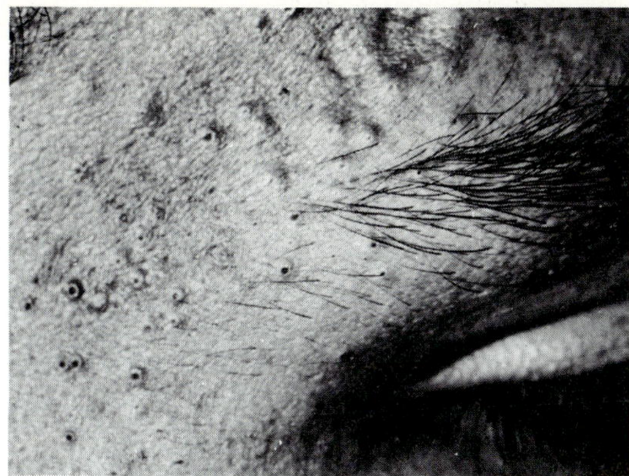

Figure 13-2 Blackheads and whiteheads on the temple. (*From JS Strauss, AM Kligman.*[19])

unique to this disease, since they may be seen under other conditions (e.g., so-called senile comedones commonly seen in the periorbital area of older persons).

Inflammatory lesions in acne vary from small papules with an inflammatory areola to pustules to large, tender, fluctuant nodules (Fig. 13-3). All these lesions show an inflammatory infiltrate in the dermis and, as indicated below, have a common pathogenesis; their appearance depends on the size and location of the infiltrate.

Pathology

Comedo development starts in the midportion of the follicle as an expanding mass of lipid-impregnated keratinous material, resulting in thinning and ballooning of the follicular wall. Gradually, more keratinous material accumulates, and, as it does, further thinning and dilatation of the follicular wall occur. The fully formed comedo has a thin wall and minute sebaceous appendages, if these can be found at all. The open comedo has a patulous orifice, and the keratinous material is arranged in a lamellar concentric fashion (Fig. 13-4). With lipid stains, it can be shown that the keratin is permeated by lipid. *P. acnes* is alo present. In cross sections, the orderly arrangement of the keratinous material consists of smaller whorls of lamellar material centered on appendageal structures such as the hairs. In fact, most comedones contain multiple hairs. The closed comedo differs from the open comedo in that the keratinous material is not as compact, as the follicular orifice is narrow and not distended (Fig. 13-5).

The fully developed open comedo usually is not the site of inflammatory changes unles it is traumatized by the patient. Inflammatory changes develop in closed comedones. Initially there is an area of inflammation along the follicular wall, which then ruptures. Once complete rupture has occurred, the entire contents of the comedo are extruded into the dermis,

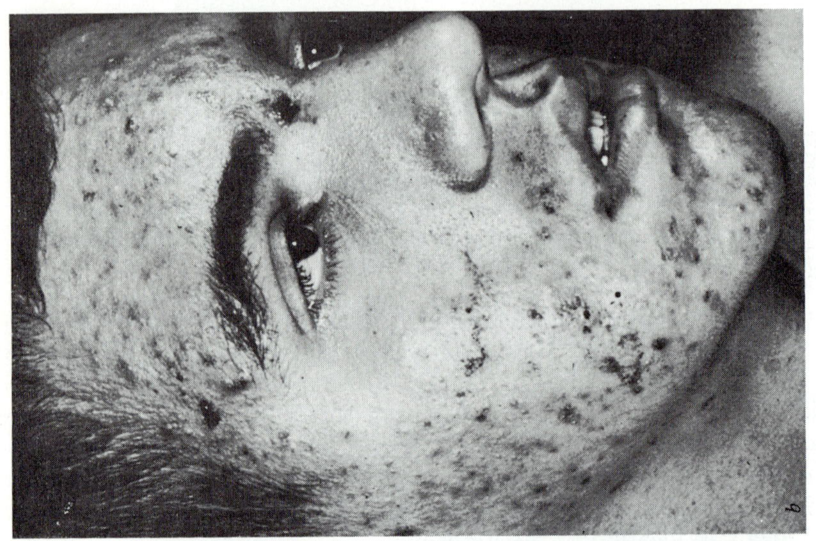

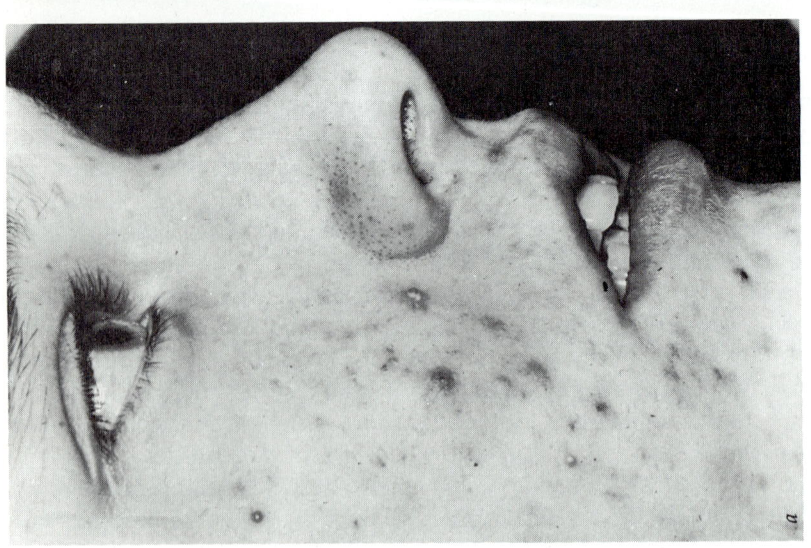

Figure 13-3 (*a*) Mild and (*b*) severe acne. In both cases many different lesions are present. [*From TB Fitzpatrick et al (eds), Dermatology in General Medicine, 3d ed, New York, McGraw-Hill, 1987, p 670.*]

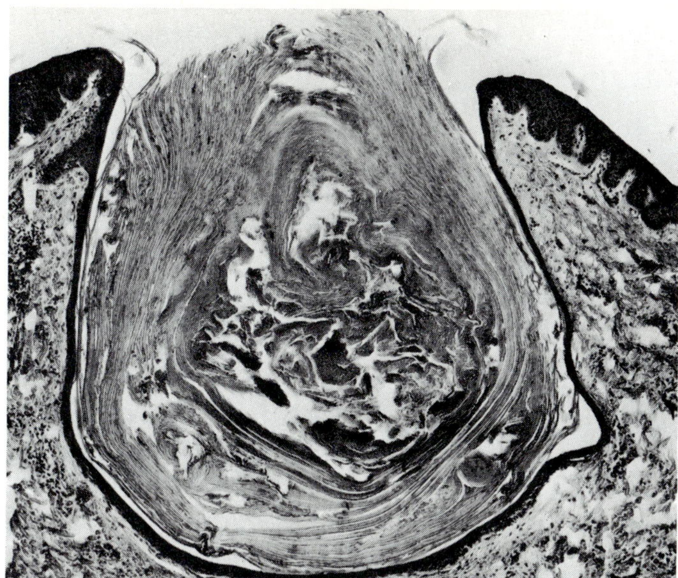

Figure 13-4 Open comedo. The mouth of the follicle is widely dilated. The comedo is composed of a lamellar keratinous mass impregnated with lipid. Bacteria are also present. The sebaceous glands have undergone atrophy. (*From JS Strauss, AM Kligman.*[19])

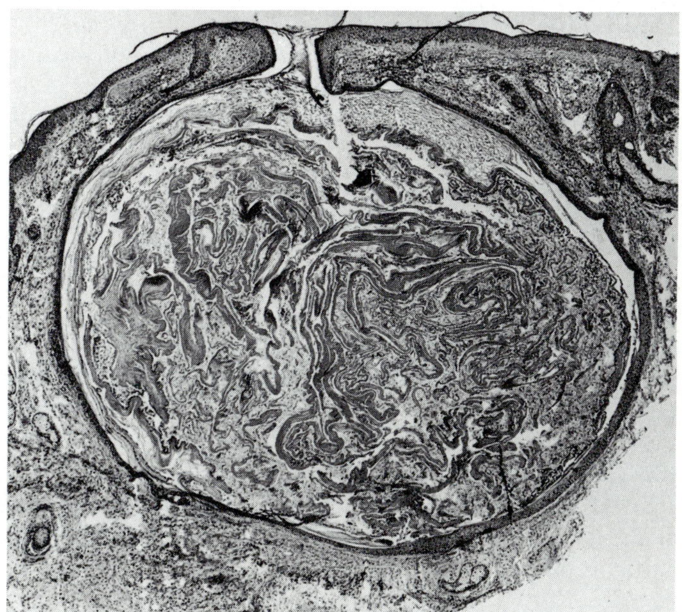

Figure 13-5 Closed comedo. The structure of the lesion is similar to that of the open comedo. However, the orifice is small and the contents of the comedo are not as compact. (*From JS Strauss, AM Kligman.*[19])

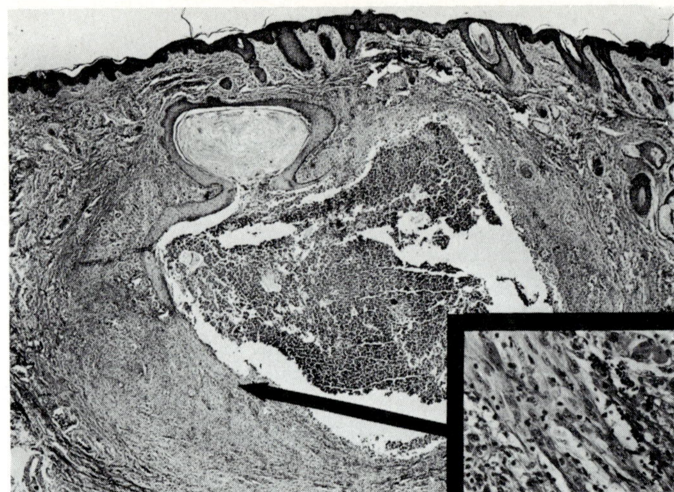

Figure 13-6 Ruptured closed comedo. In the upper portion of the lesion there is lamellar keratinous material from the comedo. Below this, necrotic material is being encapsulated by new epithelial cells. These new cells are shown in higher magnification in the insert. Multinucleated giant cells are present in the inflammatory infiltrate in the dermis. (*From JS Strauss, AM Kligman.*[19])

exciting a greater inflammatory response. Depending upon the site and extent of the inflammation, these ruptured lesions may appear as a pustule, a nodule, or a nodule surmounted by a pustule.

The sheaths of cells grow out from the epidermis and/or the appendageal structures in an attempt to encapsulate the inflammatory reaction (Fig. 13-6). This encapsulation may be complete, so that the inflammatory infiltrate appears to be within the follicle, but it often is far from complete, and further rupture may occur, leading to multichanneled tracts, as can be seen in many acne scars. Fibrous contraction also contributes to scar formation.

Therapy

There are four principles of therapy, which are based on the current knowledge of the pathogenesis of the disease. These principles are: (1) correct the pattern of altered keratinization within the follicle, (2) decrease sebaceous gland activity, (3) decrease the *P. acnes* population and/or decrease the generation of inflammatory substances by the bacterial population, and (4) produce anti-inflammatory effects. However, rigid guidelines cannot be established, since there is likely to be considerable overlap in the type of lesions in any one case, and often combination therapy is indicated.

To Correct the Defect in Keratinization

The most effective drug used to change the pattern of keratinization is topically applied vitamin A acid. Vitamin A acid is comedolytic,[20] and at an ultrastructural level the process of follicular wall keratinization returns toward normal.[21] The drug may produce irritation, and some patients cannot tolerate its use, even if it is applied as infrequently as every 2 or 3 days. Patients should be cautioned about sun exposure while using vitamin A, because the drug may cause an exaggerated sunburn. Salicylic acid also is comedolytic. Benzoyl peroxide, although predominantly an antibacterial agent, also has weak comedolytic activity.

When acne surgery is done, the comedo is extruded to the skin surface; thus this procedure can be considered an aid in changing the pattern of keratinization. If acne surgery is not performed with care, the contents of the comedo can be extruded into the dermis, resulting in increased inflammation. For this reason, this procedure should be done by a trained person and not by the patient.

To Decrease Sebaceous Gland Activity

Suppression of sebaceous gland activity is important in treating acne, especially inflammatory acne. It is known that pharmacologic dosages of estrogens will inhibit sebaceous glands,[4] and estrogens, usually given as oral contraceptives containing high concentrations of estrogen, may be used in the management of acne.[5] Estrogens are not indicated for routine use; they should be given to women with recalcitrant acne, and the physician must assess the risk/benefit ratio carefully before starting any patient on therapy. Since estrogens do not have any known effect on existing lesions but appear to work by limiting the contribution of sebum to the inflammatory process in new lesions, their clinical effect is delayed while the preexisting lesions undergo their natural involution.

There are new developments in the use of antiandrogens in the management of acne. Cyproterone acetate, used in conjunction with estrogen (an oral contraceptive combination available in Europe), is more effective in suppressing sebum production and improving acne than estrogen alone in women[22]; cyproterone acetate given alone is effective in men, although it has many side effects.[23] While cyproterone acetate is not available in the United States, spironolactone, which also has locally acting antiandrogenic properties, has been shown to be useful in the management of severe acne.[24]

There is evidence that a few patients with acne have partial hydroxylase blocks that influence adrenal steroid metabolism, leading to increased androgen production.[25] In these patients, excess androgen production can be blocked by the administration of exogenous adrenocorticosteroids through a feedback mechanism.

Probably the most exciting development in acne therapy in recent years has been the use of the synthetic oral retinoid, isotretinoin (13-*cis*-retinoic acid). This drug has proved to be extremely effective in the control of severe nodulocystic acne.[26] Not only has it produced remarkable improvement, but the remissions after cessation of treatment have been very long.[27] While there may be long-term inhibition of sebaceous gland secretion, this is by no means seen in all patients[28] and cannot be considered the sole reason for the long-term remissions. The other possible mechanisms of action, as well as the clinical effectiveness of isotretinoin, have recently been summarized.[29] The drug also has been shown to be effective in controlling disorders of keratinization and to have anti-inflammatory effects, but these activities do not explain the protracted remissions. *P. acnes* counts are suppressed for long periods of time,[30] but it is not known whether the decrease is responsible for the long-term remissions.

The excitement surrounding the use of isotretinoin must be tempered by the many side effects produced by this drug. In essence, every patient treated with isotretinoin develops signs and symptoms of chronic hypervitaminosis A. Most of these side effects are integumentary (dry skin, dry mucous membranes, cheilitis, dermatitis, pruritus, desquamation of the palms and soles). Certain laboratory abnormalities, such as a reversible hypertriglyceridemia accompanied by a decrease in high-density lipoproteins, are also common. Other side effects, such as skeletal hyperkeratosis and pseudotumor cerebri, both of which are part of the hypervitaminosis A syndrome, have also been reported. Of greatest importance, however, is the fact that the drug, while not mutagenic, has marked teratogenic effects on organogenesis during early fetal development. Retinoid embryopathy is severe.[31] The problem is a serious one,[32] and because of this, there are strict guidelines* for its use in women of childbearing age.[33] These guidelines must be followed, and those physicians who are not well informed and well trained in the use of isotretinoin should not use the drug under any circumstances.

Superficial x-ray therapy can produce temporary inhibition of the sebaceous glands. Although it was used in the past for the treatment of acne, it is not used now.

To Reduce the P. acnes Population

P. acnes is probably responsible for the generation of inflammatory substances; therefore, the suppression of the intrafollicular bacterial population is important in controlling inflammatory acne. Benzoyl peroxide is an extremely effective topical antimicrobial agent,[34] and preparations containing benzoyl peroxide are the most popular agents for the topical control of the follicular *P. acnes* population. Topical antimicrobials are used for the same purpose.

Orally administered antibiotics are widely used in the treatment of acne. In fact, 10 percent of all tetracycline sold in the United States is used for the treatment of acne. Since acne is not a bacterial disease per se, the therapeutic response is not fast, as in true bacterial infections such as cellulitis. Improvement may take a month or more, since that much time is required for the existing lesions to undergo involution. While tetracycline is the most commonly used antibiotic for acne, erythromycin is equally effective. Minocycline is probably the most effective antibiotic for control-

**Guidelines are also provided by the manufacturer in the package insert.*

ling the inflammatory component of acne, but its comparative cost at this time precludes its use unless the patient does not respond to other antibiotics. In addition, pigment deposition may occur in the skin during minocycline therapy.

A rare complication of antibiotic therapy is the development of a gram-negative folliculitis.[35] With prolonged antibiotic therapy, gram-negative organisms may proliferate in the anterior nares and spread out onto the surrounding skin. The clinical lesions of gram-negative folliculitis are either multiple pustules with an intense inflammatory areola or deep, indolent nodules. This complication may easily be overlooked and is suggested by a sudden inflammatory flare with pustules or nodules in a patient who is otherwise improving on antibiotic therapy. Culture is necessary, and appropriate antibiotic therapy should be governed by the results of sensitivity studies.

To Produce an Anti-inflammatory Effect

The anti-inflammatory effect of adrenocorticosteroids may be utilized in the treatment of acne. It is preferable to use them intralesionally in order to prevent the side effects that may follow high-dose oral therapy. If proper attention is given to the concentration of the drug as well as to the total dosage used, intralesional steroids are safe and highly effective in severe nodulocystic acne.

Since inflammatory lesions develop in closed comedones and closed comedones are removed during acne surgery, this form of therapy can be considered to have an anti-inflammatory effect.

OTHER ACNE-LIKE DISEASES

Acne Conglobata

Acne conglobata is generally considered a separate entity from acne vulgaris because of its occurrence at a later period and its chronic, unremitting course. Patients with acne conglobata have a mixture of comedones, papules, pustules, nodules, abscesses, cysts, and scars on the back, buttocks, chest, and, to a lesser extent, the abdomen, shoulders, neck, face, upper arms, and thighs. The comedones often have multiple openings. The inflammatory lesions are large, tender, and dusky colored, and they discharge a foul-smelling serous, purulent, or mucoid material. Subcutaneous dissection with the formation of multichanneled sinus tracts is common. Healing results in depressed or keloidal scars.

While some lesions may be sterile or show only the presence of resident coagulase-negative staphylococci and anaerobic diphtheroids, it is common to isolate coagulase-positive staphylococci. Occasionally, β-hemolytic streptococci are found. The presence of a chronic infection may be reflected by the presence of a normochromic, normocytic anemia, an elevated white blood count with an increased percentage of neutrophils, and an increased sedimentation rate. There is no evidence that these patients have decreased gamma globulins, and the gamma globulins may even be elevated. The fasting blood sugar and glucose tolerance tests are usually normal.

Since lesions may occur in the axillary and inguinal regions, the disease may resemble hidradenitis suppurativa. In fact, the latter disease has been considered to form part of a triad with dissecting perifolliculitis of the scalp. It would appear, however, that these are separate entities, especially since both dissecting perifolliculitis of the scalp and hidradenitis suppurativa may occur alone.

The management of these patients is a very difficult problem, and even if there is improvement, it often is temporary. Therapy with the appropriate systemic antibiotic as determined by in vitro sensitivity studies is indicated, as are injections of corticosteroids directly in the lesions on frequent occasions. Systemic corticosteroids are useful; however, recurrence of the disease is common when they are discontinued. Surgical debridement, surgical incision, and surgical excision are also useful adjuncts to therapy, although the extent of involvement may make this an overwhelming task. The oral retinoids often are of use in these patients, but the precautions about their use, discussed earlier in this chapter, should be observed.

Miscellaneous Acne-like Diseases

In addition to the types of acne described above, there are other miscellaneous acneform disorders. Acne can be seen in newborns as a result of stimulation of the sebaceous glands in utero. Adrenocorticosteroids may induce acne, which often is very prominent on the back and chest. In contrast to acne vulgaris, comedones are almost always absent and the lesions are all papulopustular. Other drugs that may produce acne are halogens, isonicotinic acid, diphenylhydantoin, and lithium carbonate. Acne may occur from industrial exposure to coal tar derivatives, cutting oils, and chlorinated hydrocarbons. A highly inflammatory, severe form of acne, similar to acne conglobata, may be seen particularly on the trunk in individuals living in the tropics. Acne can be produced by certain cosmetics and pomades, from overwashing, and from repetitive rubbing (e.g., from a chin strap of a football helmet).

Rosacea

Rosacea is a chronic disorder of the face in middle-aged and older persons, characterized by a vascular component (erythema and telangiectases), with or without an acneform component (papules, pustules, nodules). The onset of rosacea is insidious; most patients cannot state when it started. Initially, there is transient vascular dilatation with varying erythema. Primary involvement occurs over the blush area of the cheeks and nose. The chin and central portion of the forehead also may be involved. While the lesions are intermittent initially, eventually persistent erythema accompanied by telangiectases appears. The areas of erythema blanch on diascopy. There is no adequate explanation for the vascular dilation.

The acneform component is similar to acne vulgaris. The predominant lesions are papules and pustules, although in rare instances nodules may also appears. In contrast to acne vulgaris, comedones are rare.

Rosacea may be accompanied by hyperplasia of the soft tissues of the nose, a condition known as rhinophyma. Rhinophyma is more common in men. The lower portion of the nose is involved first. There is irregular thickening of the skin, and the follicular orifices are enlarged. The color of the skin, which is not uniform, varies from bright to purplish red. The amount of thickening varies and, in some instances, the adjacent portions of the cheeks are involved.

Ocular lesions, including blepharitis, conjunctivitis, episcleritis, iritis, and keratitis, may be seen in patients with rosacea. The incidence of eye disease depends on the source of the patient population. Thus, in 134 rosacea patients seen in a general hospital, there were only 4 with ocular lesions; in contrast, 99 of 104 rosacea patients seen in an eye hospital had ocular lesions.[36] Blepharitis and conjunctivitis are most common. Keratitis, while less common, is more serious, since ulceration and ultimate impairment of vision often occur.

In general, the acneform component of this disease is treated similarly to acne vulgaris. The systemic administration of broad-spectrum antibiotics has been of great help in the management of the acne-like lesions and also has been reported to be of benefit in diminishing the erythema. It is reported that rosacea keratitis may be improved by tetracycline therapy.[37] Topical corticosteroids may be used for the inflammatory component, but treatment should be of short duration, as corticosteroids may accentuate the telangiectases. There is recent evidence that metronidazole, administered either orally[38] or topically,[39] is helpful in managing patients with acne rosacea. There is no definite treatment for the erythema, but theoretically it is advisable to avoid vascular stimuli such as heat, cold, excessive sunlight, and ingestion of hot liquids, highly seasoned foods, and alcoholic beverages. Rhinophyma can be treated surgically.

REFERENCES

1. Ebling FJ: Hormonal control and methods of measuring sebaceous gland activity. *J Invest Dermatol* 62:161, 1974.
2. Shuster S, Thody AJ: The control and measurement of sebum secretion. *J Invest Dermatol* 62:172, 1974.
3. Pochi PE, Strauss JS: Endocrinologic control of the development and activity of the human sebaceous gland. *J Invest Dermatol* 62:191, 1974.
4. Pochi PE, Strauss JS: Sebaceous gland suppression with ethinyl estradiol and diethylstilbesterol. *Arch Dermatol* 108:210, 1973.
5. Strauss JS, Pochi PE: Effect of cyclic progestin-estrogen therapy on the sebum and acne in women. *JAMA* 190:815, 1964.
6. Greene RS et al: Anatomical variation in the amount and composition of human skin surface lipid. *J Invest Dermatol* 54:240, 1970.
7. Ramasastry P et al: Chemical composition of human skin surface lipids from birth to puberty. *J Invest Dermatol* 54:139, 1970.
8. Strauss JS, Pochi PE: The quantitative gravimetric determination of sebum production. *J Invest Dermatol* 36:293, 1961.

9. Harris HH et al: Sustainable rates of sebum secretion in acne patients and matched normal control subjects. *J Am Acad Dermatol* 8:200, 1983.
10. Knutson DD: Ultrastructural observations in acne vulgaris: the normal sebaceous follicle and acne lesions. *J Invest Dermatol* 62:228, 1974.
11. Plewig G: Follicular keratinization. *J Invest Dermatol* 62:308, 1974.
12. Pochi PE, Strauss JS: Sebum production, casual sebum levels, titratable acidity of sebum, and urinary fractional 17-ketosteroid excretion in males with acne. *J Invest Dermatol* 43:383, 1964.
13. Kligman AM et al: Comedogenicity of human sebum. *Arch Dermatol* 102:267, 1970.
14. Strauss JS, Pochi PE: Intracutaneous injection of sebum and comedones. *Arch Dermatol* 92:443, 1965.
15. Strauss JS et al: Acne: perspectives. *J Invest Dermatol* 62:321, 1974.
16. Morello AM et al: Octadecadienoic acids in the skin surface lipids of acne patients and normal subjects. *J Invest Dermatol* 66:319, 1976.
17. Downing DT et al: Essentially fatty acids and acne. *J Am Acad Dermatol* 14:221, 1986.
18. Leyden JJ et al: Propionibacterium levels in patients with and without acne vulgaris. *J Invest Dermatol* 65:382, 1975.
19. Strauss JS, Kligman AM: The pathologic dynamics of acne vulgaris. *Arch Dermatol* 82:779, 1960.
20. Kligman AM et al: Topical vitamin A acid in acne vulgaris. *Arch Dermatol* 99:469, 1969.
21. Plewig G, Braun-Falco O: Kinetics of epidermis and adnexa following vitamin A acid in the human. *Acta Derm Venereol (Stockh)* 55 [Suppl 74]:87, 1975.
22. Colver GB et al: Cyproterone acetate and two doses of oestrogen in female acne; a double-blind comparison. *Br J Dermatol* 118:95, 1988.
23. Misch KJ et al: Response of male acne to antiandrogen therapy with cyproterone acetate. *Dermatologica* 173:139, 1986.
24. Goodfellow A et al: Oral spironolactone improves acne vulgaris and reduces sebum excretion. *Br J Dermatol* 111:209, 1984.
25. Rose LE et al: Adrenocortical hydroxylase deficiencies in acne vulgaris. *J Invest Dermatol* 66:324, 1976.
26. Farrell LN et al: The treatment of severe cystic acne with 13-cis-retinoic acid: evaluation of sebum production and the clinical response in a multiple-dose trial. *J Am Acad Dermatol* 6:602, 1980.
27. Peck GL et al: Isotretinoin versus placebo in the treatment of cystic acne: a randomized double-blind study. *J Am Acad Dermatol* 6:735, 1982.
28. Strauss JS, Stranieri AM: Changes in long-term sebum production from isotretinoin therapy. *J Am Acad Dermatol* 6:751, 1982.
29. Shalita AR et al: Isotretinoin revisited. *Cutis* 42:1, 1988.
30. Leyden JJ et al: Qualitative and quantitative changes in cutaneous bacteria associated with systemic isotretinoin therapy for acne conglobata. *J Invest Dermatol* 86:390, 1986.
31. Lammer EJ et al: Retinoic acid embryopathy. *N Engl J Med* 313:837, 1985.
32. Stern RS: When a uniquely effective drug is teratogenic: the case of isotretinoin. *N Engl J Med* 320:1007, 1989.
33. Pochi PE et al: Guidelines for prescribing isotretinoin (Accutane) in the treatment of female acne patients of childbearing potential. *J Am Acad Dermatol* 19:920, 1988.
34. Fulton JE Jr et al: Studies on the mechanism of action of topical benzoyl peroxide and vitamin A acid in acne vulgaris. *J Cutan Pathol* 1:191, 1974.
35. Leyden JJ et al: Gram-negative folliculitis: a complication of antibody therapy in acne vulgaris. *Br J Dermatol* 88:533, 1973.
36. Borrie P: Rosacea with special references to its ocular manifestations. *Br J Dermatol* 65:458, 1953.
37. Knight A, Vickers CFH: A follow-up of tetracycline-treated rosacea with special reference to rosacea keratitis. *Br J Dermatol* 93:577, 1975.
38. Saihan EM, Burton JL: A double-blind trial of metronidazole vs oxytetracycline therapy for acne. *Br J Dermatol* 102:443, 1980.
39. Bleicher PA et al: Topical metronidazole therapy for rosacea. *Arch Dermatol* 123:609, 1987.

14

Normal and Abnormal Eccrine Sweat Gland Function

Kenzo Sato, Minoru Ohtsuyama, Yuichi Suzuki, and Fusako Sato

In humans, thermoregulation is achieved primarily through evaporated heat loss, which is regulated by perspiration (eccrine sweating). In tropical environments or under extremely hot industrial conditions, a person can perspire as much as 10 liters/day. Because profuse sweating causes an obligatory loss of water and electrolytes, conservation of electrolytes by ductal reabsorption, with resultant secretion of hypotonic sweat, is a vital role that the eccrine sweat gland plays in adaptation to heat.

Inadequate capacity to perspire properly leads to heat intolerance (e.g., in patients with anhidrotic ectodermal dysplasia or poorly acclimatized individuals suddenly exposed to a high ambient temperature). Likewise, patients with cystic fibrosis, whose eccrine sweat ducts are variously defective in reabsorbing NaCl, are intolerant of a hot environment because they lose excessive amounts of salts in sweat. Miliaria, or prickly heat, is a condition that is caused by interference with the delivery of sweat to the skin surface. Hyperhidrosis is a troublesome condition in which perspiration is far in excess of the physiological need. It usually involves the palms, soles, and axillae but can also occur in other areas of the body.

While the role of the eccrine sweat gland in the pathophysiology of the skin is still poorly understood, it is of interest that two major organic molecules excreted in sweat are lactate and urea, which are known to be efficacious for ichthyotic or dry skin when applied topically as dermatologic preparations. Excessive dry skin and the resultant asteatotic dermatitis are common occurrences in winter months. Epidermal growth factor and interleukins have also been identified in human sweat, although their roles in cutaneous pathophysiology remain to be studied. It has been shown that, like the kidney, the sweat gland potentially performs an excretory function. It excretes urea, ammonia, other organic metabolites, drugs, immunoglobulins, and mediators of inflammation such as histamine, kallikrein, interleukins, and prostaglandins.[1-6]

The eccrine sweat gland is one of the target organs in cystic fibrosis, the most frequent semilethal recessive disease affecting the Caucasian population. An increased NaCl concentration in sweat is still regarded as one of the most reliable diagnostic criteria for cystic fibrosis. Two recent observations made in cystic fibrosis sweat glands, namely, chloride impermeability of the sweat duct[7] and defective β-adrenergic function of the secretory coil,[8] have triggered renewed interest in cystic fibrosis research.

The eccrine sweat gland is perhaps the most active exocrine gland in terms of fluid and electrolyte secretion. Due to its accessibility for in vivo and in vitro studies in humans, the eccrine sweat gland is potentially an excellent model system for studying either the mechanism of stimulus secretion coupling or membrane transport.

GROSS AND FINE MORPHOLOGY OF ECCRINE AND APOECCRINE SWEAT GLANDS

There are three histologically distinguishable types of sweat glands: the eccrine, apocrine, and apoeccrine glands.[9,10] In humans, 2 to 3 million eccrine sweat glands are distributed throughout the skin on all parts of the body except the lips and the inner surface of the foreskin. The number of sweat glands remains unchanged throughout life. Apocrine glands are present mainly in the axillae, pubis, umbilicus, and external ear canals, whereas apoeccrine glands are present in the axillae.[9]

The eccrine sweat gland consists of two components: the secretory coil, which secretes a nearly isotonic sweat, and the duct, through which NaCl is reabsorbed in excess of water, producing hypotonic sweat on the skin surface. The size of the sweat gland varies as much as fivefold among different individuals, which largely correlates with individual (and perhaps regional) differences in the rate of sweating (the maximal sweat rate ranges from 2 to 20 nl/min per gland).[11]

The secretory coil is composed of three distinct cell types: clear, dark (mucoid), and myoepithelial.[12] The fine morphology of the clear cell is characterized by the presence of intricate basal infoldings and the intercellular canaliculi (Fig. 14-1). The basal infoldings stain densely with ouabain-sensitive, Na-K–dependent paranitrophenyl phosphatase[13] (which reflects the catalytic activity of Na-K-ATPase) and bind labeled ouabain.[14] In contrast, the intracellular canaliculus, which is actually a pouch made up of the luminal membrane opening into the lumen, is free of both ouabain binding and paranitrophenyl phosphatase activity.[13] This supports

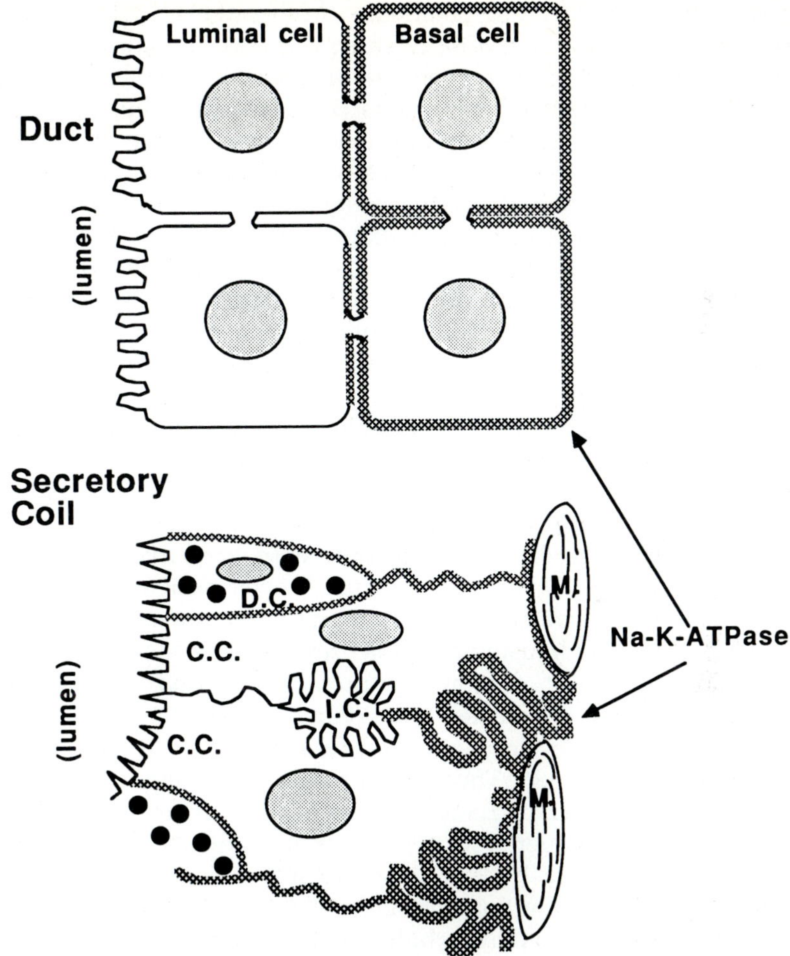

Figure 14-1 Schematic illustration of the ultrastructure of the eccrine sweat gland. The hatched thick tracings of the cell membrane indicate the localization of Na-K-ATPase. *Upper panel,* duct; *lower panel,* secretory coil. DC = dark cell; CC = clear cell; M = myoepithelial cell; IC = intercellular canaliculus.

the notion that the basolateral membrane, but not the luminal membrane, is the Na-pump site. The presence of abundant mitochondria in clear cells is consistent with the thesis that clear cells are mainly responsible for secretion of water and electrolytes.

The secretory coils' dark cells are easily discernible because of the presence in the cytoplasm of many electron-dense *dark cell granules.* Although the function of the dark cells is unknown, secretion of periodic acid-Schiff (PAS)-positive sweat glycoproteins may be one of their functions.[15]

Myoepithelial cells are located at the periphery of the secretory tubule and are filled with dense myofilaments. Myoepithelial cells are spindle-shaped and contract in response to cholinergic but not adrenergic stimulation.[16] The function of the myoepithelium may be to provide mechanical support for the secretory coil wall against the increase in luminal hydrostatic pressure rather than simply to pump out preformed sweat.[16]

The duct is composed of two layers of cells: basal and luminal ductal cells. Although ductal cells all look alike at the light-microscopic level, basal (or peripheral) cells are morphologically and functionally distinct from luminal cells. The basal ductal cells are replete with mitochondria, and the entire circumference of their cell membranes is rich in ouabain-sensitive, Na-K–dependent paranitrophenyl phosphatase activity[13] (Fig. 14-1), suggesting that the entire cell membrane is involved in Na^+ pumping for ductal Na^+ absorption. In contrast, the luminal ductal cells have fewer mitochondria, much less ouabain-sensitive paranitrophenyl phosphatase activity, and a dense layer of tonofilaments near the luminal membrane (which is often referred to as the *cuticular border* because of its resemblance to the cuticle at the light-microscopic level). The cuticular border thus provides structural resilience to the otherwise very friable tubule. The entire structural organization of the duct is well designed for the most efficient Na^+ absorptive function, the luminal membrane serving as the absorptive surface by housing both Na^+ and Cl^- channels, and the basal ductal cells serving Na^+ pumping by providing the maximally expanded Na^+ pump sites and the efficient energy metabolism.

The morphology, development, and function of the apoeccrine gland are described elsewhere.[9,10] The apoeccrine gland develops during puberty from eccrine-like precursor glands and is consistently present in the adult axillae. Its relative frequency varies widely in different adults. However, in patients with axillary hyperhidrosis, as many as 50 percent of all the axillary glands are of the apoeccrine type, whereas in some individuals with no history of axillary hyperhidrosis, this percentage is much lower. Like eccrine glands, apoeccrine glands have long ducts that open directly onto the skin surface (unlike apocrine glands, which open directly into hair follicles).

The gross morphology of the apoeccrine gland differs widely even in the same individual. Basically, its secretory tubule consists of a segment of small diameter (as in the eccrine secretory tubule, i.e., less than 80 μm in diameter) and a segment of uniform or irregular dilatation to as much as 500 μm in diameter (Fig. 14-2). That these tubules are functionally connected to each other was shown by micropuncture study.[9] Ultrastructurally, the thick segment is very similar to the apocrine gland, whereas the thin segment is indistinguishable from the eccrine secretory coil (Fig. 14-3). Like the eccrine gland, the apoeccrine gland is predominantly cholinergic, and its secretory rate is as much as 10 times that of the eccrine gland, mainly because of its large size,[10] suggesting that the apoeccrine gland may play a role in axillary hyperhidrosis.

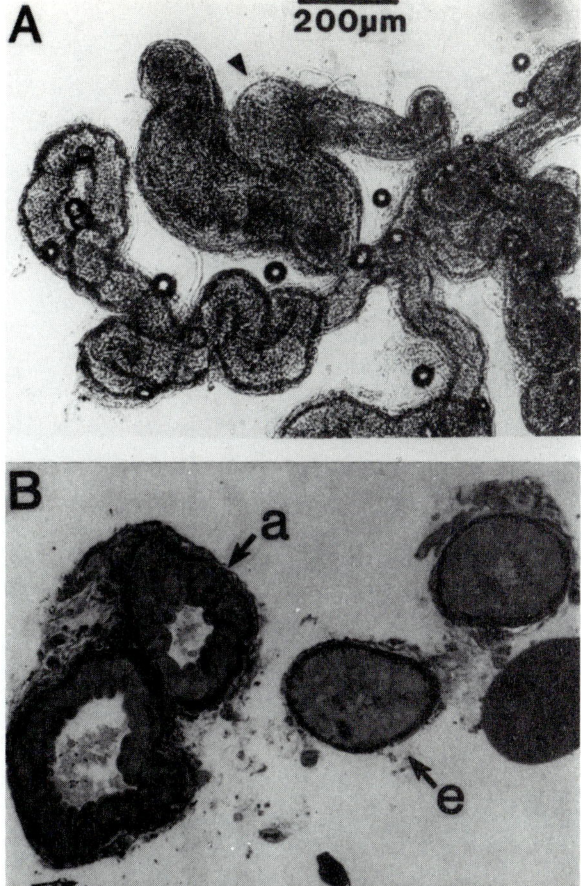

Figure 14-2 Apoeccrine sweat gland. (*A*) Note the segmental dilatation of the secretory tubule (arrowhead). This gland also shows a rare bifurcation of the secretory segment. (*B*) A 1-μm-thick section of an apoeccrine gland showing the apocrine-like segment (a) and the eccrine-like segment (e).

CENTRAL AND PERIPHERAL CONTROL OF SWEATING

Sweat Center and Temperature Set Point

Comprehending the function of the sweat center and the temperature set point (T_{se}) is instrumental in understanding the pathogenesis of abnormal sweating, such as in episodic hypothermia with hyperhidrosis (diencephalic epilepsy or Hines-Bannick syndrome), where the pathological episodic decrease of T_{se} is followed by a decrease in body temperature and the onset of profuse sweating.[17]

The sweat center is most likely located in the preoptic region–anterior

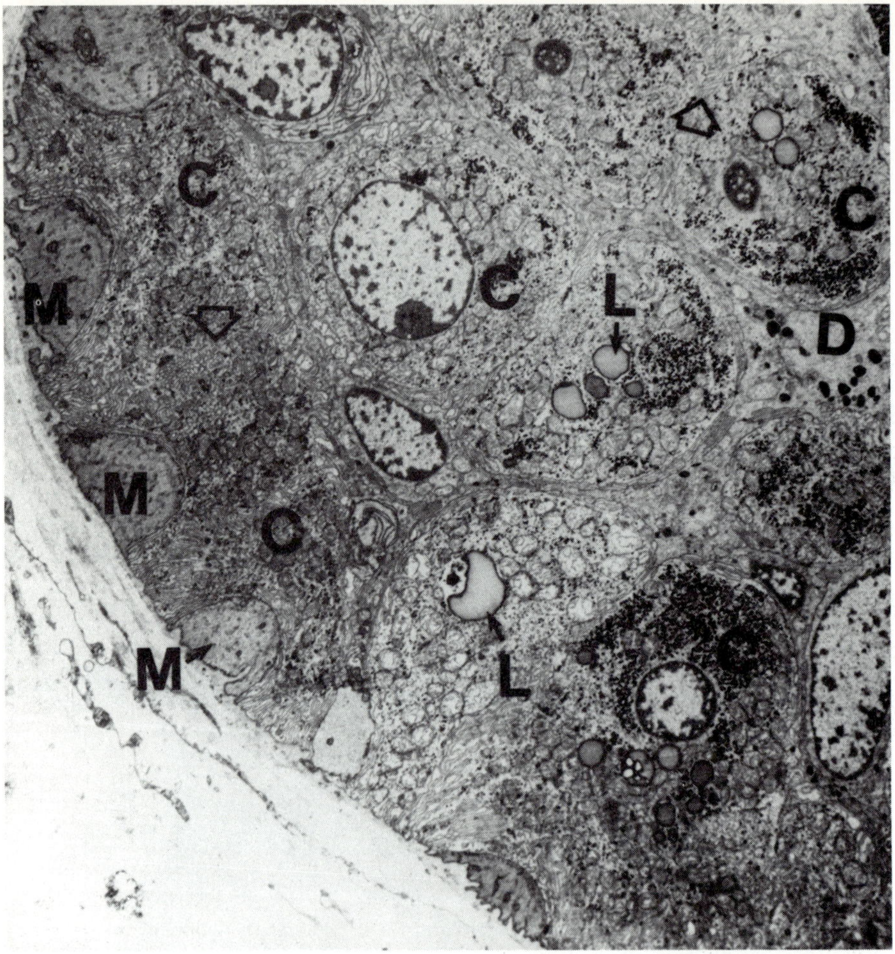

Figure 14-3 Electron micrograph of the eccrine-like tubule from the secretory portion of an apoeccrine gland (segment e in Fig. 14-2). C = clear cell; L = lipofuscin granules; M = myoepithelial cell; D = dark cell. Large empty arrows indicate intercellular canaliculi. ×5400 in the original magnification.

hypothalamus, where thermosensitive neurons are abundant.[18] In fact, preoptic heating causes sweating, panting, vasodilatation, and various behaviors that enhance heat loss.[19,20] Sweat center temperature is not the only mechanism by which the sweating rate is controlled. Sweating appears to respond as if controlled by a weighted sum of central (or core) and peripheral (or skin) temperatures.[21,22] If skin temperature is relatively constant, the rate of sweating is linearly related to core temperature above T_{se}. As skin temperature rises, the relation between sweating and core temperature shifts in the direction of lower core temperature (Fig. 14-4).

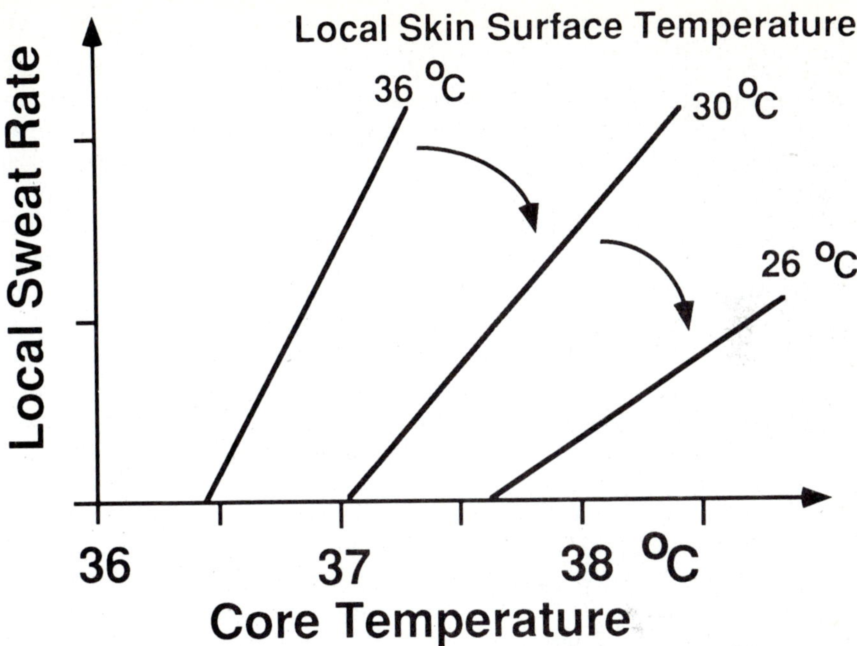

Figure 14-4 Dependence of local sweating rate on the core temperature and local skin surface temperature. (*Modified from ER Nadel et al.*[21,22])

On a degree-to-degree basis, an increase in core temperature is about nine times more efficient than an increase in mean skin temperature in stimulating the sweat center and thus the sweating rate. It remains to be studied whether the effect of local temperature on sweating is due to the increased release of periglandular neurotransmitters or to glandular metabolism, or both. Furthermore, in certain studies,[21,22] the periglandular temperature was not determined. In normal subjects, T_{se} changes with acclimatization, with different homeostatic states, and with exercise or heat exhaustion. For example, infusion of hypertonic NaCl (by 15-20 m*M*) into the brains of experimental animals increases the body temperature by about 1°C.[23] During exercise, elevating the plasma Na concentration [Na] in humans slows the onset of sweating and raises the plateau level of the core temperature, whereas increasing the plasma [Ca] has the opposite effect.[24] Isotonic hypovolemia also reduces the sensitivity of the sweating response, increases the threshold core temperature for the onset of the sweating response, and increases the threshold core temperature for the onset of cutaneous vasodilation.[25] Thus it is tempting to speculate that the paradoxical anhidrosis that is seen frequently in heat stroke is mediated in part by the altered function of the sweat center caused by the deranged plasma homeostasis following prolonged sweating.

Periglandular Neurotransmitters

The nerves surrounding the sweat glands are the sympathetic postganglionic fibers, consisting of unmyelinated class C nerve fibers. In contrast to the ordinary sympathetic innervation, acetylcholine is the principal terminal neurotransmitter. In addition, catecholamine,[26,27] vasoactive intestinal peptide (VIP),[28,29] natriuretic peptide (ANP), calcitonin gene-related peptide (CGRP) and galanin,[29,30] and adenosine triphosphate (ATP)[31] are localized in the periglandular nerves. The significance of these peptides or neurotransmitters for sweat gland function is not fully understood. Since immunoreactivity for ANP, CGRP, and galanin is also noted in the cutaneous sensory nerves, the specificity of their function on the sweat gland is less convincing. In contrast, VIP is not only a stimulant of sweat secretion in a cyclic AMP–mediated fashion but also a synergistic amplifier of the isoproterenol-stimulated cyclic AMP accumulation in the isolated eccrine sweat gland.[32] Interestingly, such amplified intracellular cyclic AMP accumulation is further augmented synergistically by acetylcholine, which by itself has no effect on the cyclic AMP level. Although the role of the synergistically amplified cyclic AMP level is not clear, it is possible to speculate that cyclic AMP may be involved in regulation of intracellular [Ca].[33] The function of periglandular ATP is also unknown.

DISORDERS OF THE SYMPATHETIC NERVOUS SYSTEM

After acute disruption of sympathetic nervous transmission (by sympathectomy, trauma, infection, etc.), the physiological sweating that occurs in response to thermal or emotional stimuli disappears immediately, whereas the sweating response to intradermal cholinergic agents lasts for a few weeks when the damage occurred at the postganglionic level but for several months when the sympathectomy occurred at the preganglionic level.[34] Thus, in theory, it is possible to differentiate the localization of nerve damage by periodically following the patient's sweating response to intradermal cholinergic agents (e.g., 0.01 to 0.1 percent pilocarpine or methacholine) as well as to heat exposure (e.g., in a sauna or simply by immersing both legs in water at 42°C to raise the body temperature by 1°C) (Fig. 14-5). A complete history and physical examination, including sensory, motor, and autonomic function tests, must be included wherever appropriate. These include examinations for Horner's signs (to rule out disturbance of the cervical and thoracic sympathetic trains); pupillary responses to light, accommodation, 2.5 percent methacholine, and 1 percent phenylephrine (to rule out tonic pupil); Schirmer's test for lacrimation (to rule out familial dysautonomia and sensory neuropathy with anhidrosis); salivation test, blood pressure responses to upright position, cold immersion of hands, apneic face immersion in cold water, and the Valsalva maneuver (to rule out orthostatic hypotension and/or systematic autonomic dysfunction); and an intradermal histamine test and nerve conduction tests (to search for peripheral sensory and motor neuropathy).[35]

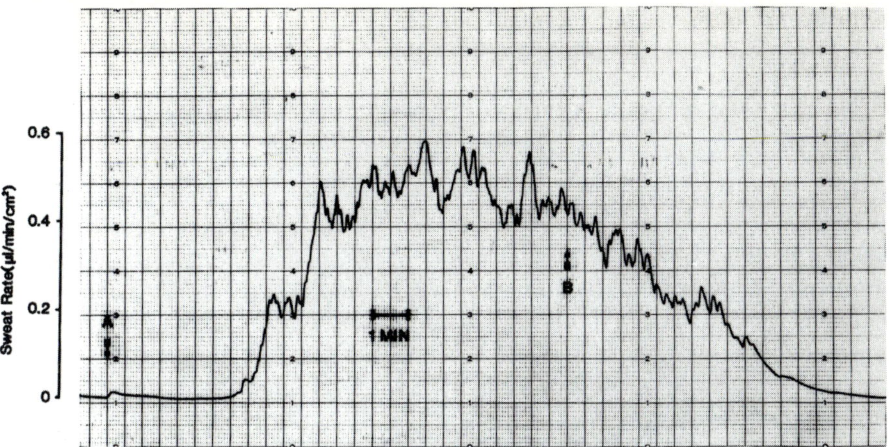

Figure 14-5 Thermal sweating induced by immersing both feet in a bath kept at 42°C. (A) Bathing on; (B) bathing off. The pulsatile output of sweating is characteristic of thermal sweating (pharmacological sweating is relatively smooth, as shown in Fig. 14-6) and may reflect the pulsatile central sympathetic discharges. Sweating from the feet was continuously monitored using a Meeco electrolytic moisture analyzer.

It is also important to ascertain that a lack of sweating is not due to other causes, such as poral occlusion, absence or atrophy of the sweat glands, or direct damage to the glands by trauma or inflammation of the skin. An increase in the number of patent pores after Scotch tape stripping (to remove poral plugging; stripping must be repeated 20 times) is evidence for involvement of superficial poral occlusion as the mechanism of anhidrosis, although this method is insufficient to detect poral occlusion below the stratum corneum. Skin biopsy may help determine the absence or atrophy of the glands in many reported cases of anhidrosis, although the lack of apparent morphological abnormality does not rule out glandular dysfunction.

Occasionally, multiple skin biopsy specimens and serial horizontal sections may be needed to determine more accurately the morphology and density of the sweat gland. In order to rule out definitively deep poral occlusion or altered pharmacological receptor function, in vitro sweat induction from isolated sweat glands[36] may be necessary. Nerve biopsy specimens have been reported to be helpful in establishing the diagnosis of congenital sensory neuropathy with anhidrosis.[37] In reality, however, interpretation of the neurological examination for sweating disorders is extremely perplexing and confusing. The difficulty is caused in part by our insufficient knowledge of the adaptive mechanism of the nervous system after damage, such as degeneration and regeneration of severed autonomic fibers, sprouting of new neurons and the misdirected reinnervation of new fibers, and postdenervation hypersensitivity of pharmacological receptors in the sweat glands, among others. It is not surprising, therefore, that most of the reported cases of abnormal sweating are based on incomplete experimental protocols and/or inadequate data.

PHARMACOLOGICAL RESPONSIVENESS OF THE ECCRINE SWEAT GLAND

Human eccrine sweat glands respond to intradermal injection of acetylcholine or epinephrine, but the adrenergic sweat rate is less than 10 percent of the cholinergic sweat rate. Hyperhidrosis during the crisis of pheochromocytoma can be abolished by anticholinergic agents, suggesting that such perspiration in these patients may be cholinergic (again, the reported cases are not based on quantitative data). The same holds true for emotionally triggered sweating, which is inhibited by atrophine and is thus cholinergic. The sweating response to intradermally injected isoproterenol in humans is transient, peaking at about 2 to 4 min after injection (Fig. 14-6), whereas isoproterenol-induced sweating in vitro is more persistent in both the monkey[38] and the human.[39] The reason for this differing β-adrenergic responsiveness in vivo and in vitro is unknown. α-adrenergic stimulation also induces sweat secretion, but to a much lesser extent than does β-adrenergic stimulation.

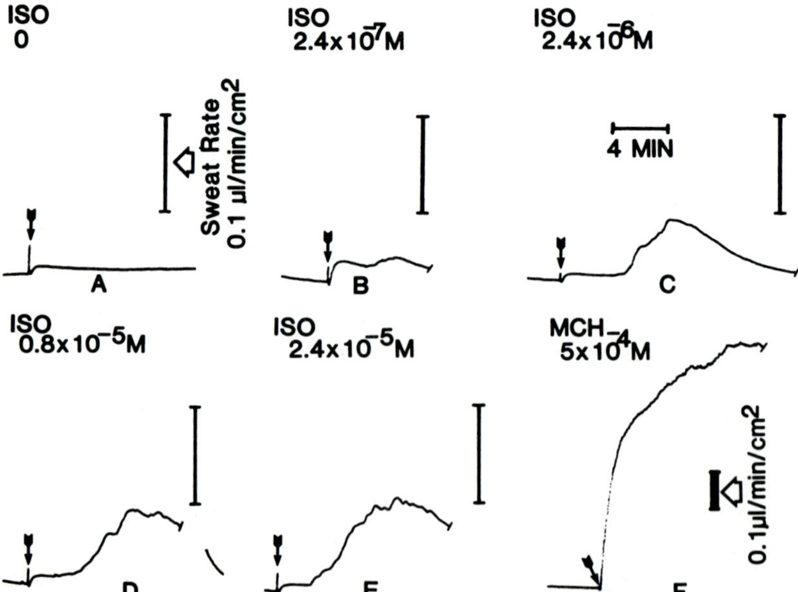

Figure 14-6 Sweating response to intradermally injected isoproterenol (ISO) as determined by a moisture analyzer. All ISO solutions contain 10 m*M* theophylline and 0.14 m*M* atropine. Repeated injection of ISO into the same test site failed to restart sweating (not shown). Note the normal methacholine (MCH) response.

Prostaglandins E_1 and E_2 stimulate sweat secretion in vitro, but their physiological role in eccrine sweating in vivo remains unknown. Histamine, serotonin, and substance P fail to induce sweat secretion in vitro. VIP, which is present in the periglandular nerves, is a strong stimulant of sweat secretion, although the sweating response is transient.[32] ATP, another sympathetic cotransmitter, transiently stimulates sweating in vitro, but its maximal sweat rate is less than 10 percent of the cholinergic sweat rate. Puzzlingly, ATP at 1 m*M* elevates intracellular [Ca] to the level normally induced by maximal cholinergic stimulation,[40] providing the basis for questioning whether intracellular [Ca] alone is a sufficient stimulus for sweat secretion. It remains to be studied whether ATP is involved as a regulator of other receptor functions or of glandular metabolism. Determination of the pharmacological responsiveness of the sweat gland in vivo is especially informative in cystic fibrosis, where stimulation with β-adrenergic agonists fails to induce sweating both in vivo and in vitro[39] (Fig. 14-7). Another convenient use for the intradermal cholinergic sweat test is to provide a measure of overall glandular function; that is, the higher the sweat $rate_{max}$, the larger the gland and the higher the pharmacological sensitivity.[41]

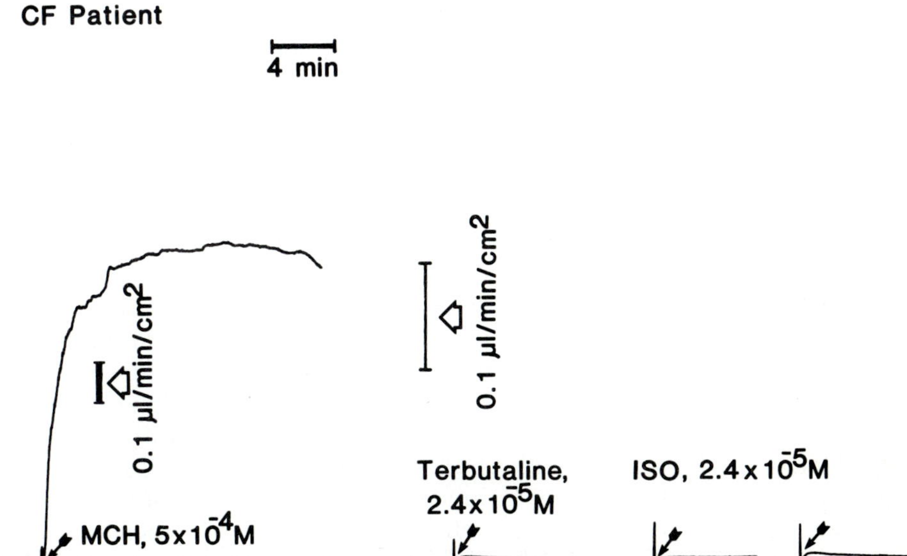

Figure 14-7 Absence of β-adrenergic sweating response to terbutaline and isoproterenol (ISO) in patients with cystic fibrosis in vivo. An illustrative example. Note the normal methacholine (MCH, injected intradermally) responsiveness (the first trace). CF = cystic fibrosis.

STIMULUS–SECRETION COUPLING IN ECCRINE SWEAT SECRETION

The term *stimulus–secretion coupling* refers to the observation[42] that Ca ion is required for catecholamine secretion from chromaffin cells after stimulation with various physiological secretagogues as well as diverse nonphysiological chemicals. In stimulus–secretion coupling, Ca^{2+} is viewed as the link in the chain of events initiated at the cell membrane by the action of acetylcholine and other stimulants that trigger the release of secretory products. A similar link has been postulated in the eccrine sweat gland, with Ca^{2+} being an intracellular mediator of cholinergic stimulation.[43] Some of the supporting evidence includes the following facts: cholinergic sweating is absolutely dependent on extracellular [Ca]; a Ca ionophore, A23187, which transports Ca^{2+} across the cell membrane, induces sweat secretion as profusely as does acetylcholine; a blocker of Ca^{2+} transport, such as D600 or verapamil, abolishes sweat secretion; and strontium ion, which substitutes for Ca^{2+} but diffuses into the cell, bypassing agonist–receptor interaction, induces profuse spontaneous sweat secretion. More recently, the increase in intracellular [Ca] after cholinergic, but not β-adrenergic, stimulation has been directly demonstrated using fluorescent probes such as quin 2[33] and fura 2[44] (Fig. 14-8).

In contrast, sweat secretion induced by the β-adrenergic agonist isoproterenol is relatively insensitive to Ca^{2+} removal from the external medium; however, the resting level of intracellular [Ca] may still be necessary for β-adrenergic sweating because prolonged chelation of Ca^{2+} with ethylene glycol tetraacetic acid (EGTA) in a Ca^{2+}-free medium may eventually abolish β-adrenergic sweating. Cyclic AMP is accumulated in the sweat gland during stimulation with isoproterenol but not with acetylcholine. External Ca^{2+} is not required for the isoproterenol-induced cyclic AMP response. Furthermore, sweat secretion can be induced by theophylline (a phosphodiesterase inhibitor that enhances endogenous cyclic AMP) or by dibutyryl cyclic AMP.[45] Intracellular [Ca] is not raised by isoproterenol or other cyclic AMP–elevating agents. The data are thus consistent with the thesis that cyclic AMP may be an intracellular mediator of β-adrenergic stimulation. Despite the lack of increase in intracellular [Ca], the role of intracellular [Ca] has been the subject of controversy. For example, in the salivary gland, the isoproterenol-activated K^+ and Cl^- current are inhibited by Ca^{2+} chelation, not mimicked by cyclic AMP and other cyclic AMP–elevating agents such as forskolin. Cook et al. thus postulated that Ca^{2+}, rather than cyclic AMP, is the intracellular mediator of β-adrenergic stimulation,[46] although, as indicated earlier, the effect of complete Ca^{2+} chelation may not be physiological and thus the data should be interpreted with caution. In the sweat gland, the increase in intracellular [Ca] is associated with net efflux of K^+ from the secretory coil cells.[47,48] However, K^+ efflux (Fig. 14-9) by cyclic AMP–elevating drugs is absent or diminishingly small, further suggesting that the role of Ca^{2+} in isoproterenol-induced sweat secretion

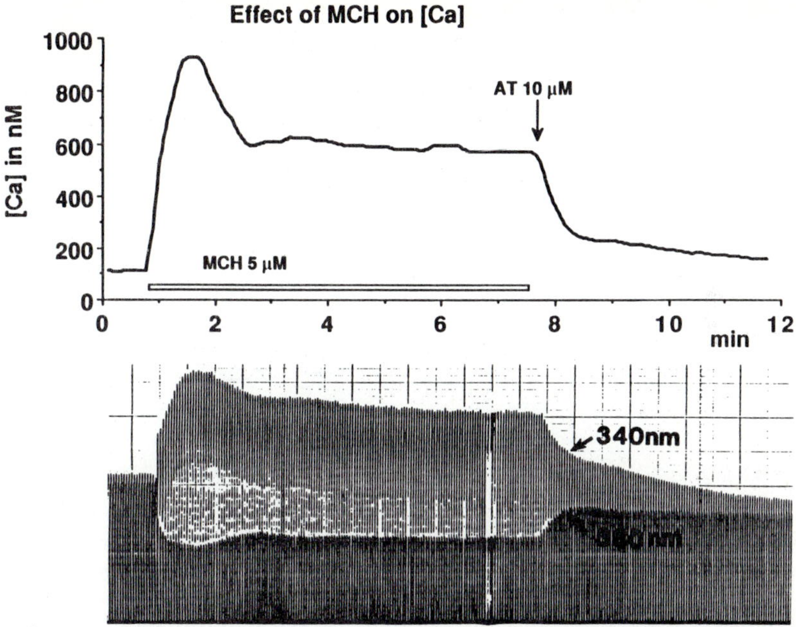

Figure 14-8 Elevation of intracellular calcium [Ca] by methacholine (MCH) in a dissociated eccrine clear cell of the monkey palm eccrine sweat gland, as determined by the fura 2 method using microfluorometry. Note the inhibition of MCH-induced [Ca] by atropine (AT). The lower panel shows the emission at 500 nm due to the two excitation wavelengths, 340 and 380 nm, and [Ca] calculated with a computer from the ratios according to Ref. 44.

is very limited or absent. To make the matter more complex, the role of cyclic AMP is also questioned in isoproterenol-induced mucin secretion in rat salivary glands.[49] Nevertheless, we surmise that cyclic AMP (and thus the subsequent cyclic AMP–dependent protein phosphorylation) is still important during isoproterenol-induced sweat secretion, but in some tissues a minute elevation of cyclic AMP in the critical intracellular compartment may suffice. β-adrenergic stimulation may also require the basic (if not the elevated) level of Ca^{2+}, that is, in the 50- to 100-n*M* range. Thus the complete chelation of Ca^{2+}, as done by Cook et al.,[46] could abolish the effects of β-agonists, as well as those of cyclic AMP, in some tissues.

Cyclic GMP was once viewed as the intracellular mediator of cholinergic stimulation in some tissues. In the sweat gland, cyclic GMP does not appear to be directly involved as a mediator of cholinergic sweating because the tissue cyclic GMP level reaches a peak at 2 min and returns to the baseline level by 5 min after methacholine stimulation, whereas the sweating response starts within seconds of stimulation and persists for hours.[51] Figure 14-10 summarizes our hypothetical schema for the mechanism of stimulus–secretion coupling in the clear cell, the cell mainly involved in secretion of water and electrolytes.

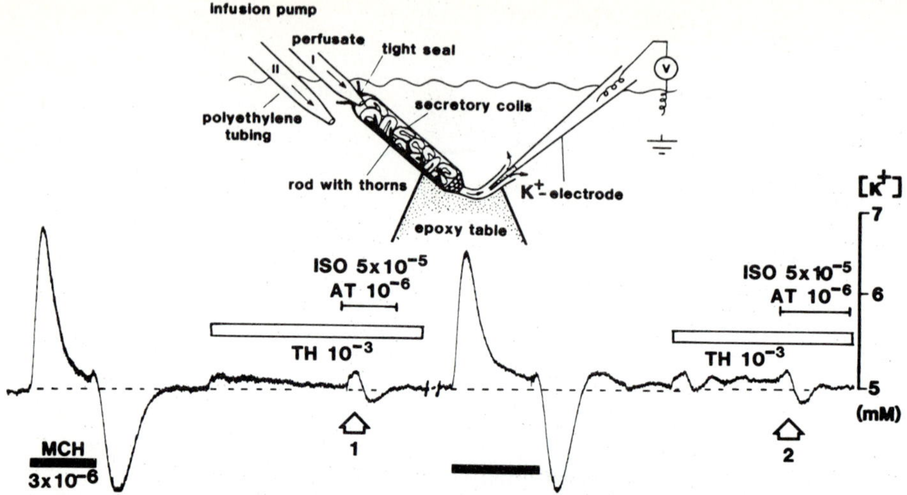

Figure 14-9 Effects of methacholine (MCH) and isoproterenol (ISO) on K^+ efflux from the isolated sweat secretory coils. The insert shows the method of superfusing the secretory coils. K^+ efflux from the coils is continuously monitored with a K^+-sensitive electrode. The K^+ trace is shown in the lower panel. Note the massive K^+ efflux during the initial 2 min of MCH stimulation. On cessation of stimulation, K^+ is taken up by the gland, as shown by the downward deflection of the curve. In contrast, very little K^+ is lost during stimulation with ISO. Arrow 2 indicates the second ISO stimulation. TH = theophyllin; AT = atropine.

STIMULATION OF MEMBRANE TRANSPORT DURING SWEAT SECRETION

Although the movement of ions in the clear cells during cholinergic sweat secretion was once assumed to conform to the Ussing's leak-pump model[52] (Fig. 14-11), this model was abandoned and replaced by the more recent modified Na-K-Cl cotransporter model with addition of parallel exchangers, as shown in the left panel of Fig. 14-11. The Na-K-Cl cotransport model was originally postulated to occur in Ehrlich ascites tumor cells[53] and was subsequently widely adapted to a number of transporting epithelia, including the tracheal epithelium, the rectal mucosa, and the salivary acini.[54] Some of the observations in the sweat secretory coil that lead us to adopt the Na-K-Cl cotransport model (Fig. 14-11, cell B in the left panel) include the following[5]: (1) Na-K-ATPase (and thus the Na^+ pump) is present in the basolateral membrane; (2) the luminal electrical potential in the secretory coil decreases from −1 mV at rest to −6 mV during methacholine stimulation; (3) K^+ channels as well as K^+ conductance are present in the basolateral membrane; (4) Cl^- channels are present (presumably in the luminal membrane) and are activated because the luminal membrane depolarizes during cholinergic stimulation; (5) sweat secretion is inhibited by the loop diuretics such as furosemide and bumetanide; and (6) sweat secretion depends on the presence of Cl^- and Na^+ in the bath.[55-58]

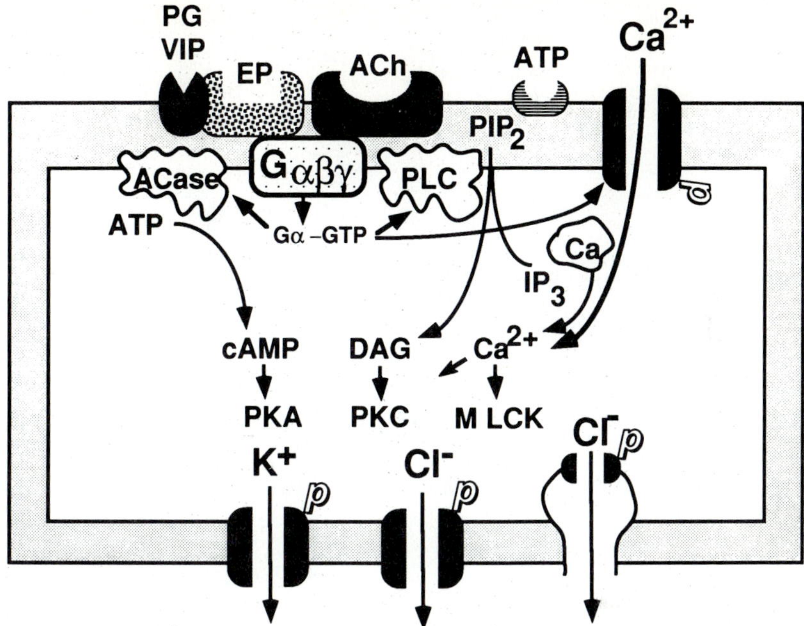

Figure 14-10 A hypothetical schema for stimulus–secretion coupling in the eccrine clear (secretory) cell. Based on the sweating response in vitro, we assumed the presence of receptors for acetylcholine (ACh), adenosine triphosphate (ATP), epinephrine (EP, which acts through both α and β receptors), prostaglandins (PG), and vasoactive intestinal peptide (VIP). Stimulation of all or many of these receptors may be transduced by G proteins (α, β, γ) by analogy to other tissues. Stimulation with cyclic AMP-elevating agents such as PG, VIP, or ISO (a β agonist) results in activation of adenylate cyclase (ACase), whereas cholinergic stimulation results in activation of phospholipase C (PLC), which hydrolyzes phosphatidylinositol bisphosphate (PIP_2) to generate diacylglycerol (DAG) and inositol 1,4,5-triphosphate (IP_3). IP_3 releases stored Ca^{2+}, but its significance in the sweat gland is limited (unpublished data). The major source of Ca^{2+} is therefore extracellular. It enters through the Ca^{2+} channels that are presumably activated by the activated G protein(s) or by phosphorylation of the Ca^{2+} channels. Likewise, introduction of Ca^{2+} by means of Ca^{2+} ionophores such as A23187 or ionomycin also stimulates sweat secretion in vitro for relatively short periods. We also speculate that cyclic AMP, DAG, and Ca^{2+} may activate ion channels or putative regulatory proteins of channels through protein kinases such as kinase A (PKA), kinase C (PKC), or myocin light chain kinase (M LCK).

According to this cotransport model, one Na ion, one K ion, and two Cl ions enter the cell in an electrically neutral fashion via the cotransporter. Na ions do not accumulate in the cell because they are pumped out in exchange for K ions. K ions that enter the cell via both the cotransporter and the Na^+ pump exit the cell through the K^+ channels across the basolateral membrane. This K^+ diffusion out of the cell generates the K^+ diffusion potential that helps keep the electrical potential of the cell's interior always negative, which in turn facilitates cellular Cl^- crossing of the luminal membrane through the Cl^- channels by providing the necessary

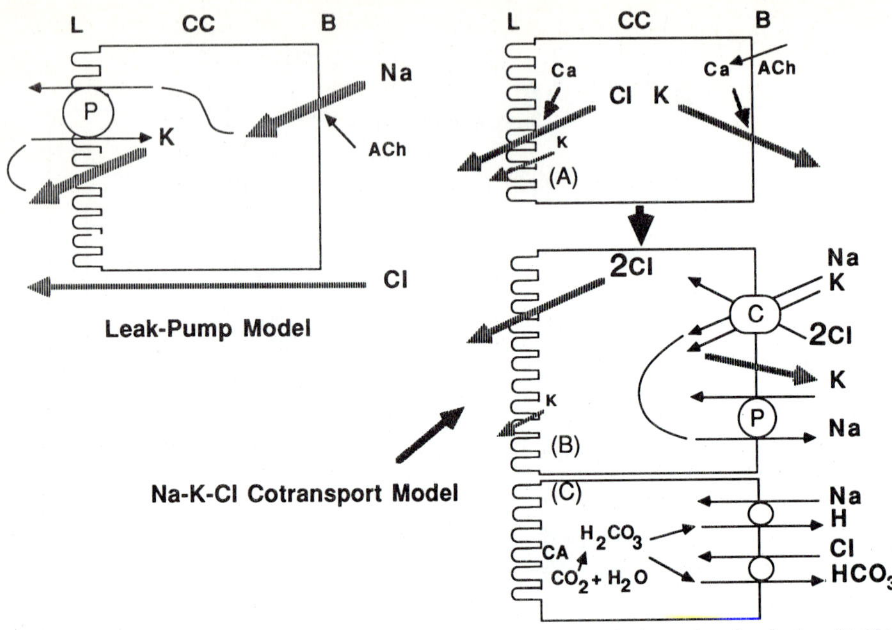

Figure 14-11 Transport models for sweat secretion during cholinergic stimulation (ACh). The left panel shows the old model of sweat secretion, adopting Ussing's leak-pump model, whereby ACh directly increases Na^+ permeability in the basal membrane. The right panel shows the most recent model of sweat secretion, involving the Na-K-Cl cotransporters as well as the parallel exchangers. Cell A in the left panel shows the hypothetical scheme during the transient period of ACh stimulation whereby K^+ leaves the cell across the basal membrane and Cl^- across the luminal membrane following activation of K^+ and Cl^- channels. K^+ and Cl^- channels are most likely controlled by Ca^{2+}. The net KCl loss results in cell volume shrinkage. Cell B is the original Na-K-Cl cotransport model, which may be the major mechanism of ionic movement during the steady state of cholinergic sweat secretion. Note that both K^+ and Na^+ recycle across the basal membrane, and only Cl^- traverses the cell to enter the lumen. Na^+ is assumed to enter the lumen across the intercellular junction. Cell C illustrates the parallel Na^+/H^+ and Cl^-/HCO_3^- exchangers (*solid circles*) that may also be involved during the steady state of cholinergic sweating. L = lumen; CC = clear cell; B = basal side; P = ouabain-sensitive Na-K exchange pump mediated by Na-K-ATPase; C = Na-K-Cl cotransporter sensitive to loop diuretics such as bumetanide or furosemide; CA = carbonic anhydrase. Hatched thick arrows indicate passive movement of ions. At present, the ionic mechanism of sweat secretion during β-adrenergic sweating is poorly understood.

electrical driving force for Cl^-. Thus, after each transport cycle, two Cl ions are transported into the lumen across the cell, but both K^+ and Na^+ are recycled across the basolateral membrane. Although this cotransport model apparently explains the movement of Na, K, and Cl ions during the steady state of sweat secretion, the question remains as to how each transporter is activated and regulated at the onset of cholinergic sweating. Several consequences of cellular response can be predicted: (1) if it is the Na^+ pump that is initially stimulated after cholinergic stimulation, then the cellular Na concentration [Na] initially decreases but the cellular K concentration [K] increases; (2) if the Na-K-Cl cotransporter is initially stimulated, cellular [Na], [K], and [Cl] all increase; if not, the cellular volume increases (without a detectable change in cellular ion concentrations); (3) if Cl^- and K^+ channels alone are initially stimulated by cholinergic stimulation presumably mediated by an increase in cellular [Ca], cellular [KCl] decreases; if not, the cell volume shrinks (without a change in cellular KCl concentration).

After stimulation of the cell with methacholine, there is a sudden decrease of cellular [K], an increase of [Na], a decrease of [Cl], outflux of as much as 50 percent of cellular KCl from the perfused secretory coils, and cell shrinkage by about 25 percent of the initial cell volume[55-62] (Fig. 14-9). These observations are partially consistent with consequence 3 predicted above but are not fully explained without invoking an additional mechanism such as simultaneous stimulation of the cotransporter (consequence 2) and/or stimulation of the parallel exchangers. At present, the functional significance of the cell volume shrinkage (which is presumably due secondarily to KCl efflux) is unknown (cell A in Fig. 14-11). On the other hand, the decrease in cellular KCl concentration during methacholine stimulation provides a favorable chemical gradient for the influx of K^+ and Cl^- from the basal medium via an Na-K-Cl cotransporter (which utilizes the downhill chemical gradients of Na^+). Ca^{2+}-dependent activation of Cl^- channels across the luminal membrane depolarizes this membrane, generates the lumen's negative transepithelial potential, and causes Cl ions to flow into the lumen, which attracts Na^+ from the bath into the lumen across the paracellular pathway that is permeable to Na^+. Water can readily enter the lumen so as to maintain the near isotonicity of the luminal fluid (i.e., primary sweat).

Although the cotransport model may be the most prominent ionic mechanisms for sweat secretion, some modifications of the model may be necessary. For example, we have observed that methacholine-induced KCl efflux from the secretory coil is significantly inhibited by removal of HCO_3^- from the bath, inhibitors of parallel Na^+/H^+ and Cl^-/HCO_3^- exchangers,[48] and the NH_4Cl loading (a maneuver that increases the intracellular pH) but was stimulated during the washout period after NH_4Cl loading (a maneuver that decreases the intracellular pH). These additional observations have lead us to modify the original Na-K-Cl cotransport model by adding parallel Na^+/H^+ and Cl^-/HCO_3^- exchangers as shown in the cell (C) of Fig. 14-11.

PATHOPHYSIOLOGY OF THE ECCRINE SWEAT GLAND

Heat Stroke

Heat stroke tends to occur in the elderly and in poorly acclimatized individuals after sudden exposure to a hot environment. During the summer heat wave of 1980, most of the 1265 fatalities involved elderly people and young children. Heat intolerance of patients with anhidrotic ectodermal dysplasia is well known. Patients usually present with hyperthermia, dry skin, mental disorientation, or even generalized convulsive seizures, followed by hypotension, oliguria, metabolic acidosis, jaundice, and hyperkalemia. It has been debated whether the failure of sweating that usually precedes the onset of hyperthermia is caused by the dysfunction of the sweat glands or by that of the hypothalamus/sweat center. Although the genesis of heat stroke may well be multifactorial, the abnormal regulation of T_{se} in the hypothalamic sweat center may also play a critical role, as discussed earlier (see "Sweat Center and Temperature Set Points").[5]

Cystic Fibrosis (Mucoviscidosis)

Cystic fibrosis is the most common recessively inherited lethal or semilethal disease of whites, affecting primarily exocrine glands. The incidence of cystic fibrosis in the white population is about 1 per 1600. In 1989, cloning of the cystic fibrosis gene was reported and a three-base deletion that removes phenylalanine 508 from the 1480 amino acid coding region was identified as the mutation that causes cystic fibrosis in at least 70 percent of cases.[63]

Despite the breathtaking discoveries in the molecular genetics of cystic fibrosis, the elevated sweat NaCl concentration (e.g., 65 to 120 m*M* in cystic fibrosis vs. <<65 m*M* in non–cystic fibrosis) will continue to be used as the diagnostic criterion for cystic fibrosis at least during the 1990s. Since the mid-1960s, it has been established that the elevated sweat NaCl concentration in cystic fibrosis sweat is due to the decreased ductal NaCl absorption because the NaCl concentration in the primary sweat is nearly isotonic to plasma in both control groups and cystic fibrosis patients.[64] The electrical potential of the sweat ductal lumen is about twice as negative in cystic fibrosis ducts (−60 mV) as in normal ducts (−30 mV) both in vivo and in vitro[7]; this has been proved to be due to impermeability of Cl^- across the luminal membrane.[65] However, our recent electrophysiological analysis of the membrane permeability of the isolated cystic fibrosis duct suggests that Cl^- permeability is abnormally low not only across the luminal membrane but also across the cellular junction and across the basolateral membrane.[66]

It was soon reported that the abnormal Cl^- permeability is the universal basic defect in cystic fibrosis. Investigators in two different laboratories, using patch clamp techniques, found that cultured cystic fibrosis tracheal cells failed to show Cl^- channel activities when stimulated with isoproterenol in intact cells.[67,68] However, when the membrane patches were excised and exposed to the Ca^{2+}-containing bathing media, Cl^- channels were activated in cystic fibrosis cells as well as in normal cells, suggesting that Cl^- channels are present but may be abnormally regulated in cystic fibrosis tracheal cells.[68]

The secretory portion of the cystic fibrosis sweat gland has long been regarded as normal and, in fact, shows an entirely normal cholinergic sweating response. However, when its β-adrenergic sweating response was studied, the cystic fibrosis secretory portion failed to show sweating responses to a combination of isoproterenol and theophylline in vivo as well as in vitro, despite the fact that the cystic fibrosis sweat gland accumulated cyclic AMP normally in response to the β-adrenergic agents.[8] They speculated that the pathogenesis of the defective β-adrenergic responsiveness of the cystic fibrosis sweat secretory cells may be distal to cyclic AMP production in the cyclic AMP cascade. Since Cl^- channels are present in the luminal membrane and may play a critical role in eccrine sweating (Figs. 14-10 and 14-11), cyclic AMP–mediated phosphorylation of Cl^- channels may be abnormal in cystic fibrosis. At present, the role of Cl^- channels in β-adrenergic sweating is still unknown. In contrast, the

Table 14-1

HYPERHIDROSIS

Affecting a relatively large area (>>100 sq. cm)

- In patients with a history of spinal cord injuries
  - Due to autonomic dysreflexia
  - With orthostatic hypotension
  - Due to posttraumatic syringomyelia
- Associated with peripheral neuropathies
  - In familial dysautonomia (Riley-Day syndrome)
  - Due to congenital autonomic dysfunction, with universal pain loss
  - On exposure to cold
- Associated with probable brain lesions
  - Episodic, with hypothermia (Hines-Bannick syndrome)
  - Episodic, without hypothermia
  - Olfactory
- Associated with intrathoracic neoplasms or lesions
- Associated with systemic illnesses
  - Pheochromocytoma, Parkinson's disease, thyrotoxicosis, diabetes mellitus, congestive heart failure, anxiety, menopause, etc.
- Night sweats

Affecting a relatively small area

- Idiopathic, unilateral, circumscribed
- Gustatory sweating associated with
  - Encephalitis, syringomyelia, diabetic neuropathies, herpes zoster parotitis, parotid abscesses, thoracic sympathectomy
  - Auriculotemporal (Frey's) syndrome
- Reported to be associated with
  - Blue rubber bleb nevus, glomus tumor, POEMS syndrome, burning feet syndrome (Gopalan's), causalgia, pachydermoperiostosis, pretibial myxedema

Table 14-2

HYPOHIDROSIS OR ANHIDROSIS

Affecting a relatively large area
- Due to poral occlusion
  - In papulosquamous, dermatitic, or ichthyosiform lesions
  - In xerosis (including xerosis of atopics)
  - Acquired generalized anhydrosis (tropical anhidrotic asthenia?)
- Due to absence of the sweat gland
  - Anhidrotic ectodermal dysplasia (Christ-Siemens-Touraine syndrome)
- Due to paucity, atrophy, or dysfunction of the sweat gland
  - In systemic sclerosis
  - ?In Fabry's disease
- Due to neuropathy
  - Congenital sensory neuropathy
    - Type III (Riley-Day syndrome)
    - Type IV (congenital insensitivity to pain with anhidrosis)
  - Progressive segmental anhidrosis with Adie's tonic pupils (Ross' syndrome)
  - ?Progressive isolated segmental anhydrosis without tonic pupils
  - ?Autonomic insufficiency syndrome (postural hypotension and anhidrosis)
  - ?Chronic idiopathic anhidrosis
  - Others: diabetic neuropathy, Guillain-Barré syndrome, Fabry's disease (?)

Affecting a relatively small area
- Damage to the glands by infection, trauma, tumors, morphea, scars, or inflammatory infiltrate
- ?Denervation
  - Incontinentia pigmenti
  - Dermatomal vitiligo
- Miscellaneous
  - Follicular atrophoderma (Bazex's syndrome)
  - Sjögren's syndrome (? due to inflammatory infiltrate)

Ca^{2+}-mediated regulation of the Cl^- channels may be normal in cystic fibrosis, as predicted from the normal sweating response of the cystic fibrosis sweat glands to Ca^{2+}-elevating agents.

Disorders of Eccrine Sweating: A Preliminary Attempt at Classification

Disorders of eccrine sweating have recently been reviewed.[5,6] The study of sweat gland function in patients is a formidable task in most clinical settings. It is thus understandable that most authors often rely on subjective means, such as visual inspection of skin moisture or the history of the

Table 14-3

SWEAT RETENTION SYNDROMES

Miliarias
Miliaria crystallina
Miliaria rubra (prickly heat)
Miliaria pustulosa
?Transient acantholytic dermatoses (Grover's disease)
?Dyshidrosis (Pompholyx)

patient, to judge the presence or absence of hyper- or hypohidrosis instead of employing more reliable qualitative or quantitative methods for analysis of the patient's sweat gland function. In this chapter a working classification of disorders of eccrine sweating based on the possible pathogenesis is presented. Tables 14-1 to 14-3 are designed to serve as a working guide for future investigations using more accurate analytical methods. These tables may also be useful for clinicians who wish to provide a differential diagnosis for patients who present with abnormal sweating. The disorders of eccrine sweating have been divided into three groups: hyperhidrosis (Table 14-1), hypo- or anhidrosis (Table 14-2), and sweat retention syndromes (Table 14-3). In classifying them, we have avoided using the terms *local* and *generalized* because most of the so-called generalized sweating disorders often involve only a part of the trunk or the extremities and because the description of the abnormal areas was not clearly shown.

ACKNOWLEDGMENTS

This research has been supported in part by NIH grants DK 27857 and HL 32731 and by Cystic Fibrosis Foundation Grant R013-9-1. John G. Seyfried and Sue Cavallin helped in the preparation of the manuscript.

REFERENCES

1. Sato K: The physiology, pharmacology and biochemistry of the eccrine sweat gland. *Rev Physiol Biochem Pharmacol* 79:51, 1977.
2. Sato K: The physiology and pharmacology of the eccrine sweat gland, in L Goldsmith (ed), *Biochemistry and Physiology of the Skin*. London, Oxford University Press, 1983, p 596.
3. Benzinger TH: Heat regulation: homeostasis of central temperature in man. *Physiol Rev* 49:659, 1969.
4. Hammel HT: Regulation of internal body temperature. *Annu Rev Physiol* 30:6341, 1968.
5. Sato K et al: Biology of sweat glands and their disorders. I. Normal sweat gland function. *J Am Acad Dermatol* 20:537,1989.
6. Sato K et al: Biology of sweat glands and their disorders. II. Disorders of sweat gland function. *J Am Acad Dermatol* 20:713, 1989.
7. Quinton PM, Bijman J: Higher bioelectric potentials due to decreased chloride absorption in the sweat glands of patients with cystic fibrosis. *N Engl J Med* 308:1185, 1983.

8. Sato K, Sato F: Defective beta adrenergic response of cystic fibrosis sweat glands in vivo and in vitro. *J Clin Invest* 73:1763, 1984.
9. Sato K et al: Morphology and development of an apoeccrine sweat gland in human axillae. *Am J Physiol* 251 (*Regul Integrative Comp Physiol* 21):R166, 1987.
10. Sato K, Sato F: Sweat secretion by human axillary apoeccrine sweat gland in vitro. *Am J Physiol* 251 (*Regul Integrative Comp Physiol* 21):R181, 1987.
11. Sato K, Sato F: Individual variations in structure and function of human eccrine sweat gland. *Am J Physiol* 245 (*Regul Integrative Comp Physiol* 14):R203, 1983.
12. Ellis RA: Eccrine sweat glands, in J Jadassohn (ed), *Handbuch der Haut und Geschlechtskrankheiten.* 1 Band, *Nomale und Pathologische Anatomie der Haut.* Berlin, Springer-Verlag, 1967, p 224.
13. Saga K, Sato K: Ultrastructural localization of ouabain-sensitive, K-dependent *p*-nitrophenyl phosphatase activity in monkey eccrine sweat gland. *J Histochem Cytochem* 36:1023, 1988.
14. Quinton PM, Tormey JM: Localization of Na-K-ATPase sites in the secretory and reabsorptive epithelia of perfused eccrine sweat glands: a question to the role of the enzyme in secretion. *Membr Biol* 29:383, 1976.
15. Yanagawa S et al: Origin of periodic acid-Schiff–reactive glycoprotein in human eccrine sweat. *J Appl Physiol* 60:1615, 1986.
16. Sato K et al: Mechanical properties and functions of the myoepithelium in the eccrine sweat gland. *Am J Physiol* 237:C177, 1979.
17. Le Witt PA et al: Episodic hyperhidrosis, hypothermia, and agenesis of corpus callosum. *Neurology* 33:1122, 1983.
18. Boulant JA: Hypothalamic mechanisms in thermoregulation. *Fed Proc* 40:2843, 1981.
19. Smiles KA, Robinson S: Regulation of sweat secretion during positive and negative work. *J Appl Physiol* 30:409, 1971.
20. Adair ER: Skin, preoptic and core temperatures influence behavioral thermoregulation. *J Appl Physiol* 42:559, 1977.
21. Nadel ER et al: Importance of skin temperature in the regulation of sweating. *J Appl Physiol* 31:80, 1971.
22. Nadel ER et al: Peripheral modifications to the central drive for sweating. *J Appl Physiol* 31:828, 1971.
23. Greenleaf JE: Hyperthermia and exercise. *Int Rev Physiol Environ Physiol* 20:157, 1979.
24. Nielsen B: Effect of changes in plasma Na and Ca ion concentration on body temperature during exercise. *Acta Physiol Scand* 91:123, 1974.
25. Fortney SM et al: Effect of blood volume on sweating rate and body fluids in exercising humans. *J Appl Physiol* 51:1594, 1981.
26. Uno H: Sympathetic innervation of the sweat glands and piloerector muscle of macaques and human beings. *J Invest Dermatol* 69:112, 1977.
27. Uno H, Montagna W: Catecholamine-containing nerve terminals of the eccrine sweat glands of macaques. *Cell Tissue Res* 158:1, 1975.
28. Lundberg JM et al: Vasoactive intestinal polypeptide in cholinergic neurons of exocrine glands: functional significance of coexisting transmitters for vasodilatation and secretion. *Proc Natl Acad Sci USA* 77:1651, 1980.
29. Vaalassti A et al: Vasoactive intestinal polypeptide (VIP)-like immunoreactivity in the nerves of human axillary sweat glands. *J Invest Dermatol* 85:246, 1985.
30. Tainino H et al: The distribution of substance P-, CGRP-, galanin- and ANP-like immunoreactive nerves in human sweat glands. *Histochem J* 19:375, 1987.
31. Burnstock G: Past and current evidence for purinergic nerve hypothesis, in HP Baer, GI Drummond (eds), *Physiological and Regulatory Functions of Adenosine and Adenine Nucleotide.* New York, Raven, 1979, p 3.
32. Sato K, Sato F: Effect of VIP on sweat secretion and cAMP accumulation in isolated simian eccrine glands. *Am J Physiol* 253 (*Regul Integrative Comp Physiol* 22):R935, 1987.
33. Sato K, Sato F: Relationship between quin 2-determined cytosolic [Ca^{++}] and sweat secretion. *Am J Physiol* 254 (*Cell Physiol*):C310, 1988.
34. Faden AI et al: Progressive isolated anhidrosis. *Arch Neurol* 39:172, 1982.

35. Johnson RH, Spaulding JMK: *Disorders of the Autonomic Nervous System.* Philadelphia, FA Davis, 1974, p 179.
36. Sato K: Sweat induction from an isolated eccrine sweat gland. *Am J Physiol* 225:1147, 1973.
37. Ishii N et al: Congenital sensory neuropathy with anhidrosis. *Arch Dermatol* 124:564, 1988.
38. Sato K, Sato F: Pharmacological responsiveness of isolated single eccrine sweat glands. *Am J Physiol* 240:R44, 1981.
39. Sato K, Sato F: Defective beta adrenergic response of cyclic fibrosis sweat glands in vivo and in vitro. *J Clin Invest* 73:1763, 1984.
40. Sato K et al: Roles of Ca, cAMP, and kinase C for stimulus secretion coupling in the eccrine sweat gland. *Pediatr Pulmonol,* in press.
41. Sato K, Sato F: Individual variations in structure and function of human eccrine sweat gland. *Am J Physiol* 245 (*Regul Integrative Comp Physiol* 14):R203, 1983.
42. Douglas WW, Rubin RP: The mechanism of catecholamine release from the adrenal medulla and the role of calcium in stimulus–secretion coupling. *J Physiol* (*Lond*) 167:288, 1963.
43. Sato K, Sato F: Role of calcium in cholinergic and adrenergic mechanisms of eccrine sweat secretion. *Am J Physiol* 241:C113, 1981.
44. Grynkiewicz GM et al: A new generation of Ca^{2+} indicators with greatly improved fluorescence properties. *J Biol Chem* 260:3440, 1985.
45. Sato K, Sato F: Role of cyclic AMP in beta adrenergic mechanisms of sweat secretion. *Pflugers Arch* 390:49, 1981.
46. Cook DJ et al: Ca^{2+} not cyclic AMP mediates the fluid secretory response to isoproterenol in the rat mandibular gland: whole-cell patch clamp studies. *Pflugers Arch* 413:67, 1988.
47. Saga K, Sato K: Electron probe X-ray microanalysis of cellular ions in the eccrine secretory coil cells during methacholine stimulation. *J Membr Biol* 107:13, 1988.
48. Kang WH et al: Effects of transport inhibitors and ions on K^+ efflux from monkey secretory coils during cholinergic stimulation. *Clin Res* 36:660A, 1988.
49. Bradbury NA et al: Introduction of cyclic AMP phosphodiesterase into rat submandibular acini prevents isoproterenol-stimulated cyclic AMP rise without affecting mucin secretion. *Biochem Biophys Res Commun* 161:661, 1989.
50. Sato K, Sato F: Stimulation-induced changes in cytosolic calcium in a single dissociated eccrine secretory cell by use of fluorescent dye fura 2. *Clin Res* 37:354A, 1989.
51. Sato K, Sato F: Cyclic GMP accumulation during cholinergic stimulation of eccrine sweat glands. *Am J Physiol* 247 (*Cell Physiol* 16):C234, 1984.
52. Ussing HH: Transport of electrolytes and water across the epithelia. *Harvey Lect Ser* 59:1, 1965.
53. Geck P et al: Electrically silent cotransport of Na^+, K^+ and Cl^- in Ehrlich cells. *Biochim Biophys Acta* 600:432, 1980.
54. O'Grady SM et al: Characteristics and functions of Na-K-Cl cotransport in epithelial tissues. *Am J Physiol* 253 (*Cell Physiol* 22):C177, 1987.
55. Saga K et al: K^+ efflux from the monkey eccrine secretory cell during the transient stimulation with agonists. *J Physiol* 405:205, 1988.
56. Saga K, Sato K: Electron probe X-ray microanalysis of cellular ions in the eccrine secretory coil cells during methacholine stimulation. *J Membr Biol* 107:13, 1988.
57. Saga K, Sato K: Ultrastructural localization of ouabain sensitive K-dependent *p*-nitrophenyl phosphatase activity in monkey eccrine sweat gland. *J Histochem Cytochem* 36:1023, 1988.
58. Sato K, Sato F: Effect of periglandular ionic composition and transport inhibitors on rhesus monkey eccrine sweat gland function in vitro. *J Physiol* (*Lond*) 393:195, 1987.
59. Takemura T et al: Evidence that cholinergic stimulation is associated with cell volume decrease in eccrine secretory cells as evidenced by X-ray microanalysis and light microscopy. *Clin Res* 37:640A, 1989.
60. Suzuki Y et al: Ionic basis for cellular volume regulation in dissociated sweat secretory cells during pharmacological stimulation. *Clin Res* 37:618A, 1989.

61. Ohtsuyama M et al: Stimulation of Cl channel activity by Ca and cAMP elevating agents in dissociated eccrine clear cells as determined by cell volume analysis. *Clin Res* 38:420A, 1990.
62. Sato K, Sato F: Characteristics of Na, K, and Cl channels in the clear cells membrane of the eccrine sweat gland as studied by the patch clamp techniques. *Clin Res* 37:369A, 1989.
63. Kerem B et al: Identification of the cystic fibrosis gene: genetic analysis. *Science* 254:1073, 1989.
64. Di Sant'Agnese PA, Davis PB: Research in cystic fibrosis. *N Engl J Med* 295:481, 1976.
65. Reddy MM, Quinton PM: Localization of Cl^- conductance in normal and Cl^- impermeability in cystic fibrosis sweat duct epithelium. *Am J Physiol* 257:C727, 1989.
66. Sato K: Membrane potential and permeability properties of isolated perfused sweat duct of patients with cystic fibrosis. *Clin Res* 35:390A, 1987.
67. Welsh MJ, Liedtke LM: Chloride and potassium channels in cystic fibrosis airway epithelia. *Nature* 3222:467, 1986.
68. Frizzell RA et al: Altered regulation of airway epithelial cell chloride channels in cystic fibrosis. *Science* 233:558, 1986.

15

Hair Follicles and Pathophysiology of Certain Disorders of Hair

Howard P. Baden

Two types of human hair have been described: terminal hair, represented by scalp hair, and vellus hair, the fine, short, soft type found on the so-called hairless areas of the body. Hair growth is not continuous but rather cyclic, with alternating periods of growth (anagen) and rest (telogen).[1] The catagen phase marks the transition from anagen to telogen and is relatively short. The length of each phase is characteristic of different areas of the body. In the scalp, the anagen phase is about 6 years and the telogen phase is about 4 months. The growth of scalp hair is asynchronous, and the rate of growth is about 0.4 mm/day. About 90 percent of the more than 100,000 scalp hairs are growing, so that 50 to 100 hairs are shed daily. The newly emerging hair has a tapered end but then continues to grow with a rather constant diameter. Scalp hair varies considerably in shape, color, curl, and diameter, both among different individuals and in the same individual. For this reason, it is not possible to use the microscopic appearance of hair for individual identification; however, genetic control of hair is readily appreciated by noting the significant racial difference in hair shape.[2]

STRUCTURE AND COMPOSITION OF HAIR FOLLICLE COMPONENTS

The hair follicle consists of the hair surrounded by an epithelial sheath continuous with the epidermis, the sebaceous gland, and the arrector pili

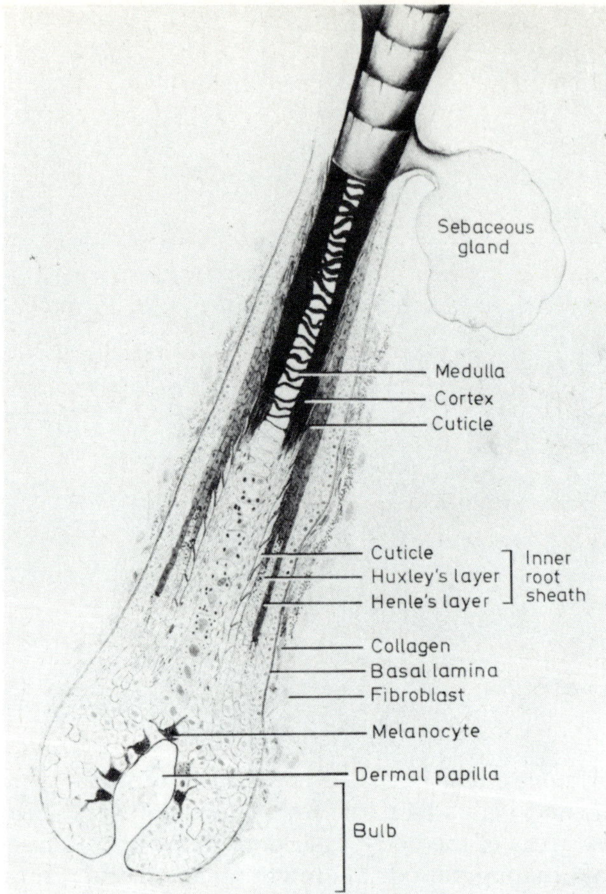

Figure 15-1 Drawing of a hair follicle. Only the cuticle, cortex, and medulla are present in the hair emerging from the scalp. [*From PF Parakkal, Katagen und Telogenphase, in CE Orfanos (ed), Haar und Haarhankheiter, Stuttgart, Gustav Fischer Verlag, 1979, p 78.*]

muscle. Hair is a complex tissue that includes a number of cells with various modes of differentiation (Fig. 15-1). Except for the dermal papilla, which contains connective tissue and blood vessels, the remainder of the hair is formed from modified epidermal cells.

The bulb is the thickest part of the follicle at its lower end and contains the proliferating pool of undifferentiated cells that give rise to the various layers. Differentiation begins at the constriction above the bulb and continues halfway up the follicle where the cells begin to cornify, the so-called keratogenous zone. The hair is fully hardened as it emerges from the skin surface.

The outer root sheath is continuous with the superficial epidermis but differs in appearance at different levels in the canal. Although keratinization in this layer is similar to that in the epidermis, differences do exist in keratohyalin, membrane-coating granules, and cornification at different depths of the follicle.

Moving inward, the next layer is the inner root sheath, which is composed of Henle's layer, Huxley's layer, and the cuticle, in that sequence. These cells contain trichohyalin granules and 70- to 80-Å filaments.[3] Differentiation starts in Henle's layer and proceeds inward. The trichohyalin granules appear first and are formed from a precursor protein of about 200 kd that is rich in the amino acids arginine, lysine, and glutamine.[4] The internal root sheath cells later develop the epithelial-type keratin filaments that are closely associated with the granules.[5] As the number of filaments increases, the trichohyalin granules disappear, the protein becoming the matrix material. This protein undergoes two types of posttranslation modification. The first is the conversion of arginine to citrulline in peptide linkage,[6] which causes the protein to develop a negative charge and may be responsible for the dispersion of the granules. The second is the formation of ε-(γ-glutamyl) lysine cross-links.[7] This may be responsible for the hardened and homogeneous appearance of the internal root sheath in its final stages of differentiation. All three layers disintegrate in the follicle at about the level of the entrance of the sebaceous gland, and the main function of the inner root sheath may be to give rigidity to the developing hair shaft, since it is the first to cornify.

The outside of the hair shaft is covered by cuticle cells that overlap one another and develop within the follicle (Fig. 15-2). In the viable layer, tonofilaments are visible that are of both the epithelial and the hair type. When the cells cornify, a number of distinct layers are discernible, as shown in Fig. 15-3, including a marginal band that is likely equivalent to the cornified envelope of the epidermis. The marginal band and exocuticle are almost completely insoluble and rich in cystine. Desmosomes are not present in the cuticle, and the attachment of cuticle cells to one another results from invaginations and infoldings of adjacent cells.

The cortex is the major component of the hair fiber and consists of

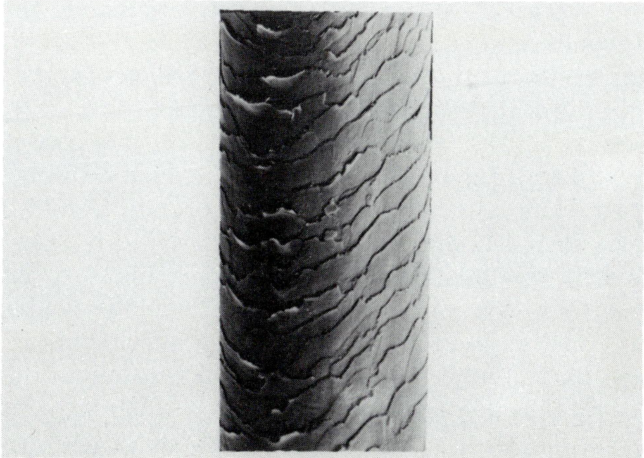

Figure 15-2 Scanning electron micrograph of hair showing the overlap of cuticle cells. ×960 in the original magnification.

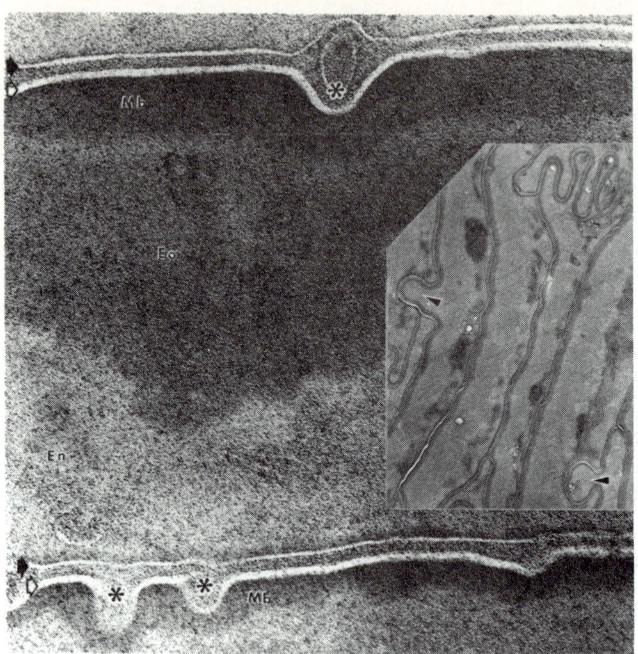

Figure 15-3 Cuticle of the cortex. On high magnification of completely keratinized cuticle cells, a thickened outer cell membrane *(open arrows),* marginal band (Mb), exocuticle (Eo), and endocuticle (En) are apparent. The inner cell membrane *(solid arrows)* is not thickened. Wedge-shaped invaginations *(arrowheads)* and interdigitation (*) of the lateral borders of adjoining cells are apparent. ×120,000, inset ×14,350 in the original magnification. [*From RL DeVillez (ed), Clinics in Dermatology. Philadelphia, Lippincott, vol 6, p 14, with permission.*]

elongated cells that run parallel to the fiber axis. Within these cells are located the 70- to 80-Å tonofilaments and interfilamentous matrix material that are responsible for most of the physicochemical properties characteristic of whole hair (Fig. 15-4). The filaments are composed of fibrous proteins that have a helical content of about 50 percent, and the matrix material consists of nonhelical proteins very rich in cystine.[8,9] Synthesis of these proteins occurs in the lower end of the follicles, and conversion of cysteine to cystine is the last stage in this process.

The properties of the structural proteins of the cortex have been elucidated by extracting samples of cut hair with alkaline buffers containing urea and a reducing agent. The solubilized protein is then treated with iodoacetic acid to block the cysteine groups by converting them to *S*-carboxymethyl (SCM) derivatives. As shown in Table 15-1, the two groups of proteins have rather different amino acid analyses, particularly in cysteine content (expressed as SCM cysteine), which is very high in the matrix protein. The fibrous proteins consist of a number of polypeptides, as shown by urea polyacrylamide electrophoresis (Fig. 15-5), but the matrix proteins run as a single band in this system. However, with other techniques, multiple matrix polypeptides can be observed.

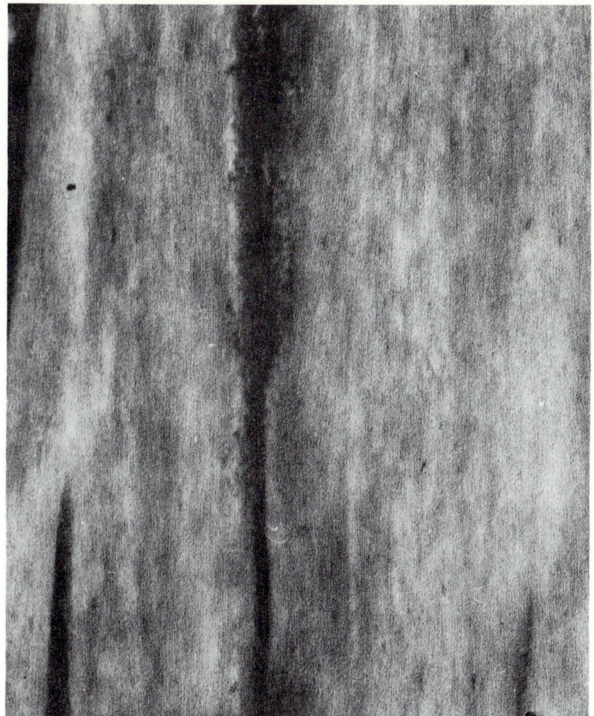

Figure 15-4 Electron micrograph of longitudinal section of hair cortex showing filaments *(white)* embedded in matrix *(black)*. ×84,000 in the original magnification.

In order to study the fibrous proteins of hair (trichocytic) in their more native state, the lower ends of hair shafts were isolated where the keratins exist in the reduced state and can be isolated without having to modify them. Using two-dimensional electrophoresis, it was found that the keratins consist of four major acid and basic polypeptides and one minor acidic and basic polypeptide (Fig. 15-6). These are different from the epithelial ones, principally in their nonhelical segments, and are present in the hair follicle only in the cuticle and cortex of the shaft (Fig. 15-7).

Although the available data do not permit a definitive model to be constructed for the 80-Å filaments seen by electron microscopy, a reasonable

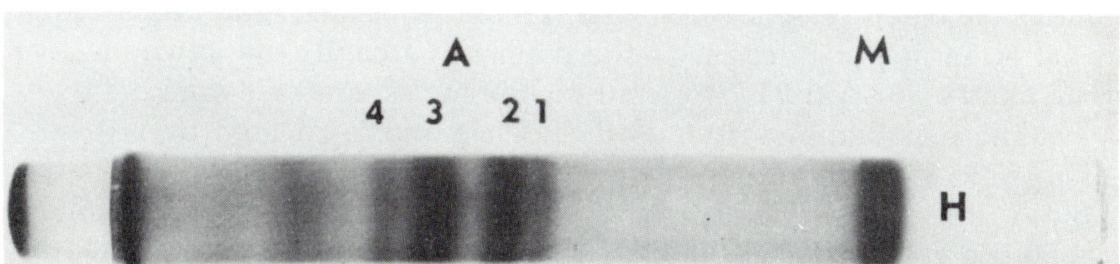

Figure 15-5 Polyacrylamide gel electrophoresis pattern of SCM solubilized hair proteins. A = fibrous components (1–4); M = matrix; H = hair proteins.

Table 15-1

AMINO ACID COMPOSITION OF α-FIBROUS AND MATRIX HAIR PROTEINS

	Hair	
Amino Acid	α	Matrix
Lysine	2.9	1.0
Histidine	0.6	0.8
Arginine	7.0	0.8
Aspartic acid	8.4	3.2
Threonine	5.9	9.9
Serine	10.5	13.1
Glutamic acid	17.1	10.1
Proline	5.6	10.9
Glycine	5.3	3.9
Alanine	6.0	2.3
Valine	5.3	4.8
Methionine	0.6	0.3
Isoleucine	3.0	1.8
Leucine	9.8	3.7
Tyrosine	2.8	1.6
Phenylalanine	2.1	1.3
S-carboxymethyl cysteine	7.1	25.0

hypothesis is that the filaments are composed of groups of double-stranded helices. The matrix protein is thought to surround the filaments and to be connected to them by disulfide bonds. What appears to be matrix by electron microscopy may include some nonhelical part of the fibrous protein.

The central portion of the hair is composed of cells with a unique type of differentiation; this region is called the medulla. The proteins of the medulla are resistant to most solvents, including alkali, and are similar in composition to those of the internal root sheath in that they contain ϵ-(γ-glutamyl) lysine cross-links and citrulline.

The dermal papilla is the connective tissue component inside the hair bulb, and its size is correlated with that of the bulb.[10] It contains variable numbers of blood vessels, fibroblasts, ground substance, and fine collagen fibers. A narrow stalk connects the papilla to a basal plate of connective tissue, and a 500-Å-thick basement membrane separates it from the bulb. A hyaline membrane surrounds the follicle and is covered by layers of collagen fibers.

Blood vessels arise from the hypodermal arterial plexus and follow straight down to the pore of the dermal papilla. These are connected by numerous shunts around the lower third of the follicle and form a rich plexus. The dermal papilla contains a large tuft of capillaries that arises

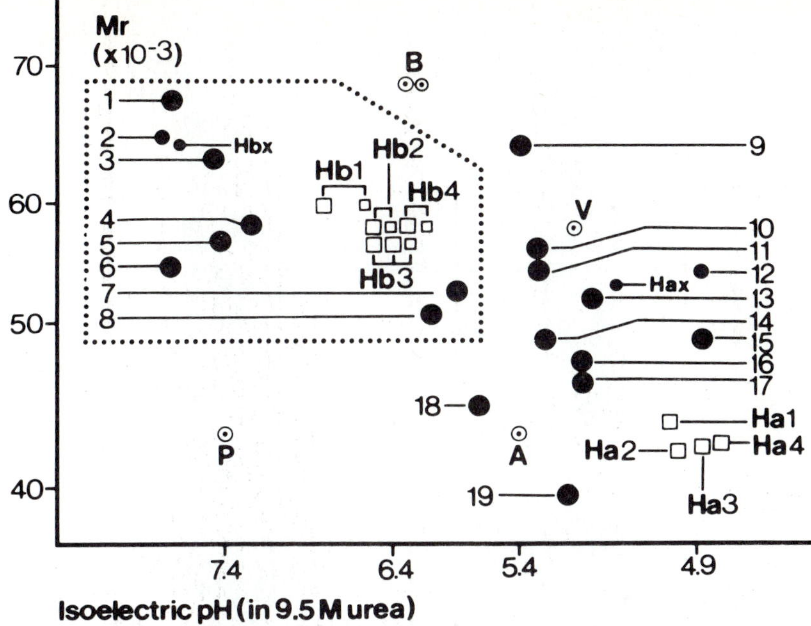

Figure 15-6 Schematic catalog of the trichocytic and epithelial human cytokeratins arranged according to their position after separation by two-dimensional gel electrophoresis, showing the 19 epithelial cytokeratins *(filled circles)*, the 8 major trichocyte cytokeratin polypeptides *(open squares)*, and the 2 minor trichocyte cytokeratin polypeptides, Hbx and Hax *(small filled circles)*. Designations are according to the Moll catalog; the polypeptides of the basic (type II) subfamily, including component Hbx, are circumscribed by a dotted line (5). A, B, P, and V are standard markers. Hb = hair basic; Ha = hair acidic; Mr = relative molecular weight. *(From HW Heit et al: Patterns of expression of trichocytic and epithelial cytokeratins in mammalian tissues. I. Human and bovine hair follicles. Differentiation 37:137, 1988, with permission.)*

from the longitudinal vessels and extends to the inner surface of the bulb. Numerous sensory nerves surround the whole length of the hair follicle. Some run parallel to it and others surround it.

When hairs go into the telogen phase, the follicle becomes smaller and ascends to a higher position in the dermis (Fig. 15-8). The architecture of the growing follicle is largely lost, and we are left with a fully hardened hair connected to the epithelial sac around it. This sac is made of the remaining inner and outermost sheaths, and has at its base a bag of quiescent epithelial cells and below this the dermal papilla cells. Regeneration of the follicle occurs from proliferation of these two structures down into the skin, with reconstruction of an anagen follicle.

DETERMINATION OF THE PHYSICOCHEMICAL PROPERTIES OF HAIR

The physical properties of hair are related to its chemical composition.[11,12] Rapid swelling in water up to about 40 percent of the dry weight is a

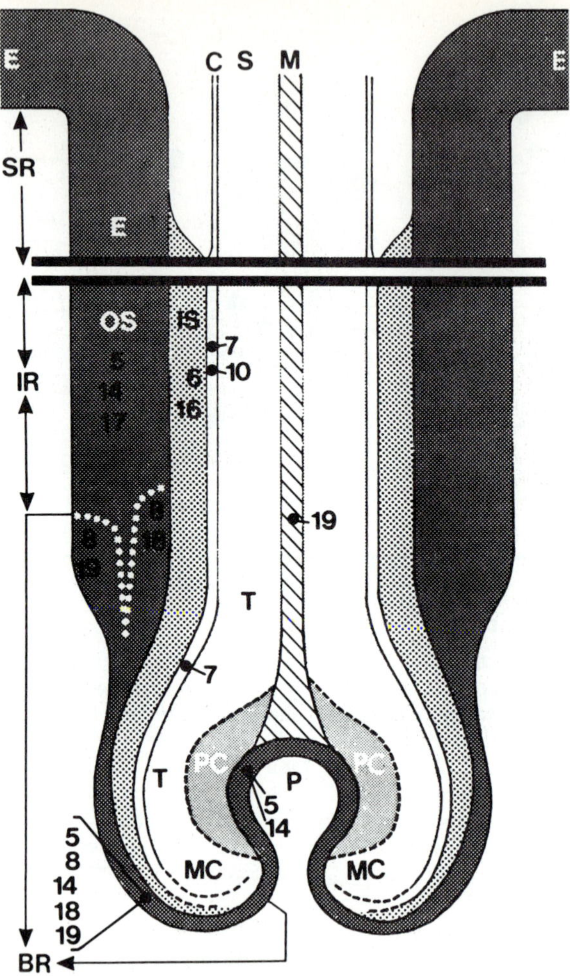

Figure 15-7 Histological scheme of a human hair follicle showing the major tissue layers and cell types and the localization of the cytokeratins. M = medulla; S = shaft matrix and cortex; C = cuticle; IS = inner root sheath; OS = outer root sheath; E = epidermis; SR = supraductal region, i.e., above the ostium of the sebaceous gland duct *infundibulum;* IR = intermediate region *isthmus;* BR = bulbar region; MC = matrix cells; PC = peripapillary cone; P = dermal papilla; T = trichocytes. The numbers of the epithelial cytokeratins are placed in tissue regions where these proteins have been localized. The trichocytic cytokeratins occur abundantly in the shaft (S), the cortex, the C, and in certain MC (5). *(From HW Heid et al: Patterns of expression of trichocytic and epithelial cytokeratins in mammalian tissues. I. Human and bovine hair follicles. Differentiation 37:137, 1988, with permission.)*

reflection of the hair's low lipid and almost pure protein content. The high birefringence of hair results from oriented filaments that run parallel to the long axis. The tensile properties of hair have been studied extensively as a means of defining the function of specific components and identifying abnormalities in them. When hair is stretched at a constant rate, there is

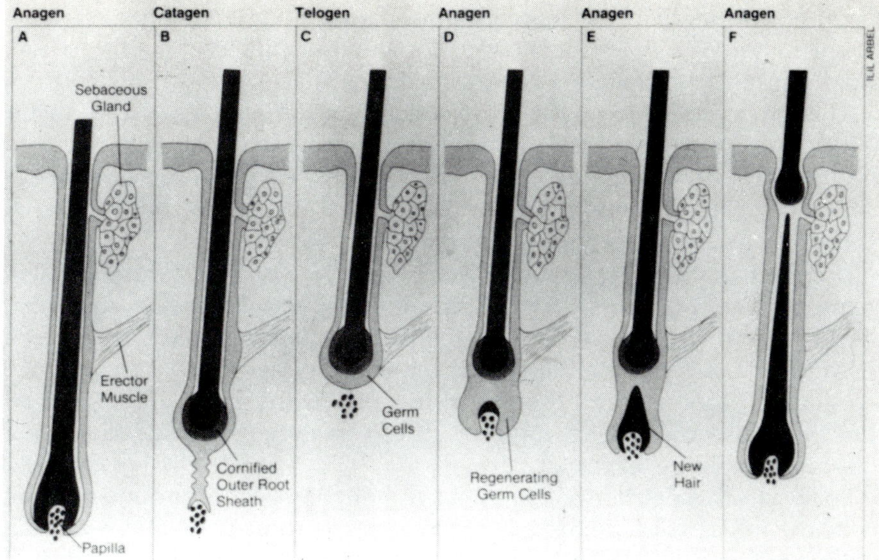

Figure 15-8 The normal hair cycle.

a linear relationship between stress and strain up to 2 percent elongation (Hookean region), and the slope is the modulus of the fiber (Fig. 15-9). The modulus is dependent on the water content and is thought to be accommodated by the microfibrillar framework. Following this Hookean region, there is a yield zone with a flatter slope in which the polypeptide

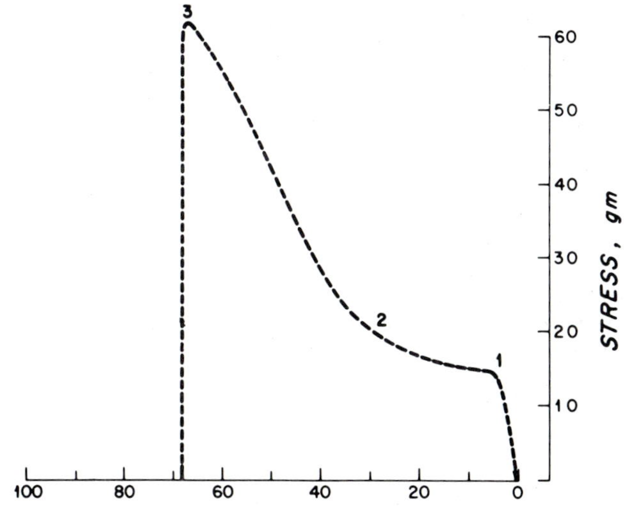

Figure 15-9 Stress strain curve of wet hair. 0–1 = Hookean region; 1–2 = yield zone; 2–3 = post-yield zone; 3 = breaking point.

chains extend to a β form. This continues up to about 30 percent elongation, at which there is a sharp increase in slope that results from configurational limitation to the exchange of disulfide bonds that occurs so readily in the yield zone. At the end of this post-yield zone the hair breaks. Reduction of disulfide bonds or oxidation by chemicals and ultraviolet light decreases the modulus, increases the length of the yield zone, and decreases the breaking strength. Under constant conditions, therefore, these tests can be used to define alterations in the structural proteins.

Chemical analyses of the hair include determination of specific elements or measurement of the structural proteins and amino acids. A number of sensitive techniques have been developed for determination of the metal content,[13] but environmental contamination and the effect of treatment of the sample seriously limit the usefulness of the analyses. Under properly controlled circumstances, however, these analyses may be of value in detecting heavy metal toxicity.

Analysis of the structural proteins of hair has been done most readily by using polyacrylamide disc electrophoresis of solubilized and *S*-carboxymethylated proteins.[14] This has proved to be of most value in studying genetic disorders of keratinization but can also be useful in detecting irreversible damage to hair. Amino acid analysis of hair is ordinarily of limited value because hair is heterogeneous, consisting of a number of components of varying composition. However, analysis of cystine content may be of help in recognizing abnormalities of the matrix proteins.

DISORDERS OF THE HAIR

In order to evaluate abnormalities of the hair, it is necessary to examine the hair in various areas of the body, as well as the skin from which it is growing. One should note the distribution of hair loss (alopecia) and whether hair is totally gone, broken, or abnormal. After shaving a small area of the scalp and marking out a 1-cm square, one can determine the hair density, which on the side of a normal scalp is about 150 hairs per square centimeter. A few hairs should be removed by gently pulling and the scalp ends examined with magnification to see if there is a normal club-shaped or a tapered, dystrophic end. Hairs can be plucked with rubber-tipped needle holders to determine the percentage of anagen hairs (normally <20 percent). A biopsy specimen of the scalp can be obtained to determine histopathologic changes in the skin.

Male Pattern Hair Loss

Male pattern hair loss is seen in virtually all adult males and cannot be considered a pathological condition. However, the amount of loss varies greatly from one individual to another and with age. In an attempt to quantitate the loss, several classification schemes have been developed that may be useful[15,16] (Fig. 15-10). The initial loss is in the frontal region, with recession of the hairline. As this progresses, alopecia also develops

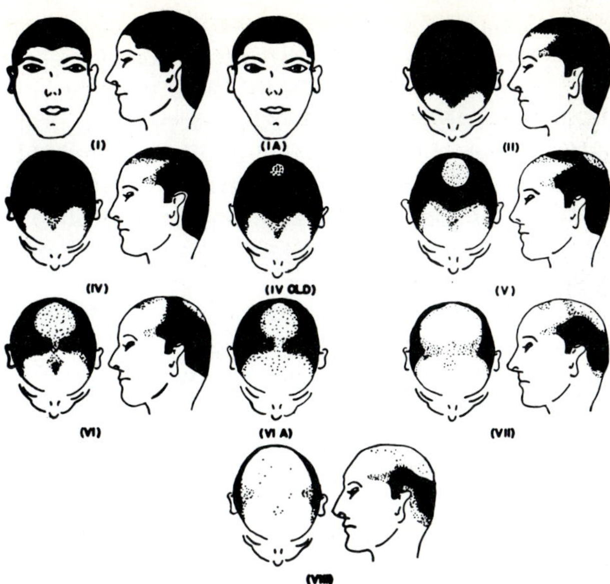

Figure 15-10 Schematic representation of the progression of hair loss in male-pattern alopecia. *(From JB Hamilton.*[15]*)*

on the vertex. The end stage of this process is a horseshoe-shaped rim of hair around the scalp. In addition to the pattern of loss, there is a decrease in the length that the hair can attain, as well as in the thickness of the hair in the balding areas. The follicles, however, are not lost.

The cause of balding in males has not been established, but several factors have been identified.[17] It has been suggested that baldness is inherited in an autosomal dominant fashion. More recently, a multifactorial or polygenic form of inheritance has been suggested, which means that there is an interaction of several genes combined with environmental factors.

Androgens have been shown to play an essential role in male pattern hair loss, but how they affect the hair has not been established. There is no difference, however, in the excretion of 17-ketosteroids or in the blood level of testosterone between normal balding and nonbalding individuals. Since it had been shown that conversion of testosterone to dihydrotestosterone occurs in target tissues, attention was turned to this conversion process in hair follicles. Schweikert and Wilson[18] studied the 5α reduction of testosterone in plucked hair follicles from various body areas and found no relation between androgen-mediated growth of hair and the capacity to form the 5α metabolites. The scalp hair of women, for example, performed the reduction to the same extent as male beard hair. The authors did find that the frontal anagen hairs of bald men had significantly more 5α-reductase activity than those of nonbalding individuals. Because the sparse hair remaining in balding individuals may represent a special population, those results could be a consequence of the process rather than a cause of it. True differential androgen responsiveness of hair roots, therefore, may be determined by something other than steroid metabolism. This possibility led to a study of cyclic AMP–dependent protein kinase in human hair roots, which is known to be inhibited indirectly by androgen. The similarity in the properties of the enzymes isolated from scalp hair and beard hair indicates that this enzyme is not responsible for the effect. Further studies of androgen metabolism in the hair cell are necessary to demonstrate its mechanism of action.

Recognizing that the amount of loss is the primary consideration in dealing with male balding, the prevalence of the different classes of balding has been determined at different ages in two studies.[15,16] There is a progressive increase with age in the number of individuals with hair loss of types IV through VII (Fig. 15-10), which is defined as balding. It is not possible, however, to use this information in any precise way to predict the rate of loss or eventual outcome for an individual. But individuals with marked balding consistently report type IV or higher hair loss starting in their twenties.

The histopathology of male pattern alopecia shows the conversion of terminal to vellus follicles, and these are present in greatest number in the most advanced stages of alopecia[19] (Fig. 15-11). The thickness of the dermis is significantly reduced, as is that of the epidermis and subcutaneous tissue. The capillaries in the upper corium appear relatively normal. Connective tissue streamers consisting of connective tissue sheaths, blood vessels, nerves, and cells are present beneath all vellus follicles. Staining for alkaline phosphatase shows the blood supply to the follicles to be normal in early male pattern alopecia, but the vessels of the smaller vellus follicles are reduced in size.

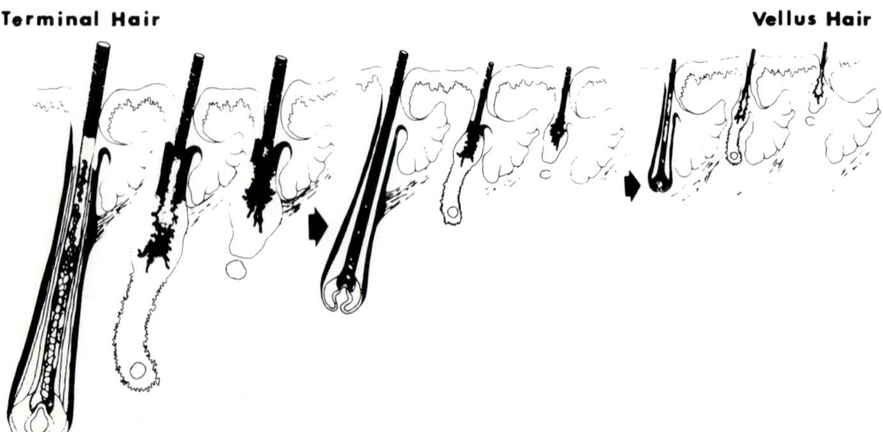

Figure 15-11 The gradual conversion of terminal to vellus hair in male pattern hair loss. *(From W Montagna, PF Parakkal, The Structure and Function of Skin, 3d ed, New York, Academic, 1974, p 250.)*

Based on clinical, chemical, and histopathologic studies, the most likely hypothesis to explain male pattern alopecia is that certain follicles are programmed to become progressively smaller in size and to have shorter periods of growth. In the end stage only vellus follicles are present, and most of these are in telogen or catagen. Although this process is androgen dependent, genetic factors are very important. It is not known how the androgens work or even whether the target tissue is the hair bulb or the supporting dermal components. It has been presumed that the process is irreversible, but there is no evidence to support this contention. In fact, the topical application of minoxidil has been found to cause growth of hair in some balding individuals.[20] The response was best in younger individuals with lesser degrees of balding.

Female Pattern Hair Loss

The findings in female pattern alopecia are rather consistent (Fig. 15-12). The frontal hairline is relatively normal, but some recession with varying numbers of short, fine hairs may be observed. There is obvious diffuse thinning over the vertex and parietal areas, which can also be found in the temporal regions when the hair is pushed aside. The occipital zone, however, appears to be spared. The normal retention of the frontal hairline relative to the amount of diffuse thinning is very striking. There

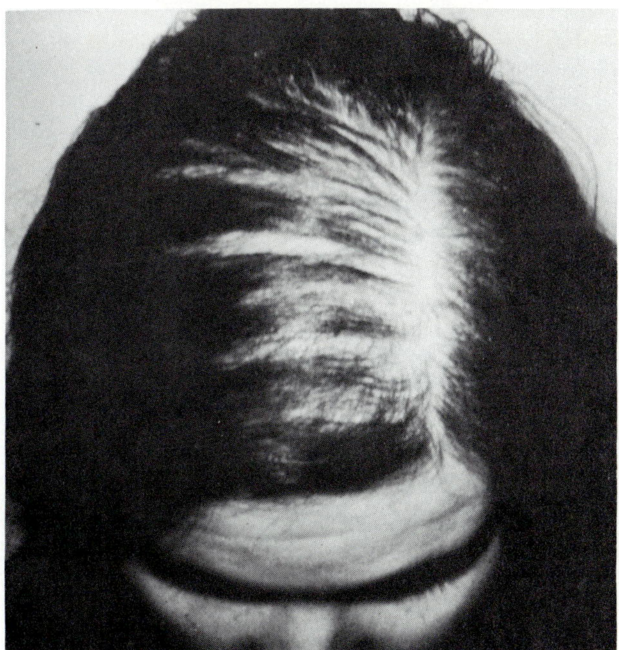

Figure 15-12 Female pattern hair loss showing thinning on top of scalp with a relatively normal hairline.

is often a difference between the physician's perception of the hair loss and the patient's, since a considerable amount of hair can be lost without it being obvious.

Female pattern alopecia has been recognized as a distinct entity for only about the past 20 years.[21,22] There is still some question as to whether the increase in the number of women seeking help for this problem reflects an increase in the incidence of the disorder. Alternatively, women may be seeking help more frequently for a variety of reasons, such as general changes in grooming habits and more concern about appearance.

The cause of female pattern alopecia has not been established. However, there is a growing belief that it has the same basis as male pattern alopecia but is modified in appearance by female genes. Many women with marked diffuse alopecia have a bald father as well as other bald male relatives, and women with masculinizing syndromes related to androgen-producing tumors may show considerable diffuse alopecia.

There are no studies of 5α-reductase activity in the plucked hair bulbs of balding women comparable to those of men. There is no evidence at present, therefore, that there is an increased conversion of androgens to a more active form in normal women with hair loss. If the pathogenesis at the cellular level proves to be the same as in men, there still remains the problem of why hair loss is diffuse in women. The progression of hair loss in women suggests that aging may be an additional factor, particularly since the degree of alopecia is more marked as women get older.

The amount of hair loss in women is generally considerably less than in men, and one rarely observes a totally bald scalp. However, alopecia in women is a more significant cosmetic liability and can cause considerable problems at hair densities that might be accepted by men.

Excessive production of androgens may cause significant alopecia in women that is largely irreversible. The disorders that may do this are listed in Table 15-2. These can be diagnosed by measuring the levels of circulating male hormones.

Alopecia Areata

Alopecia areata is an inflammatory disorder of the follicle that produces reversible injury to the growing hair. The effect may be transient, with the hair shaft showing thinning and breakage followed by regrowth (anagen effluvium), or more severe, causing the hair to enter the resting phase. The frequency of alopecia areata is less than 0.1 percent in the general population and between 1 and 4 percent in dermatology clinics. Most studies involving large numbers of patients have come from medical centers that see patients with more severe forms of the disease.[23,24] These findings may be biased, therefore, and may not reflect the true prevalence of the disease in the general population.

There is no sex difference in the incidence of the disease. Younger age groups are more severely affected, with about one-third of the cases

Table 15-2

SOURCES OF EXCESS ANDROGENS

Adrenal Cortex Disease

Congenital adrenal hyperplasia (most forms)
Adult adrenal hyperplasia
Adrenal adenoma or carcinoma
Cushing's syndrome (various causes)

Ovary Disease

Stein-Leventhal syndrome
Hyperthecosis
Leydig cell hyperplasia
Ovarian tumors
- Arrhenoblastoma
- Adrenal rest tumor
- Hilar cell tumor
- Cystadenoma or cystic carcinoma
- Several others (occasionally)

Exogenous

Testosterone therapy
Anabolic steroids
Some oral progestogens

Source: Modified from AC Brown (ed), *The First Human Hair Symposium.* New York, Medcom, 1974, p 99.

starting by age 20 and only 25 percent after age 40. Familial occurrence is between 10 and 20 percent and seems to be associated with a worse prognosis. Identical twins have been found to be affected, but the degree of concordance is not known. The disease is characterized by an irregular relapsing course, with only about 20 to 30 percent of affected individuals having a solitary episode. Regrowth of hair within several months is common, and perhaps 60 percent have regrowth by 1 year, but often it is incomplete and is followed by repeated episodes of hair loss. Some involvement of the scalp is seen in 95 percent of cases of alopecia areata, and the beard may be involved in about 10 percent of men.

Psychiatric disease of both an acute and a chronic nature has been described repeatedly in many patients with the disease, often preceding the hair loss.[25] However, there does not appear to be any correlation between the severity of the emotional problems and the extent of loss or regrowth of hair. No specific endocrine disorder has been found in these patients, although an increased incidence of thyroid diseases of various types has been reported.[23] Treatment of the thyroid disease, however, has no effect on the course of the alopecia. Pregnancy has no consistent effect

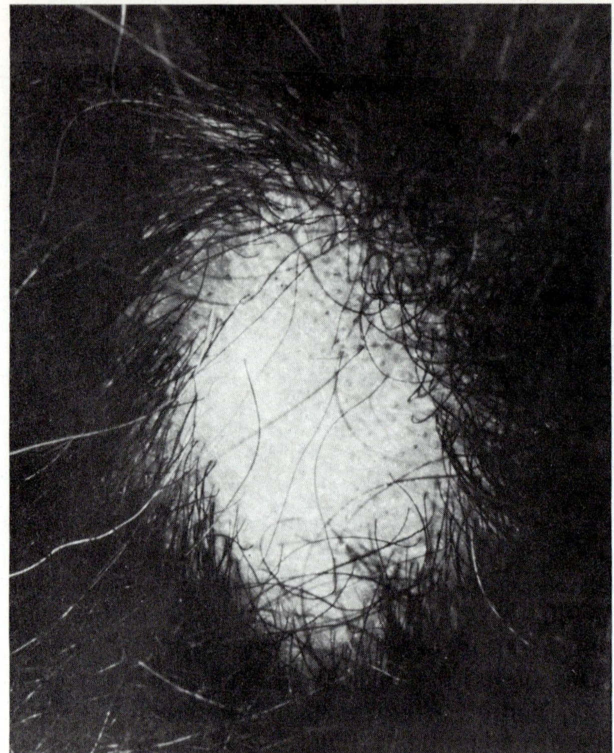

Figure 15-13 Alopecia areata shows circumscribed area of hair loss.

on the disease, although some patients report increased growth. In Down's syndrome there appears to be an increased frequency of alopecia areata, and in one large series 60 percent of the individuals were affected.[26]

Alopecia areata is rarely associated with any symptoms. The initial patch is most frequently located on the scalp but can be anywhere (Fig. 15-13). It is usually round in shape and clearly circumscribed, with a smooth white surface containing scattered small, stubby hairs. Exclamation point hairs, which have a blunt distal end and taper proximally, may be found in the periphery (Fig. 15-14), and hairs are easily plucked from the apparently normal margin of the bald area. Some of the plucked hairs are normal telogen hairs with a club-shaped end, and others are tapered as a result of breakage at abnormal regions in the shaft produced by interference with growth during the anagen phase (Fig. 15-15). Because the course of the disease is very variable, extension of the patch and development of new ones cannot be accurately predicted.

In older stable areas of alopecia, typical exclamation point hairs and easily plucked hairs are not seen. However, short, stubby hairs or fine white hairs may be found. It is usually possible to recognize the empty follicle, but occasionally in long-standing cases follicular openings may be

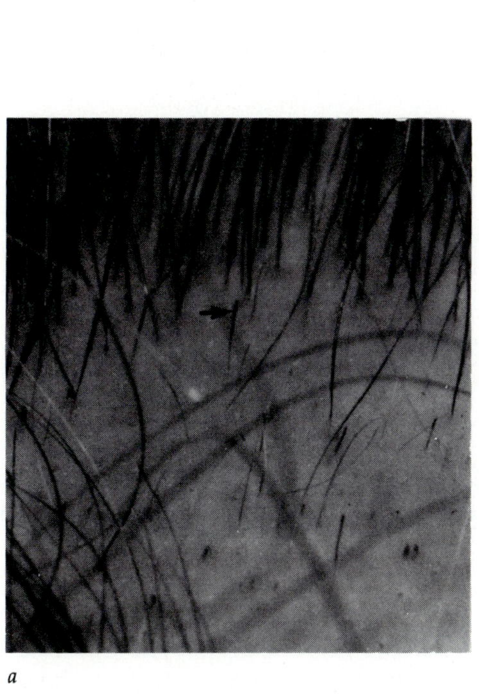

a

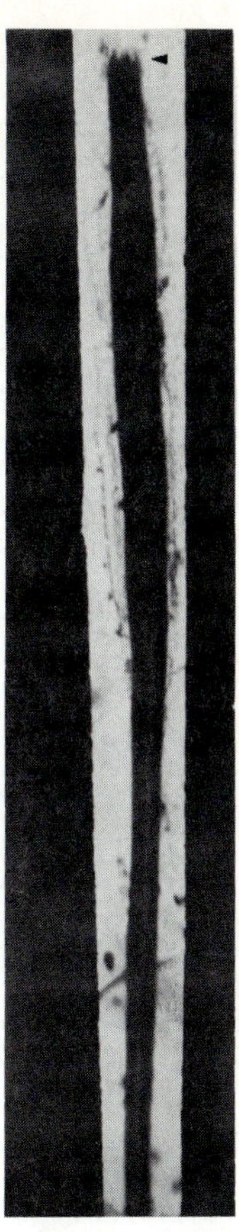

b

Figure 15-14 Exclamation point hair. (*a*) The typical hair is indicated by the arrow. (*b*) As a result of a disturbance in the bulb, an imperfect region of hair is formed that eventually breaks and produces the irregular end (*arrow*). This is followed by the growth of relatively normal hair until a new wave of abnormal growth causes thinning.

difficult to recognize, which can make one think that the scalp is scarred. When the hair regrows, it is frequently white and has a tapered distal end, indicating the initiation of a new hair cycle. The hair usually, but not always, returns to its original color. Alopecia totalis results in the loss of all scalp hair and may occur suddenly or follow partial alopecia. Loss of total body hair, called alopecia universalis, may also occur suddenly or follow long-standing partial alopecia.

Involvement of nails, most commonly the fingernails, has been reported, with a frequency of 10 to 60 percent. Pitting is the most common finding, but shedding of nails has also been described. Vitiligo is also seen in about 4 percent of patients. Atopic dermatitis also appears to occur with increased frequency.

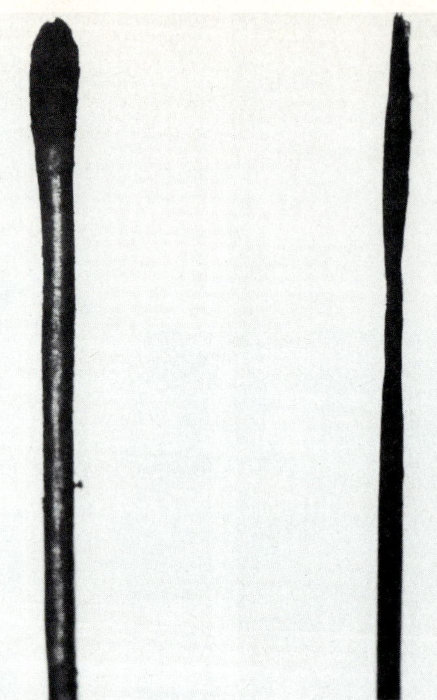

Figure 15-15 Comparison of club (*left*) and tapered dystrophic (*right*) hairs, which may be obtained by gently pulling at edge of a lesion of alopecia areata.

The early histopathologic changes are a lymphocytic infiltrate around the hair bulb, as well as within the matrix and outer root sheath of the upper portion of the hair bulb. The infiltrate consists of T lymphocytes primarily bearing the CD4 (helper/inducer) phenotype.[27] In long-standing cases the follicles appear very small and high up in the dermis. They are believed to represent arrested anagen follicles.

In most patients, the physical findings are so characteristic that the diagnosis is obvious. Alopecia areata may be confused with telogen effluvium because in both conditions hairs are shed in large quantities, but only in the former are dystrophic hairs present. Telogen effluvium is a disorder in which a large number of hairs enter the resting state and are subsequently shed. The most common causes of telogen effluvium are termination of pregnancy, major illness, severe emotional stress, rapid weight loss, and certain drugs (e.g., anticoagulants). There is no hair loss at the time the hairs enter the resting phase but rather about 4 months later, when a new hair cycle starts. Hairs come out with gentle pulling, and all are normal clubs. A hair pluck reveals that more than 40 percent of the hairs are in telogen.

The cause of alopecia areata is unknown, but an autoimmune cause has been suggested because of association of the alopecia with vitiligo, endocrinopathies, and other disorders.[28] Furthermore, the histopathologic changes with lymphocytic involvement of the follicle are suggestive. Studies of autoantibodies to thyroid cells, gastric parietal cells, smooth muscle, mitochondria, and nuclei, as well as rheumatoid factor, showed no consistent differences between affected individuals and matched controls.[29] Immunofluorescence studies have revealed no evidence of bound antibody, and no circulating antibodies to hair follicles have been demonstrated. These results, however, do not rule out the possibility of an immunologic mechanism, and the newer techniques of studying cell-mediated immunity need to be utilized.

REFERENCES

1. Montagna W, Parakkal PF: The pilary apparatus, in *The Structure and Function of Skin,* 3d ed. New York, Academic Press, 1974, p 172.
2. Hardy D: Quantitative hair form variation in seven populations. *Am J Phys Anthropol* 39:7, 1973.
3. Birbeck MSC, Mercer EH: The electron microscopy of the human hair follicle. III. The inner root sheath and trichohyalin. *J Biophys Biochem Cytol* 3:223, 1957.
4. Rothnagel JA, Rogers GE: Trichohyalin, an intermediate filament-associated protein of the hair follicle. *J Cell Biol* 102:1419, 1986.
5. Heid HW et al: Patterns of expression of trichocytic and epithelial cytokeratins in mammalian tissues. I. Human and bovine hair follicles. *Differentiation* 37:137, 1988.
6. Rogers GE et al: The origin of citrulline-containing protein in the hair follicle and the chemical nature of trichohyalin, an intracellular precursor. *Biochim Biophys Acta* 495:159, 1977.
7. Rogers GE, Harding HWJ: Molecular mechanisms in the formation of hair, in T Kobori, W Montagna (eds), *Biology and Disease of the Hair.* Tokyo, University of Tokyo Press, 1976, p 411.
8. Thompson EOP, O'Donnell IJ: Studies on reduced wool. V. A comparison of the two major components. *Aust J Biol Sci* 18:1207, 1965.
9. Gillespie JM, Inglis AS: A comparative study of high-sulphur proteins from α-keratins. *Comp Biochem Physiol* 15:175, 1965.
10. Montagna W, Parakkal PF: The pilary apparatus, in *The Structure and Function of Skin,* 3d ed. New York, Academic Press, 1974, p 215.
11. Alexander P, Hudson RF: *Wool. Its Chemistry and Physics.* New York, Reinhold, 1954, p 1.
12. Robbins CR: *Chemical and Physical Behavior of Human Hair.* New York, Van Nostrand, 1979, p 1.
13. Eatough DJ et al: Level of selected trace elements in human hair, in AC Brown (ed), *The First Human Hair Symposium.* New York, Medcom, 1974, p 377.
14. Baden HP et al: A genetic electrophoretic variant of human hair polypeptides. *Am J Hum Genet* 27:472, 1975.
15. Hamilton JB: Patterned loss of hair in man: types and incidence. *Ann NY Acad Sci* 53:708, 1951.
16. Norwood OTT: Male pattern baldness: classification and incidence. *South Med J* 68:1, 1359, 1975.
17. Ebling FJ et al: Male pattern alopecia, in A Rook et al (eds), *Textbook of Dermatology,* 4th ed. Oxford, Blackwell Scientific, 1986, p 1971.
18. Schweikert HU, Wilson JD: Regulation of human hair growth by steroid hormones. I. Testosterone metabolism in isolated hairs. *J Clin Endocrinol Metab* 38:811, 1974.
19. Lattanand A, Johnson WC: Male pattern alopecia: a histological and histochemical study. *J Cutan Pathol* 2:58, 1975.

20. Olsen EA et al: Long-term follow-up of men with male pattern baldness treated with topical minoxidil. *J Am Acad Dermatol* 16:688, 1987.
21. Sulzberger MB et al: Diffuse alopecia in women: its unexplained apparent increase in incidence. *Arch Dermatol* 81:556, 1960.
22. Ludwig E: Classification of the types of androgenic alopecia (common baldness) occurring in the female sex. *Br J Dermatol* 97:247, 1977.
23. Muller SA, Winkelmann RK: Alopecia areata. *Arch Dermatol* 88:106, 1963.
24. Gip L et al: Alopecia areata. *Acta Derm Venereol (Stockh)* 49:180, 1969.
25. Mehlman RD, Griesemer RD: Alopecia areata in the very young. *Am J Psychiatry* 125:605, 1968.
26. Carter DM, Jegasothy BV: Alopecia areata and Down syndrome. *Arch Dermatol* 112:1397, 1976.
27. Herzer P et al: Immunological studies in patients with alopecia areata. *Int Arch Allergy Appl Immunol* 58:212, 1979.
28. Cochran REI et al: An auto-antibody profile in alopecia totalis and diffuse alopecia. *Br J Dermatol* 95:61, 1976.
29. Muller HK et al: Immunohistology and autoantibody studies in alopecia. *Br J Dermatol* 102:609, 1980.

16

Pathophysiology of Nails (Onychopathophysiology)

Joseph C. Kvedar and Howard P. Baden

ANATOMY AND PHYSIOLOGY

Nails are situated on the dorsum of the distal end of the fingers and toes. They protect the terminal phalanxes and assist with grasping small objects. Like hair, the nail is a keratinized appendage of the skin. Four structures make up the nail unit: (1) nail plate, (2) nail matrix, (3) nail bed, and (4) periungual tissue (Fig. 16-1).

Nail Plate

The nail plate is the rectangular, cornified, hard, translucent product of the matrix. Its pink color comes from the vascular bed on which it rests. Usually in the thumbs but occasionally in other fingers, a white, crescent-shaped lunula is seen projecting from under the proximal nail fold. As the nail plate emerges from the matrix, its proximal and lateral edges are enveloped by folds of skin—the proximal and lateral nail folds. The skin under the free border of the nail is referred to as hyponychium and is contiguous with the skin of the fingertip. The dorsal surface of the nail is rather smooth, but its ventral surface is deeply grooved in the longitudinal axis, which allows interdigitation with the nail bed (Fig. 16-2). The nail becomes thicker in growing from its proximal origin to its distal free edge, where it varies in thickness from 0.3 to 0.65 mm.[1] The plate is mainly composed of cells firmly cemented together that are filled with structural proteins.

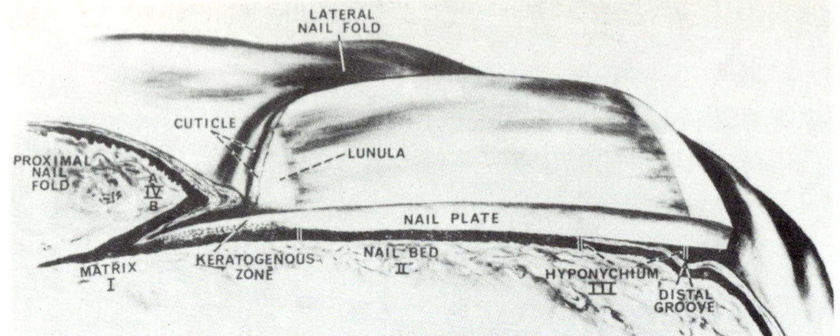

Figure 16-1 Diagrammatic drawing of adult normal fingernails. *(From TB Fitzpatrick et al, Dermatology in General Medicine, 2d ed, New York, McGraw-Hill, 1979, p 418.)*

Nail Matrix

The nail matrix represents the root of the nail and cannot be seen by physical examination except as the lunula. The matrix lies primarily beneath the proximal nail fold but extends to the outer edge of the lunula on some digits. The white color of the lunula is the result of the scattering of light by the thick layer of cells. The matrix shows cell division along its entire length, and autoradiographs of nail following incorporation of tritiated glycine indicate that the proximal matrix gives rise to the dorsal surface of the nail and the distal regions give rise to the deeper portions. As in the epidermis, the upper layers of the matrix flatten, die, lose their nuclei,

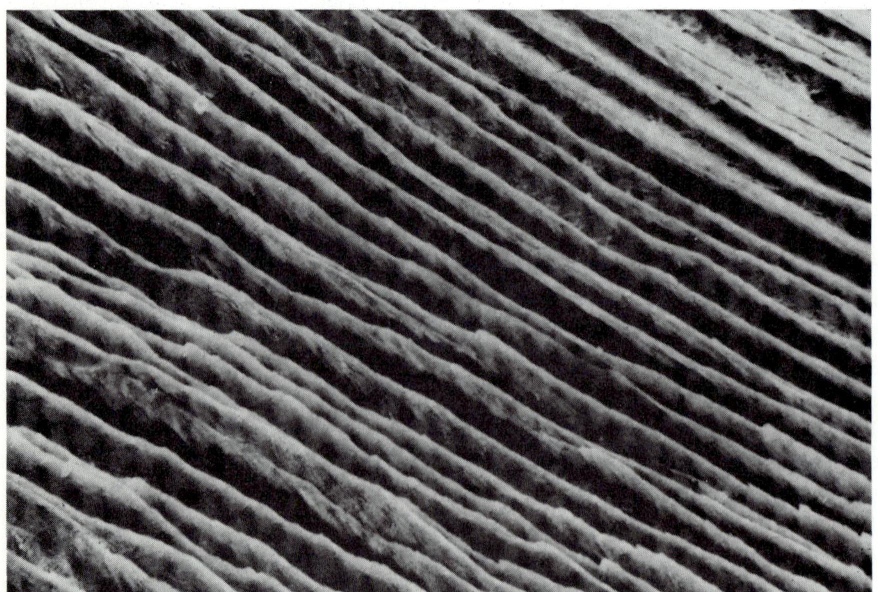

Figure 16-2 Scanning electron micrograph of the longitudinal grooves. *(From W Montagna, PF Parakkal, The Structure and Function of Skin, 3d ed, New York, Academic, 1974, p 275.)*

and cornify.[2] The long axis of the cell lies perpendicular to the axis of the digit.

In the black race, melanocytes are normally present in the matrix epithelium, and the color of the nail plate varies from off-white to gray. The nail plate can be pigmented diffusely or longitudinal bands of pigment may be present.[3]

Nail Bed

The nail bed extends from the nail fold or lunula to the hyponychium. The ventral surface of the nail bed strongly adheres to the undersurface of the nail by means of ridges, as depicted in Fig. 16-2. In the adult nail apparatus, the nail bed does not participate in the formation of the nail.[2] Cell division does not normally occur in the nail bed epidermis, which is formed from the distal end of the matrix. The bed epidermis also does not have a granular layer.[4]

Periungual Structures

The hyponychium extends from the nail bed to the distal groove and usually is not seen, but it can be observed on the fingers of people who bite their nails. The epidermis of the hyponychium is similar to that of plantar and palmar skin and contains a granular layer. The stratum corneum of the hyponychium normally is seen accumulating under the distal free edge of the nail plate.

The proximal nail fold covers the proximal nail and lies superficial to the matrix. The fold consists of two layers of epidermis. The dorsal portion is an extension of the epidermis of the skin on the dorsum of the finger, and the ventral portion overlies the newly formed nail plate. The horny layer of the ventral section adheres to the surface of the newly formed nail plate and moves distally for a short distance. This horny region is known as the cuticle and is depicted in Fig. 16-1.

Dermis

The dermis of the nail organ is limited by the underlying phalanx, no subcutaneous tissue being present. In the nail bed the dermal ridges fit into parallel, longitudinal grooves of the epidermis. The capillaries of the nail bed run in these parallel dermal ridges, and injury causes longitudinal splinter hemorrhages. The nail bed is richly supplied with glomus bodies that probably help to regulate the blood supply to the extremities in cold weather. There is also a rich supply of lymphatics.

Embryology

The nail is first recognized at about 9 to 10 weeks and gives rise to the mature nail as a result of complex interactions between epidermis and dermis. By 20 weeks of gestation the formation of the fingernails is largely completed.[5] The development of toenails lags about a month behind.[6]

Blood Supply

The blood supply of the nail arises from two arterial arches formed by anastomoses between the lateral digital arteries. One arch is parallel to the lunula, and the other follows the free margin of the nail and the region of the hyponychium.

Growth

Unlike hair growth, nail growth is continuous throughout life. Fingernails grow faster than toenails and show a mean growth rate in the adult of approximately 0.1 mm/day. Bean has recorded his own thumbnail growth for 35 years by etching a groove into the nail just distal to the proximal nail fold and recording it when it reached the free edge[7] (Fig. 16-3). Growth shows considerable variation, depending on the individual, the handedness (if right-handed, right fingernails will grow faster), the length of the finger (the middle finger grows the fastest), nutrition, illness, age (peak growth in the second and third decades, with a slight decline thereafter), and temperature (increased growth during summer and decreased growth during winter).

An increased growth rate is said to occur in males, during pregnancy, and in association with some forms of chronic trauma. Contrary to popular belief, the ingestion of gelatin does not encourage nail growth or increase nail strength.[8–10] Since the nail plate is made up of dead, cornified cells produced by the matrix, the thickness of the nail plate is directly proportional to the size of the matrix.

CHEMICAL COMPOSITION

The nail plate is composed primarily of structural proteins that are similar to those of the hair. There are fibrous and matrix components that differ in amino acid composition, the latter being richer in cystine[11] (Table 16-1). The water content of the nail ranges from 7 to 12 percent and the lipid content is only 0.15 to 0.76 percent, which is mainly cholesterol. The mineral content is low and includes phosphorus, calcium, zinc, magnesium, copper, iron, silica, lead, aluminum, and silver.[12,13] The nail appears to be a very porous structure, having a diffusion constant of water that is 100 times that of stratum corneum.[14]

The fibrous proteins of nail, which are keratin intermediate filament proteins, have been studied by several authors using electrophoretic and immunologic techniques.[15–21] Species examined include the human (both adult and fetal tissues) and the cow. The bovine hoof has been used because it is a plentiful source of tissue and bears a resemblance in its gross structure to the human nail.[15–17] These studies have demonstrated several interesting points. While hair and epidermis both have unique keratin polypeptides,[18–20] hoof and nail contain a mixture of hair and epidermal keratins.[17,18,20,21] When the keratin polypeptides are examined

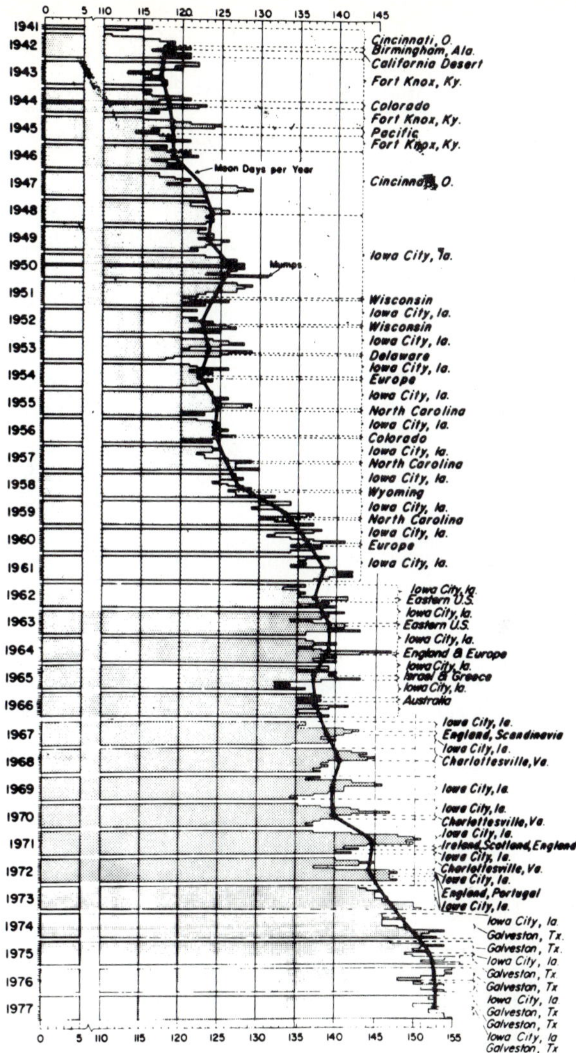

Figure 16-3 Nail growth over a period of 36 years. Abscissa gives the total days of growth. Growth is indicated by the number of days required for the mark to reach the edge of the underlying matrix. *(From WB Bean.[7])*

in a two-dimensional system that separates them by both charge and molecular weight, one can identify a group of four low-molecular-weight acidic keratins and two to four higher-molecular-weight basic keratins that are common to nail epithelia and hair bulb keratinocytes. These proteins are not found in epidermis and are higher in sulfur content than epidermal keratins. They are thus termed hard keratins.[18] Expression of these keratins is seen in suprabasal cells in both the bed and matrix regions of hoof and nail.[17,20,21] As shown in Fig. 16-4, the biochemical characteristics of these

Table 16-1

AMINO ACID ANALYSIS OF THE α-FIBROUS AND MATRIX PROTEINS OF HAIR, NAIL, AND STRATUM CORNEUM

	Hair		Nail		Stratum Corneum
Amino Acid	α	Matrix	α	Matrix	α
Lysine	2.9	1.0	2.8	0.7	4.3
Histidine	0.6	0.8	0.7	1.1	1.0
Arginine	7.0	6.3	7.1	5.0	4.8
Aspartic acid	8.4	3.2	10.4	3.7	9.5
Threonine	5.9	9.9	3.9	10.4	3.9
Serine	10.5	13.1	9.4	13.0	11.7
Glutamic acid	17.1	10.1	14.8	8.7	13.7
Proline	5.6	10.9	5.3	12.8	2.3
Glycine	5.3	3.9	8.8	6.9	18.6
Alanine	6.0	2.3	8.3	2.5	5.6
Valine	5.3	4.8	3.9	4.3	3.7
Methionine	0.6	0.3	Trace	1.1	1.5
Isoleucine	3.0	1.8	2.9	1.9	3.2
Leucine	9.8	3.7	10.7	4.6	8.5
Tyrosine	2.8	1.6	3.0	1.6	3.2
Phenylalanine	2.1	1.3	2.5	1.4	3.4
S-carboxymethyl cysteine	7.1	25.0	5.5	20.3	1.0

Note: The values are expressed as residues per 100 residues, with half of the cystine as *S*-carboxymethyl cysteine.
Source: Baden et al.[11]

keratins are quite similar in both the bovine and human species. The greater tensile strength of hair and nail compared with stratum corneum can be explained in part by the presence of these unique keratins, which are cystine rich and highly cross-linked. The cystine-rich matrix protein is also likely responsible in part for these physical properties.

DISORDERS OF NAILS

Patterns of Nail Disturbances

Physical examination should evaluate the following patterns of nail changes: (1) thickening or thinning, (2) pitting or ridging, (3) discoloration of the nail, (4) separation of the plate from the bed, (5) subungual accumulation of stratum corneum (hyperkeratosis), (6) abnormal configuration or shape of the nail, (7) loss or shedding of the nail plate, and (8) nail fold inflammation. One should attempt to relate the clinical appearance to the anatomic site of the pathological change.

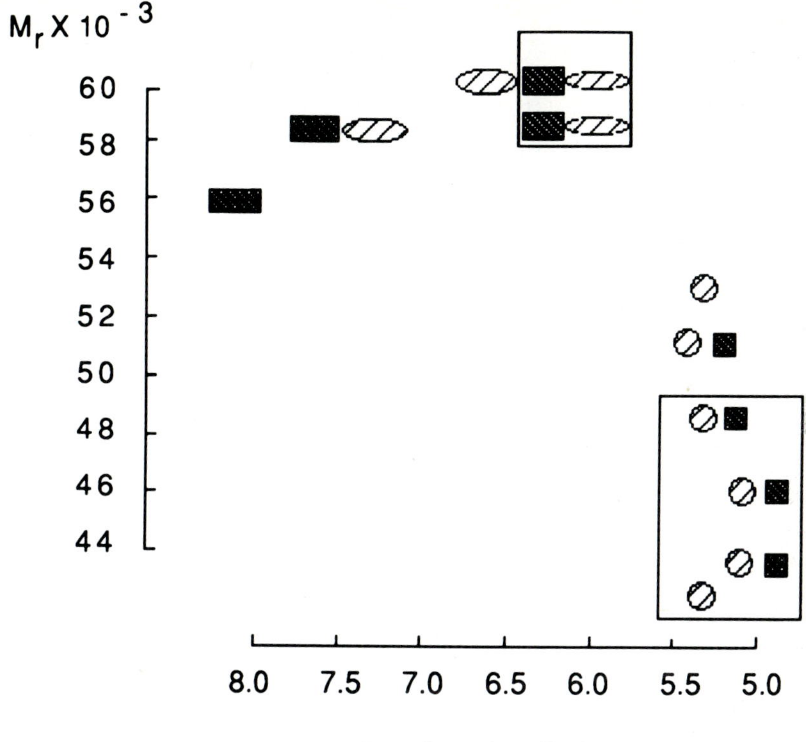

Figure 16-4 Schematic representation of the two-dimensional electrophoretic patterns of the keratins seen in the human nail (■) and bovine hoof (⊘). The spots surrounded by a box represent keratins that are present in hair and nail but absent in epidermis. M_r = relative molecular weight. [*Adapted from HP Baden, JC Kvedar: The nail, in LA Goldsmith (ed), Biochemistry and Physiology of the Skin, 2d ed, New York, Oxford University Press, in press.*]

Matrix (Plate) Defects

Abnormalities of the matrix produce changes in the nail plate. Atrophy or destruction of the matrix causes thinning (onychatrophia) or loss (anonychia) of the nail plate. Permanent splits result from any acute trauma that severs the matrix, and permanent ridging is produced by less severe injuries. Nail and cuticle biting and cuticle picking are common practices causing chronic trauma. Nail biting usually is manifested by short, irregular nails, and cuticle biting induces recurrent attacks of paronychia. A characteristic deformity is produced in the thumbnail by picking the cuticle with the index finger of the same hand. The resultant damage takes the form of a depression about 2 mm wide down the center of the nail from the cuticle to the tip, and within it are multiple cross-ridges (Fig. 16-5).

Beau's lines are transverse depressions that occur because of an arrest or retardation of the functioning matrix. Common causes are infection (syphilis, gonococcal arthritis, scarlet fever), malnutritional states, myo-

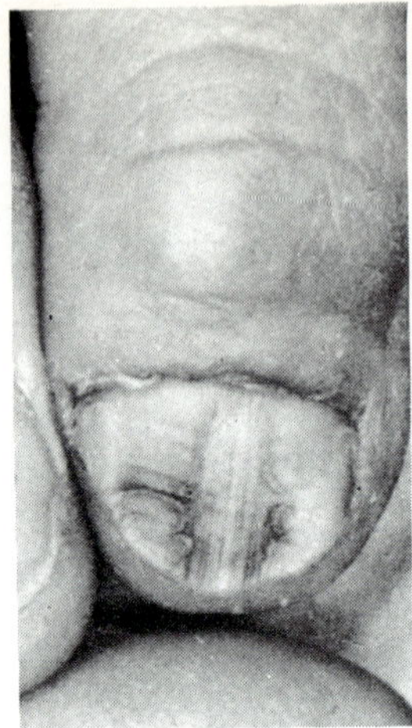

Figure 16-5 Central defect of the thumbnail because of picking.

cardial infarction, diabetes, and malabsorption disorders. Hypertrophy of the matrix causes thickening of the plate (onychauxis).

A defect in keratinization characterized by an accumulation of nucleated cells (parakeratosis) is manifested by white spots in the nail. If these areas are severely affected they disintegrate, leaving pits in the nail plate. This frequently occurs in psoriasis (Fig. 16-6).

Longitudinal striations (onychorrhexis) are a common feature in old nails, resulting from irregular growth and maturation along the matrix (Fig. 16-7).

The definition of clubbing is that the angle made by the proximal nail fold and the nail plate exceeds 180° (Fig. 16-8). This anatomic site is also known as Lovibond's angle[22] (Fig. 16-9). There is a bulbous enlargement of the distal portion of the digits associated with a noticeable mobility of the matrix due to hyperplasia in the fibrovascular tissues between the matrix and the phalanx. Clubbing has long been recognized as a sign of

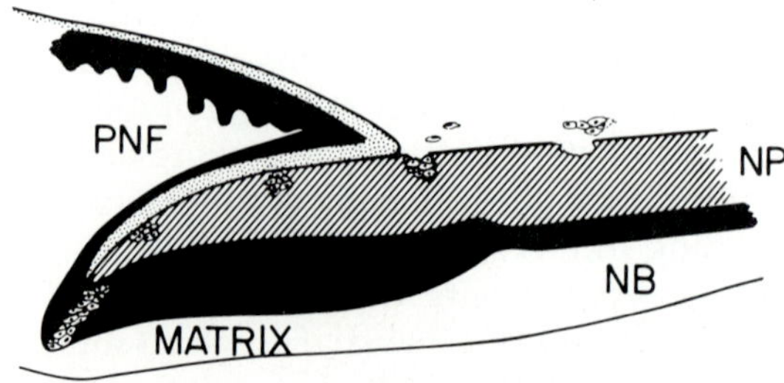

Figure 16-6 Diagrammatic drawing of the longitudinal section of a finger through psoriatic matrix lesion, showing various stages in the formation of a pit. PNF = proximal nail fold; NB = nail bed; NP = nail plate. *(From TB Fitzpatrick et al, Dermatology in General Medicine, 3d ed, New York, McGraw-Hill, 1987, p 654.)*

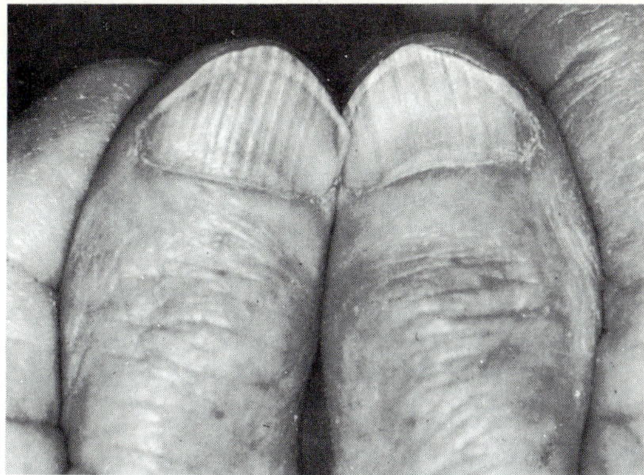

Figure 16-7 Onychorrhexis—"old nails." *(From TB Fitzpatrick et al, Dermatology in General Medicine, 3d ed, New York, McGraw-Hill, 1987, p 653.)*

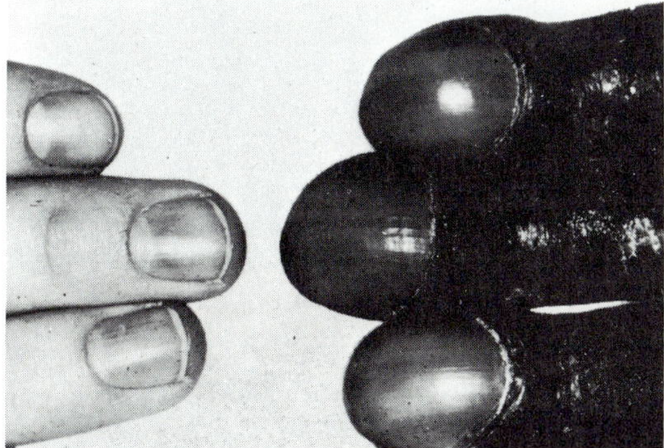

Figure 16-8 The changes of clubbed nails (*right*) contrasted with normal fingers and nails (*left*). *(From TB Fitzpatrick et al, Dermatology in General Medicine, 3d ed, New York, McGraw-Hill, 1987, p 660.)*

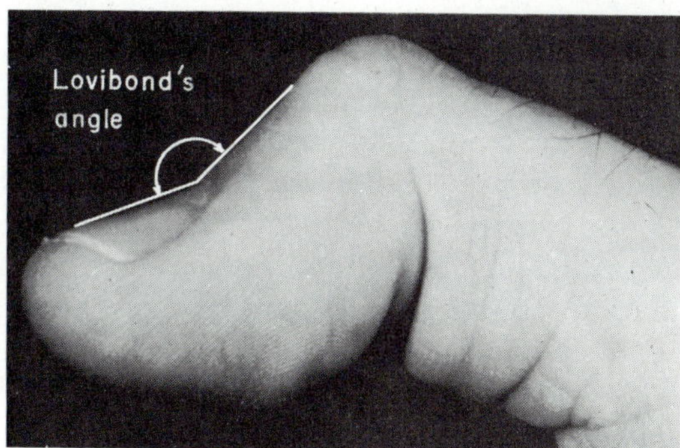

Figure 16-9 The angle formed by the dorsal surface of the distal phalanx and the nail plate (Lovibond's angle) is less than 180° in normal persons. *(From TB Fitzpatrick et al, Dermatology in General Medicine, 3d ed, New York, McGraw-Hill, 1987, p 660.)*

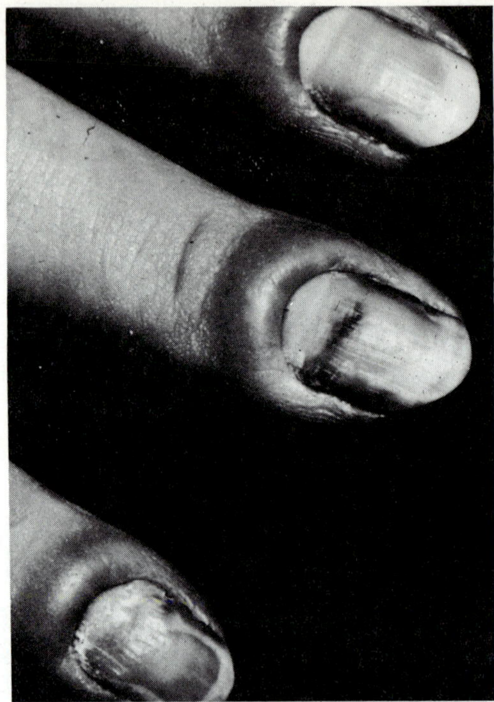

Figure 16-10 Chronic *Candida albicans* paronychia with periungual swelling and separation of nail fold from nail plate. *(From TB Fitzpatrick et al, Dermatology in General Medicine, 3d ed, New York, McGraw-Hill, 1987, p 653.)*

underlying diseases, including lung carcinoma, chronic lung diseases, cardiovascular disease, cirrhosis, and chronic malabsorptive disorders.

Nail Fold Disorders

Paronychia is an infection of the nail fold with bacteria, fungi, or yeast and is manifested by erythema, swelling, exudation, and separation of the nail fold from the plate. In most cases the initial change is a loss of cuticle, usually due to maceration from water but occasionally the result of trauma or manicure. The loss of cuticle allows a portal of entry for colonization by organisms; various bacteria, including staphylococci, streptococci, *Escherichia coli, Pseudomonas aeruginosa,* and/or *Candida,* are frequently involved. Chronic inflammation occurs in the surrounding dermis. In the early stages the nail plate is unaffected, but cross-ridging and discoloration occur later (Fig. 16-10). Eventually the size of the nail is reduced, and considerable swelling and induration of the surrounding soft tissues occur.

Neoplasms of the nail fold region include verruca vulgaris, glomus tumors, squamous cell carcinomas, pyogenic granulomas, and myxoid cysts.

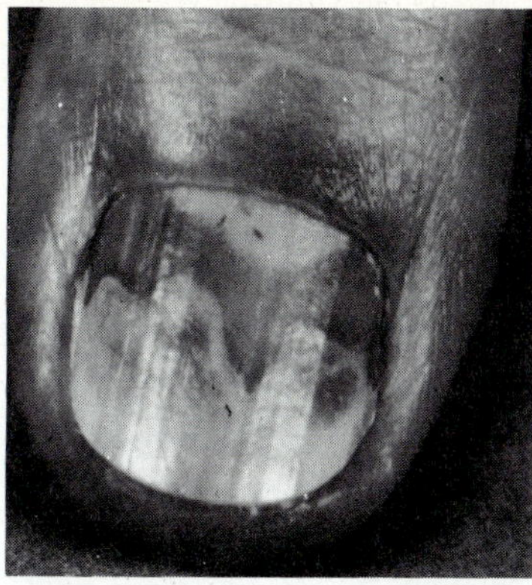

Figure 16-11 Onycholysis. *(From TB Fitzpatrick et al, Dermatology in General Medicine, 3d ed, New York, McGraw-Hill, 1987, p 653.)*

Disorders of the Nail Bed

Onycholysis is separation of the nail plate from the nail bed at its distal and lateral attachments (Fig. 16-11). Onychomadesis is the term used when the entire nail separates and is shed. Underneath the nail plate, horny scales or dirt may collect. The air layer between the plate and the bed scatters light, making the detached plate particularly evident because of its yellowish-white color. Normally, the nail bed epidermis contributes several horny cells to the underside of the plate that attach the nail plate to the nail bed. Injury to the nail plate–bed cohesion causes onycholysis, common causes being trauma, defective peripheral circulation, mycotic infections, psoriasis, *Pseudomonas* infection, thyroid disease, drugs, and contact sensitivity to nail lacquers and hardeners.[23,24] The pathogenesis of onycholysis in all of these disorders is an abnormal keratinization of the bed that results in loss of cohesion of the bed and plate and their separation.

Splinter hemorrhages are red linear defects in the nail bed due to rupture of the venules or capillaries (Fig. 16-12). The unique architecture of this region allows bleeding to occur along the epidermal-dermal ridges. The portion of the hemorrhage that remains in the dermis is reabsorbed, but the portion within the epidermis remains attached to the nail plate and moves distally with it. These defects are characteristic signs of subacute bacterial endocarditis but are not specific. Minor trauma can also cause splinter hemorrhages—even immersion in hot water. Other disease states causing this condition include mitral stenosis, hypertension, vasculitis, renal disease, trichinosis, cirrhosis, psoriasis, and fungal infections.

Tumors affecting the nail bed include Bowen's disease, squamous cell carcinoma, and malignant melanoma.

Nail Discoloration

Special attention to the color of the nails may aid in recognition of systemic disease.[25]

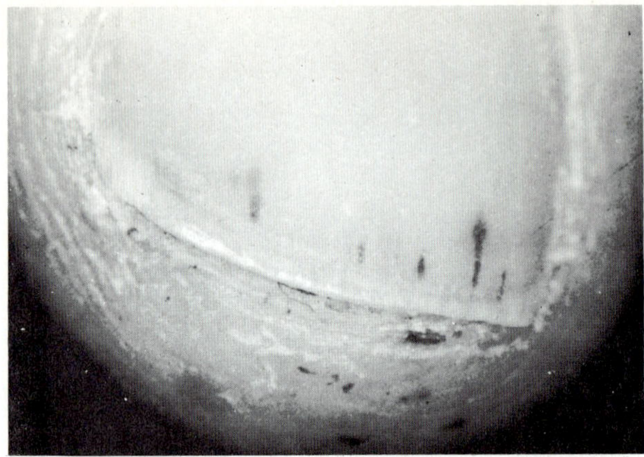

Figure 16-12 Splinter hemorrhages. *(From TB Fitzpatrick et al, Dermatology in General Medicine, 3d ed, New York, McGraw-Hill, 1987, p 654.)*

In anemia the nail bed appears pale due to the decreased hemoglobin concentration apparent through the translucent plate. The patient may also have white palmar creases.

In chronic renal failure the proximal portion of the nail bed may be white, being sharply demarcated from the distal red, pink, or brown portion—the so-called half-and-half nail. In various forms of cirrhosis, the proximal nail bed becomes white.

Discoloration of the nails is produced by systemic absorption of many drugs, notably arsenic, silver, chloroquine, and cancer chemotherapeutic agents. Arsenic causes white bands in the nail plate (Mee's lines).[26] These lines seem to be due to a sudden arrest of plate growth at the level of the lunula due to a toxic effect. Silver may produce blue discoloration of the lunula due to actual deposition of silver in the lunula, nail plate, and

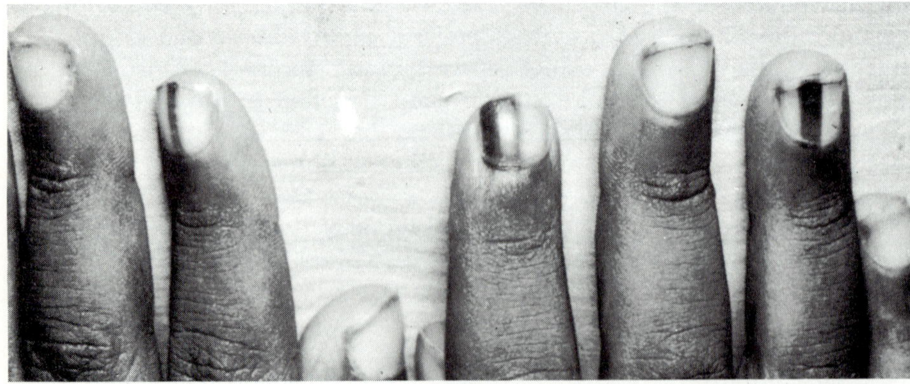

Figure 16-13 Junctional nevi in a black woman showing black streaks in the nail plates. *(From TB Fitzpatrick et al, Dermatology in General Medicine, 3d ed, New York, McGraw-Hill, 1987, p 664.)*

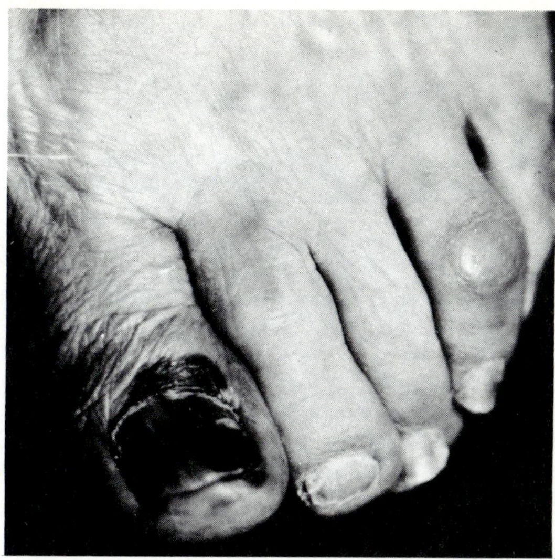

Figure 16-14 Ungual melanoma showing paronycheal pigment. *(From TB Fitzpatrick et al, Dermatology in General Medicine, 3d ed, New York, McGraw-Hill, 1987, p 665.)*

matrix. Chloroquine causes blue-brown discoloration of the nail bed and plate, probably due to melanin and drug deposition in these areas. Some of the cancer chemotherapeutic agents known to cause blue, brown, or black changes in the nail plate, bed or lunula include bleomycin, busulfan, cyclophosphamide, doxorubicin, 5-fluorouracil, hydroxyurea, and melphalan. The mechanism of the color change is postulated to be melanin deposition.

Junctional nevi may cause a black streak in the nail plate due to nests of nevus cells in the matrix. This is not uncommon in black persons (Fig. 16-13).

From 2 to 3 percent of melanomas are ungual. The thumb and large toe are the most frequently affected digits. In early lesions there is a brown to black discoloration of the matrix and nail bed. In later stages the lesion may become nodular, ulcerate, or deform the nail. A characteristic sign of ungual melanoma, melanotic whitlow of Hutchinson, consists of leakage of pigment into the paronychial area (Fig. 16-14).

In *Pseudomonas* infection a green discoloration of the nail plate may result from pyocyanin pigment.

REFERENCES

1. DeNicola P et al: Anatomy and physiology, in *Nail Diseases in Internal Medicine*. Springfield, Ill, Charles C Thomas, 1974, p 6.
2. Zaias N, Alvarez J: The formation of the primate nail plate: an autoradiographic study in squirrel monkey. *J Invest Dermatol* 51:120, 1968.
3. Zaias N: Anatomy and physiology, in *The Nail in Health and Disease*. Jamaica, NY, Spectrum, 1980, p 3.

4. Zaias N: Anatomy and physiology, in *The Nail in Health and Disease.* Jamaica, NY, Spectrum, 1980, p 4.
5. Zaias N: Embryology of human nail. *Arch Dermatol* 87:37, 1963.
6. Zaias N: Embryology, in *The Nail in Health and Disease.* Jamaica, NY, Spectrum, 1980, p 21.
7. Bean WB: Nail growth: thirty-five years of observation. *Arch Intern Med* 140:1, 1980.
8. Samman PD: Principle nail symptoms, in *The Nails in Disease.* London, Heinemann, 1978, p 14.
9. Zaias N: Anatomy and physiology, in *The Nail in Health and Disease.* Jamaica, NY, Spectrum, 1980, p 6.
10. DeNicola P et al: Anatomy and physiology, in *Nail Diseases in Internal Medicine.* Springfield, Ill, Charles C Thomas, 1974, p 23.
11. Baden HP et al: A comparative study of the physicochemical properties of human keratinized tissues. *Biochim Biophys Acta* 322:269, 1973.
12. DeNicola P et al: Anatomy and physiology, in *Nail Diseases in Internal Medicine.* Springfield, Ill, Charles C Thomas, 1974, p 18.
13. Zaias N: Anatomy and physiology, in *The Nail in Health and Disease.* Jamaica, NY, Spectrum, 1980, p 6.
14. Baden HP: The physical properties of nail. *J Invest Dermatol* 55:115, 1970.
15. Baden HP, Kubilus J: Fibrous protein of the bovine hoof. *J Invest Dermatol* 81:220, 1983.
16. Baden HP, Kubilus J: A comparative study of the immunological properties of hoof and nail fibrous proteins. *J Invest Dermatol* 83:327, 1984.
17. Kvedar JC et al: Cytokeratins of the bovine hoof: classification and studies on expression. *Biochim Biophys Acta* 884:462, 1986.
18. Lynch MH et al: Acidic and basic hair/nail ("hard") keratins: their colocalization in upper cortical and cuticle cells of the human hair follicle and their relationship to "soft" keratins. *J Cell Biol* 103:2593, 1986.
19. Heid HW et al: Patterns of expression of trichocytic and epithelial cytokeratins in mammalian tissues. I. Human and bovine hair follicles. *Differentiation* 37:137, 1988.
20. Heid HW et al: Patterns of expression of trichocytic and epithelial cytokeratins in mammalian tissues. II. Concomitant and mutually exclusive synthesis of trichocytic and epithelial cytokeratins in diverse human and bovine tissues (hair follicle, nail bed and matrix, lingual papilla, thymic reticulum). *Differentiation* 37:215, 1988.
21. Moll I et al: Patterns of expression of trichocytic and epithelial cytokeratins in mammalian tissues. III. Hair and nail formation during human fetal development. *Differentiation* 39:167, 1988.
22. Lovibond JL: Diagnosis of clubbed fingers. *Lancet* 1:363, 1938.
23. Ray LF: Onycholysis: a classification and study. *Arch Dermatol* 88:181, 1963.
24. Jawny L, Spada FJ: Contact dermatitis to a new nail hardener. *Arch Dermatol* 95:199, 1967.
25. Daniel CR, Osment LS: Nail pigmentation abnormalities: their importance and proper examination. *Cutis* 25:595, 1980.
26. Mees RA: Een verschijnsel bij polyneuritis arsnenicosa. *Nederl T Geneesk* 1:393, 1919.

SECTION FIVE

DISORDERS OF MELANOCYTES

17

Biology and Pathophysiology of the Melanin Pigmentary System

Thomas B. Fitzpatrick, George B. Fitzgerald, and Michael M. Wick

Much of the diversity in appearance among humans is the result of variations in the coloration of skin. Although human skin color is determined by a number of factors[1]—such as the reflection coefficient of the skin surface; absorption coefficient of epidermis and dermis; scattering coefficient of epidermis and dermis; thickness of the various layers (stratum corneum, epidermis, and dermis); content of ultraviolet- and visible light-absorbing components [keratin, elastin, melanin in melanosomes and macrophages, nucleic acid, urocanic acid, carotenoids, hemoglobin (oxidized and reduced), and lipids]; and number, size, type, and pattern of distribution of melanosomes in the epidermis as secreted by melanocytes[2]—melanin distribution is the most important determinant.

The epidermal melanin unit[3] is a functional and structural system composed of specialized dendritic, pigment-producing cells called *melanocytes.* These cells are associated with a cluster of keratinocytes that are supplied with pigment particles by this single melanocyte (Fig. 17-1). The pigment particles, called *melanosomes,* are secreted into the keratinocytes by a process, apparently unique in biology, in which a cell secretes into another cell and is therefore called *cytocrine.*[2]

In the hair and skin of humans, characteristic coloration is determined not by variations in the number of melanocytes but by the number and distribution of melanosomes and by their melanin content. Melanin, formed from tyrosine by the action of the enzyme tyrosinase, is deposited on

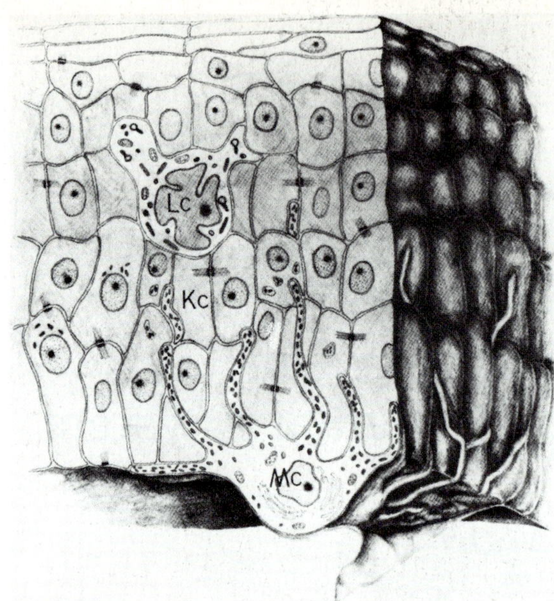

Figure 17-1 Epidermal melanin unit, consisting of a melanocyte (Mc) and associated pool of keratinocytes (Kc). Note Langerhans cell (Lc). *(From Scriver CR et al, The Metabolic Basis of Inherited Disease, 6th ed, New York, McGraw-Hill, 1989, p 2909.)*

melanosomes within the melanocyte. The color of the skin is related to the number of these melanized melanosomes present in the keratinocytes. In certain human disorders, for example, with a defect in melanosome transfer, melanocytes may contain many heavily melanized melanosomes, but the skin looks white (hypomelanosis) because of the reduction in the number of melanosomes in the keratinocytes.

The level of melanin pigmentation in humans is determined by genes,[4] exposure to sunlight, and pituitary hormones [melanocyte-stimulating hormone (MSH) or ACTH]. Genetic factors fix the basic level of skin color, called *constitutive* skin color, which is the major factor in racial pigmentation. When the skin is exposed to sunlight, or when high levels of MSH or ACTH are present (as in Addison's disease), the basic level of skin color increases; this is called *facultative* skin color and is also under genetic control, as there is considerable variation in the depth of pigmentation inducible in different persons. The additive interaction of three or four gene pairs is believed to be adequate to account for the variation in skin color in the various races. These few interacting loci probably explain the wide variation in constitutive skin color throughout the world.

FUNCTION

In humans, melanocytes, by means of their production and transfer of the pigment melanin, provide defense against the biologic damage caused by ultraviolet radiation (UVR) and visible radiation. Melanin in the uveal tract and in the retinal pigment epithelium protects the eye from visible and longer-wavelength [ultraviolet A (UVA)] radiant energy inasmuch as ultraviolet B (UVB) is largely filtered by the cornea; UVA enters the eye but is absorbed by the lens. Melanized human epidermis shields the epidermis and dermis by effectively reducing the transmission of UVB and UVA radiant energy.

In humans, furthermore, this defense against UVR is highly developed in that exposure of skin to this portion of the electromagnetic spectrum causes the activation of an integrated mechanism for the formation of dense organelles containing chromoprotein (melanosomes) and the delivery of these to epidermal cells. Within the epidermal cells, melanosomes scatter and absorb UVR and remove the damaging free radicals[5] that are generated in the skin after exposure to UVR. The production of melanosomes, therefore, is probably triggered by epidermal cells that respond to ultraviolet injury by mitosis, thus creating a new demand for melanosomes.

In a heavily pigmented skin, the epidermal cells and the stratum corneum are filled with myriads of melanosomes. Melanosomes contain about 30 percent melanin and, because of their density and universal absorption of UVR, can protect against solar damage. The perinuclear localization of melanosomes in epidermal cells may serve to protect the vulnerable DNA-containing nuclei by reducing the direct impact of the photons. In addition to absorption of UVR and dissipation of the absorbed energy in the form of heat, which is less harmful, melanin can undergo photooxidation, seen clinically as immediate pigment darkening; it is not known whether this effect has any protective role.

The role of melanin in protecting against the damaging effects of UVR is generally accepted. Blacks and dark-skinned whites are far less susceptible to acute and chronic actinic damage than fair-skinned whites. There is a reciprocal relationship between the degree of solar elastosis and skin color.[6] Sun-induced skin cancer on the exposed areas of the face and upper extremities is rare in black people living in geographic regions with high UVB flux; by contrast, black albinos living in these areas are very susceptible to skin cancer, and develop solar keratoses and skin cancer in childhood. Finally, since many of these deleterious biologic processes are involved in aging, melanin may well provide protection against environmentally induced premature aging.

STRUCTURE

Melanin Biosynthesis

The relationship of melanocyte, melanosome, tyrosinase, and tyrosine is shown in Fig. 17-2, which presents the components of the cellular and biochemical elements based on levels of organization. Clinical pigmentation can be considered at the levels of tissue (epidermal melanin unit), cell (melanocyte), organelle (melanosome), macromolecule (tyrosinase), and

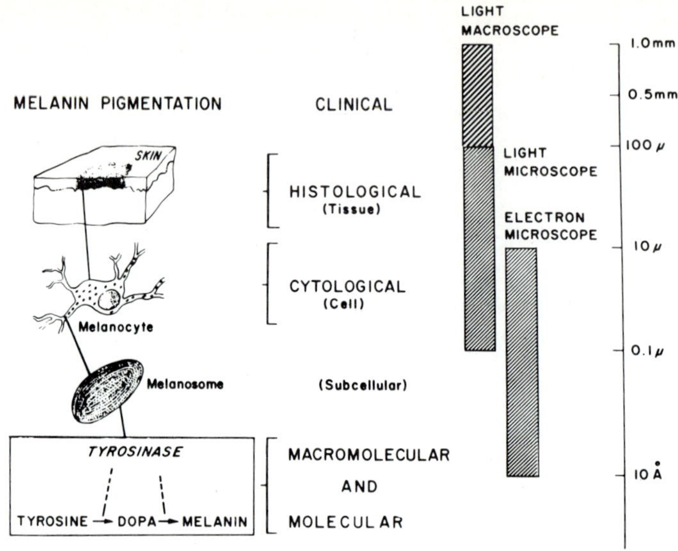

Figure 17-2 Levels of organization of the melanin pigmentary system. *(From TB Fitzpatrick et al, Dermatology in General Medicine, 3d ed, New York, McGraw-Hill, 1987, p 252.)*

molecule (tyrosine). Mechanisms of change in melanin pigmentation in various disease states have been elucidated by study of the skin with light microscopy, the histochemical dopa reaction, and electron microscopy.

Under the light microscope, melanin is seen as a brown particle, but not all black or brown pigments are melanin. In humans, black or brown cytoplasmic particles are present in a variety of cells—in the neurons of the central nervous system (substantia nigra), in the cells of the chromaffin system (adrenal medulla, sympathetic ganglia, etc.), and in the cells composing the melanin system. Neuromelanin, the pigment found in the pigmented nuclei of the brainstem (substantia nigra) and in the chromaffin system, is derived from tyrosine by the action of an enzyme, tyrosine hydroxylase, whereas melanin in the skin and hair bulb is formed from tyrosine by the action of a copper-containing aerobic oxidase, tyrosinase. Brown-black melanin produced in the melanocytes is called *eumelanin* and is a high-molecular-weight polymer. A reddish-brown macromolecular pigment called *phaeomelanin* is also produced in melanocytes; it is formed by the tyrosinase oxidation of tyrosine and subsequent reaction with cysteine. The biosynthesis of phaeomelanin is a deviation from the pathway leading to eumelanin, the key step being the reaction of cysteine with dopaquinone[7] (Fig. 17-3).

In the conversion of tyrosine to melanin, tyrosine is oxidized to dopa and then to dopaquinone, which then cyclizes to leukodopachrome. The first two steps in the reaction require enzymic catalysis; both are catalyzed by the aerobic oxidase tyrosinase. Leukodopachrome is oxidized to do-

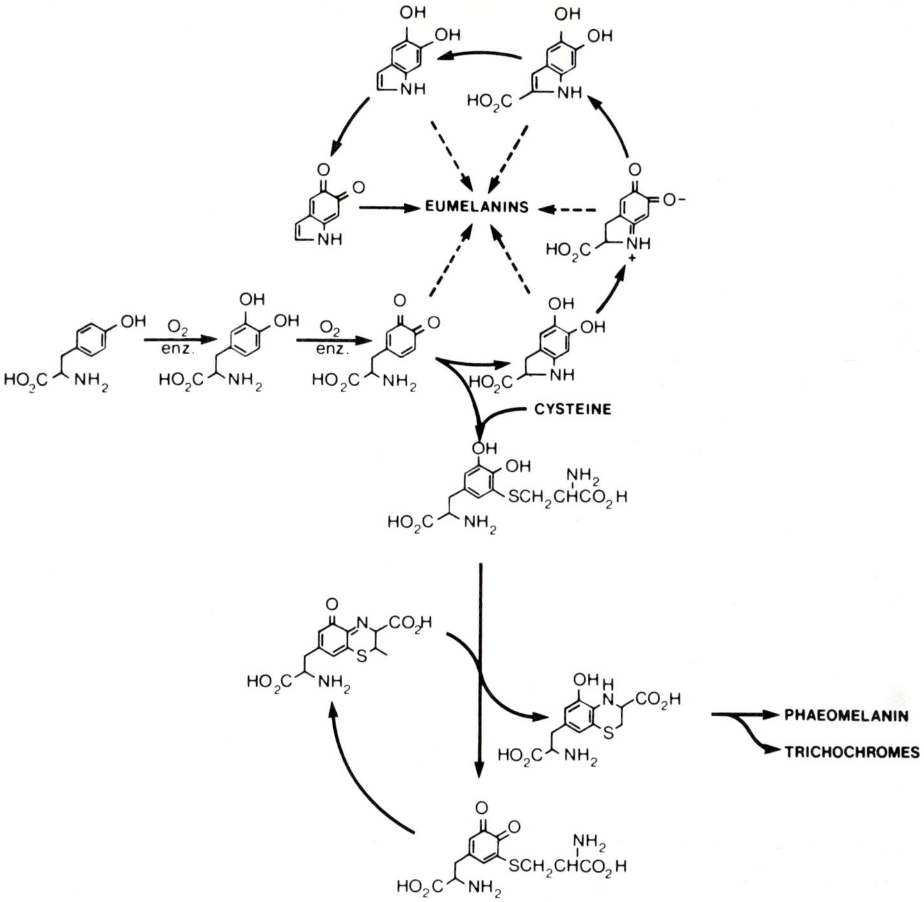

Figure 17-3 Metabolic pathway of eumelanin and phaeomelanin biosynthesis, each of which begins with the enzymatic conversion of tyrosine to dopa or dopaquinone. *(From TB Fitzpatrick, NA Soter, Pathophysiology of Skin, in LH Smith Jr, SO Thier, Pathophysiology: The Biological Principles of Disease, Philadelphia, Saunders, 1981, vol 1, p 1761.)*

pachrome, which rearranges with loss of carbon dioxide to 5,6-dihydroxyindole-4; these steps are not enzymatic. The actual mechanism of the oxidative polymerization by way of indole-5,6-quinone or its semiquinone is not known. Melanin is a huge, extremely stable, dense polymer that shows general absorption with no characteristic maxima in the range from 200 to 2400 nm; only the infrared spectra (in the range from 2.5 to 10 μm) show maxima absorption at 2 or 6 μm.

The formation of melanosomes entails the assembly and organization of four elements, including structural proteins, tyrosinase, "membranes," and, possibly, certain auxiliary enzymes. The structural proteins and enzymes are synthesized according to genetic programs and segregated within the membrane-limited vacuoles that may arise from either Golgi vesicles, the Golgi-associated endoplasmic reticulum, or the general endoplasmic reticulum. Within the membrane-limited early melanosomes, the segregated proteins assemble to form a matrix consisting of several concentrically arranged protein sheets.

Of the several hypotheses about the formation of melanosomes, the most plausible one is that the structural proteins and tyrosinase are not incorporated simultaneously into the melanosome but that tyrosinase accumulates in a particular area of the Golgi apparatus and condenses in coated vesicles, which then transfer to the dilated tubules of the smooth endoplasmic reticulum where the structural protein matrices (lamellae) are aggregated. Four steps of melanosome development are currently recognized (Fig. 17-4).

The various melanosomal components are under genetic control, the key regulatory steps being associated with the transcription and translation of information coded within "pigmentary" genes. The qualitative attributes of melanosomal components are specified by the nucleotide sequence within DNA; transcriptional and translational control mechanisms may interplay to affect not only the number of melanosomes synthesized but also certain qualitative attributes of individual melanosomes.

Melanocytes among all cells in the body are uniquely capable of synthesizing tyrosinase, which, when incorporated within melanosomes, initiates events leading to the synthesis of melanin.[8] Melanocytes are not of epidermal origin but are derived from the neural crest; the melanocyte

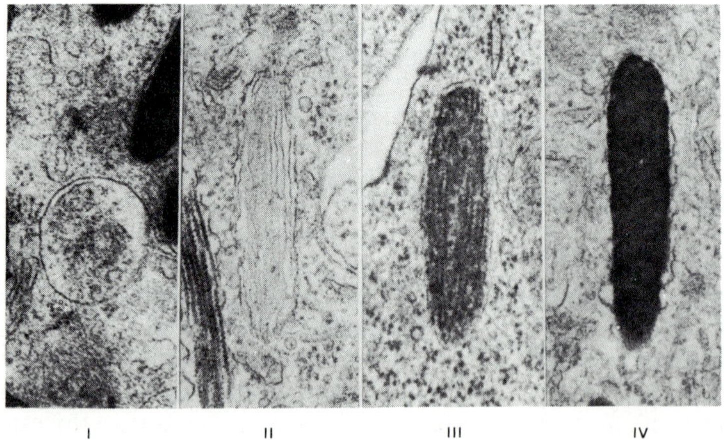

Figure 17-4 Ontogeny of melanosomes. *(Stage I)* A spherical, membrane-delineated vesicle that may be called a melanosome is shown to contain tyrosinase by electron microscopy combined with histochemistry or contains filaments that have a distinctive periodicity. *(Stage II)* The organelle is oval and shows numerous membranous filaments, with or without cross-linking, having a distinctive periodicity. *(Stage III)* The internal structure, characteristic of stage II, has become partially obscured by electron-dense melanin. *(Stage IV)* The oval organelle is electron-opaque, without a discernible internal structure. *(From TB Fitzpatrick et al, Dermatology in General Medicine, 3d ed, New York, McGraw-Hill, 1987, p 229.)*

system comprises melanocytes not only of the skin and mucous membrane but also of the eye (the uveal tract and retinal pigment cells), the ear (the stria vascularis), and the central nervous system (leptomeninges). All melanocytes other than the epidermal and hair melanocytes form measurable amounts of melanin, for the most part only in embryonic life. Hair bulb melanocytes are active during the anagen stage of the hair growth cycle; epidermal melanocytes form melanin all the time but increase production in response to appropriate stimuli, such as exposure to ultraviolet light or to pituitary hormones.

Melanocytes have dendritic processes that permit them to secrete melanosomes into keratinocytes. It is now believed that keratinocytes may play an active role in the phagocytizing of portions of the melanosome-laden dendrites of melanocytes. The transferred melanosomes exist in keratinocytes, either singly (nonaggregated) or as two or more particles within membrane-limited vesicles (aggregated). Whether melanosomes become aggregated or remain discrete depends on their size; small, ellipsoid melanosomes aggregate within the phagosomes in the keratinocytes and undergo degradation, while larger melanosomes appear to do neither. Keratinocytes in the skin of African and American blacks and of Australian aborigines contain large, single melanosomes (nonaggregated); those in the skin of Asiatics, whites, and American Indians contain small melanosomes, predominantly aggregated in membrane-limited organelles. In these phagolysosomes, the melanosomes undergo degradation by the action of acid phosphatase and probably other enzymes.

Melanocyte Regulation

The regulation of melanogenesis and melanin pigmentation is controlled by three major determinants: genes, hormones, and ultraviolet radiation. These factors may act independently or in combination. In addition, certain intrinsic factors within the melanin unit, including tissue-specific chalones and glycopolypeptides, may markedly affect melanogenesis and melanin pigmentation by exerting negative feedback control and regulating the mitotic activity of melanocytes and keratinocytes. Recently, several other factors have been suggested to have a substantial influence in determining the level of pigmentation. Korner and Pawelek[9] have proposed the existence of conversion factors that can either promote or block the synthesis of eumelanin subsequent to the action of tyrosinase. However, Palumbo et al.[10] have argued that the results reported to demonstrate such regulatory factors[11,12] can be explained by the action of certain metal ions, such as copper, iron, and zinc, that can also induce the rearrangement of dopachrome.

Another possible controlling element has been suggested by recent findings of Slominski et al.,[13] which indicate that tyrosine and, to a lesser extent, levodopa may regulate the expression of the tyrosinase gene(s), resulting in increased tyrosinase activity. In addition, tyrosine's influence on melanogenesis may also include stimulation of melanosome synthesis and control of the subcellular distribution of tyrosinase.

A reanalysis of a well-known side effect of pigmented metastatic melanoma, i.e., the excretion of cysteinyldopa, has led to a novel hypothesis about the way in which melanocytes control pigmentation. The formation of cysteinyldopa arises from the interaction of dopaquinone with either cysteine or glutathione. Although glutathionedopa has not been observed under normal physiological conditions, it has been detected using animal models following injection of large doses of dopa.[14] Furthermore, since glutathione is the major sulfhydryl compound found in cells and is known to form adducts readily with dopaquinone, it seems likely that it would contribute to the formation of cysteinyldopa. Most likely, certain enzymes[15] enzymatically hydrolyze glutathionedopa to cysteinyldopa. Prota[7] has suggested that the extent to which a melanocyte can convert glutathionedopa to cysteinyldopa plays a large role in determining the level of pigmentation, since glutathionedopa, but not cysteinyldopa, acts as a reservoir of the melanin precursor dopaquinone. In support of this hypothesis, Prota has presented evidence that links the level of glutathione reductase, an enzyme that is important in maintaining the high intracellular level of glutathione, and the level of pigmentation in both animal models and human skin.[7] The involvement of various hormones in the control of pigmentation of melanocytes has been a subject of considerable controversy.[16,17] However, research in this field has benefited greatly from a recent development in tissue culture technology that now enables normal melanocytes to be grown in the laboratory.[18,19] Results suggest that one of the first hormones implicated in pigmentation, the pituitary-derived MSH, does not affect tyrosinase activity in normal human melanocytes.[20] However, β-estradiol and, to a lesser extent, the vitamin D–derived secosteroid 1,25-dihydroxyvitamin D_3 have been shown to stimulate tyrosinase activity in foreskin-derived melanocytes.[20]

Recent studies have demonstrated a reciprocal relationship between melanogenesis and the metabolism of melanocytes. Specifically, the high oxygen consumption associated with the synthesis of melanin stimulates the hexose monophosphate shunt, producing reduced nicotinamide-adenine denucleotide phosphate (NADPH). Moellmann et al.[21] have suggested that the level of NADPH relative to its oxidized form ($NADP^+$) may regulate the activity of tyrosinase, as well as other steps in melanogenesis.

The study of the regulation of pigmentation has revealed that while melanin synthesis appears to be a relatively simple process, readily duplicated in the laboratory, it is in fact governed by a complex regulatory mechanism. The reason for this level of complexity is unclear. However, given that pigmentation generates a variety of potentially cytotoxic reactants (e.g., free radicals and quinones), it would seem reasonable that a pigment-producing cell would evolve a number of mechanisms for controlling melanogenesis.

PATHOPHYSIOLOGY OF PIGMENTARY DISORDERS

The morphologic and metabolic pathway of melanin pigmentation as presented in Fig. 17-5 depicts the specific site of pathologic change of the various pigment disorders.[22] These disorders (e.g., albinism) may have intrinsic significance because they profoundly vitiate the functional role of melanin or have indirect significance (e.g., brown spots in neurofibromatosis) by providing an important clue for diagnosis of a systemic disease.

Disturbances of melanin pigmentation can be divided on the basis of color change into three types: hypomelanosis (white or lighter than normal), brown hypermelanosis, or gray and blue hypermelanosis. Disturbances in melanogenesis (production of melanized melanosomes) and in melanin pigmentation (transfer of melanosomes to keratinocytes) therefore can result in an increase or decrease of pigmentation of skin or hair.

The precise localization of the defect or defects in the morphologic and metabolic pathway of human epidermal melanin pigmentation is not known except in a few instances. In some, these are still speculative (e.g., piebaldism); in others (e.g., albinism), they are reasonably well understood.

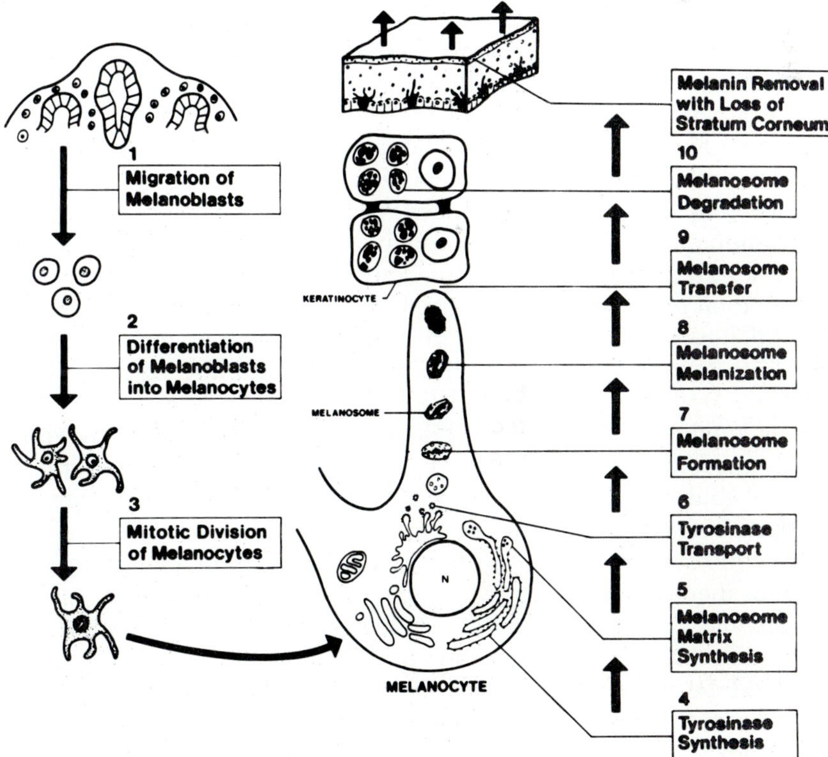

Figure 17-5 Morphological and metabolic pathway of epidermal melanin pigmentation. *(From TB Fitzpatrick et al, Dermatology in General Medicine, 3d ed, New York, McGraw-Hill, 1987, p 226.)*

Steps 1 and 2: Migration and Differentiation of Melanoblasts into Melanocytes

In human piebaldism, an autosomal dominant trait, a white spotting occurs in the skin in a regular pattern. This hypomelanosis results from a virtual absence of melanocytes in the skin and hair. It is presumed that in piebaldism, the melanoblasts migrate from the neural crest to the skin and fail either to survive or to differentiate into melanocytes. In mice, specific genes are known to influence pigment patterns by their action at the neural crest level, and other genes act at the tissue environment (skin) level and create a hostile environment so that melanoblasts fail to survive.

Step 3: Mitotic Division of Melanocytes

Melanoblasts arise from the neural crest and migrate to the skin during neonatal life, there differentiating into melanocytes, which can undergo mitotic division. Mature melanocytes can be stimulated to undergo mitosis, for example, by ultraviolet stimulation.

A reduction in melanocyte replication would appear to be the best explanation for the graying or whitening of human hair that occurs with aging and that usually begins in the fourth or the early fifth decade of life. Premature graying may begin in the second decade and occurs in over one-third of patients with vitiligo.

Failure of replication and loss of melanocytes occur in vitiligo. Vitiligo is a common acquired, patterned, idiopathic hypomelanosis that is often familial and is characterized by pale white macules that enlarge centrifugally over time[23] (Fig. 17-6). In vitiligo there is a virtual absence of melanocytes that is demonstrated with electron microscopy. However, there may be a progressive, gradual reduction of melanocytes with an end stage characterized by total disappearance. The general health is usually not impaired, but the disfigurement, especially in darkly pigmented persons, can be socially catastrophic, notably in India, Africa, and the Middle Eastern countries.

Various medical disorders are known to be associated with vitiligo, especially thyroid disease [Graves' disease, thyroiditis, toxic goiter (1.8 to 38 percent), but also Addison's disease (2 percent), pernicious anemia (10 percent), diabetes mellitus (1 to 7 percent), and alopecia areata (16 percent)]. Three hypotheses attempt to explain the occurrence of vitiligo in such a mélange of medical disorders.

The *immune hypothesis* proposes an aberration of immune surveillance that produces melanocyte destruction or dysfunction, or both. The primary event could be an injury to melanocytes, with release of antigen and subsequent autoimmunization. The occurrence of satellite and remote hypomelanosis after sunburn, and the spontaneous and bacille Calmette-Guérin–related occurrence of uveitis, poliosis, and vitiligo, suggest an immune induction of vitiligo. Five patients have been observed with a syndrome of Addison's disease—hypoparathyroidism, mucocutaneous

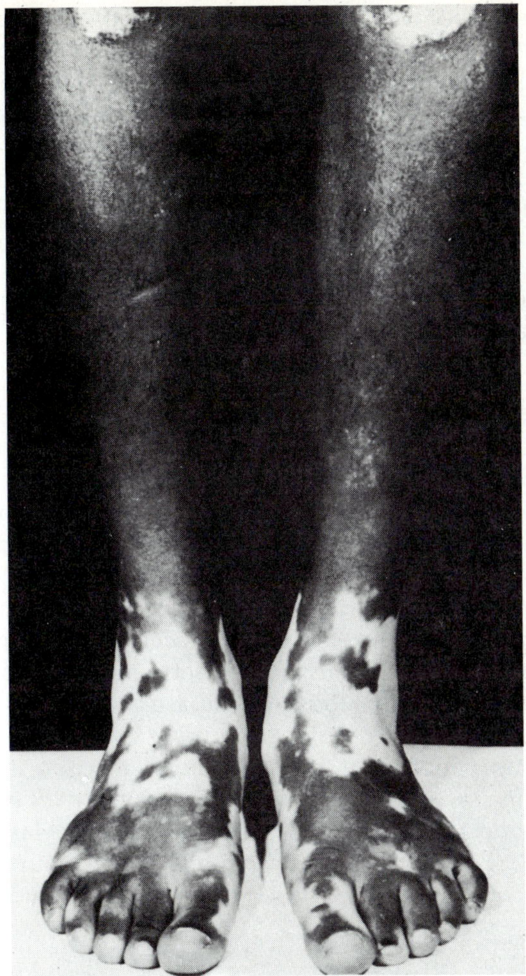

Figure 17-6 Symmetric distribution of vitiligo. There is often a striking mirror-image symmetry, as shown in this 12-year-old girl. *(From TB Fitzpatrick et al, Dermatology in General Medicine, 3d ed, New York, McGraw-Hill, 1987, p 812.)*

moniliasis, and vitiligo-like hypomelanosis; one of the patients also has alopecia areata. Antimelanocyte antibodies have been isolated in two patients with vitiligo and multiglandular deficiencies.

The *neural hypothesis* postulates a neurochemical mediator that destroys melanocytes. This is suggested by the occasional patient whose vitiligo occurs in a dermatomal distribution, by vitiligo following peripheral nerve injury, or by vitiligo with multiple sclerosis and Horner's syndrome.

The *"self-destruct" hypothesis* implicates an intermediate in melanin metabolism (tyrosine, dopa, or another intermediate) that causes destruction of melanocytes. It is of note that there are several synthetic phenol compounds that can induce depigmentation in human skin.

None of these hypotheses is entirely satisfactory. The neural hypothesis is contradicted by the observation that sympathectomy does not induce vitiligo. The autoimmune hypothesis is intriguing, but there is an absence of mononuclear infiltrate in most vitiligo macules and specific circulating autoantibodies have not been found in patients who have vitiligo except in the multiglandular syndrome (vitiligo with hypoparathyroidism, primary adrenal insufficiency, and mucocutaneous moniliasis). The response of vitiligo to potent topical corticosteroids would favor an immunologic basis for the hypomelanosis.

Step 4: Tyrosinase Synthesis

Melanocytes may be present and melanosomes may be formed and transferred to keratinocytes in a normal manner, and yet hypomelanosis can be present if melanization of melanosomes does not occur normally. This is the probable defect in oculocutaneous albinism.

Albinism (Fig. 17-7), a genetic disorder affecting humans and other mammals, is a dilution of skin, hair, and eye color based on a failure of synthesis of tyrosinase.[24] In humans, albinism occurs as six different types in which a congenital absence or dilution of skin, hair, or eye color is noted, accompanied by decreased visual acuity, nystagmus, and photophobia. The six types are distinguished from one another by both clinical and biochemical criteria, including tyrosinase activity and the presence of melanin. Tyrosinase activity varies from none to moderate, as detected by the hair bulb incubation test, a histochemical reaction in which plucked hair bulbs are incubated in the tyrosine solution for 12 h. The hair bulbs containing melanocytes darken by the formation of melanin from tyrosine through the action of tyrosinase. No autoxidation occurs, since tyrosine, without the presence of tyrosinase, does not form melanin. It is thus

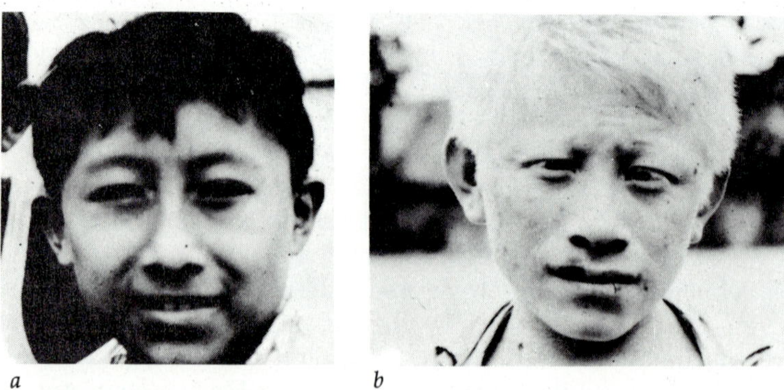

Figure 17-7 Oculocutaneous albinism in a San Blas Indian of the Cuna tribe. There is a dilution of the skin, hair, and eye color in the albino child (*b*) in comparison with the normal coloring of the Cuna child (*a*). *(From TB Fitzpatrick et al, Dermatology in General Medicine, 3d ed, New York, McGraw-Hill, 1987, p 801.)*

possible to classify the type of albinism as tyrosinase-negative or tyrosinase-positive albinism. Since melanocytes and melanosomes are present in albinism, the decreased pigmentation is the result of a reduction of tyrosinase. Tyrosinase is either completely absent or, if present, is functionally inactive.

Step 5: Melanosome Matrix Synthesis

The leukodermic macules that not infrequently occur in patients with metastatic melanoma contain, in the white macules, large melanocytes, and the total population of melanocytes is reduced. The pathogenesis of the leukoderma in metastatic melanoma is presumed to be related to an immunologic cytotoxicity of melanocytes. The large remaining melanocytes contain tyrosinase, but there are virtually no melanosomes. This could be a failure of melanosome matrix synthesis.

Step 6: Tyrosinase Transport

There is no definitive clinical example of a defect in tyrosinase transport.

Step 7: Melanosome Formation

Eumelanosome size (1.0 μm in length, 0.4 μm in diameter) and normal shape (ellipsoidal) are under genetic control in mice and in humans. In the autosomal dominant trait, von Recklinghausen's neurofibromatosis (VRN) (Fig. 17-8), melanosomes become aggregated within melanocytes (autophagocytosis), and these autophagosomes merge with secondary lysosomes to form giant pigment globules called *melanin macroglobules*[25] (Fig. 17-9). These are characteristic in the café-au-lait macules of VRN but

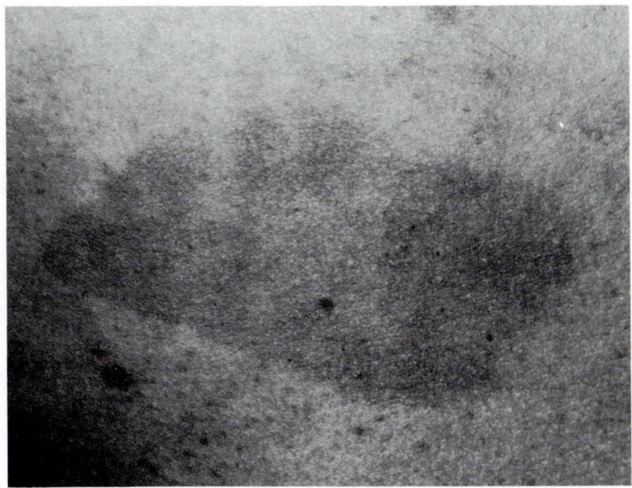

Figure 17-8 Neurofibromatosis showing a café-au-lait macule.

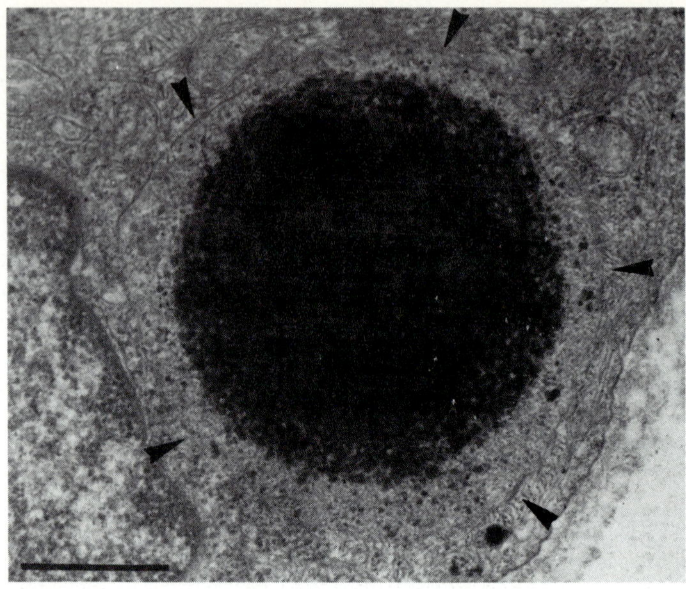

Figure 17-9 Melanin macroglobule. A very large, pigmented organelle is formed by merging of autophagosomes with secondary lysosomes. These large particles are transferred from melanocytes to keratinocytes.

also are found in lesser numbers in several disorders—dysplastic nevi, nevus spilus, X-linked ocular albinism, and xeroderma pigmentosum.[26]

Step 8: Melanization of Melanosomes

Failure of melanin deposition on melanosomes can result from absence or reduction of tyrosinase, as already described in the discussion of oculocutaneous albinism, but also from an inhibition of the tyrosine-melanin metabolic pathway. This is the explanation of the decreased melanization in the autosomal recessive disease phenylketonuria, in which there is a competitive inhibition of tyrosinase by high levels of phenylalanine and its degradation products, especially phenylpyruvic acid.

Step 9: Melanosome Transfer

As emphasized earlier, melanin pigmentation implies not only the production of melanosomes but also their transfer to keratinocytes. For melanosome transfer, two structures are necessary: dendrites to facilitate the passage of the organelle to the keratinocyte and receptive normal keratinocytes. Pathologic alterations (e.g., edema of the keratinocytes, as in eczematous dermatitis, or short, "stubby" dendrites, as in the melanocytes) often occur in chronically sun-damaged skin and result in a failure of melanosome transfer. A syndrome of immunodeficiency and hypopigmentation has been reported in France.[27] The basis for the dilution of skin and hair color was found to be a "transfer block" of melanosomes; in addition, stage IV melanosomes were "stuffed" in the melanocytes and the keratinocytes were therefore hypopigmented.

Step 10: Melanosome Degradation

Melanosomes within melanocytes are normally nonaggregated, single, discrete organelles, but rarely in normal melanocytes and in certain diseases, melanosomes can become aggregated, surrounded by a lysosomal membrane, and degraded; this is autophagocytosis and occurs, for example, in malignant melanocytes. Also, see Step 7 for a discussion of the melanosomes in von Recklinghausen's neurofibromatosis.

CONCLUSION

The melanocyte provides a model for the study of various cellular processes involved in growth and differentiation. The study of this system also is an excellent example of the impact that basic science can have on the understanding of human disease. For example, significant advances have been achieved using the principles of pigment biology in the design of specific antitumor agents directed against the malignant counterpart of the melanocyte, the melanoma cell.[28,29] With additional basic information, further progress in the treatment of human pigmented diseases can be anticipated.

REFERENCES

1. Toda K et al: Skin color: its ultrastructure and its determining mechanism, in VJ McGovern, P Russel (eds), *Pigment Cell.* Basel, S Karger, 1972, vol 1, p 66.
2. Quevedo WC et al: Biology of melanocytes, in TB Fitzpatrick et al (eds), *Dermatology in General Medicine,* 3d ed. New York, McGraw-Hill, 1987, p 225.
3. Fitzpatrick TB, Breathnach AS: Das epidermale melanin—Einheit system. *Dtsch Med Wochenschr* 147:481, 1963.
4. Silvers WK: *The Coat Colors of Mice: A Model for Mammalian Gene Action and Interaction.* New York, Springer-Verlag, 1979.
5. Mason HS et al: The free radical property of melanins. *Arch Biochem Biophys* 86:225, 1960.
6. Kaidbey KH, Kligman AM: Photoprotection by melanin—a comparison of black and caucasian skin. *J Am Acad Dermatol* 1:249, 1979.
7. Prota G: Progress in the chemistry of melanins and related metabolites. *Med Res Rev* 8:525, 1988.
8. Szabo G: The biology of the pigment cell, in EE Bittar, N Bittar (eds), *The Biological Basis of Medicine.* London, Academic, 1969, vol VI, p 59.
9. Korner AM, Pawelek J: Dopachrome conversion: a possible control point in melanin biosynthesis. *J Invest Dermatol* 75:192, 1980.
10. Palumbo A et al: A new look at the rearrangement of adrenochrome under biomimetic conditions. *Biochim Biophys Acta* 990:297, 1989.
11. Barber JI et al: Dopachrome oxidoreductase: a new enzyme in the pigment pathway. *J Invest Dermatol* 83:145, 1984.
12. Hearing VJ et al: New regulators of melanogenesis are associated with tyrosinase isozymes. *J Invest Dermatol* 79:16, 1982.

13. Slominski A et al: Positive regulation of melanin pigmentation by two key substrates of the melanogenic pathway, L-tyrosine and L-dopa. *J Cell Sci* 89:287, 1988.
14. Fehling C et al: Formation of glutathionedopa in albino rats after DOPA injection. *Acta Derm Venereol (Stockh)* 61:339, 1981.
15. Agrup G et al: Formation of cysteinyldopa from glutathionedopa in melanoma. *Acta Derm Venereol (Stockh)* 55:1, 1975.
16. Halaban R et al: Regulation of tyrosinase in human melanocytes grown in culture. *J Cell Biol* 97:480, 1983.
17. Nielsen HI, Don P: Culture of normal adult human melanocytes. *Br J Dermatol* 110:569, 1984.
18. Pittelkow MR, Shipley GD: Factor requirements of normal human melanocytes in vitro. *J Invest Dermatol* 88:513, 1987.
19. Herlyn M et al: Regulatory factors that determine growth and phenotype of normal human melanocytes. *Exp Cell Res* 179:322, 1988.
20. Ranson M et al: Human melanocytes as a target tissue for hormones: in vitro studies with 1α-25, dihydroxyvitamin D_3, α melanocyte-stimulating hormone, and β-estradiol. *J Invest Dermatol* 91:593, 1988.
21. Moellmann G et al: Regulation of melanogenesis in melanocytes. *Pigment Cell Res* 1:79, 1988.
22. Mosher DB et al: Disorders of pigmentation, in TB Fitzpatrick et al (eds), *Dermatology in General Medicine,* 3d ed. New York, McGraw-Hill, 1987, p 794.
23. Ortonne J-P et al: *Vitiligo and Other Hypomelanoses of Hair and Skin.* New York, Plenum, 1983.
24. Witkop CJ Jr et al: Albinism, in CR Scriver et al (eds), *The Metabolic Basis of Inherited Disease,* 6th ed. New York, McGraw-Hill, 1989, p 2905.
25. Jimbow K et al: Ultrastructure of giant pigment granules (macromelanosomes) in the cutaneous pigmented macules of neurofibromatosis. *J Invest Dermatol* 61:300, 1973.
26. Nakagawa H et al: The nature and origin of the melanin macromolecule. *J Invest Dermatol* 83:134, 1984.
27. Gricscelli C et al: A syndrome associating partial albinism and immunodeficiency. *Am J Med* 65:691, 1978.
28. Wick MM: An experimental approach to the chemotherapy of melanoma. *J Invest Dermatol* 74:63, 1980.
29. Lerner AB: On the etiology of vitiligo and grey hair. *Am J Med* 51:141, 1971.

18

Pathophysiology of Pigmented Melanocytic and Nevomelanocytic Nevi

Arthur R. Rhodes

Nevus is derived from the Latin word *naevus* (birthmark), a general term applied to any congenital lesion, although the same term is commonly applied to acquired lesions. *Mole* is derived from the Anglo-Saxon word *mal* (spot), a lay term often referring to a protuberant congenital or acquired nevomelanocytic nevus. In the differential diagnosis of mole, varieties of pigmented lesions may be described as melanotic (increased pigment only), melanocytic (increased number of melanocytes), nevomelanocytic (increased number of nevomelanocytes), or combinations thereof.

DERMAL MELANOCYTOSIS

It was originally believed, based on the affinity of silver for melanin, that dermal melanoblasts first appeared in the human fetus during the 10th week of uterine development, that epidermal melanocytes were visible by the 11th week in utero, and that epidermal melanocytes were numerous by the 12th to 14th weeks.[1] More recent studies using monoclonal antibody HMB-45, which binds specifically to melanoma cytoplasmic antigens, have demonstrated melanocytes in the epidermis in human embryos of at least 8 weeks estimated gestational age.[2] Dermal melanoblasts are believed to disappear gradually during gestation, so that by birth they are restricted to localized cutaneous sites as blue-gray macules known as *congenital dermal melanocytosis* or *mongolian spots* (Fig. 18-1). The term *mongolian spot*

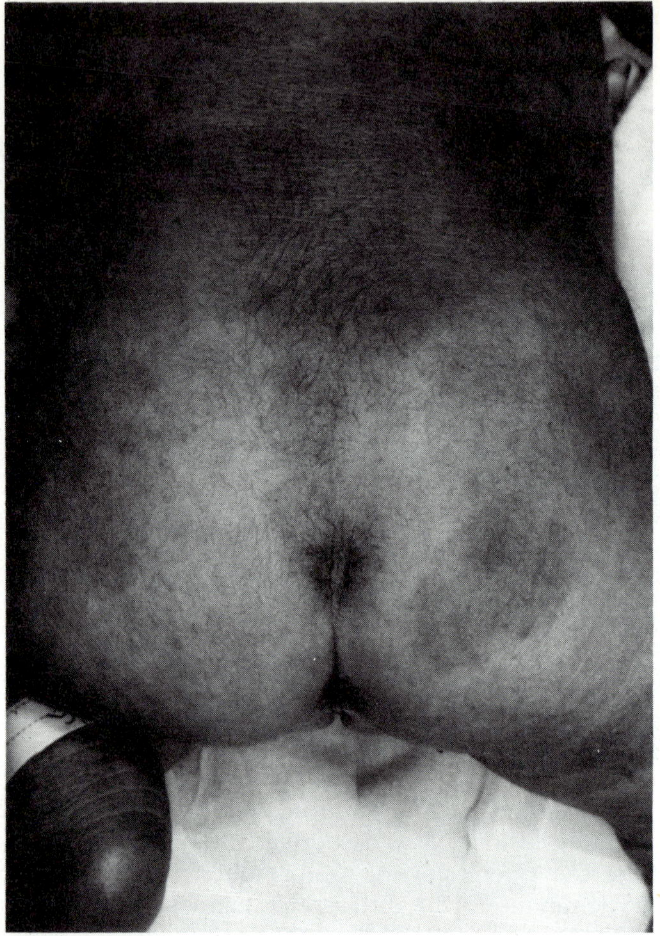

Figure 18-1 Congenital dermal melanocytosis (mongolian spots). Multiple blue-gray macules were present at birth on the buttocks and sacrum of a 48-h-old Asian baby girl.

is not entirely satisfactory, because this lesion is detected during the newborn period not only in 90 percent of Asians and AmerIndians but also in 96 percent of blacks, 46 percent of Latinos, and 9.5 percent of whites.[3] Mongolian spots may be single or multiple, usually varying from a few millimeters to 10 cm in diameter, occasionally larger. The sites most commonly involved with mongolian spots are the sacral-gluteal region (81 percent) and the shoulder (23 percent). Mongolian spots usually disappear within the first 5 years of life but occasionally persist into adulthood. Mongolian spots, which have no reported malignant potential, are characterized histologically by spindle-shaped melanocytes in the lower half of the dermis.

A localized form of dermal melanocytosis is the *blue nevus*, which occurs usually as a single, isolated, acquired papule less that 0.5 cm in diameter *(common blue nevus)* or occasionally as a relatively large, congenital, dome-shaped nodule or plaque *(congenital cellular blue nevus).* Blue nevi are more common in Asians than in whites. The prevalence rate of blue nevi in white adults is about 1 percent. Blue nevi contain abundant melanin-producing melanocytes in the dermis. Their malignant potential is relatively low, mostly associated with cellular varieties of blue nevi.[4]

Blue nevi and congenital dermal melanocytosis appear blue-gray or blue-black, the color related to the presence of melanin in the deep dermis. Ordinarily, melanin in typical nevomelanocytic nevi and other varieties of pigmented lesions (e.g., solar lentigines, lentigo simplex, and café-au-lait spots) is confined to the epidermis and superficial papillary dermis, which absorb all wavelengths of visible light, resulting in a brown or black color. In blue nevi and congenital dermal melanocytosis, visible light penetrates deeply into the dermis and is absorbed almost totally by the deeply situated melanin, except for the shorter blue wavelengths, which are reflected outward, imparting a blue cast to the dark brown or black. Blue and/or blue-gray color should be considered a suspicious feature of "typical" moles.

EPIDERMAL MELANOCYTOSIS

Solar Lentigo

The most common epidermal melanocytotic lesions are *solar lentigines* (commonly called *freckles*), which occur as circumscribed, flat, brown macules on sun-exposed skin in 75 percent of whites older than age 60 years (Fig. 18-2). Identical lesions occur in children and young adults. Solar lentigines are characterized histologically by increased numbers of melanocytes.[5–7] For instance, intraepidermal melanocytes constitute 6 percent of epidermal basal unit cells in sun-protected skin (Fig. 18-3) and 15 percent of basal unit cells in sun-exposed skin, while in solar lentigines, intraepidermal melanocytes comprise 27 percent of basal unit cells.[7] The sun-induced pigmented macules associated with xeroderma pigmentosum, an autosomal recessive disorder characterized by defective repair of ultraviolet-induced DNA damage and the early development of epidermal and melanocytic neoplasms early in life, and the pigmented macules induced by photochemotherapy, also have increased numbers of melanocytes, often associated with cellular atypia.[7,8] Another lesion relevant to solar lentigines is *lentigo maligna,* an irregularly pigmented, relatively large macule appearing uncommonly on sun-damaged sites of predominantly elderly white adults, responsible for 5 percent of cutaneous melanomas. (See below for a more detailed discussion of lentigo maligna.)

Lentigo Simplex

Lentigo simplex is a congenital or acquired circumscribed, pigmented macule, small or large, on any cutaneous surface, unrelated to sun exposure. It is characterized by a proliferation of intraepidermal melano-

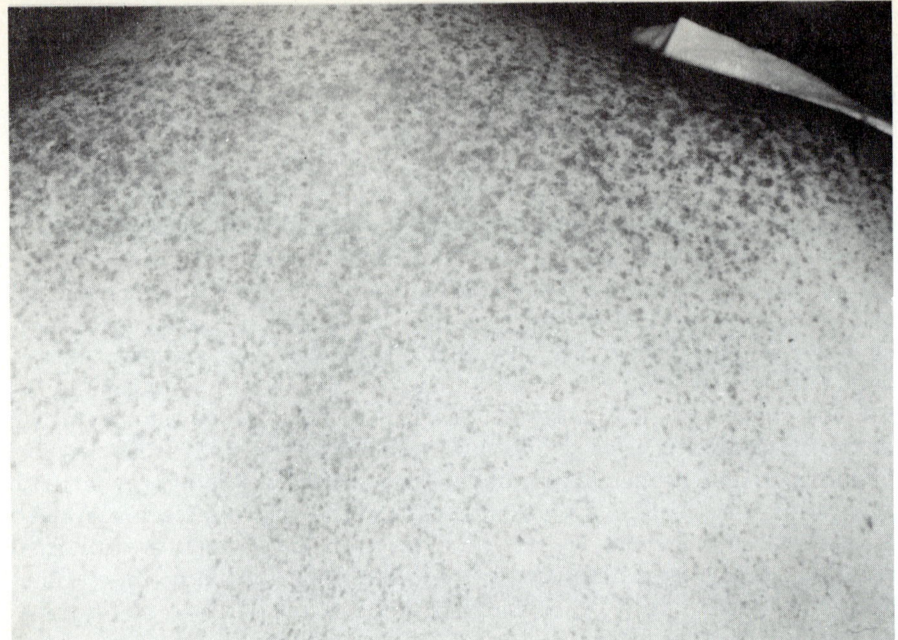

Figure 18-2 Solar lentigines. These circumscribed brown macules on the back of a 23-year-old white man were said to have appeared during early childhood many months after a sunburn.

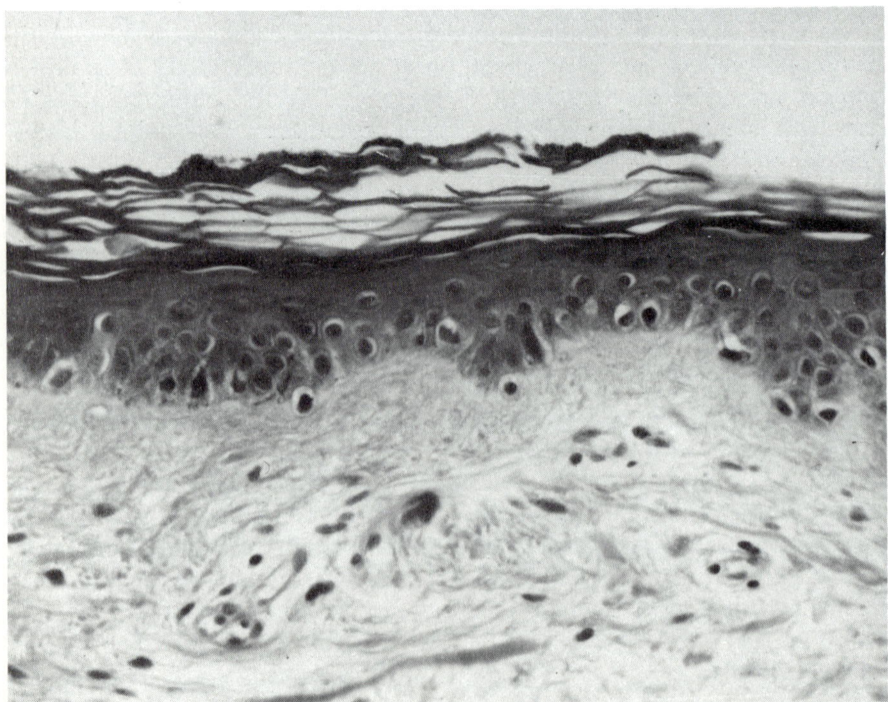

Figure 18-3 Typical intraepidermal melanocytes in the basal unit of sun-protected buttock skin of a healthy 40-year-old white adult. Dopa-incubated tissue section, cut at 6-μm thickness, stained with hematoxylin and eosin. ×600 in the original magnification.

cytes in elongated and club-shaped epidermal rete ridges. Lesions may be single or multiple. Lentigo simplex may appear as an isolated finding in healthy people or as multiple lesions in multisystemic disorders such as Peutz-Jegher syndrome (small intestinal polyposis), LEOPARD syndrome (cardiac and somatic abnormalities), and LAMB syndrome (cardiac and somatic abnormalities).[9]

NEVOMELANOCYTIC NEVI

Definition, Appearance, and Regression

Nevomelanocytic nevi (NMN) represent localized collections of nevomelanocytes. Several morphological and functional characteristics distinguish nevomelanocytes from melanocytes. Both cells have tyrosinase,[10] the enzyme responsible for melanin synthesis, and both cells contain single premelanosomes indicating intrinsic melanin production. Nevomelanocytes have short pseudoplasmic projections analogous to the dendrites of melanocytes.[11] Nevomelanocytes in the epidermis are arranged in well-formed nests, whereas ordinary intraepidermal melanocytes are distributed as single cells in the basal layer of the epidermis. It is presumed that melanocytes and nevomelanocytes are derived from the same progenitor cells in the neural crest.

NMN are classified according to the historic age of first appearance (congenital vs. acquired), gross morphological appearance (typical vs. atypical), and location of nevomelanocytes (junctional if confined to the epidermis, dermal if confined to the dermis, and compound if present in both locations). Typical acquired NMN are soft, nonkeratotic papules that are symmetrically pigmented light or medium brown. On high magnification they reveal darker speckles of darker brown on a lighter brown field. Typical acquired NMN are relatively well demarcated, round or oval, and characterized by skin markings that are normal, accentuated, or effaced evenly (Fig. 18-4). The average number of NMN per person has been reported to be 15 to 40 for whites,[12] 2 for American blacks,[13] 6 for eastern Indians,[14] and 11 for black Ugandans,[15] but gross definitions of NMN in these studies vary. The use of 7–10× magnification of the mineral oil–coated surface may be required to differentiate lightly pigmented NMN (papules or plaques—darker brown speckles on a lighter brown field) from solar lentigines (macules—reticular pigment network), café-au-lait spots (macules—hypopigmented hair follicle openings on a tan field), and seborrheic keratoses (papules or plaques—deep and superficial horn cysts).[9]

Only 1 percent of newborns have NMN at birth,[16–18] with a slightly higher prevalence in nonwhites (1.2 percent) than in whites (0.8 percent). In congenital NMN, nevomelanocytes frequently involve reticular dermal appendages, blood vessels and lymphatics, and neurovascular structures, and usually penetrate the collagen of the lower two-thirds of the reticular dermis or the panniculus. Congenital NMN are commonly associated with hamartomatous changes in blood vessels, lymphatics, neurovascular struc-

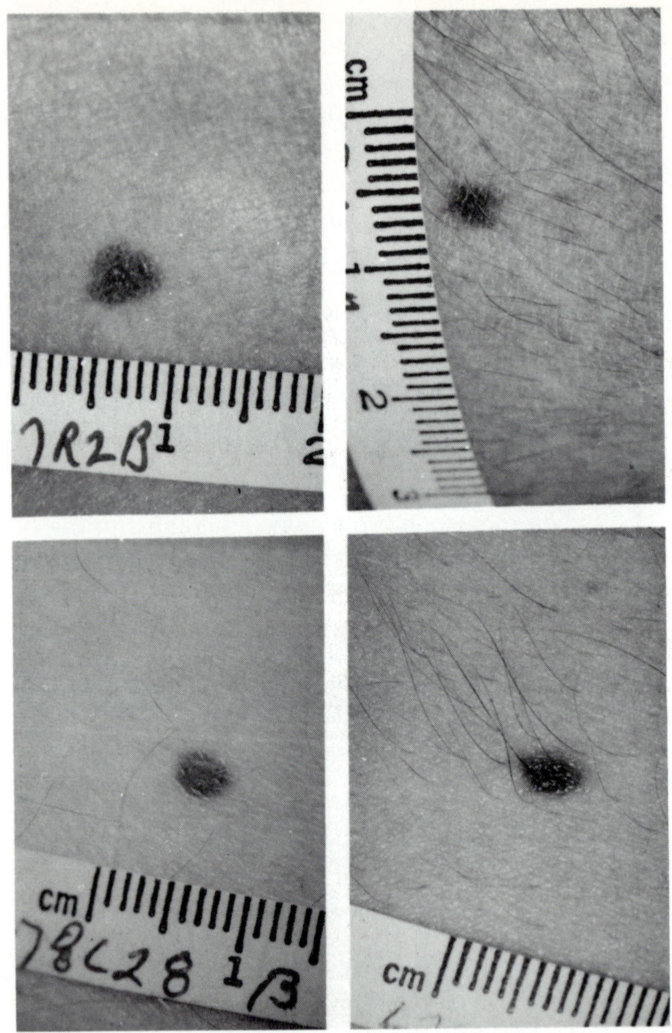

Figure 18-4 Typical acquired NMN from four healthy white adults. All of these papules are soft, relatively small, and evenly pigmented light brown or tan, with well-demarcated, regular borders.

tures, and appendages. Such findings are significantly less common in acquired NMN[19,20] (Fig. 18-5).

The congenital split NMN of the eyelid[9] is an important experiment in nature, providing an indication of when during fetal life congenital NMN develop. When the eyelid is closed, the split nevus is a single lesion, suggesting that nevus cells were in place during the period of lid fusion but before the eyelid split. In utero, human eyelids form between the 5th and 6th weeks, begin to fuse at about 8 to 9 weeks, and reopen during the 24th week. It may be presumed that congenital NMN form between

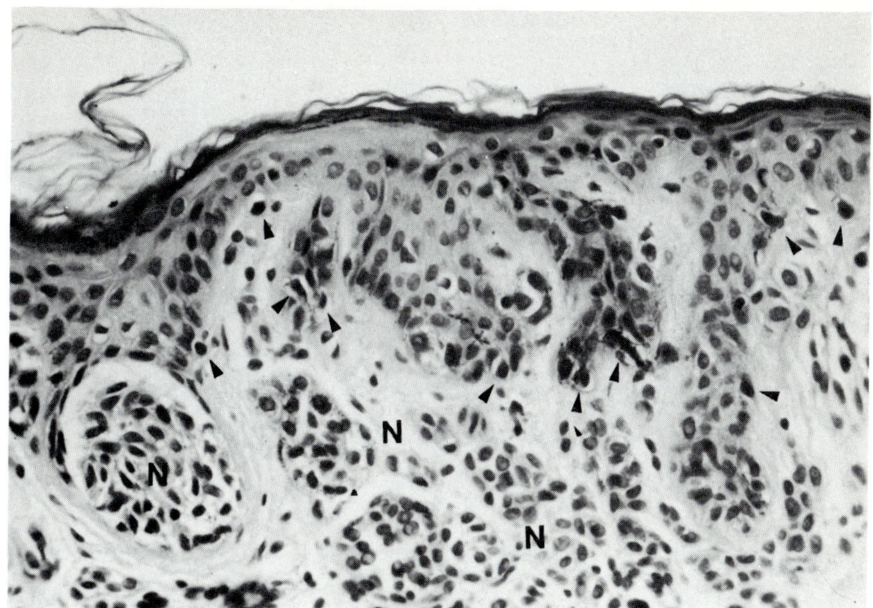

Figure 18-5 Histopathology of a typical acquired NMN on the arm of a 26-year-old white woman. Note the nevus cells (N) as well-formed nests in the epidermis and as scattered cells in the dermis, and typical dopa-reactive melanocytes (arrows) scattered singly in the epidermal basal unit. Dopa-incubated tissue section, cut at 6-μm thickness, stained with hematoxylin and eosin. ×400 in the original magnification.

the 10th week (when melanoblasts are believed to appear for the first time in the fetal dermis) and the 24th week of fetal life (when the eyelids reopen).

Congenital NMN have been arbitrarily defined as small or large on the basis of absolute surface area, relative surface area, or the difficulty of excisional surgery for a given lesion. Small lesions are easily excised and the wound defect is closed primarily, without the use of grafts or rotation flaps. The term *giant* is reserved for large lesions that involve a major portion of a single anatomic region (e.g., the head, the torso, or an extremity) (Fig. 18-6). Large congenital NMN having a greatest diameter of at least 99 mm occur in 1 of every 20,000 newborns, and giant congenital NMN are present in 1 of every 500,000 newborns.[18]

Most acquired NMN are not apparent until after the first 6 to 12 months of life. In a prevalence study of NMN that were 2 mm or larger in diameter in more than 1500 whites aged 5 to 69 years,[12] an increasing number of lesions per person was noted during the first two decades of life; the peak prevalence occurred in the mid-teens in males (average of 43 per person) and the mid-twenties in females (average of 27 per person). Thereafter, the prevalence of NMN fell progressively, so that by age 80 years, NMN were infrequent or rare.[12] The postulated mechanisms of regression for

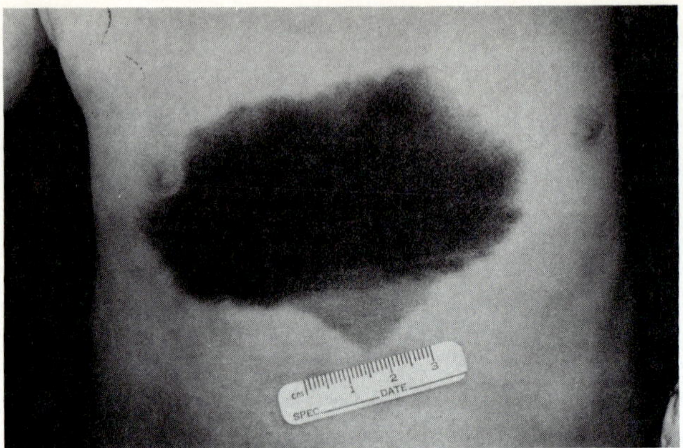

Figure 18-6 Giant congenital NMN. This irregularly pigmented plaque occupies a major portion of the anterior torso of a 6-month-old white boy.

NMN include fibrosis, fatty degeneration, and inflammatory autodestruction.

The observation that NMN are more prevalent in sun-exposed skin in whites has been interpreted to suggest that ultraviolet radiation may play a role in their evolution.[21] Periods of darkening and slight enlargement of NMN occur during puberty and ACTH therapy. NMN are also reported to appear for the first time or darken during pregnancy. In addition, NMN may have a familial pattern of distribution and number. Support for familial aggregation of NMN comes from work in which 1783 pigmented NMN among 45 pairs of monozygotic twins were noted to be similar in number for each twin pair, although nonidentical in distribution.[22] Dysplastic melanocytic nevi (see below), an important histogenic precursor and risk factor for the development of cutaneous melanoma, have a pattern of familial aggregation consistent with autosomal dominant inheritance in some kindreds.[23] Familial aggregation also has been demonstrated for congenital NMN.[24]

LESIONS ASSOCIATED WITH THE DEVELOPMENT OF CUTANEOUS MELANOMA

Lentigo Maligna

While lentigo maligna (LM) accounts for only 5 percent of all cutaneous melanomas, it is important to recognize because of the potential for lethal melanoma prevention when treated in an early phase of development. LM is a haphazardly pigmented, relatively large, irregular spot on sun-exposed skin of older people, rather like a brown varnish stain (Fig. 18-7). It consists of a disordered proliferation of variably atypical melanocytes in an atrophic epidermis overlying sun-damaged dermal collagen. LM may be regarded as a dysplasia of melanocytes (see the definition of

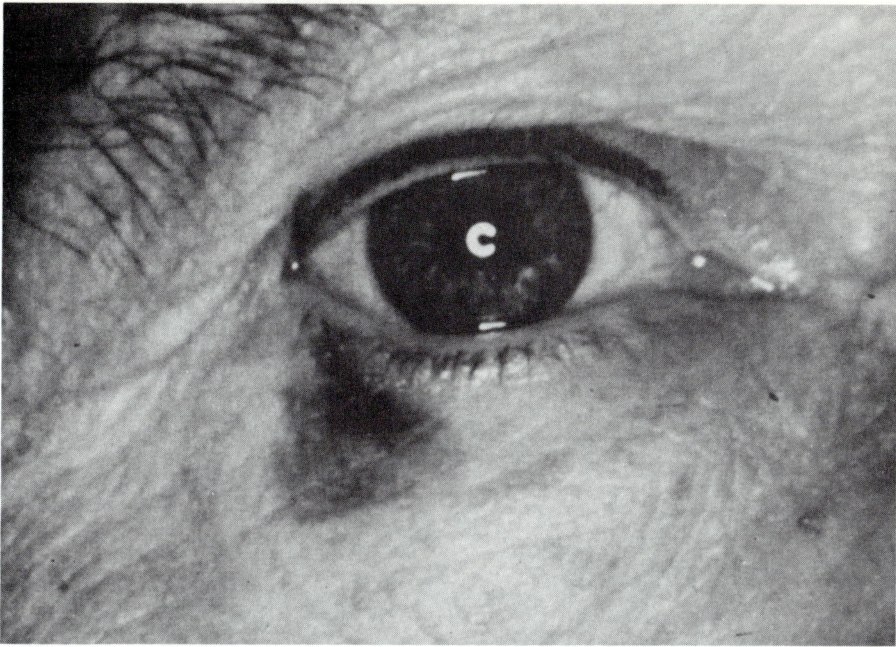

Figure 18-7 LM. This irregularly pigmented macule on the lower eyelid of a 74-year-old white man has been present for many years, slowly enlarging and becoming darker.

dysplasia in the section on dysplastic melanocytic nevi) caused by excessive sun exposure. With time, LM may remain stable or expand slowly and become more haphazardly pigmented. Invasive melanoma developing in LM, which is associated with the development of focal or diffuse elevation of the lesion surface, may result in metastatic disease and death.[9]

While it has been stated that one-third to one-half of all cases of LM develop invasive melanoma, the actual lifetime risk of melanoma in persons who have LM may well be less than 5 percent. Based on available information, it has been estimated that persons who have LM have a tenfold increased risk of developing melanoma prior to age 75 years.[25]

Dysplastic Melanocytic Nevi

Dysplastic melanocytic nevi (DMN) are usually rather large, irregularly and darkly pigmented lesions (Figs. 18-8 and 18-9), characterized histologically by the presence of intraepidermal melanocytic dysplasia. Melanocytic dysplasia in the context of DMN is defined as a proliferation of variably atypical intraepidermal melanocytes in elongated and club-shaped epidermal rete (lentiginous epidermal pattern), in contrast to LM. DMN are frequently associated with one or more dermal mesenchymal alterations (eosinophilic fibrosis and/or lamellar fibroplasia), excessive melanin-laden macrophages, lymphocytic infiltrates, and a dermal nevomelanocytic

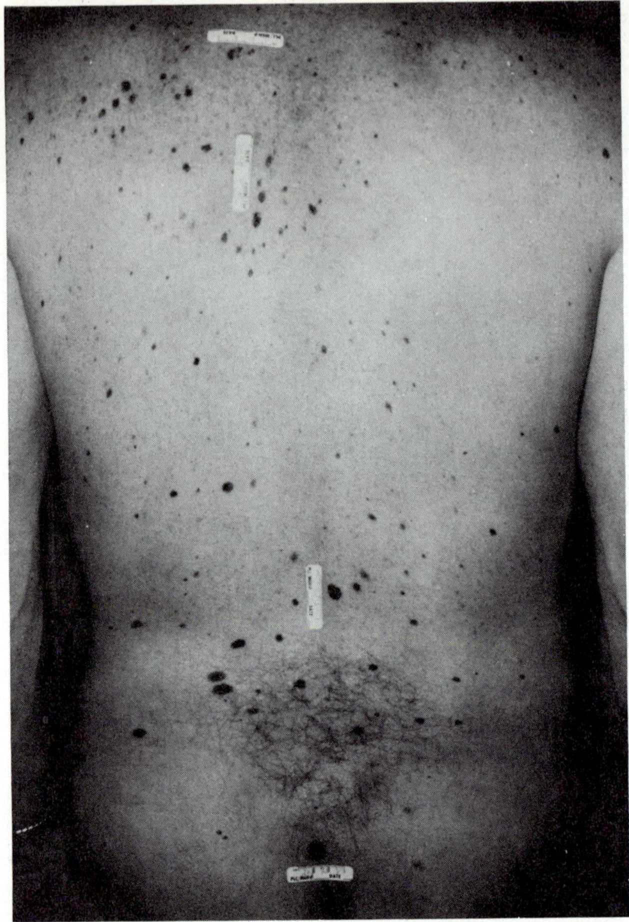

Figure 18-8 DMN. Note the numerous, relatively large, pigmented moles on the back of a 60-year-old white man. These lesions were reported to have been present since the early teenage years.

component[9] (Fig. 18-10). One or more DMN have been noted on the cutaneous surface in 90 percent of people who have familial cutaneous melanoma (two or more members affected in a given kindred), in 42 to 56 percent of nonmelanoma first-degree blood relatives in the setting of familial melanoma, and in 34 percent of white adults who have nonfamilial melanoma compared to 2 to 5 percent of white adults who do not have melanoma.[9] DMN are rare in nonwhites. They may occur anywhere on the skin surface but appear in increased numbers on the torso. DMN also may be present in increased numbers in sites not frequently associated with NMN, such as the buttocks, breasts, and scalp. Histologic features of DMN have been detected at the most lateral tumor margin in at least 22 percent of nonfamilial melanomas and in 70 to 90 percent of familial melanomas, suggesting that DMN are precursor lesions in these cases.

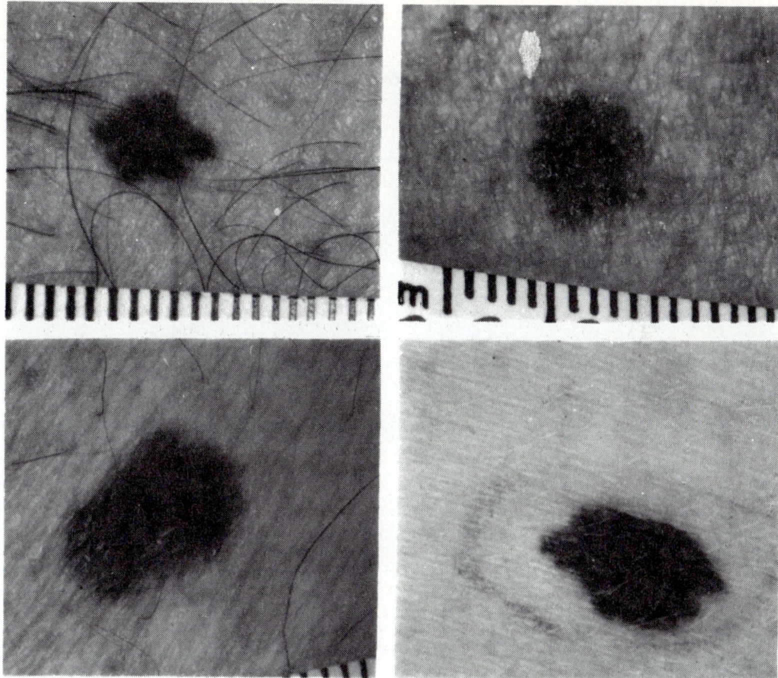

Figure 18-9 DMN. Note the haphazard or dark pigmentation, relatively large size, and fuzzy and/or irregular borders of the lesion.

Morphologic studies using the dopa histochemical technique demonstrate that melanocytes in DMN tend to be larger and more crowded than melanocytes in typical acquired NMN and solar lentigines (Fig. 18-10) but smaller and less concentrated than the intraepidermal component of melanoma (Fig. 18-11), which is defined as a continuous and side-to-side proliferation of melanocytes that show fully evolved cellular atypia, often spanning the breadth of the epidermis. Contrast the dopa-reactive melanocytes in DMN and intraepidermal melanoma with those in sun-protected skin (Fig. 18-3).

DMN, one of the most important risk factors for the development of cutaneous melanoma, ought to be sought during the cutaneous examination of older children and adults. Young children who have a large number of prominent nevi should be suspected of evolving DMN. All blood relatives of people who have DMN should be examined for DMN and early melanoma. People who have one or more DMN have an estimated 7- to 27-fold increased risk of melanoma.[9]

Congenital Nevomelanocytic Nevi

A potential risk of melanoma probably exists for all congenital NMN, regardless of their absolute or relative size. For giant congenital NMN, the risk has been estimated to be at least 6.3 percent over a lifetime.[26] Of the

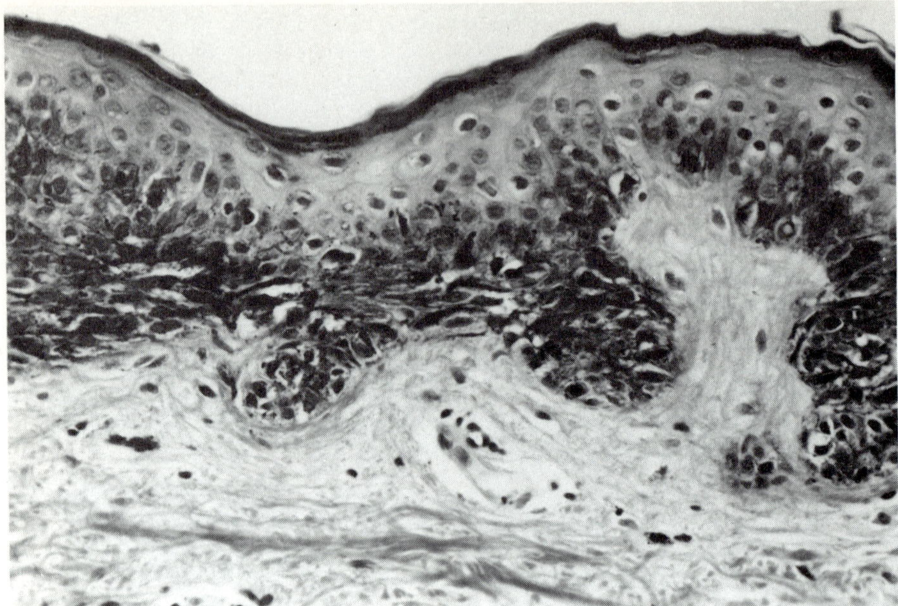

Figure 18-10 Histopathology of a DMN from the anterior torso of a 39-year-old white man. Note the increased number of relatively large, dopa-reactive melanocytes crowded haphazardly in the epidermis. Dopa-incubated tissue section, cut at 6-μm thickness, stained with hematoxylin and eosin. ×400 in the original magnification.

metastatic melanomas associated with giant congenital NMN, about one-half are diagnosed within the first 3 to 5 years of life. Also, approximately two-thirds of the melanomas associated with giant congenital NMN have a nonepidermal origin,[26] suggesting the need to seek the presence of a dermal nodule, and even metastatic melanoma in lymph nodes and viscera, when following people who have such lesions. Large congenital NMN on the head or neck regions may be associated with leptomeningeal melanocytosis (a proliferation of meningeal melanocytes), which may be asymptomatic or manifested by obstructive hydrocephalus, seizures, or even melanoma.

While there seems to be little question that at least some melanomas develop in small congenital NMN,[27] the exact risk is unknown. It has been estimated that the risk of melanoma associated with small congenital NMN in people who live to age 60 years may be as high as 4.9 percent based on history and 0.8 to 2.6 percent based on histology.[9]

Atypical Moles on Acral and Mucosal Sites

Other pigmented melanocytic lesions may be potential precursors of melanoma, including atypical varieties of melanocytic lesions on palms, soles, nail beds, and mucous membranes.[9] Benign varieties of pigmented lesions are relatively common on palms and soles, occurring in 10 percent

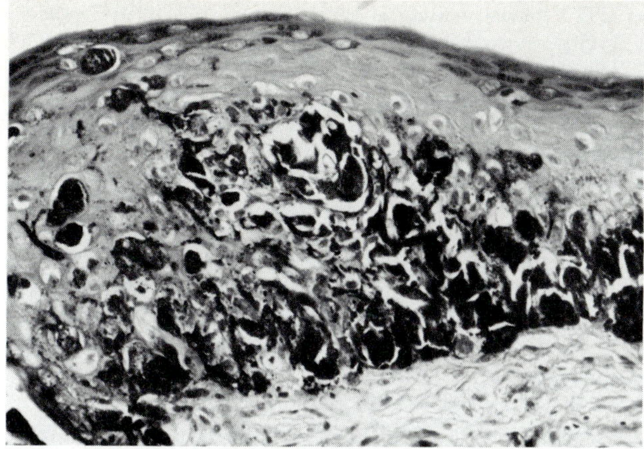

Figure 18-11 Histopathology of intraepidermal melanoma. Note the markedly enlarged, dopa-reactive melanocytes distributed singly and in dyshesive nests as a continuous and side-to-side proliferation at all levels of the epidermis. Dopa-incubated tissue section, cut at 6-μm thickness, stained with hematoxylin and eosin. ×400 in the original magnification.

of whites and in a higher percentage of nonwhites. Pigmented lesions also occur on the genitalia in 15 percent of men and women. Pigmented lesions on nail beds and conjunctivas are relatively common in nonwhites but are extremely uncommon in whites. Very darkly pigmented or irregularly pigmented lesions on palms, soles, nail beds, or mucous membranes require evaluation for biopsy or close observation, regardless of race. In whites, pigmented lesions on nail beds or conjunctivas should be considered for biopsy and histologic examination.

REFERENCES

1. Zimmerman AA, Becker SW Jr: *Melanoblasts and Melanocytes in Fetal Negro Skin.* Illinois Monographs in Medical Science. Urbana, University of Illinois Press, 1959, vol VI, part 3, p 1.
2. Holbrook KA et al: Melanocytes in human embryonic and fetal skin: a review and new findings. *Pigment Cell Res* 1(Suppl):6, 1988.
3. Cordova A: The Mongolian spot, a study of ethnic differences and a literature review. *Clin Pediatr* 20:714, 1981.
4. Hernandez FJ: Malignant blue nevus: a light and electron microscopic study. *Arch Dermatol* 107:741, 1973.
5. Hodgson C: Senile lentigo. *Arch Dermatol* 87:197, 1963.
6. Montagna W et al: A reinvestigation of solar lentigines. *Arch Dermatol* 116:1151, 1980.
7. Rhodes AR et al: The PUVA-induced pigmented macule: a lentiginous proliferation of large, sometimes cytologically atypical melanocytes. *J Am Acad Dermatol* 9:47, 1983.
8. Robbins JK, Moshell AN: DNA repair processes protect human beings from premature solar damage: evidence from studies on xeroderma pigmentosum. *J Invest Dermatol* 73:102, 1979.
9. Rhodes AR: Neoplasms: benign neoplasms, hyperplasias, and dysplasias of melanocytes, in Fitzpatrick TB et al (eds), *Dermatology in General Medicine,* 3d ed. New York, McGraw-Hill, 1987, p 877.

10. Thorne EG et al: Tyrosinase activity in dermal nevus cells. *Arch Dermatol* 104:619, 1971.
11. Gottlieb B et al: Fine structure of the nevus cell. *Arch Dermatol* 92:81, 1965.
12. Nicholls EM: Development and elimination of pigmented moles, and the anatomical distribution of primary malignant melanoma. *Cancer* 32:191, 1973.
13. Pack GT, Davis J: The relation of race and complexion to the incidence of moles and melanomas. *Ann NY Acad Sci* 100:719, 1963.
14. Reddy CRRM et al: Incidence and evolution of moles and the relationship to malignant melanoma in Eastern India. *Int Surg* 61:469, 1976.
15. Lewis MG, Johnson K: The incidence and distribution of pigmented nevi in Ugandan Africans. *Br J Dermatol* 80:362, 1968.
16. Walton RG et al: Pigmented lesions in newborn infants. *Br J Dermatol* 95:389, 1976.
17. Alper J et al: Birthmarks with serious medical significance: nevocellular nevi, sebaceous nevi, and multiple café-au-lait spots. *J Pediatr* 95:696, 1979.
18. Castilla EE et al: Epidemiology of congenital pigmented nevi; incidence rates and relative frequencies. *Br J Dermatol* 104:307, 1981.
19. Mark GJ et al: Congenital melanocytic nevi of the small and garment type: clinical, histologic, and ultrastructural studies. *Hum Pathol* 4:395, 1973.
20. Rhodes AR et al: A histologic comparison of congenital and acquired nevomelanocytic nevi. *Arch Dermatol* 121:1266, 1985.
21. Kopf AW et al: Prevalence of nevocytic nevi on lateral and medial aspects of arms. *J Dermatol Surg Oncol* 4:153, 1978.
22. Siemens HW: Untersuchungen über die Ätiologie der Naevi. *Arch Dermatol Syph (Berl)* 145:207, 1924.
23. Bale SJ et al: Mapping the gene for hereditary cutaneous malignant melanoma-dysplastic nevus to chromosome 1p. *N Engl J Med* 320:1367, 1989.
24. Rhodes AR et al: Familial aggregation of small congenital nevomelanocytic nevi. *Am J Med Genet* 22:315, 1985.
25. Weinstock MA, Sober AJ: Risk of progression of lentigo maligna to lentigo maligna melanoma. *Br J Dermatol* 16:303, 1987.
26. Rhodes AR et al: Non-epidermal origin of malignant melanoma associated with a giant congenital nevocellular nevus. *Plast Reconstr Surg* 67:782, 1981.
27. Illig L et al: Congenital nevi < 10 cm as precursors to melanoma: 52 cases, a review, and a new conception. *Arch Dermatol* 121:1274, 1985.

SECTION SIX

DISORDERS OF THE DERMAL-EPIDERMAL INTERFACE

19

Biology of the Dermal-Epidermal Interface and the Pathophysiology of Bullous Pemphigoid, Epidermolysis Bullosa Acquisita, and Lupus Erythematosus

Richard D. Sontheimer and Jo-David Fine

Basement membranes are essential structures in virtually all mammalian tissues. Separating epithelium from the underlying connective tissue, they provide a structural support or scaffold to which epithelial cells can become firmly attached.[1-6] Furthermore, specific components of basement membranes provide chemical signals that influence the migration and differentiation of cells within the adjacent epithelium. In skin, injury to or biochemical alteration of one such basement membrane, located at the dermal-epidermal junction, results in altered integrity of the epithelial–connective tissue interface; as a clinical correlate, such injury or disruption is commonly associated with the development of blisters and, in some diseases, with eventual scar formation.[2,4,5,7] In this chapter, we first discuss the ultrastructure and biochemical composition of normal skin basement membrane and then illustrate the role of this structure in the pathophysiology of disease by discussing three common disorders—bullous pemphigoid, epidermolysis bullosa acquisita, and lupus erythematosus—that are characterized by autoimmune injury to the dermal-epidermal junction.

BIOLOGY OF THE DERMAL-EPIDERMAL JUNCTION

Structure[1-6,8]

In skin, basement membranes delimit or surround three major areas—the dermal-epidermal junction (including the hair follicle), vasculature,

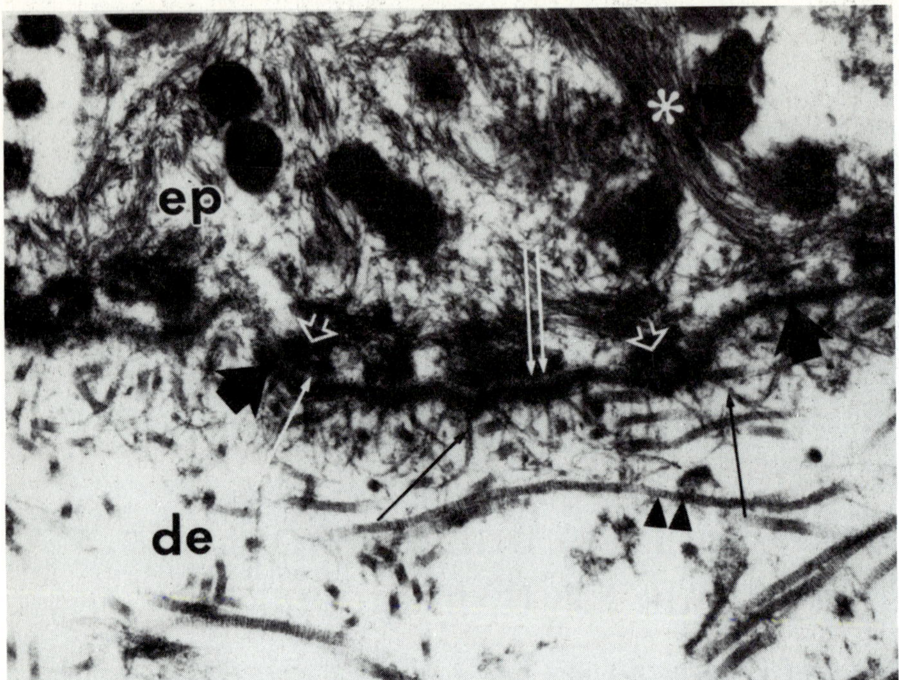

Figure 19-1 Transmission electron micrograph of the dermal-epidermal junction. The basement membrane zone in this portion of the skin is composed of a lamina lucida (white arrow), a lamina densa (heavy dark arrow), hemidesmosomes (empty white arrow), subbasal dense plate (double white arrow), anchoring fibrils (long black arrows), and anchoring filaments. The asterisk denotes keratin filaments within the lower pole of the basilar keratinocyte. Directly underneath the basement membrane zone are sparse collagen fibers (double arrowhead). ep = basilar epidermal cell; de = dermis. ×50,000 in the original magnification.

and appendages (including glandular structures, nerves, and the arrector pili muscles). Although antigenic differences exist,[9] depending on the nature of the adjacent skin structure, all of these basement membranes share common ultrastructural features. At the electron-microscopic level (Fig. 19-1), an electron-sparse region, referred to as the lamina lucida, is located parallel to and directly underlying the most basilar epithelial cells; this is analogous to the lamina rara of the glomerular basement membrane. The second major component of the basement membrane zone, the lamina densa, is an electron-dense band that is bordered superiorly by the lamina lucida and inferiorly by the upper papillary dermis. Several additional structures are considered part of the basement membrane zone of the dermal-epidermal junction. These include the hemidesmosome, anchoring filament, subbasal dense plate, and anchoring fibril. The hemidesmosome is a protein-containing, linear, electron-dense condensation located along the inner side of the inferior pole of the basal keratinocyte cytoplasmic membrane. Directly underneath the hemidesmosome, within the midportion of the lamina lucida, is a thin, electron-dense, linear structure named the subbasal dense plate. In some areas of the basement membrane zone, fine filamentous structures, accordingly named anchoring filaments, traverse the lamina lucida, presumably inserting into both the overlying hemidesmosomes and the lamina densa. Finally, fan-shaped, fibrillar structures with irregular central cross-banding, referred to as anchoring fibrils, insert superiorly into the lamina densa and connect directly with other anchoring fibrils laterally and inferiorly within the upper dermis. Condensations of the latter have been termed anchoring plaques.[10] Although nothing is known about the function or even the biochemical composition of the subbasal dense plate and anchoring filament, it is believed that the anchoring fibril somehow connects the basement membrane to larger collagen fibers within the upper dermis, thereby providing additional mechanical stability to the skin. As partial evidence of the likelihood of this hypothesis, the reduction or absence of visible anchoring fibrils in the autosomal dominant and autosomal recessive forms of a frequently severe inherited blistering disease named dystrophic epidermolysis bullosa is associated with the presence of marked mechanical fragility of skin and spontaneous or induced blister formation just beneath the level of the lamina densa.[7,9]

It is now clear that in normal skin the structurally weakest portion of the dermal-epidermal junction is the lamina lucida. For example, application of sufficient suction and/or heat, or incubation of skin with specific chemicals (i.e., sodium chloride, sodium bromide, sodium isothiocyanate, ethylene diamine tetraacetic acid) or enzymes (i.e., trypsin), results in complete separation of the epidermis from the dermis at the level of the lamina lucida. This has practical utility, since it permits a ready means of chemically isolating epidermal cells from the extracellular matrix for use in a variety of laboratory studies, including the propagation and maintenance of keratinocyte and melanocyte cell cultures. In addition, these enzymatic findings suggest a plausible mechanism (i.e., release of lamina lucida–degrading proteases from leukocytes) whereby eventual blister formation may occur in selected autoimmune disorders characterized by the presence of inflammatory cell infiltrates within the upper dermis.

Biochemistry and Antigenicity of the Dermal-Epidermal Junction

The human dermal-epidermal junction is highly complex biochemically. It contains a variety of collagenous and noncollagenous proteins, glycoproteins, and proteoglycans (Table 19-1). Although some of its components may be located in more than one ultrastructural region, each component of the skin basement membrane has a predilection for a single region or structure. Each of these basement membrane constituents differs in biochemical composition and, in many, in distribution (i.e., dermal-epidermal junction–specific vs. ubiquitous) and ultrastructural localization

Table 19-1

ANTIGENS IN HUMAN SKIN BASEMENT MEMBRANES

Antigen	Distribution in Skin BMZs	Species Specificity	Organ Specificity	Localization within BMZ
Laminin	All	None	Epitope dependent	LL and LD
Type IV collagen	All	None	None	LD
Type V collagen	DE junction, perivascular BMZs, and dermal interstitium	?	?	LD and lower basilar keratinocyte cytoplasm and membrane
Type VII collagen	DE junction	?	Skin, cornea, chorioamnion, oral mucosa, and cervix	Anchoring fibrils
Bullous pemphigoid antigen	DE junction	None	Stratified squamous epithelium	Hemidesmosomes
Cicatricial pemphigoid antigen	DE junction	None	Stratified squamous epithelium and some mucosal	LL
AA3	DE junction and adnexal BMZs	?	?	LL

GB3 (BM 600)	DE junction and adnexal BMZs	?	?	LL & LD
19-DEJ-1	DE junction and smooth muscle BMZ	Primate	Stratified squamous epithelium	Mid-LL (beneath hemidesmosome)
EB acquisita	DE junction	None	Stratified squamous epithelium and some mucosal	LD and anchoring fibrils
KF-1	DE junction	Primate	Stratified squamous epithelium	LD
Entactin (nidogen)	All	None	None	Primarily LD
HSPG	All	None	None	Primarily LD and sub-LD
C6-SPG	All	None	None	LD
LDA-1	All	Human and rabbit	None	LD/sub-LD
AF1 and AF2	DE junction	Primate	Stratified squamous epithelium	Anchoring fibrils

Abbreviations: BMZ = basement membrane zone; DE = dermal-epidermal; LL = lamina lucida; LD = lamina densa; HSPG = heparan sulfate proteoglycan; C6-SPG = chondroitin 6-sulfate proteoglycan; AF = anchoring fibril–associated antigen (all other abbreviations under "Antigen" are specific names).

in human skin, ontogeny, enzymatic sensitivities, restrictions in expression in other human organs or other mammalian species, and/or degree of expression in skin from patients with various subsets of epidermolysis bullosa.[11-14]

Although a variety of skin basement membrane constituents have been recently identified by immunohistochemical means, most notably via the monoclonal antibody technique, only a few have been well characterized biochemically. These include laminin, types IV and VII collagen, bullous pemphigoid antigen, entactin (nidogen), and heparan sulfate and chondroitin 6-sulfate proteoglycans. Laminin, a glycoprotein, is present within both the lamina lucida and the lamina densa of all basement membranes; epitopes of the laminin molecule, with rare exceptions, lack organ or species restrictions in their expression.[15,16] This cross-shaped molecule has been shown to assist in many different functional roles, including the attachment of cells to other extracellular matrix components. Types IV and VII collagen are the only known collagens exclusively confined to the basement membrane zone. Whereas type IV collagen is located within the lamina densa,[17,18] type VII collagen is the major component of the anchoring fibril,[19] and is also detectable within anchoring plaques.[10] At the light-microscopic level, type IV collagen, like laminin and heparan sulfate and chondroitin 6-sulfate proteoglycans, is a ubiquitous component of all basement membranes. In contrast, both type VII collagen and bullous pemphigoid antigen are present solely along the dermal-epidermal junction of skin and other stratified squamous epithelial tissues. Bullous pemphigoid antigen, a protein originally identified in normal human skin using antibasement membrane autoantibodies present in the sera of patients with bullous pemphigoid, is closely associated with the hemidesmosomes at the ultrastructural level.[20] As will be discussed, this particular protein plays a pivotal role in the disease mechanism of the autoimmune disorder bullous pemphigoid. In contrast, three other ubiquitous basement membrane components—heparan sulfate proteoglycan,[21,22] chondroitin 6-sulfate proteoglycan,[23] and entactin (nidogen)[22,24]—are primary constituents of the lamina densa, although at least the former proteoglycan may be detected within or closely associated with virtually every region or structure within the dermal-epidermal junction, further emphasizing the spatial and presumably functional interactions that occur among many of the biochemical components of skin basement membrane.

Several other biochemical constituents or epitopes of the dermal-epidermal junction have been recently identified and partially characterized[5,9,25,26] (Table 19-1). Although lack of complete biochemical characterization precludes proof that one or more may simply represent new epitopes present on previously isolated basement membrane components, many of these novel epitopes are noteworthy because of their apparent utility in the diagnosis, both postnatally and prenatally, of specific subsets of patients with inherited epidermolysis bullosa.[9,12-14,27-29]

PATHOPHYSIOLOGY OF SELECTED AUTOIMMUNE BULLOUS DISEASES

Bullous Pemphigoid

Bullous pemphigoid is a rather common autoimmune skin disease that occurs primarily in the elderly. In contrast to some other blistering diseases, no ethnic, racial, or histocompatibility antigen associations have been noted in bullous pemphigoid. Clinically, this disease is characterized by the development of often intensely pruritic, tense blisters that frequently arise on flexural surfaces of the skin (Fig. 19-2). Less frequently, urticarial plaques may be seen.[30,31] Healing occurs without scarring, and usually milia formation, mechanical fragility of the skin, and involvement of mucous membranes are lacking.

Histologically, bullous pemphigoid is characterized by the presence of subepidermal blister formation, associated with eosinophils within the blister cavity, along the dermal-epidermal junction, and within the upper papillary dermis. In very early urticarial lesions, the first inflammatory cell detectable is the mast cell, which can be seen in close alignment with the dermal-epidermal junction.[32] At the ultrastructural level, blister formation occurs within the lamina lucida in the absence of any evidence of epidermal cell injury or death. Direct immunofluorescence studies performed on

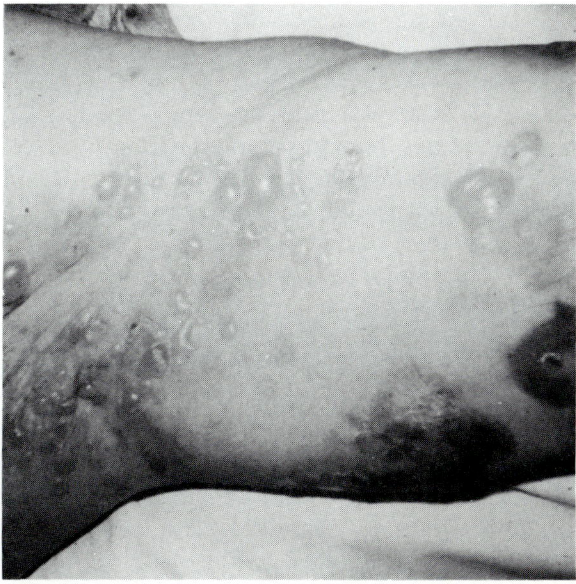

Figure 19-2 Multiple tense bullae distributed over the upper extremity in an individual with bullous pemphigoid. (*From NA Soter, HP Baden, Pathophysiology of Dermatologic Diseases. New York, McGraw-Hill, 1984, p 241.*)

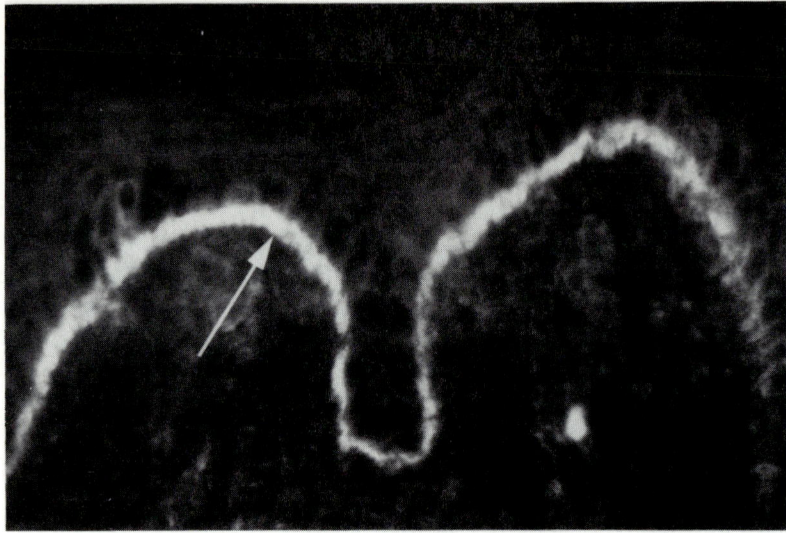

Figure 19-3 Direct immunofluorescence of perilesional skin from a patient with bullous pemphigoid demonstrating the presence of tissue-bound IgG (arrow) in linear array along the dermal-epidermal junction. ×312.5 in the original magnification.

perilesional skin reveal the presence of tissue-bound IgG and C3 in a linear, homogeneous array along the dermal-epidermal junction (Fig. 19-3). Such tissue-bound immunoreactants can be shown to reside within the lamina lucida if direct immunoelectron microscopy is performed. Similarly, in approximately 80 percent of patients, indirect immunofluorescence studies performed with patients' sera demonstrate the presence of circulating autoantibodies that bind along the dermal-epidermal junction and to the epidermal portion of separated basement membrane of intact and sodium chloride–split human skin, respectively. In contrast to one other autoimmune bullous disease (pemphigus vulgaris), however, no correlation usually exists between the titer (level) of bullous pemphigoid autoantibodies and the extent of disease activity present in any given patient.

Bullous pemphigoid autoantibodies have been isolated and purified, and subsequently utilized in a variety of studies aimed at better elucidation of the mechanism of this disease. In general, attempts to reproduce blisters in experimental animals with such autoantibodies have been unrewarding,[33] although a rabbit cornea model has been proposed.[34] Similarly, with the possible exception of one dog strain, no animal lines have been identified in which a disease analogous to bullous pemphigoid has been found to arise spontaneously. In contrast, an excellent in vitro model, referred to as the leukocyte attachment assay, has been described for this disease.[35] Specifically, if purified bullous pemphigoid autoantibodies, complement, and neutrophils are coincubated with freshly prepared cryosections of normal human skin, IgG and C3 bind along the dermal-epidermal junction, chemotaxis of neutrophils to this region occurs, and microvesiculation subsequently develops at the level of the basement membrane zone. Further studies have shown that this model is autoantibody, neutrophil, and complement dependent.

A series of biochemical studies have now demonstrated that bullous pemphigoid antigen is a normal constituent of the dermal-epidermal junction and that it is a biosynthetic product of basilar keratinocytes.[36,37] Although proteins with several different molecular weights have been immunoprecipitated or immunoblotted with bullous pemphigoid autoantibodies, it appears that the major protein identified by such autoantibodies has a molecular weight of approximately 230 kd.[38] Most recently, the gene encoding for this protein has been partially characterized from cDNA prepared from human keratinocytes.[39]

One plausible mechanism for blister formation in bullous pemphigoid is depicted in Fig. 19-4.[7,40,41] Although the actual triggering event is still unknown, bullous pemphigoid antigen is recognized as foreign by the patient's immune system. Autoantibodies against this antigen are produced, which then bind to the dermal-epidermal junction and fix complement. Mast cells are attracted and release one or more chemical mediators (such as eosinophil chemotactic factor of anaphylaxis). Chemotaxis of eosinophils to the dermal-epidermal junction occurs, neutral proteases and eosinophil granular basic proteins are released, and then intralamina lucida cleavage and subsequent frank subepidermal blister formation develop.

Epidermolysis Bullosa Acquisita[42,43]

Epidermolysis bullosa (EB) acquisita is a relatively common blistering disorder that can occur at any age. It is estimated that up to 5 percent of

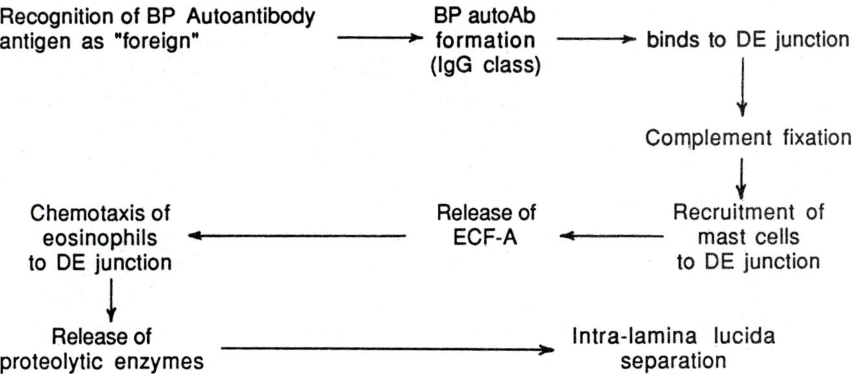

Figure 19-4 Schematic representation of the proposed mechanism for blister formation in bullous pemphigoid (BP). ECF-A = eosinophil chemotactic factor of anaphylaxis; DE = dermal-epidermal.

all patients previously diagnosed as having bullous pemphigoid actually have EB acquisita. In contrast to bullous pemphigoid, there is a very strong association between the presence of the HLA-DR2 haplotype and EB acquisita.[44]

There may be several different clinical presentations of EB acquisita, further confusing the diagnosis. In classical EB acquisita, tense blisters arise in association with mechanical fragility of the skin, milia formation, scarring, and often severely debilitating mucosal involvement (particularly of the oral cavity, ocular tract, and gastrointestinal tract), the last at times resembling that seen in pemphigus vulgaris or dominant dystrophic EB. Rare patients may even die as a result of secondary overwhelming systemic bacterial infections. Pruritus or a burning sensation in the skin is a frequent complaint. In contrast, other patients may present with clinical features morphologically reminiscent of or indistinguishable from those observed in cicatricial pemphigoid, bullous pemphigoid, or porphyria cutanea tarda.

Similarly, several different histological patterns may be seen. For example, although all patients with EB acquisita have subepidermal blister formation, the composition of dermal inflammatory cells, when present, may vary considerably. Most commonly, however, neutrophils are noted, initially in linear array along the dermal-epidermal junction. Electron-microscopic findings vary, depending on the age of the lesion, the presence or absence of inflammatory cells, and the duration of disease activity. For example, intralamina lucida cleavage is commonly seen early in the course of the disease in association with the presence of leukocytes (particularly neutrophils) within the inflammatory cell infiltrate.[45] In contrast, much later in the course of disease, sublamina densa cleavage may be observed, especially in the absence of inflammatory cells within the dermis and in association with the marked disruption of anchoring fibrils. In addition, variable amounts of electron-dense, amorphous material may be noted just beneath the level of the basement membrane zone.

Direct immunofluorescence studies of perilesional skin usually demonstrate the presence of multiple tissue-bound immunoreactants (especially IgG, IgA, and/or C3) in rather broad linear array along the dermal-epidermal junction in a pattern somewhat reminiscent of that seen in some patients with lupus erythematosus. The majority of patients with EB acquisita have detectable circulating antibasement membrane (dermal-epidermal junction–specific) autoantibodies, especially when sodium chloride–split skin is used as the tissue substrate. On the latter tissue, EB acquisita autoantibodies bind exclusively to the dermal portion of the separated basement membrane, clearly differentiating them from autoantibodies that develop in patients with bullous pemphigoid and bind to the epidermal portion.[46] Indirect immunoelectron-microscopic studies confirm the binding localization of EB acquisita autoantibodies to the level of the lamina densa and anchoring fibrils.

No animal models exist for EB acquisita. However, findings similar to those of bullous pemphigoid have been noted with EB acquisita autoantibodies when the leukocyte attachment assay has been employed, suggesting that this disease is also autoantibody, cell, and complement dependent.[47] Most recently, this model has been used to demonstrate the role of cytokines in promotion of leukocyte chemotaxis and attachment following the binding of EB acquisita autoantibodies along the dermal-epidermal junction.[48] Presumably the major mechanistic differences between bullous pemphigoid and EB acquisita are differences in (1) the specific basement membrane antigens involved, (2) the types of inflammatory cells present (i.e., mast cells and eosinophils in bullous pemphigoid; polymorphonuclear leukocytes, mononuclear cells, or possibly even no inflammatory cells in some subsets of EB acquisita), and (3) the influence of HLA class II alleles.

Biochemical studies have demonstrated that EB acquisita autoantibodies identify a protein, referred to as the EB acquisita antigen, that is extractable from the dermal portion of sodium chloride–split skin and has two molecular weight subunits (290 and 145 kd).[49] Identical autoantibodies have been now identified in some patients with the bullous eruption of systemic lupus erythematosus. Most recently, it has been shown that the EB acquisita antigen is in fact a portion of type VII collagen,[50] thereby explaining its rather unique ultrastructural localization.

Lupus Erythematosus

Lupus erythematosus (LE) is an extremely heterogeneous clinical entity that often involves the skin, either alone or in combination with one or more internal organs (joints, kidneys, brain, heart, lungs, blood elements, systemic vascular tree). There is a high female preponderance with the primarily systemic form of the disease (systemic LE or SLE); however, this is much less marked in certain cutaneous varieties of the disorder, such as discoid LE (DLE). When the epidemiology of LE is examined, cutaneous disease is often found to be second only to joint inflammation in cumulative frequency of overall clinical expression. In addition, skin disease is frequently found to be the second most common initial disease symptom following arthralgia/arthritis.

LE is most commonly classified among the autoimmune connective tissue (or rheumatic) diseases that share the feature of humoral autoimmunity. Although the etiology of this multifaceted inflammatory disease process is currently unknown, most authorities believe that it will ultimately be proven to result from a genetically predisposed state of autoimmunity that can be exacerbated by both environmental insults and endocrine abnormalities[51] (Fig. 19-5).

The focus of this discussion will be on the cutaneous manifestations of this disorder. For a more in-depth overview of LE in general, the reader is referred to several comprehensive monographs,[52,53] several recent thorough reviews that focus on the cutaneous manifestations of this disorder,[54–56] and several discussions of the underlying humoral autoimmune response that is seen in this disease process.[57,58]

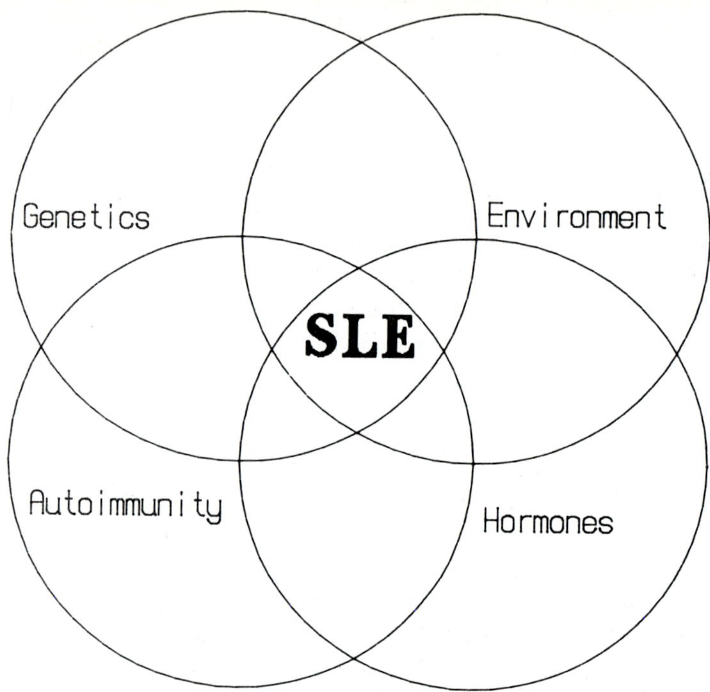

Figure 19-5 Etiological and pathogenetic factors in LE. Genetic factors such as certain HLA phenotypes, complement component deficiency states, and C3bi receptor deficiency predispose patients to develop polyclonal or oligoclonal B-cell autoimmune responses. The resulting state of humoral autoimmunity can then be exacerbated by environmental insults such as exposure to ultraviolet light, drugs, and infections, as well as disorders of estrogen metabolism.

Clinical and Laboratory Features

A convenient paradigm for conceptualizing this heterogeneous disorder is to visualize LE as a disease continuum or spectrum of clinical illness in which patients can present with variable patterns of organ involvement and in which variable degrees of involvement can develop within the same organ system. For example, some patients develop only one of several clinical types of LE skin disease, whereas others present with one of several varieties of glomerulonephritis. The potentially fatal outcome of this illness is primarily a function of the severity and degree of irreversibility of vital organ dysfunction (i.e., nephritis, vasculitis, central nervous system dysfunction) and the side effects of immunosuppressive medical intervention required to control the disease activity. Although most LE patients today do not die from their illness, many do suffer both emotional and occupational disability from chronic smoldering disease activity in the cutaneous and/or musculoskeletal systems.

Since some of these patterns of clinical illness occur in close association with certain autoantibody specificities, it has become fashionable to divide

Table 19-2

CLASSIFICATION OF LE-RELATED SKIN DISEASES

Specific
Acute cutaneous LE
SCLE
Annular
Papulosquamous (psoriasiform)
Chronic cutaneous LE
Classical DLE
Localized
Generalized
Hypertrophic (verrucous) LE
LE profundus (panniculitis)
Lupus tumidus
Palmar/plantar LE
Mucosal LE
Nonspecific
Leukocytoclastic vasculitis

the disease population into more limited groups of patients who share common clinical, pathological, and/or laboratory features. Several LE subgroups have somewhat predictable prognostic outcomes, thereby allowing the physician to tailor more rationally the medical management of this disorder. Moreover, certain LE subgroups are marked by the presence of clinically characteristic skin lesions. One classification of the many types of skin lesions that can occur in LE patients is shown in Table 19-2.[56,59]

The LE-related skin lesions can be subdivided into those that are and are not histopathologically specific for LE. LE-specific skin lesions are those, such as acute cutaneous LE, subacute cutaneous LE (SCLE), and chronic cutaneous LE, that contain the basic elements of the set of histopathological changes recognized as diagnostic of the LE process as it is expressed in the skin (Fig. 19-6). Other lesions, such as leukocytoclastic vasculitis, which also have characteristic but different histopathological features, can also be seen in LE patients and are in other ways related to the underlying autoimmune abnormalities. Such lesions, however, can be seen in a number of other disease states and thus are not specific for LE.

Acute cutaneous LE (i.e., malar or generalized photosensitive erythema reactions) is seen almost exclusively in patients with active SLE who are at risk for life-threatening complications such as diffuse proliferative glomerulonephritis. Patients who present with the most common form of chronic cutaneous LE, classical DLE, and those who express predominantly SCLE lesions represent two of the more homogeneous cutaneous LE subsets. Classical DLE is characterized by chronic, circumscribed, coin-shaped (discoid) lesions having adherent hyperkeratosis, follicular plug-

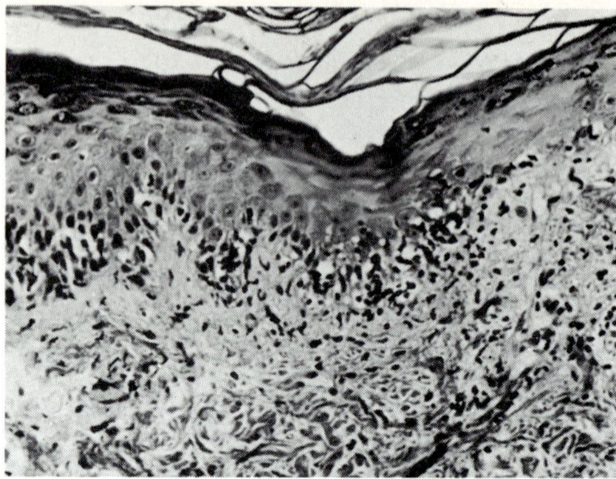

Figure 19-6 Histopathological manifestations of LE-specific skin disease. A mononuclear cell infiltration containing numerous melanophages and activated T cells is present at the dermal-epidermal interface, as well as around blood vessels and cutaneous appendages. The epidermal basal cell layer, in a state of disarray, is undergoing a vacuolar or liquefactive pattern of degeneration. In addition, there is hyperkeratosis and basement membrane thickening (basal lamina reduplication). (*Photomicrograph by Wallace H. Clark, Jr., M.D.*)

ging, peripheral hyperpigmentation, central depigmentation, and telangiectasia. As these lesions progress, central atrophic scarring characteristically develops. A patient is said to have localized DLE when he or she has lesions on the head and neck only. The scalp, ears, and central face are most frequently involved. Patients who present with localized DLE and show no involvement for the first 2 years of the disease course have no more than a 5 to 10 percent risk of developing severe manifestations of SLE later in their illness. The term generalized DLE indicates that the patient has more widespread lesions, particularly on the upper back and shoulders, v-area of the upper chest and neck, and extensor surfaces of the upper extremities. Patients with generalized DLE have a somewhat higher risk of developing SLE. Otherwise typical DLE lesions can be seen in as many as 20 to 30 percent of SLE patients at some point in their disease course as well. There are several other less common forms of chronic cutaneous LE (e.g., verrucous or hypertrophic LE, lupus tumidus, palmar/plantar LE) that do not appear to be clinically significant with respect to a linkage with an increased risk of associated underlying systemic disease. Mucous membrane LE (conjunctivae, nasal mucosa, and oral mucosa) and LE profundus (panniculitis) are clinical variants that are associated with a higher risk (50 percent) of SLE. Evidence of humoral autoimmunity (antinuclear and anti-double-stranded DNA antibodies, antibodies to precipitating ribonucleoproteins such as Ro/SS-A [Ro], La/SS-B, U1RNP, and Sm) is usually negative in localized DLE patients even though such patients may have some of the same circulating B- and T-cell abnormalities present in SLE patients.[60] It has been suggested that SLE patients who develop DLE lesions have a somewhat better prognosis than those who do not. It cannot be denied, however, that some patients who suffer fatal outcomes from SLE have been found to have otherwise typical DLE lesions at the time of their death.

SCLE is a more widespread and confluent form of photosensitive cutaneous LE that characteristically does not produce atrophic scarring.[61] This variety of LE-specific skin disease occurs predominantly in two clinical forms—annular/polycyclic and papulosquamous/psoriasiform. The lesions of SCLE also lack the adherent hyperkeratosis and follicular plugging that are characteristic of classical DLE. Although approximately 50 percent of SCLE patients have four or more of the American Rheumatism Association's criteria for the classification of SLE, most often these are the less serious expressions of the systemic illness such as serological abnormalities and musculoskeletal complaints. Vital internal organ dysfunction such as renal and central nervous system disease occurs in only 10 percent of patients. Circulating antinuclear antibodies detectable on human antinuclear antibody substrates and precipitating anti-Ro autoantibodies are seen in 70 to 80 percent of SCLE patients. Precipitating anti-La/SS-B antibodies also occur, but at a lower frequency. SCLE patients also have a characteristic HLA haplotype (HLA-B8, DR3, DQ1-2, DRW52). This is the same HLA association seen in Sjögren's syndrome, and recent studies have documented that some patients have overlapping features of SCLE and Sjögren's syndrome.[62]

The reader is referred to Refs. 54, 56, 61, 63, and 64 for a more detailed discussion of the clinical, pathological, and laboratory correlations of acute cutaneous LE, SCLE, and chronic cutaneous LE.

Histopathology and Immunopathology

The histopathological manifestations of LE-specific skin disease (Fig. 19-6) can best be summarized as representing a cell-poor lichenoid tissue reaction.[65,66] Differences do exist between the pathological changes seen in different clinical forms of LE-specific skin lesions.[67] Classical DLE lesions have more prominent hyperkeratosis, basement membrane thickening, and perifollicular and perivascular dermal inflammation compared to SCLE lesions, which have comparatively more prominent epidermal atrophy. These pathological differences do correlate with a disparity in the clinical appearance of the lesions. The keratin-plugged follicles and prominent dermal/subcutaneous atrophy that are characteristic of classical DLE do not occur in SCLE lesions.

A granular, continuous, band-like array of immunoglobulin and complement (including components of the membrane attack complex[56-59]) can be seen on direct immunofluorescence examination of both lesional and nonlesional skin in LE patients[56] (Fig. 19-7). These immunoreactants, the specificities of which have never been clearly identified, have been noted by immunoelectron-microscopic studies to be deposited on the subbasal lamina connective tissue and the reduplicated basal lamina material that comprises the thickened basement membrane seen on routine histopath-

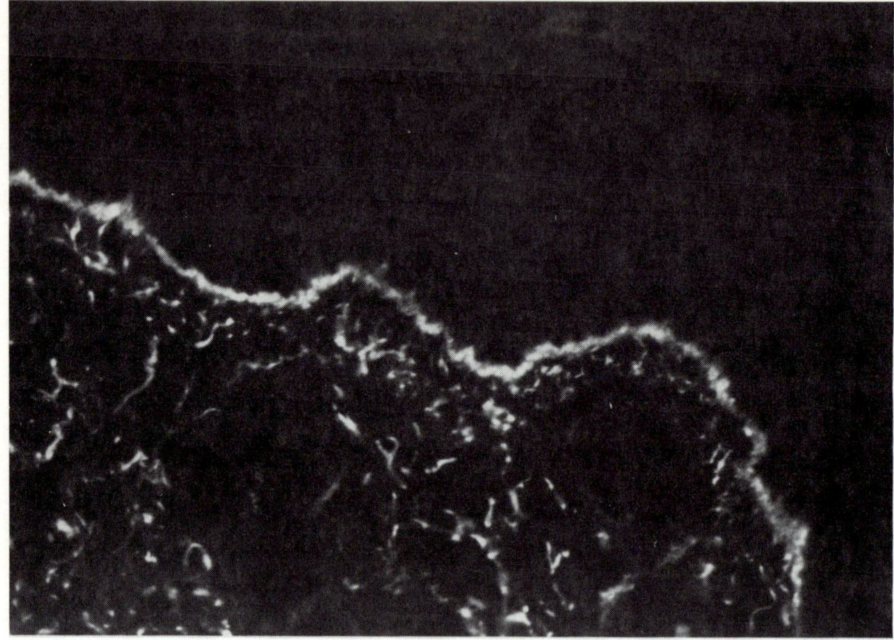

Figure 19-7 Immunopathology of cutaneous LE. Direct immunofluorescence examination of a nonlesional skin biopsy specimen from a patient with SLE reveals a continuous granular band of IgG at the dermal-epidermal junction.

ological examination. This phenomenon, which is commonly referred to as the lupus band, is more frequently seen in lesional skin, particularly DLE lesions on the head and upper trunk (80 to 90 percent). This finding is less common in SCLE lesions (50 to 60 percent). The presence of a lupus band in nonlesional skin has been referred to as a positive lupus band test. The presence of three or more individual immunoglobulin classes or complement components at the dermal-epidermal junction of nonlesional skin is highly specific for SLE.[68] Sun-exposed skin regions have a higher frequency of lupus band test positivity than do sun-protected sites. A positive lupus band test in skin regions that have not been actinically damaged has prognostic significance with respect to the risk for LE nephritis,[69] however; this finding appears to have relatively little incremental value over the presence of circulating anti-double-stranded DNA antibodies and hypocomplementemia. Recent studies have suggested that a more specific pattern of "dust-like" IgG epidermal deposition focused at the basal cell layer can be seen in SCLE lesions. Some observers have found this pattern of IgG deposition to be directly related to the presence of circulating anti-Ro autoantibodies,[70] although others have not noted a statistically significant association with this autoantibody specificity.[71]

Immunological Abnormalities and Pathogenesis

It is logical to attempt to relate the humoral immune findings present at the dermal-epidermal junction to the pathogenesis of cutaneous LE. The argument between those who believe that these immune deposits represent preformed circulating immune complexes that become bound to the dermal-epidermal junction and others who think that they result from free antibodies that bind to autoantigens normally found at the dermal-epidermal junction has never been fully resolved. Elution studies of lupus band immunoreactants in SLE patient skin have suggested that they do contain antinuclear and antibasement membrane zone antibody activity.[72] In addition, idiotypes that are commonly shared by antibodies to native DNA have been shown to be present in lupus band immunoglobulin deposits.[73] More recent studies have suggested that antibodies to type VII procollagen (a component of the basal lamina–anchoring fibril complex) that are characteristic of EB acquisita can be seen in the occasional SLE patient who develops dermatitis herpetiformis–like manifestations of vesiculobullous cutaneous LE.[74] Some workers have argued that these dermal-epidermal junction immunoreactants result from the binding of free autoantibodies to epidermal cell-derived nuclear antigens such as double-stranded[75] or ultraviolet-altered DNA[76] that have a special binding affinity for the dermal-epidermal junction. In addition, there is the suggestion that the epidermal basement membrane zone normally contains a binding receptor for the third component of complement that might serve to localize complement-fixing immune complexes to this site.[77]

Several lines of investigation, however, argue that dermal-epidermal junction immunoreactants may not be primarily involved in the pathogenesis of LE-specific skin inflammation. Some work has suggested that cationized antibodies or immune complexes of any specificity could become nonspecifically bound to the dermal-epidermal junction through charge-charge interactions[78] with the anionic binding sites that are normally present within the dermal-epidermal junction.[79] Studies have failed to identify circulating antibodies in the large majority of both cutaneous and SLE patients that bind specifically to the constituents of normal human skin. In addition, dermal-epidermal junction immunoglobulin deposition has been observed to follow by as much as 6 weeks the first appearance of inflammatory changes in ultraviolet light–challenged nonlesional skin of DLE patients.[80] Thus, it is possible that the lupus band immunoreactants may represent only an epiphenomenon.

A great deal of circumstantial evidence (Table 19-3) points to the possibility that autoantibodies to constituents of the saline-extractable Ro ribonucleoprotein particle might play a direct pathogenetic role in the pattern of cutaneous inflammation seen in SCLE and neonatal LE skin lesions.[55,56,81] This hypothesis suggests that Ro antigen can be aberrantly induced on the surface of viable epidermal keratinocytes by the action of

Table 19-3

EVIDENCE FAVORING AND OPPOSING A DIRECT ROLE FOR ANTI-RO AUTOANTIBODIES IN THE PATHOGENESIS OF SCLE AND NEONATAL LE*

Favoring

1. Circulating anti-Ro antibodies are seen in 70–80% of SCLE and virtually 100% of neonatal LE patients.
2. Ro antigen is expressed in human adult, neonatal, and fetal cutaneous and cardiac tissue.
3. In neonatal LE patients, the duration of cutaneous inflammation closely parallels the presence of placentally transferred maternal IgG anti-Ro in the newborn's circulation.
4. When human Ro antibodies are infused into nude mice bearing explants of normal human skin, preferential binding of the human anti-Ro to the human epidermal cells has been observed and UVB light exposure appears to potentiate this pattern of anti-Ro antibody binding.
5. UVB light and estrogen pretreatment, which are relevant to the clinical manifestations of LE, have been shown to perturb the intracellular distribution of Ro antigen in human keratinocytes, inducing translocation of this antigen to the cell surface, where it may be bound by anti-Ro antibodies present in the interstitial fluid.
6. Anti-Ro immunoblobulins are of a type (predominantly IgG1) that are capable of triggering ADCC in vitro.
7. The lichenoid pattern of tissue injury seen in SCLE and neonatal LE skin lesions is also compatible with an in vivo ADCC reaction.

Opposing

1. Studies have failed to demonstrate a positive correlation between circulating anti-Ro antibody levels and SCLE skin disease activity.
2. Patients with primary Sjögren's syndrome have serum levels of anti-Ro antibody that are equal to those of SCLE patients but infrequently develop photosensitive cutaneous LE lesions.
3. Only a very small percentage of infants who are exposed to Ro antibody from their mothers' circulation during fetal development develop neonatal LE or congenital heart block.
4. Although the anti-Ro antibody that is passively infused into nude mice bearing grafts of normal human skin does bind preferentially to the human epidermal cells, no pathological injury can be detected as a result of this binding.
5. Although human IgG can be demonstrated in the cutaneous and cardiac tissues of newborn guinea pigs whose mothers have been injected with anti-Ro-containing serum, neither skin nor heart pathology has been found.

* Primary data cited in Refs. 55, 56, and 81.

ultraviolet B (UVB) light or estrogen exposure. Ro antibody bound to this surface Ro antigen could then target this cell type for destruction by the mononuclear lymphoid cells present in the inflammatory infiltrate through effector mechanisms such as antibody-dependent, cell-mediated cytotoxicity (ADCC). The results of other studies, however, are not consistent with this hypothesis (Table 19-3).

There is increasing evidence to suggest that antigen-specific T cells may be involved in the production of autoantibodies to self antigens such as Ro and La/SS-B.[82,83] This raises the interesting possibility that Ro-specific T cells may exist in SCLE patients and participate directly in the cutaneous injury pattern seen in these patients, a possibility supported by the predominance of activated T lymphocytes and macrophages in the cellular infiltrate of LE-specific skin lesion. The recent cloning of several genes that encode human Ro proteins will make it possible to synthesize large amounts of pure, nontoxic peptide antigen. This material, coupled with our current capability to expand T cells clonally from cutaneous tissue and peripheral blood, should soon make it possible to identify such Ro antigen–specific T cells in the skin lesions and circulation of SCLE patients if in fact they do exist.

The idea that cutaneous autoantigen-specific T cells may participate in the pathogenesis of LE-specific skin disease is also supported by several other lines of evidence. Whereas the mononuclear cell infiltrate seen in the pathology of SCLE and neonatal LE lesions is consistent with an ADCC immune effector mechanism, the experimental models that most closely reproduce the lichenoid histopathology of LE-specific skin disease are systems in which activated T cells are reacting to class I or II histocompatibility antigens in the skin, such as graft-versus-host skin disease[84] and experimental murine lichen planus.[85] Abnormalities in the number and distribution of epidermal Langerhans cells have also been demonstrated in cutaneous LE lesions.[86] In addition, HLA-DR antigen expression has been detected on the surface of epidermal keratinocytes in LE skin lesions. This phenomenon can be reproduced in vitro by treating cultured normal human keratinocytes with T-cell-derived cytokines such as γ interferon. Cytokine-induced expression of lymphoid cell adhesion molecules such as intercellular adhesion molecule-1 (ICAM-1) on epidermal keratinocytes could also exacerbate the process of keratinocyte destruction by facilitating the binding of aggressor lymphocytes to this cell type. In addition, proinflammatory cytokines such as IL-1 and IL-6 that might be secreted by keratinocytes as a result of ultraviolet light exposure could also enhance the inflammatory milieu in such lesions.

Any hypothesis put forward to explain the pathogenetic mechanism(s) of LE-specific skin disease must also be able to account for certain clinical observations related to the induction of exacerbation of LE skin lesions. In addition to ultraviolet light exposure (both UVB and UVA), physical trauma of any kind to nonlesional LE skin can trigger LE-specific cutaneous inflammation (the Koebner or isomorphic response). In addition, extreme emotional stress has also been observed to cause certain forms of cutaneous LE, such as SCLE, to flare.

ACKNOWLEDGMENTS

Supported in part by grants (AR19101, AR36629, N01 AR62271) from the National Institutes of Health and the Medical Research Service of the Veterans Administration.

REFERENCES

1. Vracko R: Basal lamina scaffold: anatomy and significance for maintenance of orderly tissue structure. *Am J Pathol* 77:314, 1974.
2. Briggaman RA: The epidermal-dermal junction and genetic disorders of this area, in LA Goldsmith (ed), *Biochemistry and Physiology of the Skin.* New York, Oxford University Press, 1983, p 1001.
3. Hay EB: Cell–matrix interaction in the embryo: cell shape, cell surface, cell skeletons, and their role in differentiation, in RC Trelstad (ed), *The Role of the Extracellular Matrix in Development.* New York, Alan R. Liss, 1984, p 1.
4. Katz SI: The epidermal basement membrane zone—structure, ontogeny, and role in disease. *J Am Acad Dermatol* 11:1025, 1984.
5. Fine JD: The skin basement membrane zone, in *Advances in Dermatology,* Chicago, Year Book Medical, 1986, vol 2, p 283.
6. Eady RAJ: The basement membrane: interface between the epithelium and the dermis: structural features. *Arch Dermatol* 124:709, 1988.
7. Spiers EM, Fine JD: Immunopathogenesis of bullous diseases, in DJ Demis (chief ed), *Clinical Dermatology.* Philadelphia, Harper & Row, 1987, Unit 6-1, p 1.
8. Holbrook KA: Structure and function of the developing human skin, in LA Goldsmith (ed), *Biochemistry and Physiology of the Skin.* New York, Oxford University Press, 1983, p 64.
9. Fine JD: Antigenic features and structural correlates of basement membranes: relationship to epidermolysis bullosa. *Arch Dermatol* 124:713, 1988.
10. Keene DR et al: Type VII collagen forms an extended network of anchoring fibrils. *J Cell Biol* 104:611, 1987.
11. Fine JD et al: The appearance of four basement membrane zone antigens in developing human fetal skin. *J Invest Dermatol* 83:66, 1984.
12. Fine JD: Altered skin basement membrane antigenicity in epidermolysis bullosa, in KD Wuepper and T Gedde-Dahl Jr (eds), *Biology of Heritable Skin Diseases.* Basel, Karger, 1987, p 111.
13. Eady RAJ et al: Approaches to the study of epidermolysis bullosa, in KD Wuepper and T Gedde-Dahl Jr (eds), *Biology of Heritable Skin Diseases.* Basel, Karger, 1987, p 127.
14. Fine JD: Pathology and pathogenesis of epidermolysis bullosa, in DM Carter and AN Lin (eds), *Epidermolysis Bullosa, Basic and Clinical Aspects.* Springer-Verlag, in press.
15. Timpl R et al: Laminin: a glycoprotein from basement membranes. *J Biol Chem* 254:9933, 1979.
16. Horiguchi Y et al: Epitope mapping of the laminin molecule in murine skin basement membrane zone: demonstration of differences in ultrastructural localization. *J Invest Dermatol* 92:447A, 1989.
17. Miller EJ, Gay S: The multiple types and forms of collagen. *Methods Enzymol* 82A:3, 1982.
18. Yaoita H et al: Localization of the collagenous component in skin basement membrane. *J Invest Dermatol* 70:191, 1978.
19. Sakai LY et al: Type VII collagen is a major structural component of anchoring fibrils. *J Cell Biol* 103:1577, 1986.
20. Westgate GE et al: Bullous pemphigoid antigen localization suggests an intracellular association with hemidesmosomes. *J Invest Dermatol* 86:218, 1985.

21. Horiguchi Y et al: Organ specificity, ontogeny, and ultrastructural localization of the core protein of heparan sulfate proteoglycan, a new component of human skin basement membrane zone. *J Histochem Cytochem* 37:961, 1989.
22. Caughman SW et al: Nidogen and heparan sulfate proteoglycan: detection of newly isolated basement membrane components in normal and epidermolysis bullosa skin. *J Invest Dermatol* 89:547, 1987.
23. Fine JD, Couchman JR: Chondroitin-6-sulfate-containing proteoglycan: a new component of human skin dermoepidermal junction. *J Invest Dermatol* 90:283, 1988.
24. Carlin B et al: Entactin, a novel basal lamina-associated sulfated glycoprotein. *J Biol Chem* 256:5209, 1979.
25. Verrando P et al: The new basement membrane antigen recognized by the monoclonal antibody GB3 is a large size glycoprotein: modulation of its expression by retinoic acid. *Biochim Biophys Acta* 942:45, 1988.
26. Fine JD et al: Detection and partial characterization of a mid-lamina lucida-hemidesmosome–associated antigen (19-DEJ-1) present within human skin. *J Invest Dermatol* 92:825, 1989.
27. Fine JD, Couchman JR: Chondroitin 6-sulfate proteoglycan but not heparan sulfate proteoglycan is abnormally expressed in skin basement membrane from patients with dominant and recessive dystrophic epidermolysis bullosa. *J Invest Dermatol* 92:611, 1989.
28. Fine JD et al: 19-DEJ-1, a hemidesmosome-anchoring filament complex–associated monoclonal antibody: definition of a new skin basement membrane antigenic defect in junctional and dystrophic epidermolysis bullosa. *Arch Dermatol* 125:520, 1989.
29. Rusenko KW et al: The carboxyl-terminal domain of type VII collagen is present at the basement membrane in recessive dystrophic epidermolysis bullosa. *J Invest Dermatol* 92:623, 1989.
30. Lever WF: Pemphigus and pemphigoid. *J Am Acad Dermatol* 1:2, 1979.
31. Jordon RE: Bullous pemphigoid, cicatricial pemphigoid, and chronic bullous dermatosis of childhood, in TB Fitzpatrick et al (eds), *Dermatology in General Medicine*, 3d ed. New York, McGraw-Hill, 1987, p 580.
32. Wintroub BU et al: Morphologic and functional evidence for release of mast-cell products in bullous pemphigoid. *N Engl J Med* 298:417, 1978.
33. Gammon WR, Briggaman RA: Absense of specific histologic changes in guinea pig skin treated with bullous pemphigoid antibodies. *J Invest Dermatol* 90:495, 1988.
34. Anhalt GJ et al: Pathogenic effects of bullous pemphigoid autoantibodies on rabbit corneal epithelium. *J Clin Invest* 68:1097, 1981.
35. Gammon WR et al: An in vitro model of immune complex–mediated basement membrane zone separation caused by pemphigoid antibodies, leukocytes, and complement. *J Invest Dermatol* 78:285, 1982.
36. Stanley JR et al: Characterization of bullous pemphigoid antigen: a unique basement membrane protein of stratified squamous epithelia. *Cell* 24:897, 1981.
37. Stanley JR et al: Identification and partial characterization of pemphigoid antigen extracted from normal human skin. *J Invest Dermatol* 82:108, 1984.
38. Mueller S et al: A 230-kd basic protein is the major bullous pemphigoid antigen. *J Invest Dermatol* 92:33, 1989.
39. Stanley JR et al: Isolation of complementary DNA for bullous pemphigoid antigen by use of patients' autoantibodies. *J Clin Invest* 82:1864, 1988.
40. Sams WM Jr, Gammon WR: Mechanism of lesion production in pemphigus and pemphigoid. *J Am Acad Dermatol* 6:431, 1982.
41. Stanley JR: Pemphigus and pemphigoid as paradigms of organ-specific, autoantibody-mediated diseases. *J Clin Invest* 83:1443, 1989.
42. Briggaman RA et al: Epidermolysis bullosa acquisita of the immunopathological type (dermolytic pemphigoid). *J Invest Dermatol* 85:79s, 1985.
43. Gammon WR et al: Epidermolysis bullosa acquisita—a pemphigoid-like disease. *J Am Acad Dermatol* 11:820, 1984.
44. Gammon WR et al: Increased frequency of HLA-DR2 in patients with autoantibodies to

epidermolysis bullosa acquisita antigen: evidence that expression of autoimmunity to type VII collagen is HLA class II allele associated. *J Invest Dermatol* 91:228, 1988.
45. Fine JD et al: The presence of intra-lamina lucida blister formation in epidermolysis bullosa acquisita: possible role of leukocytes. *J Invest Dermatol* 92:27, 1989.
46. Gammon WR et al: Differentiating anti-lamina lucida and anti-sublamina densa anti-BMZ antibodies by indirect immunofluorescence on 1.0 *M* sodium chloride–separated skin. *J Invest Dermatol* 82:139, 1984.
47. Gammon WR et al: Differences in complement-dependent chemotactic activity generated by bullous pemphigoid and epidermolysis bullosa acquisita immune complexes: demonstration by leukocytic attachment and organ culture methods. *J Invest Dermatol* 83:57, 1984.
48. Gammon WR et al: Recombinant human cytokines mediate FcRlll-dependent neutrophil adherence to autoantibody-treated epithelial basement membranes. *J Invest Dermatol* 92:432, 1989.
49. Woodley DT et al: Identification of the skin basement-membrane autoantigen in epidermolysis bullosa acquisita. *N Engl J Med* 310:1007, 1984.
50. Woodley DT et al: The epidermolysis bullosa acquisita antigen is type VII procollagen. *J Invest Dermatol* 88:525, 1987.
51. Talal N: The etiology of systemic lupus erythematosus, in DJ Wallace, EL Dubois (eds), *Dubois' Lupus Erythematosus,* 3d ed. Philadelphia, Lea & Febiger, 1987, p 39.
52. Lahita RG (ed): *Systemic Lupus Erythematosus.* New York, Wiley, 1987.
53. Wallace DJ, Dubois EL (eds): *Dubois' Lupus Erythematosus,* 3d ed. Philadelphia, Lea & Febiger, 1987.
54. Gilliam JN: Systemic lupus erythematosus and the skin, in RG Lahita (ed), *Systemic Lupus Erythematosus.* New York, Wiley, 1987, p 615.
55. Lee LA, Norris DA: Mechanisms of cutaneous tissue damage in lupus erythematosus, in DA Norris (ed), *Immune Mechanisms in Cutaneous Disease.* New York, Marcel Dekker, 1989, p 359.
56. Sontheimer RD, Provost TT: Lupus erythematosus, in RE Jordon (ed), *Immunologic Diseases of the Skin.* Norwalk, CT, Appleton-Century-Crofts, in press.
57. Provost TT, Watson R: Antinuclear antibodies in systemic lupus erythematosus, in DA Norris (ed), *Immune Mechanisms in Cutaneous Disease.* New York, Marcel Dekker, 1989, p 333.
58. Tan EM: Antinuclear antibodies: diagnostic markers for autoimmune diseases and probes for cell biology. *Adv Immunol* 44:93, 1989.
59. Gilliam JN, Sontheimer RD: Distinctive cutaneous subsets in the spectrum of lupus erythematosus. *J Am Acad Dermatol* 4:471, 1981.
60. Kind P et al: Circulating T and B cell abnormalities in cutaneous lupus erythematosus. *J Invest Dermatol* 86:235, 1986.
61. Sontheimer RD: Subacute cutaneous lupus erythematosus: a decade's perspective. *Med Clin North Am* 73:1073, 1989.
62. Provost TT et al: Ro (SS-A) positive Sjögrens/lupus erythematosus overlap patients are associated with the HLA-DR3 and/or DRW6 phenotypes. *J Invest Dermatol* 91:369, 1988.
63. Prystowsky SD et al: Chronic cutaneous lupus erythematosus (DLE): a clinical and laboratory investigation of 80 patients. *Medicine* 55:183, 1975.
64. Callen JP: Chronic cutaneous lupus erythematosus. *Arch Dermatol* 118:412, 1982.
65. Romero RW et al: Unusual variant of lupus erythematosus or lichen planus. *Arch Dermatol* 113:741, 1977.
66. Pinkus H: Lichenoid tissue reactions. *Arch Dermatol* 107:840, 1973.
67. Bangert J et al: Subacute cutaneous lupus erythematosus and discoid lupus erythematosus: comparative histopathologic findings. *Arch Dermatol* 120:332, 1984.
68. Smith CD et al: The clinical utility of the lupus band test. *Arthritis Rheum* 27:382, 1984.
69. Davis BM, Gilliam JN: Prognostic significance of subepidermal immune deposits in uninvolved skin of patients with systemic lupus erythematosus: a ten year longitudinal study. *J Invest Dermatol* 83:242, 1984.

70. Lee LA et al: Pattern of cutaneous immunoglobulin G deposition in subacute cutaneous lupus erythematosus is reproduced by infusing purified anti-Ro/SS-A autoantibody autoantibodies into human skin-grafted mice. *J Clin Invest* 83:1556, 1989.
71. Nieboer C et al: Dust-like particles: a specific direct immunofluorescence pattern in subacute cutaneous lupus erythematosus. *Br J Dermatol* 118:725, 1988.
72. Landry M, Sams WM: Systemic lupus erythematosus: studies of the antibodies bound to skin. *J Clin Invest* 52:1871, 1973.
73. Isenberg D et al: Detection of cross-reactive anti-DNA antibody idiotypes on tissue-bound immunoglobulins from skin biopsies of lupus erythematosus. *J Immunol* 135:261, 1985.
74. Gammon R et al: Evidence that anti-basement membrane zone antibodies in bullous eruption of systemic lupus erythematosus recognize epidermolysis bullosa acquisita autoantigen. *J Invest Dermatol* 84:472, 1985.
75. Gilliam JN: The significance of cutaneous immunoglobulin deposits in lupus erythematosus and New Zealand mice. *J Invest Dermatol* 65:154, 1975.
76. Natali PG, Tan EM: Experimental skin lesions in mice resembling systemic lupus erythematosus. *Arthritis Rheum* 16:579, 1973.
77. Basset-Seguin N et al: C3d,g is present in normal human epidermal basement membrane. *J Immunol* 141:1273, 1988.
78. Joselow SA, Mannik M: Localization of preformed, circulating immune complexes in murine skin. *J Invest Dermatol* 82:335, 1984.
79. Manabe M, Ogawa H: Ultrastructural demonstration of anionic sites in basement membrane zone by cationic probes. *J Invest Dermatol* 84:19, 1985.
80. Cripps DJ, Rankin J: Action spectra of lupus erythematosus and experimental immunofluorescence. *Arch Dermatol* 107:563, 1973.
81. Sontheimer RD, McCauliffe DP: Pathogenesis of anti-Ro/SS-A associated cutaneous lupus erythematosus. *Dermatol Clin,* in press.
82. Craft JE, Hardin JA: Linked sets of antinuclear antibodies: what do they mean? *J Rheumatol* 14(Suppl 13):106, 1987.
83. Pham BN et al: T lymphocyte activation in systemic lupus erythematosus analyzed by proliferative response to nucleoplasmic proteins on nitrocellulose immunoblots. *Clin Exp Immunol* 77:168, 1989.
84. Charley MR et al: Murine graft-versus-host skin disease: a chronologic and quantitative analysis of two histologic patterns. *J Invest Dermatol* 81:412, 1983.
85. Shiohara T et al: Lichenoid tissue reaction induced by local transfer of Ia-reactive T-cell clones. *J Invest Dermatol* 87:33, 1986.
86. Sontheimer RD, Bergstresser JN: Epidermal Langerhans cell involvement in cutaneous lupus erythematosus. *J Invest Dermatol* 79:237, 1982.

SECTION SEVEN

DISORDERS OF THE DERMIS

20

Biology of the Dermis and Pathophysiology of Urticaria/Angioedema and Cutaneous Necrotizing Venulitis

Nicholas A. Soter

BIOLOGY OF THE DERMIS

The dermis is composed of connective tissue containing fibrous proteins—collagen, elastin, and reticulin—and ground substance. It also contains cells, the pilosebaceous unit, eccrine sweat glands, blood vessels, lymphatics, and nerves. The dermis, which is 1 to 4 mm in thickness (Fig. 20-1), comprises up to 20 percent of body weight. Most of the fibrous protein of the dermis is collagen, which has a high tensile strength. A major function of the dermis is to provide protection from mechanical injury. Its connective tissue layers are oriented in such a manner that it becomes a tissue capable of extension and relaxation according to body movement. Furthermore, the dermis binds water and serves as a reservoir for body water and electrolytes. Because it contains a complex, rich vascular network, it has a major role in thermoregulation. Its network of nerves provides the sensory contact of the body with the environment.

The dermis maintains an interaction with the epidermis during embryogenesis, morphogenesis, and wound repair by inductive interactions between the dermis and epidermis. It has been proposed that dermal inductive agents may act selectively on a series of epithelial genes and may direct the type of differentiation—for example, the thick epidermis of the palms and soles or the thin epidermis of the flexural skin.[1]

There are two major divisions of the dermis: the superficial portion, or

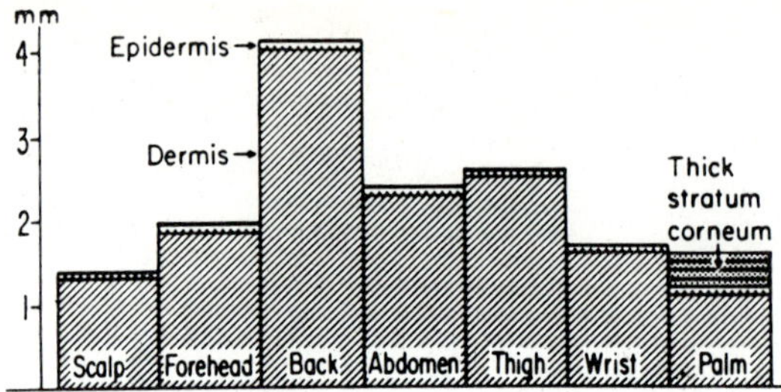

Figure 20-1 Diagrammatic representation of regional variations in thickness of skin. (*From TB Fitzpatrick et al, Dermatology in General Medicine, New York, McGraw-Hill, 1971, p 40.*)

papillary dermis, and the deeper portion, or reticular dermis (Fig. 20-2). In the papillary layer, thin collagen fibers form a loose three-dimensional network. The reticular dermis contains denser and thicker collagen fibers. These fibrous proteins are embedded in ground substance (proteoglycans), and together they make up the matrix of the dermis.

Cutaneous Microvasculature

The function of the vascular system in the dermis is predominantly temperature regulation, although it also supplies the nutrient and metabolic needs of the dermis and the epidermis. It also serves to store blood in the skin, which can be directed to the other parts of the body.

Skin blood vessels arise from undifferentiated mesodermal cells that organize into strands and form endothelial tubes. Postnatal skin is pervaded by a continuous three-dimensional network of blood vessels composed of plexuses oriented parallel to the skin surface at different levels and linked by vertically oriented communicating vessels. There is an upper plexus in the papillary dermis and a lower plexus at the junction of the dermis and subcutaneous tissue (Fig. 20-3). The bulk of the microcirculation resides in the papillary dermis below the epidermal surface.[2–5] No vessels pass the dermal-epidermal junction. The diameters of most of the blood vessels in the papillary dermis vary from 17 to 22 μm; the diameters of the deepest dermal vessels in general are 40 to 50 μm.[5]

The outside diameter of the arteriole becomes 10 to 12 μm at the beginning of the capillary bed. The external elastin layer disappears, and the basement membrane retains its homogeneous appearance. Smooth muscle cells are replaced by pericytes. These vessels are classified as arterial capillaries, and their walls vary from 2 to 3 μm in thickness. The venous capillary, which has a multilaminated vascular wall, is located between the arterial capillaries and connects with the postcapillary venule, a vessel whose external diameter increases to 35 μm. The capillary loops are perpendicular to the surface of the skin, and each dermal papilla is supplied by one capillary loop. The majority of the papillary dermal vessels are postcapillary venules.

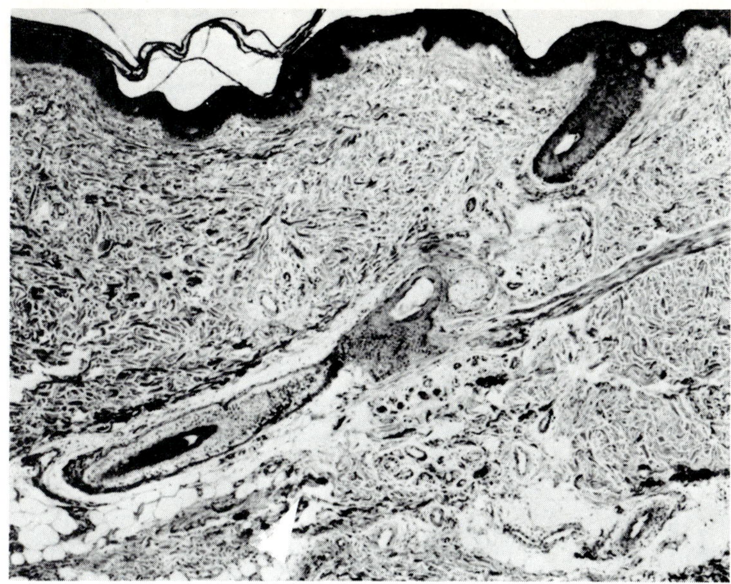

Figure 20-2 The epidermis crosses the upper portion of the micrograph. The narrow zone of dermis immediately deep to the epidermis is the papillary dermis, while most of the micrograph shows the collagen bundles of the reticular dermis. A hair with associated arrector pili muscle is present. ×40 in the original magnification. (*Micrograph by Wallace H. Clark, Jr., M.D.*)

Most of the arterioles and venules in the lower plexus are 50 μm in diameter, with layers of smooth muscle cells or pericytes in their walls. In deep dermal arterioles, collagen fibrils are embedded in the homogeneous-appearing basement membrane of the vascular wall. In the deep dermal venules, the collagen fibrils are distributed throughout the vascular wall, and the basement membrane has a laminated appearance. The arterioles and venules in the fat lobules are identical in structure and size to those of the lower horizontal plexus.

There are multiple microcirculatory units arising from the interconnecting networks of arterioles and venules that supply the glands and appendages. In various parts of the skin, differences in form, number, and distribution of blood vessels exist; for example, the microcirculation of the scalp and palms differs from that of the forearms. In addition, multiple arteriovenous anastomoses provide a direct bypass of the normal arterial-capillary-venous circuit and thus allow the blood to flow through preferential channels that shorten the distance between artery and vein. These arteriovenous anastomoses, which are particularly numerous in the digits, are composed of an ascending arteriole, the glomus (a vascular channel surrounded by smooth muscle cells), and collecting venules. They have a tendency to close if the blood pressure does not exceed a critical value. The opening

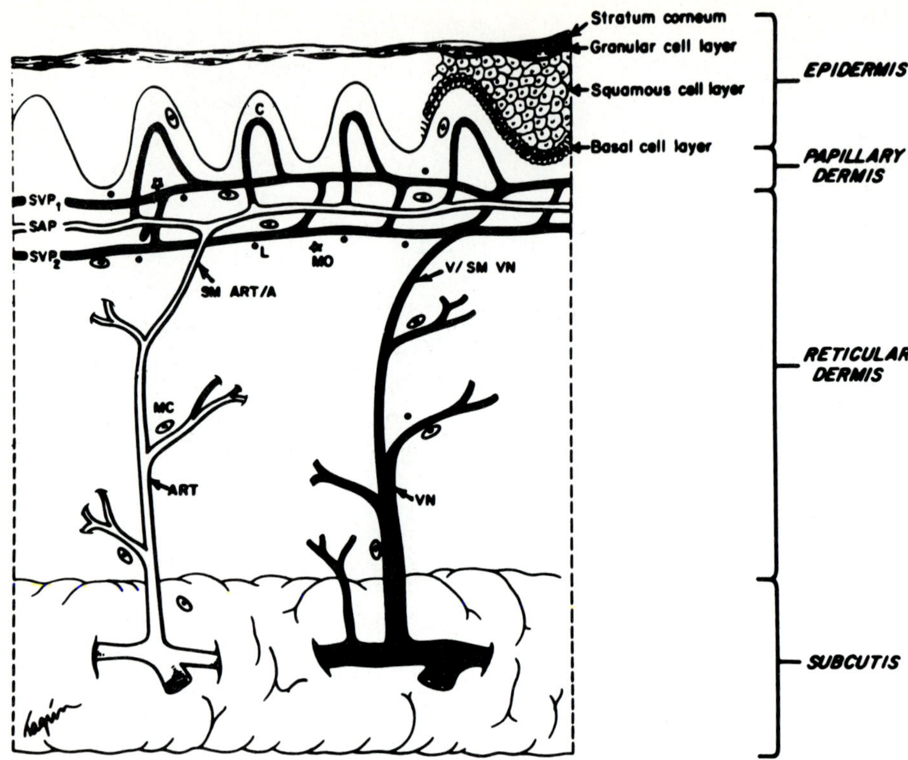

Figure 20-3 Schematic diagram of the cutaneous vasculature. L = lymphocyte; MO = monocyte-macrophage; MC = mast cell; C = capillary; SVP = superficial venular plexus; SAP = superficial arteriolar plexus; SM ART/A = small arteries and arterioles; ART = artery; V/SM VN = venules and small veins; VN = vein. (*Reprinted by permission of the publisher from NA Soter, MC Mihm Jr, Cutaneous necrotizing venulitis, in S Moschella, Dermatology Update: Reviews for Physicians, New York, Elsevier, 1979, p 434.*)

of these shunts excludes the capillary bed and permits the dermal vasculature to meet various thermal regulatory requirements.

The vasculature of the skin is developed beyond the degree necessary for the nutrition of this organ. The excess of blood vessels aids in temperature control and regulation of blood pressure. The amount of blood normally circulating through the digits is 20 to 30 times the minimum required for oxygenation of the tissue, and in vasodilation it may rise to over 100 times the minimum value.

Endothelial cells have been cultured from the microvessels of human neonatal foreskin.[6-8] These cultured cells contain Weibel-Palade bodies, a vascular endothelial cytoplasmic marker organelle, express factor VIII, generate prostaglandin E_2,[9] produce interleukin-1,[9] and do not respond to fibroblast growth factor.[6] In short-term organ cultures,[10] endothelium of postcapillary venules developed activation antigens after exposure to interleukin-1 and tumor necrosis factor.

Lymphatics

Lymphatic capillaries arise in the papillary dermis and form sinuses composed of a thin wall lined by a single layer of endothelial cells. The wall of the terminal lymphatic is a continuous type of endothelium surrounded by an indistinct and discontinuous basal lamina.[11] Lymphatic endothelium provides gaps consisting of endothelial junctions through which macromolecules can pass into its lumen. The endothelial basal lamina consists of a fine network of delicate filaments embedded in a homogeneous matrix. Identification of lymphatic endothelium using special stains shows elastic fibers and an absence of factor VIII–related antigen, which is present in blood vessels.[11] As they progress centripetally and drain into large trunks, their walls become thicker and valves develop. The large trunks of lymphatics in the subcutaneous tissue have thick walls containing muscles and valves to ensure one-way blow. Their principal role is to remove cells, water, proteins, and other macromolecules from the extracellular environment of the dermis.

Nerves

The skin is composed of a network of free and encapsulated nerve endings that convey impulses to the central nervous system. A series of mosaics of various sensitivities are spread on the skin surface. Some receptors are free nerve terminals that sense temperature (heat and cold); other free nerve terminals mediate pain and itch. Mechanoreceptors include specialized, encapsulated corpuscles (Meissner's and pacinian) and unencapsulated nerve terminals forming nets around hairs. The autonomic nerve supply of the skin appears to be entirely sympathetic. The autonomic terminals are adrenergic, cholinergic, and purinergic. Blood vessels of the arrectores pilorum muscles are supplied with cholinergic fibers, while sebaceous and apocrine glands have no detectable nerve supply.

There are no free nerve endings in the epidermis. In the superficial dermis, unmyelinated fibers predominate; the perineural sheath is lost, and the Schwann cell–axonal processes are in direct contact with collagen. The reticular dermis and subcutaneous tissue contain nerves within which there is a perineural sheath of endothelial-like cells and collagen that encloses a compartment occupied by myelinated and unmyelinated fibers and endoneural collagen.

Cells of the Dermis

The dermis contains mast cells, T lymphocytes, monocyte-macrophages, and fibroblasts. Neutrophils, eosinophils, and basophils are not present in normal skin.

Mast Cells

Mast cells are especially prominent in skin, with 12.1 ± 5.1 cells per square millimeter in a 1-μm section[12]; they vary in size and shape and often appear as elongated elements. Their cytoplasm contains spheroidal metachromatic granules that are surrounded by a membrane and contain scrolls, whorls, and crystalline lattices. In addition, human skin mast cells have the distinguishing features of villous extensions of the plasma membrane and prominent microfilaments.[13] Mast cells are not present in the epidermis. Upon activation of mast cells, exocytosis of granules occurs that involves fusion between the plasma membrane and the membranes of the granules, allowing the release of certain granule contents while the cell membrane and cytoplasm remain intact.[14]

Heterogeneous populations of mast cells exist in rodents and humans. In a still unknown way, the local tissue microenvironment determines the phenotype of the mast cell.[15,16] In rodents the more familiar type of mast cell is termed the *connective tissue mast cell;* a second type of mast cell found in the epithelial portions of the respiratory and gastrointestinal tracts is called the *mucosal mast cell.* In humans, two types of mast cells have been recognized based on their content of neutral proteases[17]; T mast cells contain tryptase, and TC mast cells contain tryptase and chymase. Human skin contains only TC mast cells.[18] The heterogeneity of human mast cells is further illustrated by the fact that cutaneous mast cells but not those from other sites release mediators in response to compound 48/80, morphine, and codeine.[19]

The tissue reactions occurring after immunologic mast cell activation are biphasic and consist of early and late phases.[20,21] Early reactions in the skin result from the release of mediators from cytoplasmic granules, the generation of mediators from membranes, and the responses of target cells. This response is recognized in the skin as a wheal and erythema reaction, with pruritus that develops within minutes. Late reactions involve the influx of inflammatory cells including various types of polymorphonuclear leukocytes and mononuclear cells. This response is recognized in skin as a deep, tender, red nodule that develops within 4 to 6 h.

Mast cells can be activated by both immunologic and nonimmunologic stimuli. Not all potential biologic products are released when the mast cell is stimulated. For example, substance P, derived from unmyelinated sensory nerve endings, will release histamine but will not generate prostaglandin D_2.[22] Human mast cells can release or generate substances with vasoactive and smooth muscle contracting abilities, chemotactic factors, enzymes, and proteoglycans (Table 20-1).

Skin mast cells release histamine at temperatures ranging from 29° to 37°C in breast tissue[23] and between 34° and 39°C in foreskin specimens.[24] The responsiveness at temperatures below 37°C in skin is noteworthy in view of the fact that peripheral skin temperatures are variable and remain uniform only over distances of millimeters[25].

T Lymphocytes

The skin contains T lymphocytes that occur predominantly around the dermal microvasculature.[26] These T cells are a mixture of $CD4^+$ (helper/

Table 20-1

HUMAN MAST CELL MEDIATORS

Mediator	Function
Vasoactive and Smooth Muscle Contracting Substances	
Histamine	H1: Increases venular permeability, contracts smooth muscle, enhances chemotaxis of neutrophils and eosinophils
	H2: Increases venular permeability, stimulates $CD8^+$ T lymphocytes, inhibits chemotaxis of neutrophils and eosinophils, augments gastric acid secretion, stimulatory cardiac effects
Prostaglandin D2	Vasodilation, vasopermeability, contracts smooth muscle, chemokinesis of neutrophils
Leukotriene C4	Increases vascular permeability, contracts smooth muscle
Platelet activating factor	Vasopermeability, bronchoconstriction, platelet aggregation and secretion, neutrophil aggregation and chemokinesis, eosinophil chemotaxis
Chemotactic Factors	
Eosinophil chemotactic factor anaphylaxis (ECF-A)	Attracts and deactivates eosinophils and (secondarily) neutrophils
Eosinophil chemotactic oligopeptides	Attracts and deactivates eosinophils and (secondarily) neutrophils
Neutrophil chemotactic factor	Attracts and deactivates neutrophils
Enzymes	
Neutral Proteases	
Tryptase	Proteolysis, C3a generation, inactivation of high-molecular-weight kininogen
Chymase	Proteolysis, angiotensin conversion
Acid Hydrolases	
Arylsulfatases	Hydrolysis of sulfate esters
N-Acetyl-β-D- glucosaminidase	Cleavage of glucosamine residues
β-Glucuronidase	Cleavage of glucuronide residues
Proteoglycan	
Heparin	Anticoagulant, antithrombin-III interaction, inhibits complement activation, augmentation of histaminase activity, binding of other mediators

inducer) and CD8$^+$ (suppressor/cytotoxic) cells. These T cells also express HLA-DR antigen and the interleukin-2 receptor. T cells possess the capacity to produce biologically active molecules known as *lymphokines* and to participate in cell-mediated or delayed-type hypersensitivity reactions. This class of response includes such entities as allergic contact dermatitis, resistance to infection with viruses and other microorganisms, resistance to tumors, and allograft rejection.

Monocyte-Macrophages

The skin contains a variety of cells of the monocyte-macrophage lineage about blood vessels of the dermis. Langerhans cells are located in the epidermis as well as in the dermis (see Chaps. 7 and 10). The Langerhans cell represents the sentinel cell in skin for delayed-type hypersensitivity reactions and is functionally similar to macrophages. Another class II antigen-expressing dendritic cell associated with the dermal microvasculature is present about the superficial vascular plexus; it expresses HLA-DR, DP, and DQ antigens.[27] Veil cells, which are of unclear lineage, surround the dermal microvasculature and demarcate the vessel from the surrounding dermis.[5]

Fibroblasts

The skin contains fibroblasts that produce collagen, elastin, and ground substance.

IMMUNOPATHOLOGIC REACTIONS

The dermis constitutes a primary site of inflammatory and immunologic reactions in the skin, which are due to the interaction of complex biologic processes that participate in the host defense against foreign substances. Immunologically induced inflammatory responses may involve immediate-type hypersensitivity, cytotoxicity, immune complex–mediated reactions, or cellular-type hypersensitivity. A variety of effector systems derived from cells and plasma may be involved. The effects of these systems reflect the biologic products of mast cells, lymphocytes, and macrophages; of the membrane-derived arachidonic acid metabolic pathways; of the complement system products; and of the Hageman factor–dependent pathways of coagulation, fibrinolysis, and kinin generation.

Pathophysiology of Urticaria/Angioedema

An immediate type of immunologic reaction (type 1, anaphylactic, or IgE-dependent hypersensitivity) results from the antigen-induced release of biologically active materials from mast cells or basophils sensitized with specific IgE antibody. The clinical signs and symptoms occur rapidly after the exposure of a sensitized individual to the appropriate antigen. The sites of clinical expression include the skin (urticaria and angioedema), the respiratory and gastrointestinal tracts, and the cardiovascular system. These sites may be involved singly or in any combination. Similar clinical manifestations may occur after nonimmunologic direct mast cell degranulation or in association with abnormalities of the arachidonic acid metabolic pathways or complement system rather than being dependent on IgE antibody. Such reactions may be associated with the release of the same chemical mediators produced by IgE-dependent mechanisms.

Circumscribed, raised, erythematous, usually pruritic, areas of edema that involve the superficial portions of the dermis are known as *urticaria* (Fig. 20-4); when the edematous process extends into the deep dermis and/or subcutaneous and submucosal layers, it is known as *angioedema*. Urticaria and angioedema may occur in any location together or individually. The lesions arise suddenly, usually persist for fewer than 24 h, and may continue to recur for indefinite periods. Episodes of lesions of less than 6 to 8 weeks' duration are considered acute, whereas those persisting longer are considered chronic.

Urticaria/angioedema includes a variety of clinical disorders and has many causes (Table 20-2). One such group of disorders is known as *physical urticaria,* in which various external stimuli such as trauma, cold, sunlight, and heat result in urticaria and angioedema. Inasmuch as certain forms of physical urticaria have provided experimental models in humans for the study of mast cell activation in vivo, a disorder from this group, acquired cold-induced urticaria, will be used as a paradigm of mast cell activation in the pathogenesis of urticaria/angioedema. In this model, the experimental physical challenge elicits a clinical symptom complex similar to that occurring during a natural attack. Such studies allow observation of

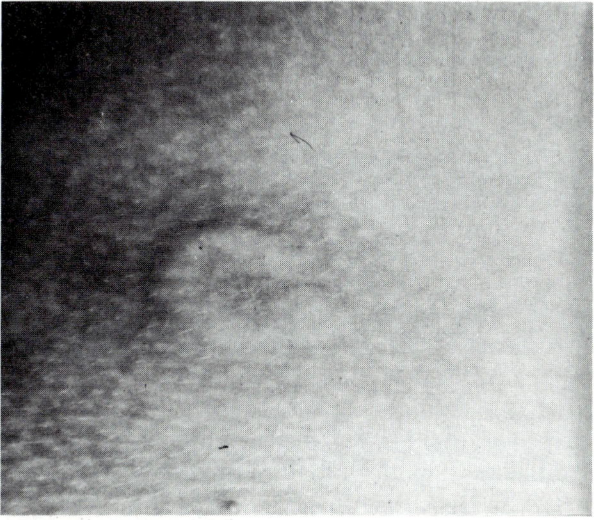

Figure 20-4 Urticaria—circumscribed edema with erythema.

Table 20-2

CLASSIFICATION OF URTICARIA/ANGIOEDEMA

IgE-mediated urticaria/angioedema
Specific antigens
Physical urticaria
Atopic diathesis
Contactants
Complement-mediated urticaria/angioedema
Serum sickness
Reactions to the administration of blood products
Necrotizing venulitis
Hereditary angioedema
Angioedema with acquired C1 inhibitor depletion and malignant disorders
Urticaria/angioedema associated with direct effects on mast cell membranes
Urticaria/angioedema associated with presumed abnormalities of arachidonic metabolism
Idiopathic urticaria/angioedema

the evolution of clinical manifestations, analysis of tissue alterations by histological techniques, the search for mediators released into the circulation, and assessment of the motility of peripheral blood leukocytes.[28]

In acquired cold urticaria, patients experience urticaria/angioedema after exposure to changes in ambient temperature or direct cold contact. Individuals with cold urticaria were subjected to experimental challenge by immersion of one arm in ice water while the unchallenged (control) arm remained at room temperature. The subjects experienced warmth, pruritus, and urticaria that evolved into angioedema within 10 min (Fig. 20-5). Histamine, prostaglandins D_2 and E_2, platelet-activating factor, and activities chemotactic for eosinophils and neutrophils were detected in the venous effluent draining the challenged arm.[29–34] The observation that these mediators appeared in the circulation with a time course similar to that of histamine suggests that the mast cell is the source of these mediators. The complement system was not involved.

Skin biopsy specimens of the experimental edematous lesions obtained over 24 h showed early mast cell degranulation with venular endothelial cell alterations; no infiltrating polymorphonuclear leukocytes of any class were observed.[32] The absence of infiltrating cells in the edematous lesion after a single experimental ice challenge is due presumably to an action of the large amounts of chemical mediators released into the venous effluent on the motility of the circulating peripheral blood leukocytes. Neutrophils obtained from the peripheral circulation of the challenged arm were

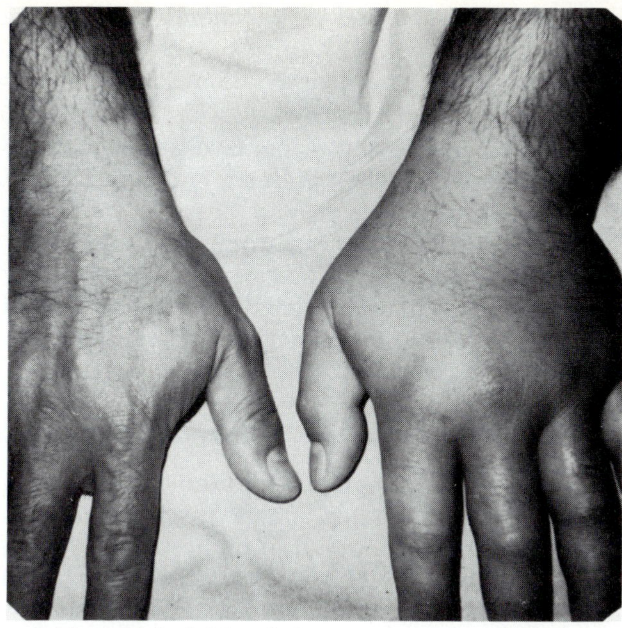

Figure 20-5 Angioedema of the left hand after experimental immersion in ice water slurry.

markedly impaired in their chemotactic responses. This defect in cell motility was attributed to mast cell activation and the release of its mediators and could be a regulatory mechanism for limiting the local tissue influx of inflammatory cells.[35]

This experimental model synthesizes observations of the clinical manifestations, histological analysis of tissue alterations, measurement of chemical mediators released into the circulation, and assessment of leukocyte motility. Such models provide evidence for the participation of mast cells in a variety of types of urticaria/angioedema.

Pathophysiology of Cutaneous Necrotizing Venulitis

Necrotizing vasculitis is a segmental inflammatory disease of the blood vessels in which the vascular alterations may be acute, subacute, or chronic and the vascular damage may be mediated by immunologic or inflammatory mechanisms. Although the term *necrotizing vasculitis* includes a variety of disorders, defined clinical syndromes are based on criteria that include the gross and microscopic appearance of the vascular lesions, the caliber of the affected blood vessels, the frequency of involvement of specific organs, and the presence of hematologic, serologic, and immunologic abnormalities. Necrotizing vasculitis of small blood vessels is termed *hypersensitivity angiitis* and in the skin involves the venules in the majority of instances. *Cutaneous necrotizing venulitis* may be the only manifestation of disease, or it may be associated with systemic involvement. The skin lesions may occur in association with coexistent chronic disorders, may be precipitated by infections or drugs, or may develop for unknown reasons (Table 20-3).

The eruption is most frequently recognized as red papules, in which the erythema does not blanch when pressed, and is called *palpable purpura* (Fig. 20-6). Palpable purpura most often appears on the lower extremities and occurs in episodes that may recur for various periods of time. An episode of cutaneous vascular lesions may be associated with fever, malaise, arthralgias, or myalgias. When associated systemic involvement occurs, the joints, muscles, gastrointestinal tract, peripheral nerves, and kidneys are frequently affected.

Animal Models and Experimental Studies in Humans

Animal Models. The participation of immune complexes is the major mechanism of tissue injury in necrotizing vasculitis. Early attempts to develop a reliable laboratory model of immune complex–mediated tissue injury included the injection of rabbits with foreign serum protein, resulting in functional and morphological alterations similar to those observed in

Table 20-3

CUTANEOUS NECROTIZING VENULITIS

Associated with coexistent disorders
- Rheumatoid arthritis
- Sjögren's syndrome
- Systematic lupus erythematosus
- Hypergammaglobulinemic purpura
- Lymphoproliferative disorders
- Cryoglobulinemia
- Ulcerative colitis
- Cystic fibrosis

Associated with recent precipitating event
- Drug-induced reactions
- Certain bacterial and viral infections

Of unknown cause
- Henoch-Schönlein syndrome
- Chronic urticaria/angioedema and variants
- Genetic C2 deficiency
- Erythema elevatum diutinum
- Nodular vasculitis
- Livedoid vasculitis
- Idiopathic

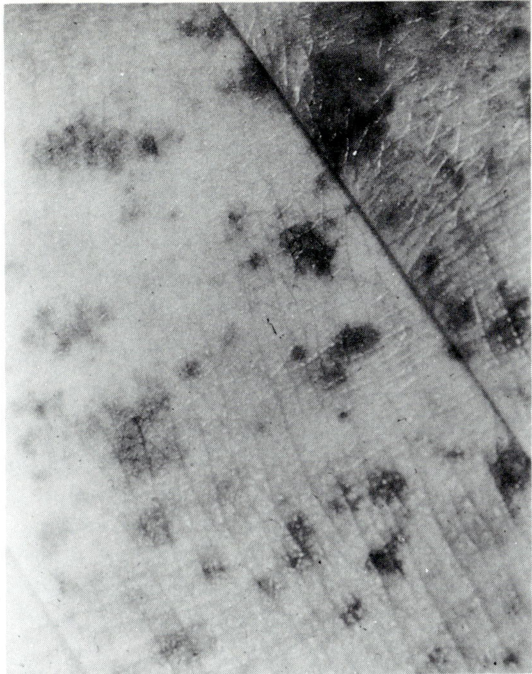

Figure 20-6 Palpable purpura in which the erythema does not blanch with pressure. Note glass in upper right corner. (*From TB Fitzpatrick et al, Dermatology in General Medicine, 3d ed, New York, McGraw-Hill, 1987, p 1302.*)

human glomerulonephritis.[36] Rabbits responding with high levels of antibody formation developed acute glomerulonephritis, whereas those responding with antibody formation barely sufficient to neutralize the antigen developed subacute and chronic glomerulonephritis. Intravenously administered colloidal carbon particles were demonstrated to deposit within vessel walls if given simultaneously with histamine or serotonin.[37] The simultaneous infusion of complexes and histamine produced deposition of the complexes in a fine granular pattern in blood vessel walls[38]. Prior treatment with Hl antihistamines prevented deposition of complexes in the animal model, presumably because vascular permeability failed to develop.[39] Only molecules larger than 19S were deposited.[40] In the rabbit model, the source of vasoactive amines appeared to be platelets[41] known to contain histamine that can be released by immune complexes.

Human Studies. Experimental studies to localize circulating immune complexes in the skin of patients with active cutaneous necrotizing venulitis have been carried out by local intracutaneous injections of histamine.[42,43]

Such injections resulted in the deposition of immunoreactive and electron-dense materials about blood vessels, as well as the development of clinical and histopathologic vascular lesions, thus confirming the role of immune complexes in this disease. In time-course analyses of the sequential development of a vascular lesion in humans, the immunofluorescence deposits peaked at 1 h and were gone by 8 h. In studies of experimental immune complex–mediated necrotizing vasculitis using direct immunofluorescence techniques in guinea pig skin,[44] immune reactants could no longer be detected at 18 h. These observations in human and guinea pig skin suggest that early lesional specimens must be obtained to search for the deposition of such immunoreactive proteins.

A unique patient with circulating immune complexes and serum hypocomplementemia, in whom the lesions of necrotizing venulitis could be induced in skin by exposure to cold or trauma, permitted a time-course study of the evolution of the vascular lesions.[12] Initially there was degranulation of mast cells and deposition of immunoglobulins and complement proteins; this was followed by a sequential influx of neutrophils, eosinophils, and basophils, with necrotic venular damage and fibrin deposition. A postulated sequence of events in the skin would be activation of mast cells by physical stimuli, deposition of circulating immune complexes, and development of cutaneous necrotizing venulitis in relation to neutrophil influx and fibrin deposition. In contrast to the Arthus reaction of vascular injury in experimental animals, the neutrophilic infiltrate did evolve into a lymphocytic cell phase in this human model of necrotizing venulitis.

Immune Complexes in Human Cutaneous Necrotizing Venulitis

The most frequently postulated mechanism for the production of cutaneous necrotizing venulitis is the deposition of circulating immune complexes or the tissue formation of immune complexes. In many patients with cutaneous necrotizing venulitis, immune complexes can be detected in the circulation and in tissues. Evidence for the presence of circulating immune complexes is derived from their detection by a variety of indirect assays, from their demonstration as cryoglobulins, and from the finding of acquired serum hypocomplementemia. In lesional tissue, the presence of immune complexes deposited in blood vessels is inferred from the demonstration of immunoreactants by direct immunofluorescence techniques and from their ultrastructural observation as electron-dense deposits.

Alterations in Serum. Patients with a necrotizing venulitis of the skin may have normal or low serum complement levels. Histopathologic examination of skin lesions in patients with serum hypocomplementemia shows necrosis of the venules and an infiltrate predominantly of neutrophils.[45] These findings are consistent with observations in animal models, where the tissue deposition of circulating complement-fixing immune complexes mediates vascular injury in association with low serum complement levels.[46] The fact that some patients may have necrosis of venules with a predominantly lymphocytic infiltrate[45] suggests that there are immune complexes able to interact with lymphocytes without activation of the complement system. Multiple types of immune complexes could therefore exist in patients with cutaneous necrotizing venulitis—those that fix complement avidly and are cleared, those that fix complement poorly in vivo and persist so as to be detected in vitro, and those that bind to lymphocyte Fc receptors and appear not to fix complement.

Putative circulating immune complexes have been sought in the serum of patients with various forms of necrotizing vasculitis by a variety of assays, such as C1q precipitation or binding, Raji cell assay, monoclonal rheumatoid factor assay, and inhibition of antibody-dependent cellular cytotoxicity. These methods for detecting immune complexes are dependent on the different physicochemical and biologic properties of the complexes, and no single assay is sufficient to recognize all types of immune complexes. Moreover, identification of the antigen has rarely been achieved. In patients with cutaneous vasculitis, 41 to 76 percent had circulating complexes detected by 18 separate assays in a study conducted by the World Health Organization.[47]

Patients with vasculitis associated with mixed-type cryoglobulins are models of immune complex–mediated tissue injury. In addition to occurring as an idiopathic syndrome, cryoglobulins may be associated with vasculitis developing in patients with collagen-vascular diseases,[48] lymphoproliferative disorders, or hepatitis B virus antigenemia.[49] When cryoglobulins contain predominantly IgG and IgM, the levels of C4 and C2 are strikingly diminished, consistent with activation of the classic complement pathway. Activated C1 molecules have been detected in the cryoprecipitate,[48] consistent with binding and activation of C1. When cryoglobulins are composed of IgG and IgA, the serum levels of C3, B, and properdin may be low in the presence of normal values of C1, C4, and C2, indicating alternative pathway activation.

Tissue Alterations. The vascular lesions of cutaneous necrotizing venulitis exhibit a perivascular infiltrate of neutrophils that may become fragmented (leukocytoclasis, karyorrhexis, or nuclear dust), variable numbers of mononuclear leukocytes, vessel wall necrosis, and fibrinoid deposits in or adjacent to the vessel wall (Fig. 20-7).

Direct immunofluorescence techniques have detected immunoglobulins and complement proteins in lesional skin biopsy specimens of patients with cutaneous venulitis. IgG is the most commonly deposited immunoglobulin, although IgM and IgA have also been detected. C3 is the only complement factor that has been sought with any frequency, and it is occasionally detected without immunoglobulin; C1q, C4, B, properdin, and C5b–9 (the membrane attack complex) have been noted. Extensive fibrin deposition about and between venules has been identified routinely.

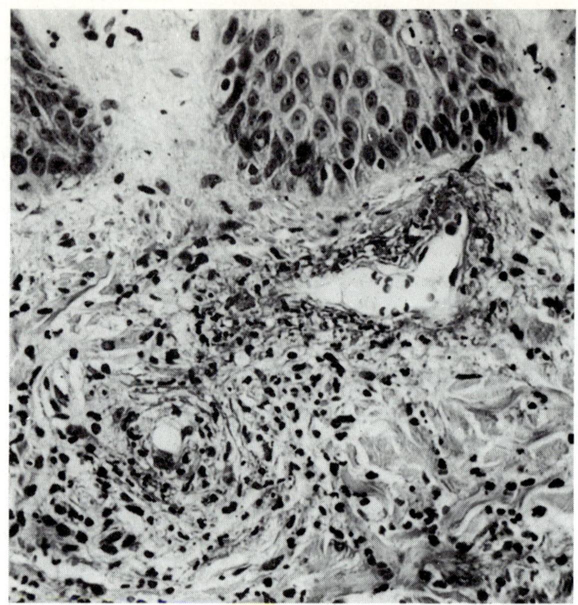

Figure 20-7 In the papillary and upper reticular dermis are venules showing the deposition of fibrillary eosinophilic material (fibrinoid) in the wall of the vessels, and the presence of neutrophils and fragmented neutrophils (nuclear dust) in and around the vessel walls. Lymphocytes and macrophages make up a portion of the inflammatory infiltrate. Extravasated erythrocytes are common. Hematoxylin-eosin. ×256 in the original magnification. (*Micrograph by Wallace H. Clark, Jr., M.D.*)

Streptococcal, staphylococcal, and mycobacterial antigens,[50] as well as hepatitis B surface antigen combined with immunoglobulins and complement proteins, have been detected in some patients. The presence of immune complexes is also inferred from the ultrastructural observation of electron-dense deposits beneath the basement membrane in lesional tissue in some patients with necrotizing venulitis of the skin.

Other types of immunopathologic mechanisms are possible but lack experimental support in animal models. Lymphocytes activated by immune complexes or through delayed-type hypersensitivity reactions can produce lymphokines that attract neutrophils, eosinophils, and basophils; degranulate basophils; and attract and retain monocyte-macrophages. Antibody-dependent cellular cytotoxicity is another possible mechanism for the production of necrotizing vasculitis, but there is no direct evidence to support this pathogenetic mechanism.

Perspective

Experimental studies in animals and humans suggest that the deposition of immune complexes in tissues is central to the pathobiologic processes that produce necrotizing vasculitis. The evidence includes the presence of circulating immune complexes associated with hypocomplementemia and activation of the classic complement pathway; the deposition of immunoreactants and the detection of electron-dense deposits in blood vessel walls; and the participation of neutrophils and other inflammatory cells. Although the identification of antigen has been accomplished infrequently, bacteria and viruses have been detected by direct immunofluorescence studies in certain instances. Some immune complexes may activate the complement system and lead to the generation of anaphylatoxins C3a, C4a, and C5a, which can degranulate mast cells. In addition, C5a can attract neutrophils that release hydrolytic enzymes during phagocytosis of complexes or generate oxygen products and damage vascular tissue. Moreover, neutrophils may generate leukotriene B4, which maintains a tissue influx of neutrophils. Other complexes may directly interact with Fc receptors on a variety of cells. Although the mechanism of localization of the circulating immune complexes to a specific vessel site remains speculative, data obtained in experimental animals and humans suggest that the localization in venules is related to vasoactive amines and vasopermeability alterations. Initial alterations in venular permeability may be due to the release of vasoactive amines from platelets, basophils, and/or mast cells. Additional factors in localization of complexes may include receptors on endothelial cell surfaces and the defective clearance of immune complexes by the reticuloendothelial system. Unexplored areas include the role of antibody-dependent cellular cytotoxicity, the participation of monocyte-macrophages and their biologic products, and the capacity of endothelial cells to produce cytokines and inflammatory mediators.

REFERENCES

1. Wessels NK: Some thoughts on embryonic inductions in relation to determination. *J Invest Dermatol* 55:221, 1970.
2. Yen A, Braverman IM: Ultrastructure of the human dermal microcirculation: the horizontal plexus of the papillary dermis. *J Invest Dermatol* 66:131, 1976.
3. Braverman IM, Yen A: Ultrastructure of the human dermal microcirculation. II. The capillary loops of the dermal papillae. *J Invest Dermatol* 68:44, 1977.
4. Braverman IM, Keh-Yen A: Ultrastructure of the human dermal microcirculation. III. The vessels in the mid and lower dermis and subcutaneous fat. *J Invest Dermatol* 77:297, 1981.
5. Braverman IM: Ultrastructure and organization of the cutaneous microvasculature in normal and pathologic states. *J Invest Dermatol* 93(Suppl):25, 1989.
6. Davison PM et al: Isolation and growth of endothelial cells from the microvessels of the newborn human foreskin in cell culture. *J Invest Dermatol* 75:316, 1980.
7. Charo IS et al: Prostaglandin I_2 is not a major metabolite of arachidonic acid in cultured endothelial cells from human foreskin microvessels. *J Clin Invest* 74:919, 1984.
8. Kubota Y et al: Role of laminin in the differentiation of human endothelial cells into capillary-like structures in culture. *J Invest Dermatol* 90:578, 1988.
9. Bull HA et al: Dermal microvascular endothelial cells are both a source of and a target for interleukin 1. *J Invest Dermatol* 90:549, 1988.
10. Messadi DV et al: Induction of an activation antigen on postcapillary venular endothelium in human skin organ culture. *J Immunol* 139:1557, 1987.

11. Ryan TJ: Structure and function of lymphatics. *J Invest Dermatol* 93(Suppl):185, 1989.
12. Soter NA et al: Cutaneous necrotizing venulitis: a sequential analysis of the morphological alterations occurring after mast cell degranulation in a patient with a unique syndrome. *Clin Exp Immunol* 32:46, 1978.
13. Trotter CM, Orr TSC: A fine structure study of some cellular components in allergic reactions. II. Mast cells in normal and atopic human skin. *Clin Allergy* 4:421, 1974.
14. Caulfield JP et al: Secretion in dissociated human pulmonary mast cells: involvement of intermediate filaments and evidence for solubilization of granule contents before discharge. *J Cell Biol* 85:299, 1980.
15. Nakano T et al: Fate of bone marrow–derived cultured mast cells after intracutaneous, intraperitoneal, and intravenous transfer into genetically mast cell-deficient W/W^v mice: evidence that cultured mast cells can give rise to both connective tissue type and mucosal mast cells. *J Exp Med* 162:1025, 1985.
16. Kobayashi T et al: Formation of mast cell colonies in methylcellulose by mouse peritoneal cells and differentiation of these cloned cells in both the skin and the gastric mucosa of W/W^v mice: evidence that a common precursor can give rise to both "connective tissue-type" and "mucosal" mast cells. *J Immunol* 136:1378, 1986.
17. Schwartz LB: Heterogeneity of mast cells in humans, in SJ Galli, KF Austen (eds), *Mast Cell and Basophil Differentiation and Function in Health and Disease*. New York, Raven Press, 1989, p 93.
18. Irani AA et al: Mast cells in cutaneous mastocytosis: accumulation of the MC_{TC} type. *Clin Exp Allergy* 20:53, 1990.
19. Benyon RC et al: Differential release of histamine and eicosanoids from human skin mast cells by IgE dependent and nonimmunological stimuli. *Br J Pharmacol* 97:898, 1989.
20. Solley GO et al: The late phase of the immediate wheal-and-flare skin reaction: its dependence on IgE antibodies. *J Clin Invest* 58:408, 1976.
21. Gleich GJ: The late phase of immunoglobulin E–mediated reaction: a link between anaphylaxis and common allergic disease. *J Allergy Clin Immunol* 70:160, 1982.
22. Church MK et al: Functional heterogeneity of human mast cells, in SJ Gallo, KF Austen (eds), *Mast Cell and Basophil Differentiation and Function in Health and Disease*. New York, Raven Press, 1989, p 161.
23. Greaves MW et al: IgE-mediated hypersensitivity in human skin studied using a new in vitro technique. *Immunology* 23:239, 1972.
24. Tharp MD et al: IgE-mediated release of histamine from human cutaneous mast cells. *J Immunol* 130:1896, 1983.
25. Crissey JT et al: Cutaneous thermography with liquid crystals. *J Invest Dermatol* 45:329, 1965.
26. Bos JD et al: The skin immune system: distribution and immunophenotype of lymphocyte populations in normal human skin. *J Invest Dermatol* 88:569, 1987.
27. Sontheimer RD et al: A macrophage phenotype for a constitutive, class II antigen-expressing, human dermal perivascular dendritic cell. *J Invest Dermatol* 93:154, 1989.
28. Soter NA: Physical urticaria/angioedema as an experimental model of acute and chronic inflammation in human skin. *Springer Semin Immunopathol* 4:73, 1981.
29. Soter NA et al: Cold urticaria: release into the circulation of histamine and eosinophil chemotactic factor of anayphylaxis during cold challenge. *N Engl J Med* 294:687, 1976.
30. Wasserman SI et al: Cold urticaria: recognition and characterization of a neutrophil chemotactic factor which appears in serum during experimental cold challenge. *J Clin Invest* 60:189, 1977.
31. Wasserman SI et al: The functional and physiocochemical characterization of three eosinophilotactic activities released into the circulation by cold challenge of patients with cold urticaria. *Clin Exp Immunol* 47:570, 1982.
32. Soter NA: High molecular weight neutrophil chemotactic factor: recognition, characterization, and role in the deactivation of neutophil leukocytes. *J Invest Dermatol* 74:354, 1980.

33. Kobza Black A et al: The release of histamine and eicosanoids in cold urticaria. *J Invest Dermatol* 84:433, 1985.
34. Grandel KE et al: Association of platelet activating factor with primary acquired cold urticaria. *N Engl J Med* 313:405, 1985.
35. Center DM et al: Inhibition of neutrophil chemotaxis in association with experimental angioedema in patients with cold urticaria: a model of chemotactic deactivation in vivo. *Clin Exp Immunol* 35:112, 1979.
36. Dixon FJ et al: Experimental glomerulonephritis: the pathogenesis of a laboratory model resembling the spectrum of human glomerulonephritis. *J Exp Med* 113:899, 1961.
37. Benacerraf B et al: Localization of colloidal substances in vascular endothelium: a mechanism of tissue damage. I. Factors causing the pathologic deposition of colloidal carbon. *Am J Pathol* 35:75, 1959.
38. Cochrane CG et al: The role of polymorphonuclear leukocytes in the initiation and cessation of the Arthus vasculitis. *J Exp Med* 110:481, 1959.
39. Kniker WT, Cochrane CG: The localization of circulating immune complexes in experimental serum sickness. *J Exp Med* 127:119, 1968.
40. Cochrane CG, Hawkins D: Studies on circulating immune complexes. III. Factors governing the ability of circulating complexes to localize in blood vessels. *J Exp Med* 127:137, 1968.
41. Waalkes TP, Coburn H: The role of platelets and the release of serotonin and histamine during anaphylaxis in the rabbit. *J Allergy* 30:394, 1959.
42. Braverman IM, Yen A: Demonstration of immune complexes in spontaneous and histamine-induced lesions and in normal skin of patients with leukocytoclastic angiitis. *J Invest Dermatol* 64:105, 1975.
43. Gower RG et al: Leukocytoclastic vasculitis: sequential appearance of immunoreactants and cellular changes in serial biopsies. *J Invest Dermatol* 69:477, 1977.
44. Cream JJ et al: Disappearance of immunoglobulin and complement from the Arthus reaction and its relevance to studies of vasculitis in man. *Br J Dermatol* 84:106, 1971.
45. Soter NA et al: Two distinct cellular patterns in cutaneous necrotizing angiitis. *J Invest Dermatol* 66:344, 1976.
46. Cochrane CG, Janoff A: The arthus reaction: a model of neutrophil and complement-mediated injury, in BW Zweifach et al (eds), *The Inflammatory Process,* 2d ed. New York, Academic, 1974, p 85.
47. Lambert PH et al: A WHO collaborative study for the evaluation of eighteen methods for detecting immune complexes in serum. *J Clin Lab Immunol* 1:1, 1978.
48. Soter NA et al: The complement system in necrotizing angiitis of the skin: analysis of complement component activities in serum of patients with concomitant collagen-vascular diseases. *J Invest Dermatol* 63:219, 1974.
49. Levo Y et al: Mixed cryoglobulinemia—an immune complex disease often associated with hepatitis B virus infection. *Trans Assoc Am Phys* 90:167, 1977.
50. Parish WE: Cutaneous vasculitis: the occurrence of complexes of bacterial antigens with antibody, and of abnormalities associated with chronic inflammation, in EH Beutner et al (eds), *Immunopathology of the Skin: Labelled Antibody Studies.* Chicago, Year Book, 1974, p 153.

21

Biology and Pathophysiology of the Extracellular Matrix in Dermis

Jouni Uitto and Michael J. Fazio

The physiological importance of human dermis is to provide tensile strength to the skin, so as to allow skin to serve as a protective organ against external trauma. The tensile properties of dermis are primarily attributable to the fibrillar components of the connective tissue, collagen and elastin, which exist in dermis in a fibrous interwoven meshwork (for additional reviews on connective tissues, see Refs. 1–4). This fibrillar meshwork is associated with other extracellular macromolecules of the dermis, such as proteoglycan-glycosaminoglycan complexes, and a number of noncollagenous glycoproteins, such as fibronectin. Also, encased in the collagenous meshwork are cells that interact with the extracellular matrix through cell-matrix receptors, such as the integrins.[5]

THE SUPRAMOLECULAR ORGANIZATION OF THE CONNECTIVE TISSUE MATRIX IN DERMIS

The dermis can be divided by morphological observations into the upper, papillary dermis, and the lower, reticular dermis. The papillary dermis interfaces with the basement membrane zone at the dermal-epidermal junction (Fig. 21-1). This association is stabilized by anchoring fibrils consisting of type VII collagen, and less well-characterized oxytalan fibers that associate with the elastic fiber network. These fibers run perpendicular to the plane of the basement membrane, thus providing stability to the

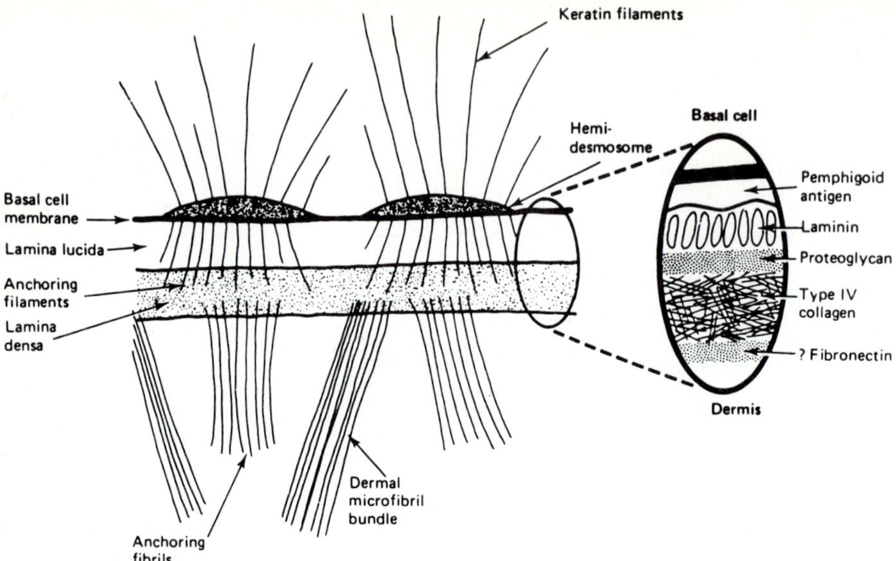

Figure 21-1 Schematic presentation of the dermal-epidermal basement membrane zone. An area on the right has been expanded to show the approximate spatial distribution of the components of the basement membrane, including type IV collagen in the lamina densa. Note the anchoring fibrils, which consist of type VII collagen. (*Adapted from J Uitto et al*[24] *with permission.*)

dermal-epidermal junction at the dermal side of the basement membrane zone. The lower part of the reticular dermis interfaces with the subcutaneous tissue in the hypodermis. The border of dermis and hypodermis in human skin is not particularly well defined, and the transition from dermis to subcutaneous tissue occurs at variable depths in different parts of the skin.

Light- and electron-microscopic examination of different levels of dermis reveals that the molecular organization of the connective tissue fibers is noticeably different in papillary dermis compared with that in mid- or lower reticular dermis.[6] Specifically, the papillary dermis contains fibers of relatively small diameter that have different histological staining properties and show a more loose packing arrangement than the fibers in the reticular dermis. These features may reflect differences in the biochemical composition of the reticular and papillary dermis. It is also clear that the extracellular matrix of the dermis consists of several biochemically distinct components whose balanced interactions and normal quantities are required for the physiologically functional skin. Differences in the interactions of these components and their relative quantities can explain some of the variation noted in the physiological properties of the skin at different body locations.

COLLAGEN BIOLOGY

Genetic Heterogeneity

The predominant fibrillar component of the dermal connective tissue is collagen, which comprises approximately 70 to 80 percent of the dry weight of the dermis.[1–3,7] During the past few years it has become clear that the collagens comprise a family of closely related but genetically distinct proteins, and as many as 25 different collageneous polypeptides have been described at this juncture, each of them being a unique gene product. These polypeptides constitute subunits of different, genetically distinct collagen types, 14 of which have been assigned a Roman numeral thus far (Table 21-1).

Currently, eight different collagen types have been detected in human skin (Table 21-2), and the corresponding genes are known to be expressed in cultured human skin fibroblasts (see Refs. 3, 8). Each of these genetically distinct collagen types has an important functional role within its compartmentalized distribution in the skin. For example, collagen types I and III are the major interstitial, fiber-forming collagens in normal human dermis, and they constitute the bulk of large collagen fibers. Utilizing immunoelectron microscopy, both type I and III collagens have been shown to be present in the same fiber structure, and it has been suggested that the addition of type III collagen molecules to the fibers interferes with the lateral growth, thus limiting the size of the fibers.[9] Since type I collagen is the predominant collagen in adult human dermis, comprising about 80 percent of the total collagen, it is clear that it plays a major role in providing tensile strength to the skin. Clinical observations on patients with the Ehlers-Danlos syndrome type IV, characterized by tissue deficiency of type III collagen, also suggest that type III collagen, which comprises some 10 percent of the total dermal collagen, also plays a major role in providing additional tensile properties to the skin.

Type IV collagen is a major constituent of the basement membrane zone in the dermal-epidermal junction. In addition, the upper dermis appears to contain basement membrane-like structures, so-called anchoring plaques, that are embedded in the interstitial collagen fiber meshwork.[10] Type VII collagen is a major constituent of the anchoring fibrils, structures that extend from the dermal-epidermal junction to the upper dermis. Type VII collagen molecules have been suggested to organize into anchoring fibrils through formation of antiparallel dimers linked through their amino-terminal ends. The large carboxy-terminal noncollagenous domains of type VII collagen are then thought to interact at one end with type IV collagen in the dermal-epidermal basement membrane and at the other end with type IV collagen in the anchoring plaques (Fig. 21-1). This type of structural organization of the anchoring fibrils could stabilize the attachment of the dermal-epidermal basement membrane to the underlying dermis. Thus, alterations in the expression, structure, or molecular interactions of type IV and/or type VII collagens could result in fragility of skin, as exemplified

Table 21-1

GENETIC HETEROGENEITY OF COLLAGEN

Collagen Type	Chain Composition	Tissue or Cell Source
I	$[\alpha 1(I)]_2\alpha 2(I)]$	Skin, bone, tendon
I trimer	$[\alpha 1(I)]_3$	Tumors, skin, tendon, liver
II	$[\alpha 1(II)]_3$	Cartilage, vitreous
III	$[\alpha 1(III)]_3$	Fetal skin, blood vessels
IV	$[\alpha 1(IV)]_2\alpha 2(IV)$	Basement membranes
V	$[\alpha 1(V)]_2\alpha 2(V)$; $[\alpha 1(V)]_3$	Ubiquitous
VI	$\alpha 1(VI)\alpha 2(VI)\alpha 3(VI)$	Aortic intima, placenta
VII	$[\alpha 1(VII)]_3$	Amnion, anchoring fibrils
VIII	$[(\alpha 1(VIII)]_3$	Endothelial cells
IX	$\alpha 1(IX)\alpha 2(IX)\alpha 3(IX)$	Cartilage
X	$[\alpha 1(X)]_3$	Cartilage
XI	$1\alpha,2\alpha,3\alpha(?)$	Cartilage
XII	?	Cartilage, fibroblasts
XIII	$[\alpha 1(XIII)]_3(?)$	HT-1080, skin fibroblasts

Source: Modified from J Uitto.[23]

Table 21-2

MOLECULAR GENETICS OF COLLAGENS PRESENT IN HUMAN SKIN

Collagen Type	Constitutent Polypeptide of Procollagen	Chromosomal Location of the Gene
I	proα1(I)	17q21–q22
	proα2(I)	7q21–22
III	proα1(III)	2q24–q33
IV	proα1(IV)	13q33–q34
	proα2(IV)	13q33–q34
V	proα1(V)	ND
	proα2(V)	2q24–q32
VI	proα1(VI)	21q223
	proα2(VI)	21q223
	proα2(VI)	2q37
VII	proα1(VII)	ND
VIII	proα1(VIII)	ND
XIII	proα1(XIII)	10q22

ND = not determined.
Source: Modified from J Uitto.[23]

by epidermolysis bullosa, a group of heritable mechanobullous disorders characterized by blistering of the skin as a result of minor trauma.[11,12]

The type V collagen gene is expressed in a variety of tissues, and it is present as a minor component in normal skin. The precise role of type V collagen in human skin is not clear, but it has been suggested that migrating epidermal cells produce type V collagen, and its continued synthesis is a prerequisite for migration of these cells.

Type VI collagen was initially thought to be a minor collagen in tissues such as the dermis. However, improvements in biochemical isolation procedures have demonstrated that type VI collagen may be an abundant collagenous component in a variety of tissues, including skin. In support of the latter suggestion is the demonstration that type VI collagen is a major gene product of cultured skin fibroblasts, as determined at the mRNA level (Fig. 21-2). In fact, molecular hybridizations with human sequence-specific cDNAs have revealed that the ratio of type I/VI collagen mRNAs in cultured skin fibroblasts is about 3:1, suggesting that type VI collagen may be even more abundant than type III collagen in the skin.[8]

Recently, type XIII collagen has been found to be ubiquitously distributed in small amounts in some, but not all, tissues that contain the major fibrillar collagens, types I and III.[13] Type XIII collagen is also found in tissues, such as epidermis, that do not contain the major fibrillar collagens. The role of type XIII collagen within these structures is currently unknown.

Molecular Structure

The individual collagen molecules consist of three polypeptide chains, so-called α-chains, which contain a variable number of amino acids in their primary sequences. In each collagen molecule, the α-chains are wrapped around each other in unique triple-helical conformation, which is responsible for the rigidity of the individual collagen molecules (Fig. 21-3).

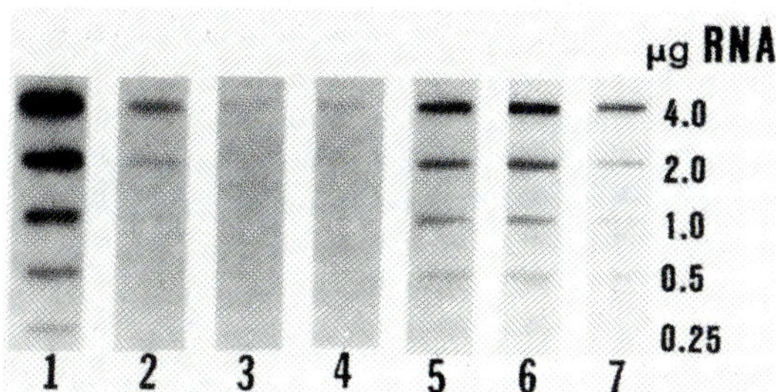

Figure 21-2 Collagen gene expression in human skin fibroblasts, as demonstrated by assay of mRNA steady-state levels. Total RNA was isolated from a fibroblast strain established from the skin of a 54-year-old individual, and varying amounts of RNA, 4.0–0.25 μg, were dotted onto nitrocellulose. Parallel filters were hybridized with α1(I) (lane 1), α1(III) (lane 2), α1(IV) (lane 3), α2(V) (lane 4), α1(VI) (lane 5), α2(VI) (lane 6), and α3(VI) (lane 7) human collagen cDNAs. The filters were hybridized and washed in parallel and exposed to X-ray film for 24 h. (*Adapted from DR Olsen et al[8] with permission.*)

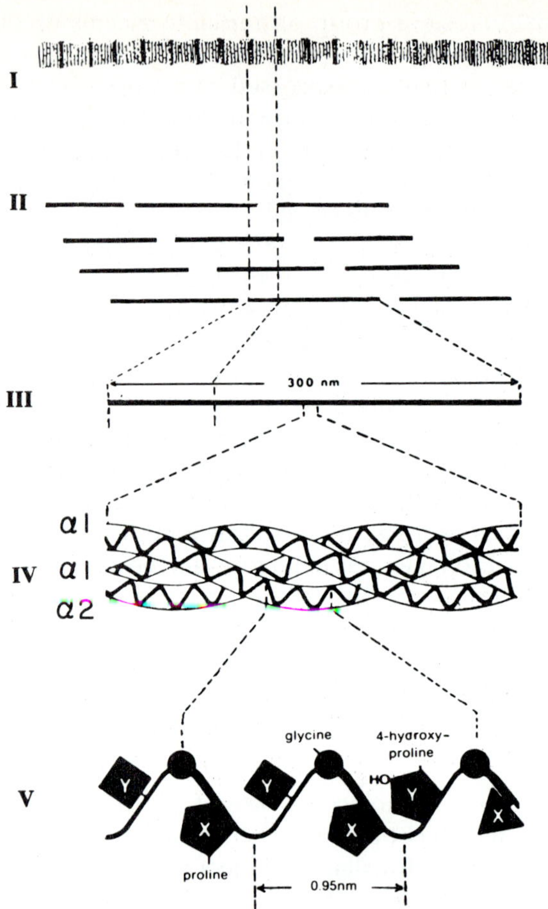

Figure 21-3 The structure of collagen. The collagen fibers (I), which on electron-microscopic examination demonstrate repeating periodicity, are composed of individual collagen molecules aligned in a quarter-stagger arrangement (II). Each collagen molecule is an approximately 300-nm-long rod-like structure (III), consisting of three individual polypeptides, so called α-chains, that are twisted around each other in a right-handed, triple-helical conformation (IV). Each α-chain is composed of amino acids in a repeating X-Y-Gly sequence (V); as indicated, the X position is frequently occupied by a prolyl residue and the Y position by a 4-hydroxyprolyl residue. The individual α-chains have a left-handed helical secondary structure with a pitch of 0.95 nm. (*Adapted from J Uitto et al*[24] *with permission.*)

Collagen is an unusual protein in that its primary amino acid sequence contains a relatively large proportion of imino acids, proline and hydroxyproline. 4-Hydroxyproline, which comprises approximately 10 percent of the total amino acid composition of the interstitial collagens, has been shown to play a critical role in stabilizing the triple-helical conformation of collagen at physiological temperature. In the absence of 4-hydroxyproline, no triple helix is formed at 37°C; instead, the individual α-chains are degraded, leading to deficient collagen formation.

Another unusual feature of collagen is the presence of a large number of glycine residues, which account for about one-third of the total amino acid composition. Sequence analyses have shown that glycine occurs in every third position of the collagenous portion of an α-chain, and this primary sequence can be described schematically as a repeating $(X\text{-}Y\text{-}Gly)_{333}$ (Fig. 21-3). The even spacing of glycine in every third position is a prerequisite for the formation of a stable triple helix.

Hydroxylysine is an amino acid that is found only in a few proteins other than collagen. Hydroxylysine, which is formed through hydroxylation of some lysyl residues in the Y position of the repeating X-Y-Gly sequence of the α-chains, participates in the formation of covalent cross-links (Fig. 21-4); as noted below, these cross-links are responsible for the tensile properties of collagen in the skin and other tissues. This fact is illustrated in patients with the Ehlers-Danlos syndrome type VI. In this condition, skin collagen is deficient in hydroxylysine due to low levels of lysyl hydroxylase activity, and this molecular defect is accompanied by loose-jointedness and hyperextensibility of the skin. The hydroxylysyl residues in collagen also serve as attachment sites for O-glycosidically linked carbohydrates in the form of galactosyl-O-hydroxylysine and glucosylgalactosyl-O-hydroxylysine (Fig. 21-4). The functional role of hydroxylysine-linked carbohydrate residues is currently unknown, but they may participate in determining the fibrillary organization of collagen in the extracellular space.

The alignment of the α-chains in the triple-helical molecule, as well as the alignment of individual collagen molecules along the microfibrils, is stabilized by covalent cross-links derived from lysine or hydroxylysine residues in the molecule. These amino acids undergo oxidative deamination, and the resulting aldehydes react with another aldehyde or with an unmodified ε-amino group on an adjacent α-chain to form the cross-links. The presence of both intra- and intermolecular cross-links is necessary for the normal tensile strength of the collagen fibers. This fact is also illustrated by experimental situations, such as lathyrism caused by feeding of animals with β-aminopropionitrile, which prevents cross-link formation. In lathyrism, inhibition of the cross-link formation results in marked fragility of the skin and other connective tissues.

The interstitial collagen types I–III are synthesized as a precursor, procollagen, which contains extension peptides at both the amino- and carboxyl-terminal ends of the molecule (Fig. 21-4). During normal collagen fibrillogenesis, these extensions are removed in the extracellular space by specific proteases. The exact role of the extension peptides and their fate after removal are not known at present. However, their removal is necessary for the formation of functional collagen fibers. This feature is illustrated by an animal disease, dermatosparaxis, in which the removal of amino-

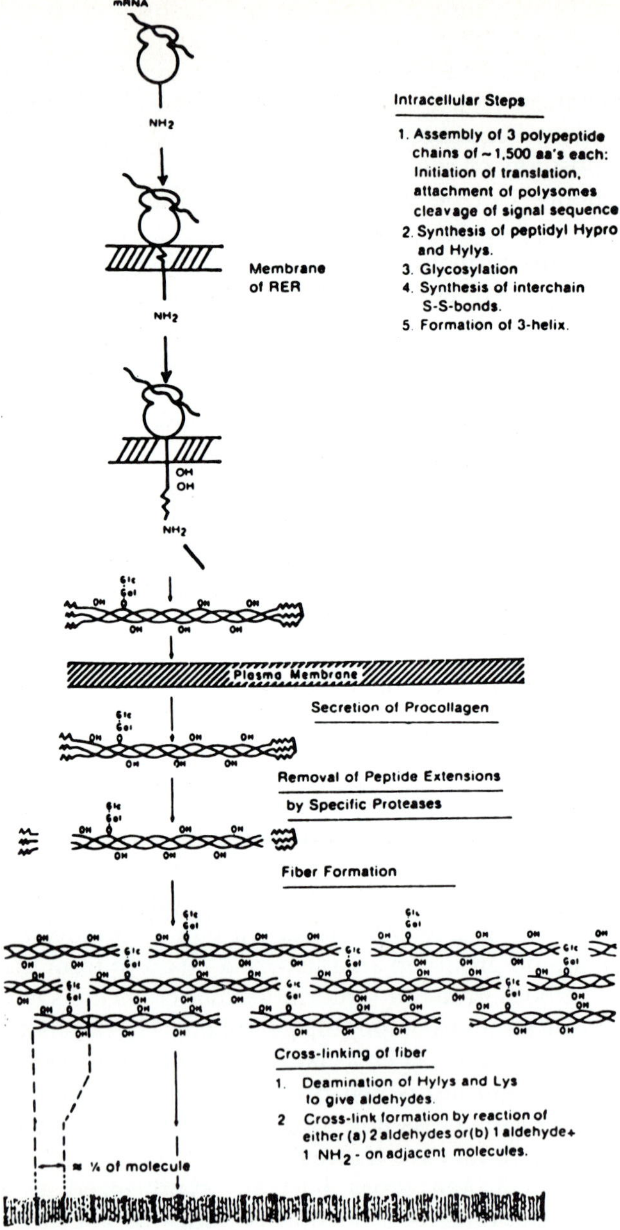

Figure 21-4 Biosynthesis of procollagen and the assembly of collagen molecules into extracellular fibers. mRNA = messenger RNA; aa's = amino acids; Hypro = hydroxyproline; Hylys = hydroxylysine; Glc-Gal = glucosyl-galactose attached to a hydroxylysyl residue; S-S bonds = disulfide bonds; Lys = lysine; NH_2- = amino terminal end of the newly synthesized polypeptide chain or the ε-amino group of either a lysyl or hydroxylysyl residue. RER = rough endoplasmic reticulum. (*Adapted from J Uitto et al*[22] *with permission.*)

terminal extensions from type I collagen is incomplete. As a result of this biochemical defect, the skin is extremely fragile and tears off easily. A human counterpart to dermatosparaxis, with similar features of connective tissue weakness, is the patient with Ehlers-Danlos syndrome type VII.

Collagen Genes

The information for the precise amino acid sequence for α-chains is coded in the collagen genes, which are diversely dispersed within the human genome.[14] Many of the collagen genes, by analogy with a variety of other eukaryotic genes, consist of several separate coding regions (exons) interspersed by noncoding, intervening sequences (introns). During the initial stages of gene expression, the information in collagen genes is transcribed into large molecular weight mRNA precursors that contain sequences complementary to both the introns and exons. The mRNA precursors then undergo a variety of posttranscriptional modification reactions, including splicing that removes the intron sequences from the primary transcript. The processed mRNAs, which contain linear coding sequences for the α-chains, then serve as a template for translation on the rough endoplasmic reticulum of the collagen-synthesizing cells, such as fibroblasts.

With the advent of the techniques of molecular biology, a wealth of information about the structure and chromosomal location of collagen genes has been developed by a large number of researchers working in the fields of connective tissue biochemistry and molecular biology (see Refs. 3, 14). In fact, the chromosomal location of most of the collagen genes within the human genome has now been defined (Table 21-2). With a few exceptions, the collagen genes are widely scattered in the human genome; for example, the two constituent polypeptide chains of type I collagen, α1(I) and α2(I), are located on separate chromosomes, 17 and 7, respectively. The precise chromosomal location of the genes coding for collagens present in human skin will allow development of linkage analyses for utilization in prenatal diagnosis of heritable cutaneous diseases.

MOLECULAR PATHOLOGY OF THE COLLAGENS

Several unique features in the biology of collagens predispose these proteins to be at fault in diseases[1–3,6,7]: For example,

1. Collagen is the most abundant protein and the major extracellular matrix component in several tissues, and collagen fibers are necessary for the physiological tensile properties of these tissues.
2. The collagens constitute a family of genetically distinct proteins that have a specific tissue distribution and that play a specialized role in providing characteristic properties to the tissues.

3. The collagenous polypeptides have a repetitive primary sequence, -glycine-X-Y-, and mutations that lead to substitution of a glycyl residue by another amino acid can result in destabilization of the collagen triple helix.

4. Collagens have a complex gene structure, and some of the collagen genes consist of as many as 53 separate coding regions, interrupted by noncoding sequences.

5. The primary gene products, preproα-chains, undergo extensive cotranslational and posttranslational modifications, many of which are enzymatically mediated.

6. The extracellular fiber assembly and the stabilization of the collagen fibers are relatively complex, multistep processes.

Based on current information about the normal biology and biochemistry of collagen fibers, we can now recognize several distinct levels at which errors could be introduced into collagen structure or metabolism in a manner that would be manifested phenotypically as a disease. In fact, several heritable connective tissue diseases with cutaneous involvement are now known to result from specific molecular defects in collagen (Table 21-3). Many of these diseases involve insertions, deletions, or subtle base substitutions in the collagen genes, which then alter the primary sequence of the protein. In several acquired diseases, the regulation of collagen gene expression is perturbed, leading to altered deposition of collagen in tissues.

This diversity of collagen pathology is exemplified by two clinical entities, namely, Ehlers-Danlos syndrome and fibrotic skin disease. The Ehlers-

Table 21-3

HERITABLE COLLAGEN DISEASES WITH CUTANEOUS INVOLVEMENT

Disease Entity	Inheritance
Ehlers-Danlos syndrome	AD, AR, XR
Osteogenesis imperfecta	AD, AR
Cutis laxa*	AD, AR, XR, NH
Marfan syndrome*	AD
Homocystinuria	AR
Menkes syndrome	XR
Focal dermal hypoplasia	XD
Tuberous sclerosis	AD
Familial cutaneous collagenoma	AD
Epidermolysis bullosa	AD, AR

AD = autosomal dominant; AR = autosomal recessive;
XD = X-linked dominant; XR = X-linked recessive;
NH = not heritable disorder.
* In these conditions, significant evidence suggests elastic fiber abnormalities in most cases.
Source: Modified from J Uitto.[23]

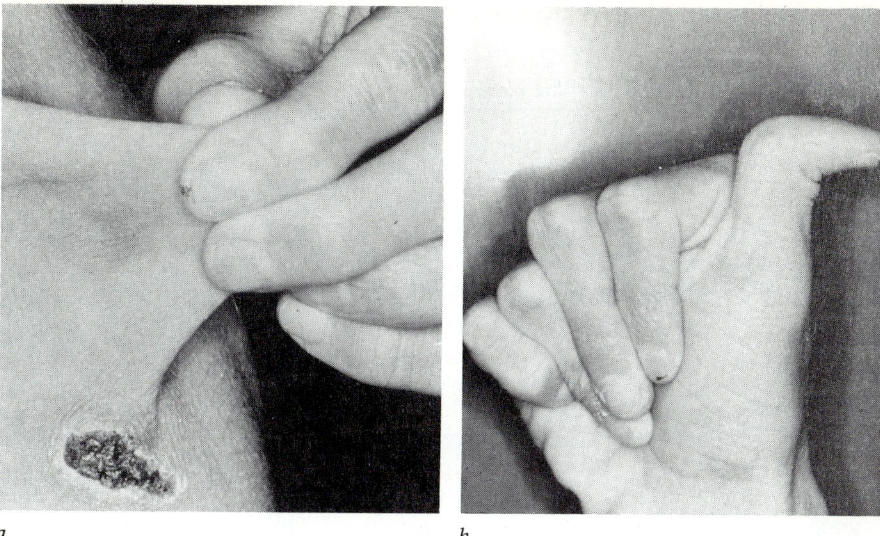

a *b*

Figure 21-5 Clinical features in a patient with the Ehlers-Danlos syndrome type IV. (*a*) Note the marked hyperextensibility of the skin at the elbow and the laseration resulting from extreme cutaneous fragility. (*b*) The patient demonstrates considerable loose-jointedness in the small joints. Also, note the presence of acrogeria, *i.e.* premature aging of the skin of hands of this 16-year old patient. *(Adapted from J Uitto et al[26] with permission.)*

Danlos syndrome illustrates a group of phenotypically similar conditions that frequently result from abnormalities in the structure of collagen (Table 21-4, Fig. 21-5). The fibrotic skin diseases exemplify conditions with altered regulation of collagen gene expression (Table 21-5).

BIOLOGY OF ELASTIC FIBERS

Fiber Structure

The elastic fibers of human skin can be visualized by special histopathologic staining techniques, such as Verhoeff-van Gieson or orcein stains. The elastic fibers are thickest in the reticular dermis, where they are oriented parallel to the surface of the skin, intertwined among the collagen bundles. In the papillary dermis, the elastic fibers, known as elaunin, are organized in an arcade-like arrangement. In the most superficial papillary dermis, even thinner elastic fibers, known as oxytalan fibers, ascend vertically to terminate at the dermal-epidermal junction.

Examination of elastic fibers by transmission electron microscopy has revealed that these fibers consist of two distinct components (Fig. 21-6). The major component is elastin, a well-characterized connective tissue protein.[15] Surrounding the elastin core are less well characterized electron-dense structures, known as elastic fiber microfibrils (Fig. 21-6). Although the precise composition of the microfibrils is currently unknown, recent

Table 21-4

GENETIC AND BIOCHEMICAL HETEROGENEITY OF THE EHLERS-DANLOS SYNDROME

Type	Inheritance	Biochemical Defect
I Gravis	Autosomal dominant	Unknown
II Mitis	Autosomal dominant	Unknown
III Benign hypermobile	Autosomal dominant	Unknown
IV Ecchymotic	Autosomal dominant or recessive	Deficiency of type III collagen in tissues
V X-linked	X-linked recessive	Unknown
VI Ocular	Autosomal recessive	Lysyl hydroxylase deficiency
VII Arthrocalasis multiplex congenita	Autosomal dominant or recessive	Defective conversion of procollagen to collagen
VIII Periodontitis	Autosomal dominant	Unknown
IX Occipital horn syndrome	X-linked recessive	Lysyl oxidase deficiency due to altered copper metabolism
X Fibronectin type	Autosomal recessive	Functionally deficient plasma fibronectin
XI Large joint hypermobility	Autosomal dominant	Unknown

Source: Modified from J Uitto.[23]

Table 21-5

HERITABLE DISEASES WITH ABNORMAL ELASTIC FIBERS

Disease	Inheritance
Pseudoxanthoma elasticum	AR, AD
Buschke-Ollendorff syndrome	AD
Cutis laxa	AD, AR, XR
Ehlers-Danlos syndrome type IX	XR
Menkes syndrome	XR
Marfan syndrome	AD
Elastoderma	?

AD = autosomal dominant; AR = autosomal recessive; XR = X-linked recessive.
Source: Modified from J Uitto et al.[21]

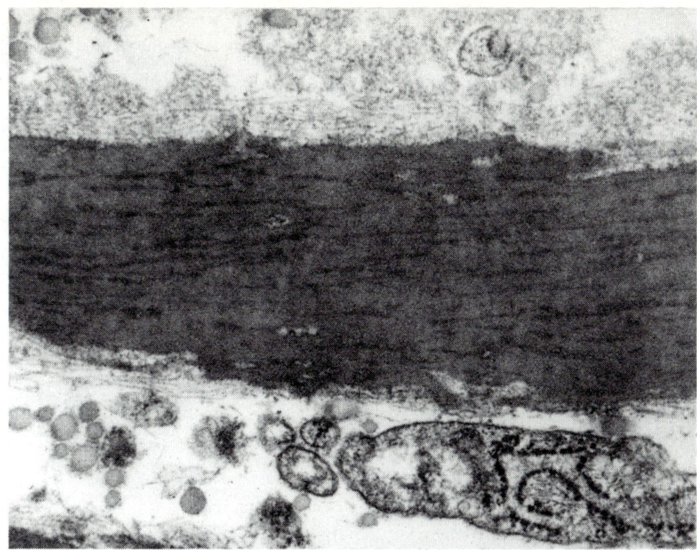

Figure 21-6 Transmission electron microscopy of the elastic fibers in normal human skin. Elastin, the electron-lucent core of the fiber, is surrounded by thin, electron-dense microfibrils. ×16,000 in the original magnification.

studies have suggested that fibrillin, another extracellular matrix protein, may be an integral part of the microfibrillar structure.

Biosynthesis and Gene Structure

Elastin is initially synthesized as a polypeptide of about 70 kd that is coded by a single-copy gene located in the long arm of human chromosome 7 (Fig. 21-7). The human elastin gene contains 34 coding segments (exons) separated by relatively large intervening sequences (introns), and they occupy a total of about 45,000 base pairs of the human genome (Fig. 21-8). During the early stages of elastin gene expression, the nucleotide sequence in the gene is transcribed to a large mRNA precursor, which is then subjected to posttranscriptional modifications, including constitutive splicing, which removes the intron sequences, resulting in mature elastin mRNAs (Fig. 21-8). An unusual variation of constitutive splicing, occurring during the processing of elastin mRNAs, is that some exon sequences are alternatively spliced, resulting in the synthesis of mRNA molecules with slightly differing primary sequences.[16,17] The significance of the alternative splicing is currently unknown, but it could provide a mechanism that would result in the synthesis of elastin molecules with slightly different physiological properties. This might explain some tissue-specific differences in elastic fibers, as noted by morphological studies.

The elastin mRNA is about 3.5 kb in size and contains an approximately 2.2-kb translatable region that encodes a polypeptide of about 750 amino

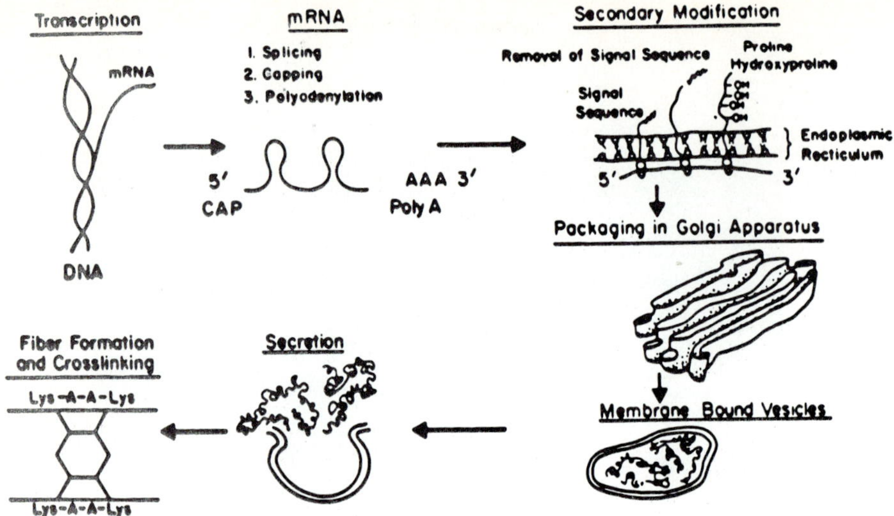

Figure 21-7 Schematic presentation of elastin biosynthesis. The elastin gene, which is located on the long arm of chromosome 7 and is about 45 kb in size (see Fig. 21-8*a*), is transcribed to an mRNA precursor. After transcription, several intranuclear reactions participate in the processing of the primary mRNA transcript, including alternative splicing. The mRNA then serves as a template for translation, and the newly synthesized polypeptide is subject to several posttranslational modifications. The elastin polypeptides are packaged in Golgi vesicles before being transferred to the extracellular space. After secretion, the individual elastin polypeptides align into the fiber structure that is stabilized by the formation of covalent cross-links, demosines, and isodesmosines (see Fig. 21-8). 5′CAP, AAA3′, and PolyA are nucleotides; Lys-A-A-Lys denotes lysine–alanine–alanine–lysine amino acid sequences in elastin polypeptides (see Fig. 21-9). (*Adapted from J Rosenbloom*[25] *with permission.*)

acids (Fig. 21-8*B*). Following translation of the elastin mRNAs on the ribosomes of the elastin-synthesizing cells, such as human skin fibroblasts, the newly synthesized polypeptides are secreted into the extracellular space (Fig. 21-7).

Fiber Formation

In the extracellular space, the individual elastin polypeptides align into a fiber structure. The fiber assembly is stabilized by the formation of unique cross-link compounds called desmosines (Fig. 21-9). The tropoelastin polypeptides contain specific cross-link domains consisting of paired lysyl residues separated by two or three amino acids, frequently alanines. Certain lysyl residues are oxidatively deaminated to the corresponding aldehydes, allysines, in a reaction that is catalyzed by lysyl oxidase, a copper-dependent enzyme. Three of the allysines and an unmodified ε-amino group of a fourth lysyl residue spontaneously fuse to form a stable cross-link, desmosine, or its isomer, isodesmosine (Fig. 21-9).

Regulation of Gene Expression

Elastin gene expression in normal situations is controlled primarily at the transcriptional level, and in general, the elastin mRNA levels correlate

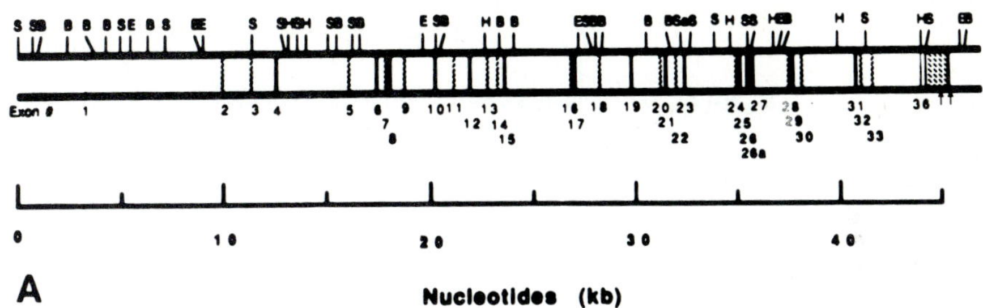

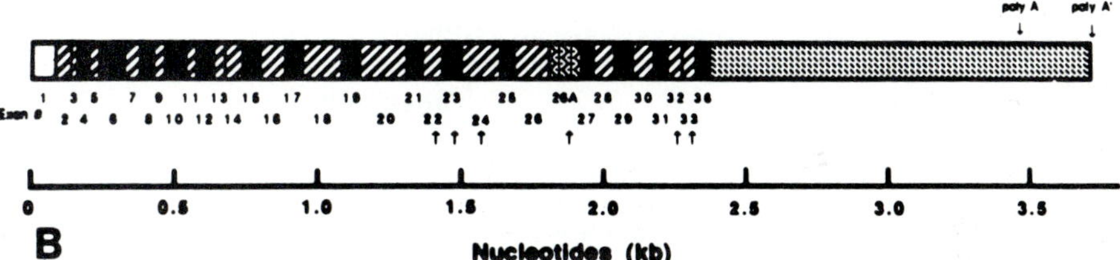

Figure 21-8 Schematic presentation of the human elastin gene (*A*) and the corresponding cDNA (*B*). (*A*) The exons have been numbered starting from the 5′-end of the gene and correspond to those shown in the cDNA (see *B*). The presence of restriction endonuclease cleavage sites: BamHI (B), EcoRI (E), HindIII (H). kb = kilobases. (*B*) The cDNA, about 3.5 kb in size, is divided into separate exons that are numbered from 1 to 36 and drawn to scale. The arrows indicate the exons that have been shown to be subject to alternative splicing. (*Adapted from J Uitto et al*[15] *with permission.*)

with the amount of elastin polypeptides being synthesized. Consequently, the elastin mRNA steady-state levels reflect the rate of elastin synthesis in tissues or cell cultures.

Human skin fibroblasts have been used as a model system to study the modulation of elastin gene expression. These studies have demonstrated that elastin gene expression, which is activated during early stages of fetal development, remains at a relatively constant level for several decades. However, after the fourth decade of life, elastin gene expression precipitously declines.[18] This observation may have relevance to the innate cutaneous aging characterized by loss of functional elastic fibers in the skin.[19]

The 5′-flanking region is crucial in the transcriptional regulation of the elastin gene. Recently, the entire human elastin gene, including the promoter sequences, has been cloned and characterized.[17,20] Analyses of the 5′-flanking region of the human elastin gene revealed several unusual features that suggest that transcriptional regulation of the elastin gene is

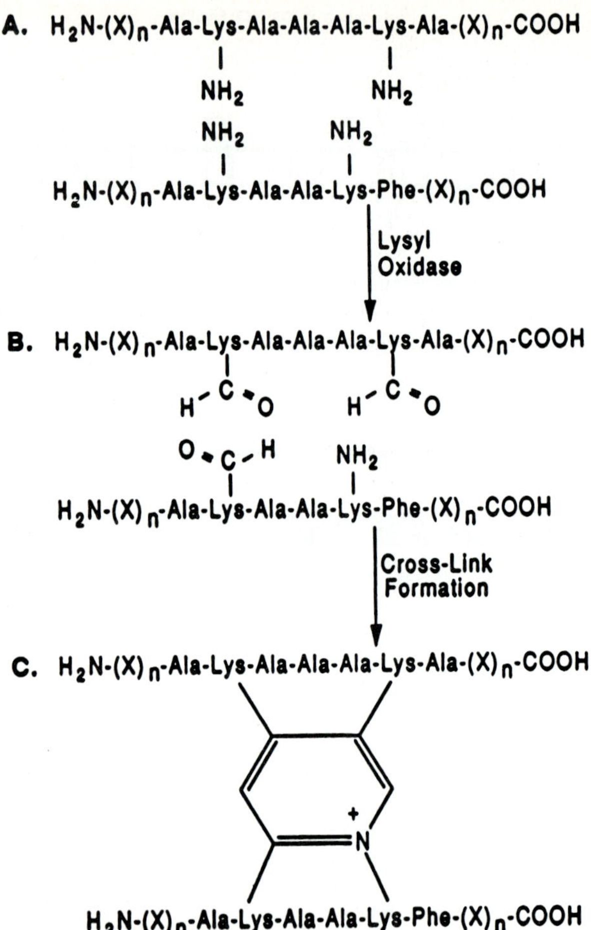

Figure 21-9 Formation of intermolecular cross-links, desmosine and isodesmosine, between two tropoelastin polypeptides. (*A*) Amino acid sequences of a potential cross-link region within the tropoelastin polypeptides. Note the ϵ-amino group (NH_2) of the four contributing lysyl residues. (*B*) Three of the lysyl residues undergo oxidative deamination catalyzed by lysyl oxidase to yield corresponding aldehyde derivatives, allysines. (*C*) Three of the allysines and the fourth unmodified lysyl residue, still containing an ϵ-amino group, fuse into a stable desmosine cross-link. (*Adapted from J Uitto et al*[15] *with permission.*)

complex. Recent construction of elastin promoter/reporter gene (CAT) plasmids[20] provides a means to study transcriptional modulation of elastin gene expression by a variety of exogenous agents, as well as in cutaneous diseases.

Degradation

Elastases comprise a family of proteolytic enzymes capable of degrading elastic fibers. Although the metabolic turnover of connective tissue proteins, especially elastin, is relatively slow, it is clear that a portion of elastic fibers

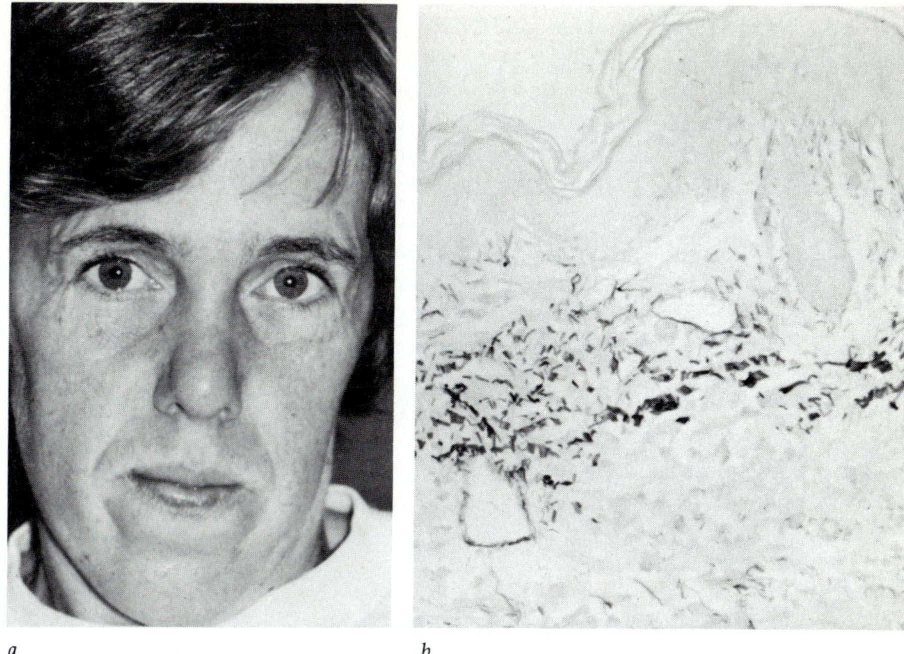

Figure 21-10 Clinical and histopathologic features of cutis laxa. (*a*) Note the loose and sagging skin and prematurely aged appearance of this 15-year old patient. (*b*) Histopathology of the dermis shows fragmentation and loss of the elastic fibers (Orcein stain) × 40 in the original magnification. *(Adapted from J Uitto, A Shamban[27] with permission.)*

is continuously degraded and replaced during early stages of development. In addition, degradation of elastic fibers is markedly increased in a variety of pathological conditions, such as some forms of cutis laxa (Fig. 21-10).[15,18]

The most powerful elastolytic enzymes are present in polymorphonuclear leukocytes, and these enzymes presumably initiate elastin degradation in inflammatory processes. The activity of these serine proteases can be inhibited by serum factors, such as α1-antitrypsin and α2-macroglobulin. In addition to serine elastases, the presence of elastase-like metalloproteases has been recently demonstrated in human serum and in different cells. These enzymes are not particularly active against insoluble elastin, but they are capable of degrading soluble elastin, as well as the oxytalan and elaunin fibers. Thus, these enzymes may contribute to the overall degradation of the elastic fiber network. Furthermore, some of the elastase-like metalloproteases have been suggested to play a role in the degradation of elastic fibers in patients with various cutaneous diseases.

ELASTIN PATHOLOGY

The complexity of gene expression and metabolic turnover of elastin can introduce errors into the biosynthetic pathway of elastic fibers in a manner that may be manifested as a clinical disease.[21,22] In fact, abnormalities in the elastic fiber network have been detected in various diseases affecting the skin (Table 21-5). The mechanisms leading to elastic fiber pathology can occur at one of several different levels of the elastin metabolic pathway. For example, the elastin gene may have aberrations in the primary structure, or the rate of elastin gene expression may be altered in heritable cutaneous disorders. Alternatively, posttranscriptional or posttranslational modifications could alter the structure of elastin, or the rate of degradation of the elastic fibers could be altered. These diseases can now be studied by biochemical and molecular biology approaches that have been developed during the past few years.[3,15] Such techniques can be utilized for precise elucidation of the underlying molecular defects in both heritable and acquired diseases affecting the elastic fibers.

ACKNOWLEDGMENTS

The original studies by the authors were supported by grants from the National Institutes of Health and the Dermatology Foundation.

REFERENCES

1. Uitto J, Perejda AJ: *Connective Tissue Diseases: Molecular Pathology of the Extracellular Matrix,* in *Series: Biochemistry of Disease,* vol 12. New York, Marcel Dekker, 1987.
2. Olsen BR, Nimni ME: *Collagen,* vol IV: *Molecular Biology.* Boca Raton, Fla, CRC Press, 1989.
3. Uitto J et al: Extracellular matrix of the skin: 50 years of progress. *J Invest Derm* 92(Suppl): 61s, 1989.
4. Goldsmith L: *Biochemistry and Physiology of the Skin,* 2d ed. New York, Oxford University Press, in press.
5. Ruoslahti E, Pierschbacher MD: New perspectives in cell adhesion: RGD and integrins. *Science* 238:491, 1987.
6. Holbrook KA, Byers P: Diseases of the extracellular matrix. Structural alterations of collagen fibers in skin, in J Uitto, A Perejda (eds), *Connective Tissue Diseases: Molecular Pathology of the Extracellular Matrix.* New York, Marcel Dekker, 1987, p 101.
7. Bauer EA, Uitto J: Collagen in cutaneous diseases. *Int J Dermatol* 18:251, 1979.
8. Olsen DR et al: Collagen gene expression by cultured human skin fibroblasts: abundant steady-state levels of type VI procollagen mRNAs. *J Clin Invest* 83:791, 1989.
9. Fleischmajer R et al: Regulatory mechanisms of collagen metabolism in scleroderma skin, in R Fleischmajer (ed), *Progress in Diseases of the Skin.* Orlando, Fla, Grune and Stratton, 1984, vol 2, p 125.
10. Keene DR et al: Type VII collagen forms an extended network of anchoring fibrils. *J Cell Biol* 104:611, 1987.
11. Kero M: Epidermolysis bullosa in Finland: clinical features, morphology and relation to collagen metabolism. *Acta Derm Venereol (Stockh),* Suppl 110, 1984.
12. Gedde-Dahl T: Clinical heterogeneity in epidermolysis bullosa: speculations on causes and consequences for research. *J Invest Dermatol* 86:91, 1986.
13. Sandberg M et al: Expression of mRNAs coding for the α1 chain of type XIII collagen in human fetal tissues: comparison with expression of mRNAs for collagen types I, II, and III. *J Cell Biol* 109:1371, 1989.
14. Chu M-L, Prockop DJ: Collagen: gene structure, in PM Royce, B Steinmann (eds), *Extracellular Matrix and Inheritable Disorders of Connective Tissue.* New York, Alan R Liss, in press.

15. Uitto J et al: Elastic fibers of the connective tissue, in L Goldsmith (ed), *Biochemistry and Physiology of the Skin,* 2d ed. New York, Oxford University Press, in press.
16. Fazio MJ et al: Cloning of full-length elastin cDNAs from a human skin fibroblast recombinant cDNA library: further elucidation of alternative splicing utilizing exon-specific oligonucleotides. *J Invest Dermatol* 91:458, 1988.
17. Bashir MM et al: Characterization of the complete human elastin gene: delineation of unusual features in the 5′ flanking region. *J Biol Chem* 269:8887, 1989.
18. Fazio MJ et al: Skin aging: lessions from cutis laxa and elastoderma. *Cutis* 43:437, 1989.
19. Uitto J et al: Molecular mechanisms of cutaneous aging: age-associated connective tissue alterations in the dermis. *J Am Acad Dermatol* 21(Suppl):614, 1989.
20. Kähäri V-M et al: Deletion analyses of 5′-flanking region of the human elastin gene: evidence for a functional promoter and regulatory *cis*-elements. *J Biol Chem* 265:9485, 1990.
21. Uitto J et al: The elastic fibers, in TK Krieg, CM Lapière (eds), *Diseases of the Connective Tissue in the Skin.* London, Dunitz, in press.
22. Uitto J et al: Heritable connective tissue diseases of the skin, in JC Alper (ed), *Year Book on Genodermatoses.* Chicago, IL, Year Book, 1990, p 287.
23. Uitto J: Molecular pathology of collagen in cutaneous diseases, in JP Callen et al (eds), *Advances Dermatol* 6. Chicago, IL, Year Book, 1991, p 265.
24. Uitto J et al: Mechanical and physical functions of skin, in AJ Thody, PS Friedmann (eds), *Scientific Basis of Dermatology.* London, Churchill Livingstone, 1986, p 6.
25. Rosenbloom J: Biology of disease. Elastin: relation of protein and gene structure to disease. *Lab Invest* 51:605, 1984.
26. Uitto J et al: The Ehlers-Danlos syndrome type IV: clinical, genetic and biochemical studies of a family, in WH Akeson, P Bornstein, MJ Glimcher (eds), *Symposium on heritable disorders of connective tissue.* St. Louis, CV Mosby, 1982, p 82.
27. Uitto J, Shamban A: Heritable skin diseases with molecular defects in collagen or elastin. *Dermatol Clin 5:63, 1987.*

22

Pathophysiology of Wound Healing

Richard A.F. Clark

Tissue repair is a necessary sequela of cutaneous injury if homeostasis of the injured skin is to be reestablished. In this chapter, a synopsis of cutaneous wound repair beginning with the initial generic injury is presented. A more comprehensive review and an extensive bibliography have recently been published.[1] Figure 22-1 presents a histological overview of early wound repair in porcine skin.

INFLAMMATION

Injury initiates inflammation by causing cell death and the disruption of blood vessels. The latter leads to extravasation of blood constituents, platelet activation,[2] blood coagulation,[3] and mediator generation. Platelets affect hemostasis by adherence to extravascular tissue structures, activation, self-aggregation, and induction of blood coagulation. In addition, platelets release biologically active materials. These include extracellular matrix molecules, fibronectin, fibrinogen, thrombospondin, and von Willebrand factor, which are necessary for platelet aggregation and binding to the tissue structure[4]; the growth factors—platelet-derived growth factor (PDGF),[5] transforming growth factor-α (TGF-α),[6] and transforming growth factor β (TGF-β),[7] which are necessary for new tissue generation; and the vasoactive substances serotonin, ADP, calcium, and thromboxin, which are necessary for blood vessel constriction to prevent hemorrhage.

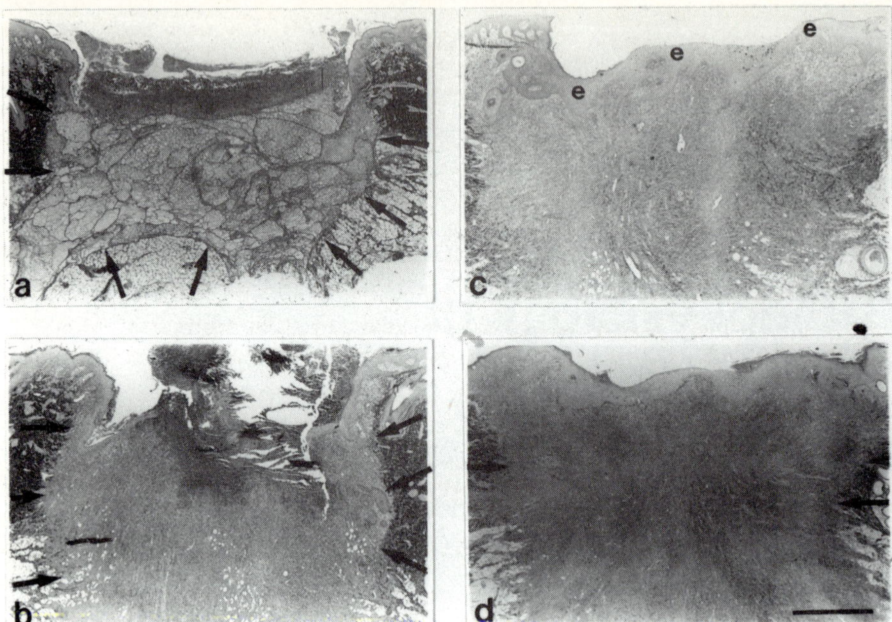

Figure 22-1 Histological overview of early wound repair in porcine skin. (*a*) Fibrin clots form within the wound space during the first few hours after injury and persist for 3 days (*arrows*). Epidermal migration over the wound surface begins by 24 h after injury and continues at a steady rate until the entire wound is reepithelialized. (*b*) Fibroblasts begin to grow into the wound space at day 4, and by day 5 an exuberant ingrowth of fibroblasts and new blood vessels has occurred (*arrows*). (*c*) By day 7 the epidermis (e) has been reestablished over the wound surface and extracellular matrix has accumulated in the neodermis (arrows). (*d*) Wound contraction is evident (*arrows*) at day 10, with a resultant compaction and reorientation of collagen bundles. Fibroblasts begin to degenerate, leading to decreased cellularity.

The initiating event of coagulation is the availability of a surface (e.g., interstitial connective tissue, membranes of activated platelets) that promotes plasma proenzyme adsorption and activation. Otherwise, these proteins are literally afloat in a sea of enzyme inhibitors. Small amounts of proenzymes are activated, in fact, under normal circumstances, but once activated, the enzymes are immediately quenched by plasma protease inhibitors. When the proenzymes have been adsorbed on a surface in a microenvironment relatively free of protease inhibitors, minute amounts of spontaneous activation are quickly amplified into the physiological response of blood clotting. Viewed from the standpoint of coagulation control, it follows that blood clotting automatically terminates when the activation surface is unavailable.

A variety of biologically active mediators are generated from the coagulation cascade, including kallikrein, thrombin, plasmin, fibrinopeptides, fibrin split products, bradykinin, and the anaphylatoxins C3a and C5a through activation of the complement cascade. Most of these factors act as chemoattractants to circulating leukocytes, bringing them to the site of injury. Thrombin and plasmin are also growth factors for parenchymal cells.[8] Dead and dying cells release a variety of substances that may be important for wound repair, such as tissue factor, lactic acid, lactate dehydrogenase, calcium, lysozomal enzymes, and fibroblast growth factor (FGF).[9] Thus, the substances from platelets, blood coagulation, and injured cells not only promote vasoregulation, blood clotting, and tissue degradation but also stimulate processes important for new tissue formation, such as cell migration and proliferation and neomatrix formation.

Several intrinsic activities of intact blood vessel endothelium[10] limit the extent of platelet aggregation and blood coagulation to the wounded area. These include production of prostacyclin, which inhibits platelet aggregation; cell surface inactivation of thrombin; cell surface activation of protein C, an enzyme that degrades coagulation factors V and VIII; and generation of plasminogen activator, which initiates clot lysis. The activated endothelium also expresses specific intercellular adhesion molecules, intercellular adhesion molecule-1 (ICAM-1), endothelial cell-leukocyte adhesion molecule (ELAM), and granule membrane protein (GMP) 140 on their surface.[11,12] The endothelial cell receptors recognize the β2 integrin family of receptors [MAC-1 (the C3bi complement receptor, CD11b/CD18), lymphocyte adhesion molecule-1 (LFA-1), and p150], which are expressed on circulating leukocytes as they are stimulated by chemotactic factors emanating from the wound site (Table 22-1). The interactions of these cell-cell receptors are responsible for leukocyte margination at the site of injury.

Subsequently, blood leukocytes diapedese through the blood vessel and invade the injured tissue. Within the first few hours, neutrophils infiltrate

Table 22-1

THE INTEGRIN SUPERFAMILY OF RECEPTORS

Receptor Function	Integrin Nomenclature
Laminin binding	$\alpha1\beta1$
Collagen binding	$\alpha2\beta1$
Generic extracellular matrix	$\alpha3\beta1$
Lymphocyte homing	$\alpha4\beta1$
Fibronectin binding	$\alpha5\beta1$
Laminin binding	$\alpha6\beta1$
Leukocyte adhesion (MAC-1)	$\alpha_m\beta2$
Leukocyte adhesion (LFA-1)	$\alpha_L\beta2$
Leukocyte adhesion (p150)	$\alpha_x\beta2$
Platelet binding to extracellular matrix	$\alpha_p\beta3$
Vitronectin binding	$\alpha_v\beta3$

the wound, followed by monocytes 24 to 48 h later. Both cell types are attracted to sites of tissue injury by a variety of chemotactic factors. The major function of neutrophils is to rid the tissue of contaminating bacteria. In doing so, they often release lysosomal enzymes and other toxic substances, which results in additional tissue destruction. Monocytes invading the wound site quickly undergo phenotypic metamorphosis to macrophages.[13] Macrophages phagocytose and kill pathogenic organisms and scavenge tissue debris, including effete neutrophils. They can also release chemotactic factors that recruit additional inflammatory cells and enzymes that augment tissue degradation. In addition, macrophages can release a second wave of growth factors, including PDGF, TGF-α, and TGF-β.[14] As mentioned before, these factors are probably critical for new tissue formation.[5–7] Since macrophages can continually produce these factors, while platelets cannot, macrophages are pivotal in the transition between wound inflammation and new tissue formation.

NEW TISSUE FORMATION

New tissue in a cutaneous wound consists of a neoepidermis and underlying granulation tissue. The granulation tissue is composed of macrophages, fibroblasts, neomatrix, and neovasculature, which together grow into the wound to form a loosely woven tissue that provides support for the neoepidermis and the origin of a neodermis.

Granulation tissue formation begins after a lag of several days when fibroblasts migrate into the wound together with new blood vessel sprouts. TGF-β, PDGF, and fragments of matrix proteins such as fibronectin and collagen promote fibroblast migration, while FGF and PDGF stimulate fibroblast proliferation.[1] Once fibroblasts have migrated into the wound, they produce and deposit exuberant quantities of fibronectin, types I and III collagen, and hyaluronate. TGF-β is currently believed to be the most important stimulus of fibroblast extracellular matrix production.[7] TGF-β also induces fibroblast surface membrane expression of collagen and fibronectin receptors in the β1 integrin family.[15] Subsequently, fibroblasts link up with each other and the extracellular matrix in radial arrays across the wound, presumably using collagen and fibronectin receptors to "grasp" the extracellular matrix (Table 22-1).[16] They develop thick actin cables along their longitudinal axes and generate tension across the wound, causing tissue contraction. PDGF, and perhaps TGF-β, stimulate the fibroblasts to contract.[17] Fibroblasts produce a variety of growth factors similar to macrophages; thus, once activated appropriately, fibroblasts may be able to sustain their own growth and/or extracellular matrix production. This possibility may have great import in fibrocontractive diseases such as scleroderma, cirrhosis, and pulmonary fibrosis. Collagen matrix appears to have a marked negative feedback on collagen production by normal cultured fibroblasts, and some evidence exists that this may also be true of cutaneous wound fibroblasts.

As mentioned above, new blood vessels form (angiogenesis) concomitantly with ingrowth of fibroblasts and neomatrix deposition (fibroplasia). Morphologically, a defined series of events occurs that results in angiogenesis.[18] Endothelial cells lining the microvasculature adjacent to a wound dissolve the intervening basement membrane and emigrate through the disrupted matrix (Fig. 22-2). Endothelial cells migrate into the newly forming granulation tissue as a cord of cells surrounded by a specialized provisional matrix.[19,20] Adjacent endothelial cell cords join together, forming arcades of new capillaries. Lumina appear within the center of the arched cords, and blood flow begins. Basement membrane rapidly forms between the capillary endothelial cells and the granulation tissue neomatrix, and thereby replaces the specialized provisional matrix from the wound margin inward toward the tips of capillary sprouts. FGF is partly responsible for angiogenesis by initiating the following cascade of events[21] (Fig. 22-2). FGF stimulates endothelial cells to secrete procollagenase and plasminogen activator. The latter enzymatically converts extravasated blood plaminogen to plasmin. Plasmin as well as plasminogen activator activates procollagenase to collagenase. Together these enzymes digest the blood vessel basement membrane. Endothelial chemoattractants, such as fibronectin fragments generated from extracellular matrix degradation and heparin released from mast cells, draw endothelial cells through the disrupted basement membrane to form a nascent capillary bud.

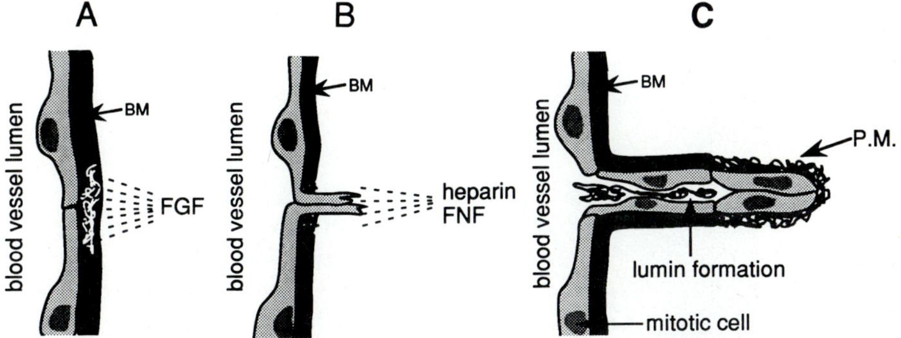

Figure 22-2 Initiation of angiogenesis. (*A*) One side of a blood vessel wall near a site of tissue injury. Fibroblast growth factor (FGF) released from injured cells stimulates the endothelial cells to release plasminogen activator and procollagenase. Plasminogen activator liberates plasmin from plasma-derived plasminogen and activates collagenase. Together these enzymes degrade the basement membrane (BM) beneath the stimulated endothelial cells. (*B*) Endothelial cell chemoattractants such as heparin and fibronectin fragments (FNF), which have been released at the site of injury, stimulate the endothelial cells to project pseudopodia through the BM defect and subsequently to migrate into the connective tissue space. (*C*) As endothelial cells migrate, they deposit a provisional matrix (PM) on which they translocate. They subsequently regenerate BM, through which they form stable connections to the neodermis. Once the capillary bud has extended some distance from the vessel of origin, a lumen forms between the endothelial cells, establishing a tube for blood flow. Endothelial cells within the vessel of origin proliferate to provide additional endothelial cells for the extending capillary.

Reepithelialization proceeds rapidly after epidermal disruption, thereby reestablishing the cutaneous barrier to the outside world. In fact, reepithelialization begins within hours after injury and is affected by the movement of epidermal cells from the wound margin and residual hair follicles over the wound surface.[22] Motility of epidermal cells across the wound surface is dependent upon epidermal cell metamorphosis. The alteration of cell phenotype includes retraction of intracellular keratin filaments, dissolution of intercellular desmosomes (structures that normally interlink epidermal cells, conferring tensile strength on the normal epidermis), and formation of peripheral cytoplasmic actin filaments to provide a motor apparatus.[23] Within a day or two, epidermal cells at the wound margin begin to proliferate, providing the migrating epidermis with a new supply of cells. Epidermal growth factor (EGF) or TGF-α likely provides the signal for this proliferation.[24,25] Migrating epidermal cells transit over a provisional matrix containing fibrin and fibronectin[26] (Fig. 22-3). Epidermal cells have the capacity to deposit fibronectin in the extracellular matrix in vivo.[27] TGF-β may stimulate the cells to do so,[28] thereby promoting translocation[29] over the surface of the wound. As reepithelialization is established, a new basement membrane forms from the wound margin inward, zippering the new epidermis to the underlying matrix.[26] Once a

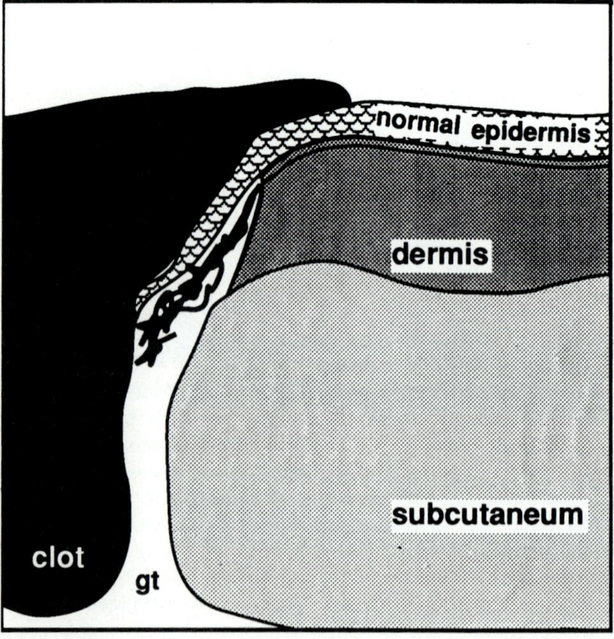

Figure 22-3 Epidermal migration over a provisional matrix within the granulation tissue (gt) begins within 24 h of injury. As reepithelialization proceeds, new basement membrane forms from the margin of the wound inward, acting as a zipper to fix the new epidermis in place on the neodermis.

new stratified epidermis covers the wound surface, the epidermal cells revert to their normal function.

TISSUE REMODELING

Tissue remodeling is the final stage of wound repair; however, it greatly overlaps the preceding tissue formation stage. In fact, as noted above, extracellular matrix remodeling, as manifested by the reestablishment of basement membranes, begins shortly after granulation tissue formation and reepithelialization. Extracellular matrix remodeling also occurs within the interstitial tissue. Most fibronectin is eliminated within a week or two after granulation tissue is established. Hyaluronate is replaced by and/or supplemented with heparin sulfate proteoglycans in basement membrane regions and with dermatan/chondroitin sulfate proteoglycans in the interstitium. Type I collagen fibers are slowly remodeled to contain less type III collagen and to form large bundles that provide the residual scar with increasing tensile strength. After much extracellular matrix remodeling, the easily traumatized granulation tissue slowly evolves into a strong, mature scar. The pathobiology of the epidermal-dermal junction and of collagen, elastin, and glycosaminoglycans is reviewed in Chaps. 19 and 21.

REFERENCES

1. Clark RAF: Cutaneous wound repair, in LE Goldsmith (ed), *Biochemistry and Physiology of the Skin*. London, Oxford University Press, in press.
2. Terkeltaub RA, Ginsberg MH: Platelets and response to injury, in RAF Clark, PM Henson (eds), *Molecular and Cellular Biology of Wound Repair*. New York, Plenum, 1989, p 35.
3. Furie B, Furie BC: The molecular basis of blood coagulation. *Cell* 53:505, 1988.
4. Ginsberg MH et al: Cytoadhesins, integrins, and platelets. *Thromb Haemost* 59:1, 1988.
5. Ross R et al: The biology of platelet-derived growth factor. *Cell* 46:155, 1986.
6. Derynck R: Transforming growth factor-α. *Cell* 54:593, 1988.
7. Sporn MB et al: Some recent advances in the chemistry and biology of transforming growth factor-beta. *J Cell Biol* 105:1039, 1987.
8. Carney DH, Cunningham DD: Role of specific cell surface receptors in thrombin-stimulated cell division. *Cell* 15:1341, 1978.
9. Folkman J, Klagsbrun M: Angiogenic factors. *Science* 235:442, 1987.
10. Chien S (ed): *Vascular Endothelium in Health and Disease. Advances in Experimental Medicine and Biology*. New York, Plenum, vol 242, 1989.
11. Tonnesen MG: Neutrophil-endothelial cell interactions: mechanisms of neutrophil adherence to vascular endothelium. *J Invest Dermatol* 93(Suppl):53s, 1989.
12. Johnston GI et al: Cloning of GMP-140, a granule membrane protein of platelets and endothelial cells: sequence similarity to proteins involved in cell adhesion and inflammation. *Cell* 56:1033, 1989.
13. Riches DWH: The multiple roles of macrophages in wound repair, in RAF Clark, PM Henson (eds), *Molecular and Cellular Biology of Wound Repair*. New York, Plenum, 1989, p 213.
14. Madtes DK et al: Induction of transforming growth factor-α in activated human alveolar macrophages. *Cell* 53:285, 1988.
15. Ruoslahti E: Fibronectin and its receptors. *Annu Rev Biochem* 57:375, 1988.
16. Welch MP et al: Temporal relationships between F-actin bundle formation, collagen and

fibronectin matrix assembly, and fibronectin receptor expression, to wound contraction. *J Cell Biol* 110:133, 1990.
17. Clark RAF et al: Platelet isoforms of platelet-derived growth factor stimulate fibroblasts to contract collagen gel matrices. *J Clin Invest* 84:1036, 1989.
18. Ausprunk DH, Folkman J: Migration and proliferation of endothelial cells in preformed and newly formed blood vessels during tumor angiogenesis. *Microvasc Res* 14:53, 1977.
19. Ausprunk DH et al: Proteoglycans in the microvasculature. II. Histochemical localization in proliferating capillaries of the rabbit cornea. *Am J. Pathol* 103:367, 1981.
20. Clark RAF et al: Blood vessel fibronectin increases in conjunction with endothelial cell proliferation and capillary ingrowth during wound healing. *J Invest Dermatol* 79:269, 1982.
21. Mignatti P et al: In vitro angiogenesis on the human amniotic membrane: requirement for basic fibroblast growth factor-induced proteinases. *J Cell Biol* 108:671, 1989.
22. Winter GD: Formation of the scab and the rate of epithelialization of superficial wounds in the skin of the young domestic pig. *Nature* 193:293, 1962.
23. Gabbiani G et al: Cytoplasmic filaments and gap junctions in epithelial cells and myofibroblasts during wound healing. *J Cell Biol* 76:561, 1978.
24. Cohen S: The stimulation of epidermal proliferation by a specific protein (EGF). *Dev Biol* 12:394, 1965.
25. Barrandon Y, Green H: Cell migration is essential for sustained growth of keratinocyte colonies: the roles of transforming growth factor-α and epidermal growth factor. *Cell* 50:1131, 1987.
26. Clark RAF et al: Fibronectin and fibrin provide a provisional matrix for epidermal cell migration during wound reepithelialization. *J Invest Dermatol* 79:264, 1982.
27. Grinwood RE et al: Fibronectin extracellular matrix assembly by human epidermal cells implanted into athymic mice. *J Invest Dermatol* 90:434, 1988.
28. Wikner NE et al: Transforming growth factor-β stimulates the expression of fibronectin by human keratinocytes. *J Invest Dermatol* 91:207, 1988.
29. Nickoloff BJ et al: Modulation of keratinocyte motility: correlation with production of extracellular matrix molecules in response to growth promoting and antiproliferative factors. *Am J Pathol* 132:543, 1988.

SECTION EIGHT

DISORDERS OF THE PANNICULUS ADIPOSUS

23

Biology and Pathophysiology of the Panniculus Adiposus

Clay J. Cockerell

The subcutaneous fat, also known as the panniculus adiposus, is that portion of the skin that lies between the lower portion of the reticular dermis and the fascia. Because of its deep location, it is not visible. However, the fullness and rounded contours of the body are largely the result of deposition or lack of fat at various sites.

Structurally, the subcutaneous fat is composed of lipocytes and fibrous tissue, both of which are mesenchymal in origin. The fibrous tissue, also known as the fibrous trabeculae or septa, represents an extension of the overlying reticular dermis.[1] In the embryo, primitive spindle-shaped stem cells migrate to a location just beneath the dermis and undergo differentiation, acquiring the ability to synthesize and deposit lipid within their cytoplasms. As a result of massive accumulation of lipid, the nuclei of the cells are compressed peripherally, leaving only a thin rim of cytoplasm. Lipocytes undergo rapid division prenatally and in infancy up until the age of 1 to 2 years. At that point, cell division ceases and any increase in fat deposition in the body occurs as a consequence predominantly of hypertrophy of cells rather than hyperplasia, although some evidence suggests that fat cell turnover may occur throughout life.[2]

Histologically, lipocytes are divided into small anatomic units. A group of lipocytes supplied by a network of capillaries is referred to as a primary microlobule. Several primary microlobules comprise a secondary lobule. Finally, a number of secondary lobules divided by fibrous trabeculae comprises the panniculus adiposus proper. Secondary lobules are supplied by one arteriole and two draining veins.[1] Because individual primary microlobules are supplied by an isolated network of capillaries without connections to other arterioles, they are relatively vulnerable to ischemic injury. This is an important concept in understanding the pathophysiology of inflammatory panniculitides.

When examined electron microscopically, individual lipocytes are shown to have prominent Golgi apparati and many ribosomes useful in the synthesis and deposition of lipid. Relatively few mitochondria are present in lipocytes with the exception of those comprising brown fat, a specialized form of fat deposited in the central upper back area. Brown fat adipocytes contain numerous mitochondria and function primarily to generate heat. Although brown fat serves an important thermoregulatory function in infants, it is thought to be largely vestigial in adults.[3]

The functions of the subcutaneous fat can be divided into biochemical and anatomic ones. Biochemically, the fat serves as a nutritional depot. Lipocytes engage in lipogenesis as well as in deposition, storage, and mobilization of lipid. Membranes of individual lipocytes possess insulin and catecholamine receptors and, in addition, contain an important hormone-sensitive lipase, the action of which is stimulated by epinephrine and lessened by decreased insulin levels. Anatomic functions of the fat are many. Classically, it serves as a heat insulator. It also serves as a shock absorber, as well as a conduit for blood vessels and nerves. In addition, it may serve as an anchoring site for hair follicles on the scalp. Wound healing is facilitated by subcutaneous fat, as demonstrated by the relatively poor healing of ulcers when they occur over areas with little panniculus. It also facilitates skin mobility over underlying structures, as demonstrated by the tautness and lack of free motion of the skin over joints and other body parts in conditions such as scleroderma. As alluded to previously, subcutaneous fat also contributes to the body's contour and generates heat in the case of brown fat.[1]

PATHOPHYSIOLOGY OF DISEASES OF FAT

Diseases of fat can be divided into inflammatory conditions or panniculitides, neoplastic processes, malformations, atrophies, and generalized hyperplasias. Probably the most important to the dermatologist are the panniculitides. These may be induced on a number of different bases, including hypersensitivity phenomena such as autoimmune diseases, physical injury such as cold, blunt trauma or injections of foreign substances, infiltrations such as deposition of abnormal material or neoplastic cells, metabolic abnormalities such as circulating lipolytic enzymes, and, finally, infectious diseases. Furthermore, on occasion, the lipid within individual lipocytes may be abnormal, resulting in inflammation of the fat such as in sclerema neonatorum.[4] Panniculitides have traditionally been divided into those that involve either the septa mostly, the lobules mostly, or both (Figs. 23-1 to 23-3).[5,6] Furthermore, the presence or absence of

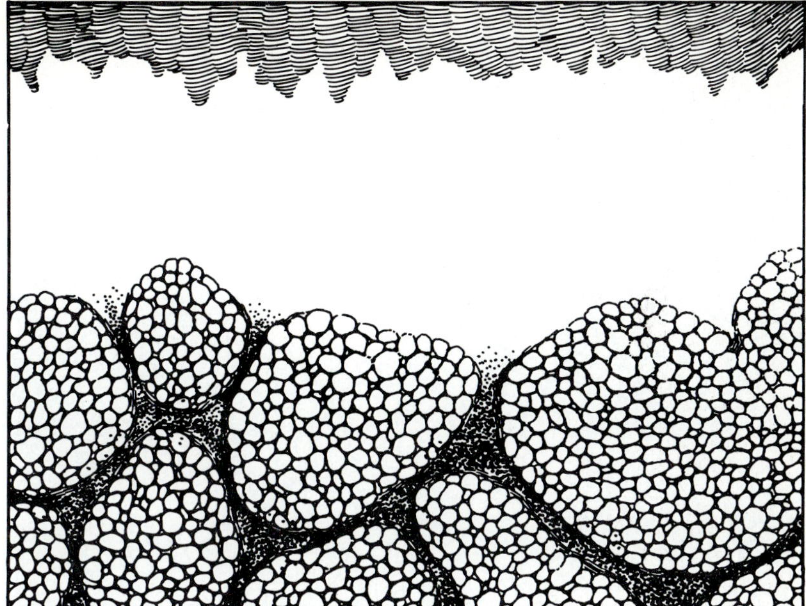

Figure 23-1 Panniculitis involving mostly the septa.

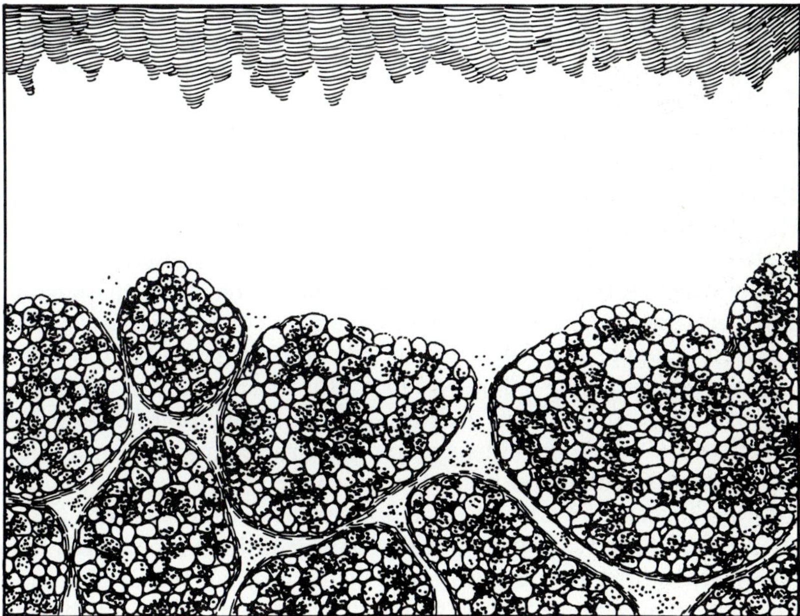

Figure 23-2 Panniculitis involving mostly the lobules.

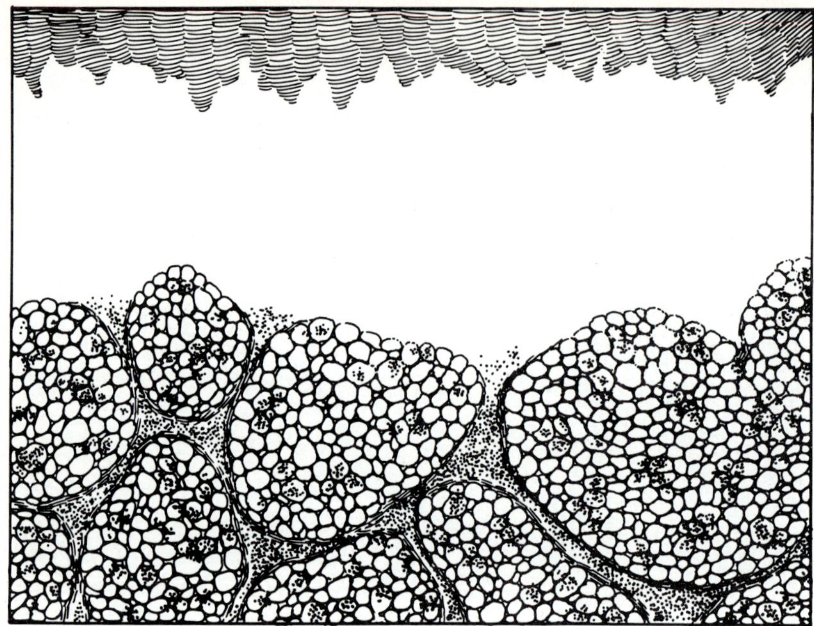

Figure 23-3 Panniculitis involving the septa and lobules equally.

vasculitis is also an important distinction to make histologically. Each histological reaction pattern can be explained pathophysiologically on the basis of one of the aforementioned mechanisms.

In addition to inflammatory diseases of the fat, however, neoplasms and malformations are quite common. One of the most common benign neoplasms of the skin is the lipoma. The rare liposarcoma is a malignant soft tissue neoplasm of fat that often has a poor prognosis. Certain malformations of fat, such as nevus lipomatosus and focal dermal hypoplasia (Goltz's syndrome), result from abnormal embryological development of the panniculus. The amount of fat in the body may be either diminished, as in certain generalized lipoatrophic conditions such as the Lawrence-Seip syndrome of lipoatrophy, insulin-resistant diabetes mellitus, and acanthosis nigricans, or excessive, as in certain metabolic diseases of increased lipocyte number such as the Michelin tire baby syndrome. Local lipoatrophy may be a consequence of a prior localized inflammatory disease or a local injection of a drug such as triamcinolone acetonide or insulin. Finally are the severe psychological problems that may underlie obesity or may be enhanced by its presence.[4,7]

Clinically, diseases of the fat have appearances that correlate well with the histological features. For example, panniculitides are usually characterized by warm, gently domed, reddish to purplish nodules or plaques in areas where subcutaneous fat is most prominent, such as the thighs, posterior portions of the lower legs, buttocks, and trunk.[7] When there is extensive ischemia as a consequence of vasculitis or when there is direct enzymatic degradation of fat, there is often overlying ulceration and drainage of an oily material that represents the breakdown products of the fat. In cases in which the subcutaneous fat is replaced by extensive thickening of the septa, the skin loses its mobility over underlying structures. In examples of lipoatrophy, there is a large depression between the surrounding normal skin and the atrophic area due to loss of substance. Finally, benign neoplasms of fat are characterized by gentle dome-shaped elevations of the skin with a spongy feel. Because the panniculitides are the most important diseases of the subcutaneous fat in dermatology, a few representative examples of them will be discussed.

PANNICULITIS WITH PREDOMINANTLY SEPTAL INFLAMMATION: ERYTHEMA NODOSUM

Erythema nodosum consists of reddish, painful, warm, dome-shaped nodules usually present on the anterior surfaces of the lower legs (Fig. 23-4). It often arises following a physiological insult such as an infectious disease, a metabolic inflammatory disease such as inflammatory bowel disease or sarcoidosis, or as a response to ingestion of certain drugs.[8,9] In

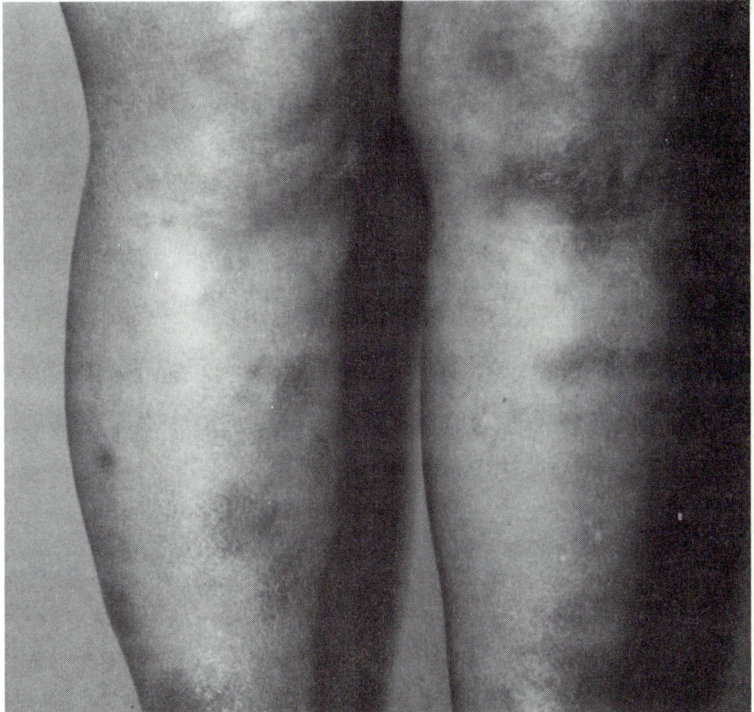

Figure 23-4 Erythema nodosum. Warm, red, tender plaques and nodules are distributed mostly on the anterior surfaces of the lower legs.

many cases, the cause may not be apparent. Although many infectious diseases may lead to the development of erythema nodosum as a sequela, the most common one is streptococcal disease, either clinical or subclinical. Streptococcal infections associated with erythema nodosum usually involve the upper respiratory tract rather than the skin or soft tissues. A serum antistreptolysin 0 titer will be elevated in most patients who had a streptococcal infection and later developed erythema nodosum, providing a valuable clinical clue to the cause of the panniculitis.[8,9] Other infectious diseases that may lead to erythema nodosum include tuberculosis, especially primary pulmonary tuberculosis, leprosy, leptospirosis, typhoid fever, yersiniosis, brucellosis, toxoplasmosis, chlamydial infections, Milker's nodule, infectious mononucleosis, and cat scratch disease. Deep fungal infections such as coccidioidomycosis and histoplasmosis also may be associated with erythema nodosum.[8,9] Thus, in a patient with erythema nodosum, it is important to exclude the possibility of an underlying serious infectious disease.

Other diseases such as sarcoidosis, especially the acute stage associated with hilar adenopathy and lacrimal gland inflammation,[10] Behcet's disease[11] and inflammatory bowel disease, both Crohn's disease and ulcerative colitis, may be associated with erythema nodosum. Although the erythema nodosum may flare when these diseases are exacerbated, the panniculitis and the underlying condition may run completely distinct courses. Finally, erythema nodosum has been associated with ingestion of drugs such as gold, sulfathiazole, and oral contraceptives.[7,8] It has also been noted to occur in pregnancy.[12]

Histologically, the septa of the subcutaneous fat are involved predominantly (Fig. 23-5). Initially, there is septal edema and an inflammatory cell infiltrate of neutrophils, eosinophils, and mononuclear cells. A few cells invariably are present in the surrounding lobules and the overlying dermis. In time, a fully developed granulomatous panniculitis develops that is characterized by marked thickening of septa with fibrosis, granulomatous inflammation, and peripheral granulation tissue where septa join fat lobules. Because of the periseptal lobular inflammation, lipocyte necrosis with "foamy" macrophages may be seen. Eventually the inflammation diminishes, the granulation tissue becomes fibrotic, and the process undergoes resolution, leaving only slightly thickened septa and slight loss of fat substance. In time, total remodeling to normal fat architecture may be observed.[5,13–15]

Although the exact pathophysiology of erythema nodosum has yet to be determined, it is almost certainly due to a hypersensitivity phenomenon. The presence of the granulomatous inflammation indicates that type IV hypersensitivity (cell-mediated immunity) is ongoing. Circulating immune complexes and deposition of C3, IgM, and fibrin within blood vessel walls have been demonstrated. Why such immune reactants should be deposited within blood vessels, with no consequent vasculitis, remains to be determined; nevertheless, deposition of immune reactants would be expected

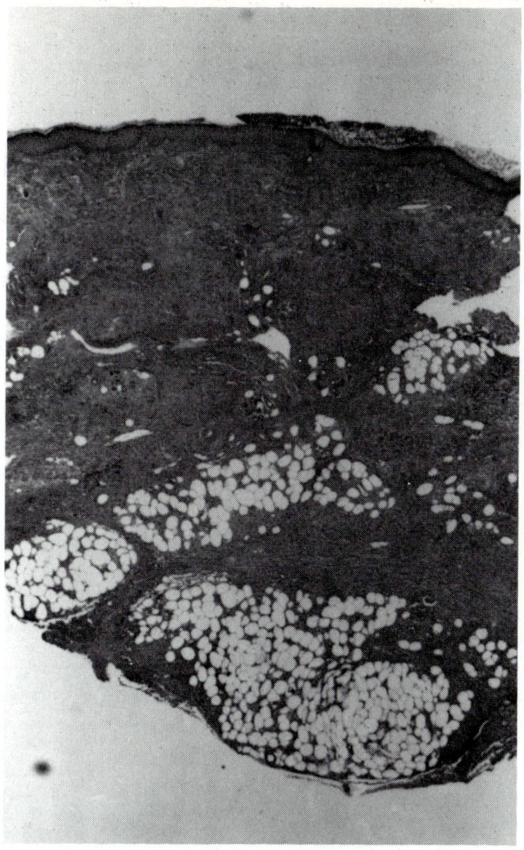

Figure 23-5 Erythema nodosum. Histologically, there is involvement predominantly of the septa of the subcutis, which are markedly widened by inflammation and fibrosis. Hematoxylin and eosin. ×10 in the original magnification.

to lead to fixation of complement, with production of chemotactic factors that result in the influx of inflammatory cells.[7,8,15] This eventually leads to the clinical manifestations of inflammation and the disease itself, namely, warm, tender, red nodules. In time, chronic inflammation supersedes the acute inflammation, resulting in a granulomatous infiltrate and fibroplasia. Because of the paucity of inflammation of the lobules, clinically, when erythema nodosum undergoes resolution, little if any residua is seen. However, there is often extravasation of erythrocytes, which may lead to a brownish discoloration with the appearance of bruising.[9]

Because erythema nodosum results from a hypersensitivity inflammatory reaction, treatment is directed at interrupting the ongoing inflammation. Nonsteroidal anti-inflammatory agents that inhibit prostaglandins are often effective alone, especially when administered early in the course of the disease. Intralesional injections of corticosteroids such as triamcinolone acetonide, as well as systemic corticosteroids, further reduce inflammation. Treatment of the underlying associated disease, if present, is also beneficial in many cases, especially with infections.[8]

LOBULAR PANNICULITIS WITH VASCULITIS: NODULAR VASCULITIS (ERYTHEMA INDURATUM)

Nodular vasculitis is characterized by an often chronic, persistent panniculitis seen most commonly in young and middle-aged women. Initially there are slightly elevated, dull red nodules that are usually only slightly tender (Fig. 23-6). Later lesions often undergo ulceration and exude an oily material that represents the breakdown products of fat. Historically, this condition was thought to be associated with tuberculosis, but it is now known to occur in patients with no history of tuberculosis or any other systemic disease.[7]

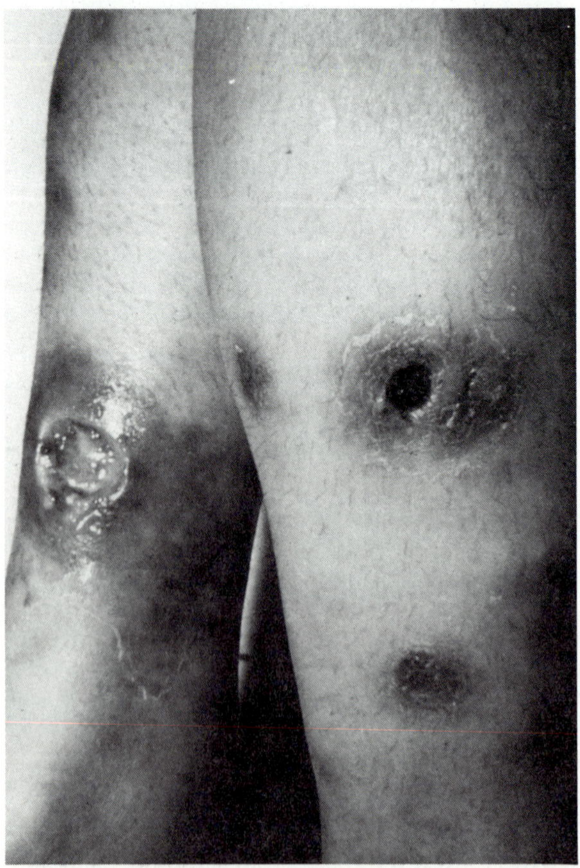

Figure 23-6 Nodular vasculitis. Located on the posterior portions of the lower legs are reddish nodules with central ulcerations.

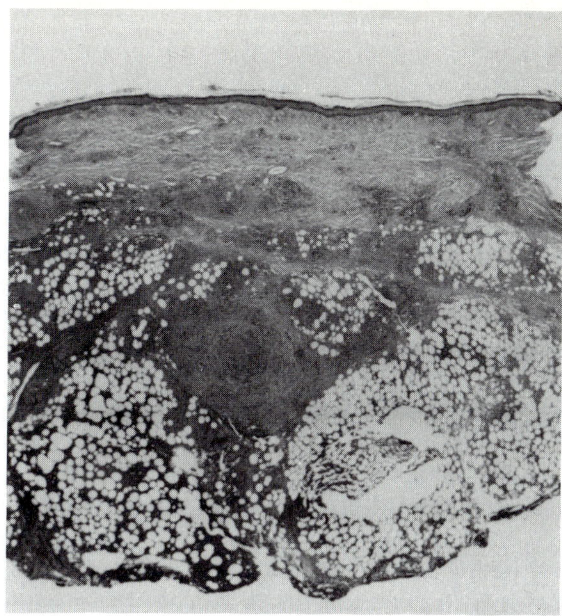

Figure 23-7 Nodular vasculitis. Histologically, there is marked inflammation of a medium-sized blood vessel centrally, with inflammation of the surrounding lobules. Note the relative sparing of the septa other than at the site of the vasculitis. Hematoxylin and eosin. ×10 in the original magnification.

The precise etiopathogenesis of nodular vasculitis remains obscure. The fact that there is a vasculitis suggests that the condition may be an immune complex–mediated process somewhat similar to that described for erythema nodosum.

Histologically, there is a medium-sized vessel vasculitis involving veins in which there are neutrophils and fibrin within the vessel wall (Fig. 23-7). There may be thrombosis. As the vascular lumen is compromised, ischemia develops distally, resulting in fat necrosis. As a consequence, there is a marked influx of polymorphonuclear leukocytes as well as mononuclear cells to the damaged fat lobules. Because degenerated lipid induces intense inflammation, a dense inflammatory infiltrate also develops in the overlying dermis that may lead to ulceration. Over time, the inflammatory response becomes more chronic, with the infiltrate consisting predominantly of mononuclear cells, especially multinucleated histiocytes, within damaged fat lobules. On resolution, dense fibrous tissue may totally replace the fat, leading to the clinical appearance of a scar and a depressed area in the skin.[5,13] Thus, the pathological changes in nodular vasculitis are all consequences of the ischemia of fat lobules resulting from the initial vasculitis. The ischemic necrosis leads to release of inflammatory mediators, resulting in a dense inflammation that is highly destructive. This sequence of events readily explains the clinical appearance of the skin lesions.

Treatment is directed at diminishing the inflammatory reaction and reversing the vasculitis. Agents such as dapsone and iodides have been used with variable success.[16] Intralesional corticosteroids as well as systemic corticosteroids also have been partially efficacious.

LOBULAR PANNICULITIS WITHOUT VASCULITIS: LUPUS ERYTHEMATOSUS PROFUNDUS

When lupus erythematosus involves the fat, a lobular panniculitis results known as lupus erythematosus (LE) profundus. It may be seen with either systemic LE or purely cutaneous forms of the disease, but up to 50 percent of patients who clinically manifest LE profundus progress to develop systemic disease. Clinically, well-circumscribed, firm, nontender subcutaneous nodules are present in a variety of locations, often on the proximal extremities and trunk as well as the face (Fig. 23-8).[17,18] When these lesions resolve, deep depressions may remain at their sites. Although individual lesions usually are not painful, there is often warmth and redness. Patients may have other cutaneous manifestations of LE, but in some cases, panniculitis may be the only clinical manifestation of the disease.[17]

The pathogenesis of LE profundus is analogous to that of other manifestations of LE, namely, immune complex–mediated disease as a consequence of the body's manufacture of autoantibodies to nucleic acids, nucleoproteins, and cytoplasmic antigens. In LE profundus, immunoglobulins and complement proteins are deposited within blood vessel walls of

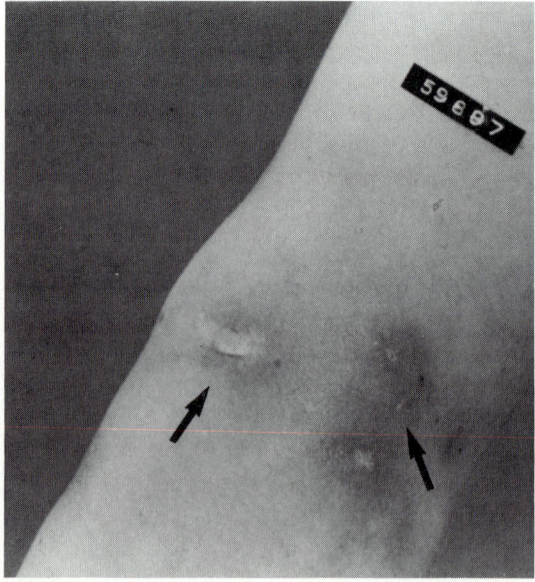

Figure 23-8 LE profundus. There are depressed areas with residual reddish-brown nodules on the arm. Often severe atrophy is a sequela.

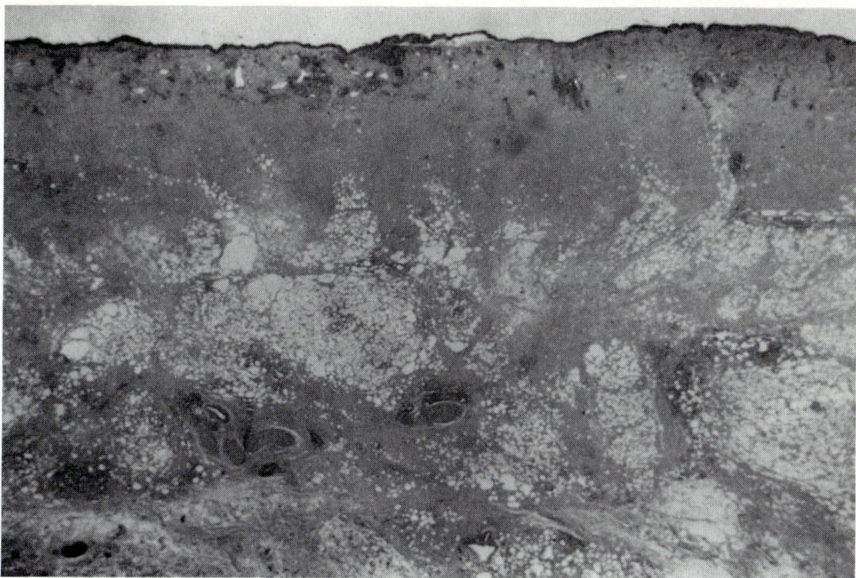

Figure 23-9 LE profundus. Histologically, there is diffuse lobular involvement with abundant degeneration of fat. There is also some inflammation of the overlying dermis. Hematoxylin and eosin. ×10 in the original magnification.

the deep dermis and subcutis and, on occasion, at the dermal-epidermal junction.[17,18] An inflammatory reaction ensues; however, rather than an influx of polymorphonuclear leukocytes, as is seen with erythema induratum and erythema nodosum initially, lymphocytes and histiocytes as well as plasma cells infiltrate the lesions of LE profundus. Plasma cells and lymphocytes may be numerous and may form aggregates within which germinal centers may form. The histological pattern is that of a diffuse lobular panniculitis with relative sparing of the septa (Fig. 23-9). Abundant fat necrosis and lipocyte "ghosts" at the sites of previously viable lipocytes are prominent features. The mummification of fat, as well as the dense inflammatory cell infiltrate of mononuclear cells, readily explains the clinical induration. In time, the fat is replaced with fibroplasia, and clinical deep atrophy manifested as "gullies" is seen.[5]

Treatment is similar to that of other forms of LE and is directed against the inflammatory response. Systemic corticosteroids, antimalarials, and other antimetabolites have all been shown to be of value.[17,18]

LOBULAR PANNICULITIS OF METABOLIC ORIGIN: PANCREATIC PANNICULITIS

Pancreatic panniculitis is not a true inflammatory panniculitis but represents tissue damage as a consequence of circulating lipases released from the pancreas damaged as a result of pancreatitis or a pancreatic

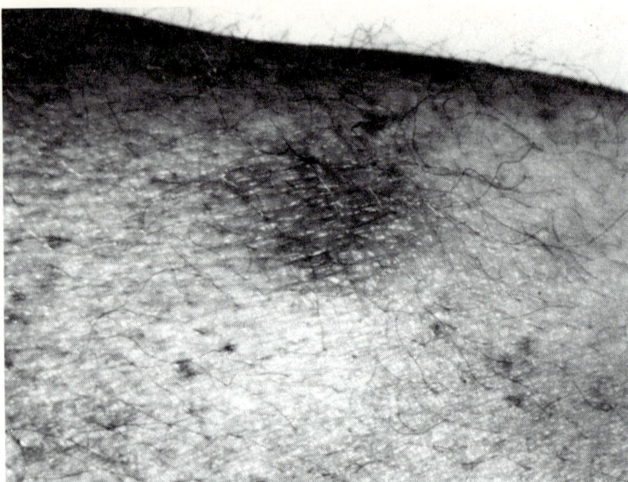

Figure 23-10 Pancreatic panniculitis. Subtle reddish, dome-shaped nodules may be the earliest manifestation.

neoplasm. Clinically, there are crops of slightly indurated, reddish, somewhat tender subcutaneous nodules present at any site of the body where subcutaneous fat is located (Fig. 23-10).[19] In time, there may be ulceration and drainage of either an oily material or a white, chalky substance. Lipases are released from the pancreas in high concentrations and are carried to the skin hematogenously. These enzymes result in dissolution

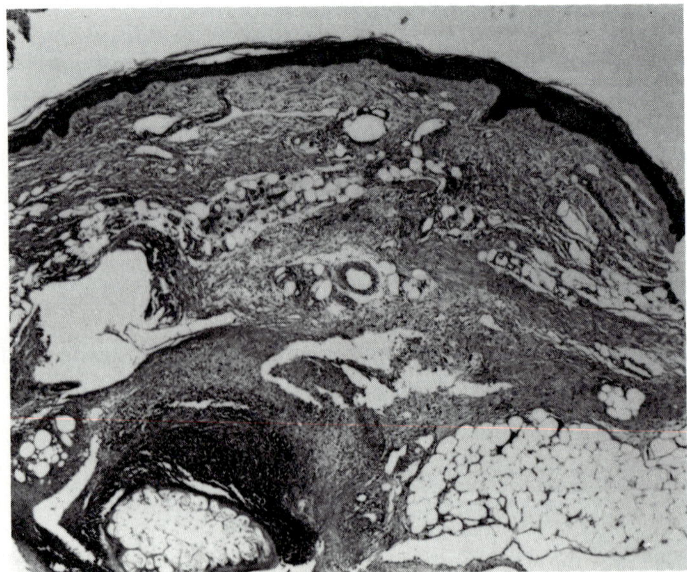

Figure 23-11 Pancreatic panniculitis. Histologically, there is focal lobular involvement and a darkly staining area corresponding to degenerated, saponified fat. Hematoxylin and eosin. ×10 in the original magnification.

of the fat and formation of free triglycerides that bind with circulating calcium ions to form soaps.[19] Histopathologically, there is characteristically massive but focal fat necrosis, adjacent to which may be normal, unaffected fat lobules (Fig. 23-11). Degenerated lipocytes appear granular and basophilic and have foci of calcification. Small, calcific, honeycomb-like structures are seen at the sites of membranes of degenerated lipocytes. Initially, little if any inflammation is present, but in time, a mixed inflammatory cell infiltrate that may be granulomatous results from the influx of inflammatory cells secondary to the damage of fat. The relative paucity of inflammation seen initially explains the relatively subtle nature of the process at its onset. In time, however, this inflammation may be dense, and ulcerations may result from degeneration of fat as well as overlying skin.[5]

Treatment is directed at the underlying pancreatic abnormality. Obviously, until the circulating enzyme level is reduced, the fat is vulnerable to its destructive action.

REFERENCES

1. Jakubovic HR, Ackerman AB: Development, morphology and physiology, in SL Moschella, HJ Hurley (eds), *Dermatology,* 2d ed. Philadelphia, Saunders, 1985, p 45.
2. Knittle JL et al: The growth of adipose tissue in children and adolescents. *J Clin Invest* 63:239, 1979.
3. Lever WF, Schaumburg-Lever G: *Histopathology of the Skin,* 7th ed. Philadelphia, JB Lippincott, 1990, p 269.
4. Fleischmajer R, Mattis NR: Diseases of the subcutaneous tissue, in SL Moschella, HJ Hurley (eds) *Dermatology,* 2d ed. Philadelphia, Saunders, 1985, p 1169.
5. Ackerman AB: *Histologic Diagnosis of Inflammatory Skin Diseases.* Philadelphia, Lea & Febiger, 1978, p 778.
6. Ackerman AB: *Histologic Diagnosis of Inflammatory Skin Diseases—Supplement.* Philadelphia, Lea & Febiger, 1988, p 37.
7. Thiers BH: Panniculitis. *Dermatol Clin* 1:4, 1983.
8. Blomgren SE: Erythema nodosum. *Semin Arthritis Rheum* 4:1, 1974.
9. Hellerstrom S: Erythema nodosum. *Acta Derm Venereol (Stockh)* 46:469, 1966.
10. Lofgren S, Lundback H: The bilateral hilar lymphoma syndrome: a study of the relation to tuberculosis and sarcoidosis in 212 cases. *Acta Med Scand* 142:265, 1952.
11. Frayha RA, Nasr FW: Erythema nodosum—arthropathy complex as an initial presentation of Behcet's disease: report of five cases. *J Rheumatol* 5:224, 1978.
12. Salvatore MA, Lynch PJ: Erythema nodosum, estrogens and pregnancy. *Arch Dermatol* 116:557, 1980.
13. Ackerman AB et al: *Differential Diagnosis in Dermatopathology.* Philadelphia, Lea & Febiger, 1982, p 66.
14. Ackerman AB, Ragaz A: *The Lives of Lesions: Chronology in Dermatopathology.* New York, Masson, 1984, p 67.
15. Winkelmann RK, Forstrom L: New observations on the histopathology of erythema nodosum. *J Invest Dermatol* 65:441, 1975.
16. Schulz EJ, Whiting DA: Treatment of erythema nodosum and nodular vasculitis with potassium iodide. *Br J Dermatol* 94:75, 1976.
17. Prystowsky SD, Gilliam JN: Cutaneous subsets of lupus erythematosus. *Dermatol Clin* 1:4, 1983.
18. Tuffanelli DL: Lupus erythematosus (panniculitis) profundus. *Hawaii Med J* 41:394, 1982.
19. Potts D et al: Syndrome of pancreatic disease, subcutaneous fat necrosis and polyserositis. *Am J Med* 58:417, 1975.

SECTION NINE

PHOTOBIOLOGY AND PHOTOMEDICINE

24

Photobiology and Pathophysiology of Cutaneous Responses to Electromagnetic Radiation

R. William Gange and Henry W. Lim

Awareness of electromagnetic radiation results from its effects on the eyes and the skin. In the retina, radiation over a narrow range of wavelengths causes specific wavelength-dependent photochemical events that provide a color map of the environment. In the skin, radiation over a wider range is absorbed, translated into thermal energy, and felt as heat.

Solar radiation also causes sunburn and tanning, which occur after a latent period of hours or days. Skin aging and skin cancer are also largely the result of solar exposure; in these instances, the changes are chronic and accumulate over decades.

In this chapter, interactions between electromagnetic radiation and biological substrates are discussed, with emphasis on the skin (Fig. 24-1). We first review the responses of *normal* skin that result in inflammation, repair of damage, and protection from further exposure to electromagnetic radiation. The pathophysiology of *abnormal* cutaneous responses will be examined, whether resulting from intrinsic abnormalities or from interactions between the skin, radiation, and exogenous photosensitizers. Finally, *therapeutic* uses of nonionizing radiation (phototherapy) will be reviewed.

ELECTROMAGNETIC RADIATION

Electromagnetic radiation is best understood as having the properties of both waves and particles. Electromagnetic radiation has the character of

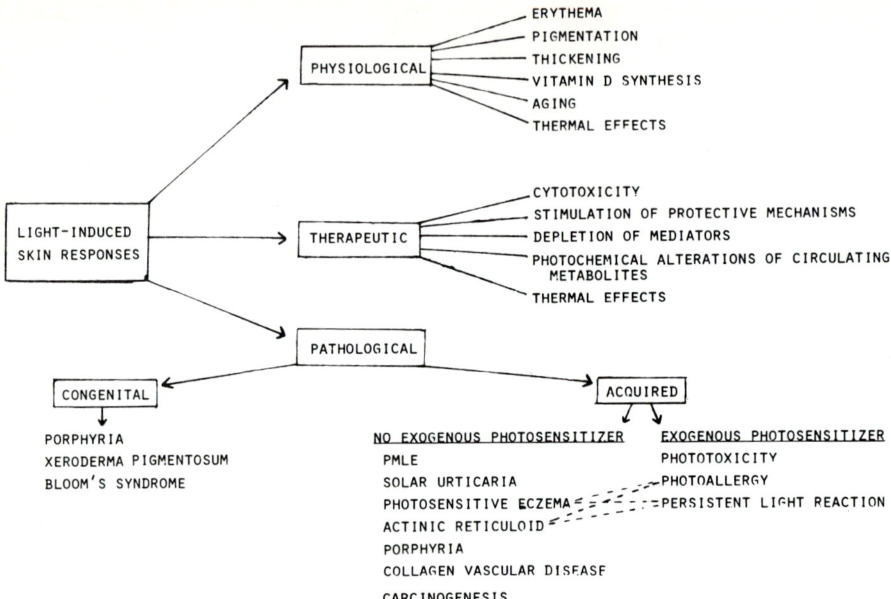

Figure 24-1 Interaction of nonionizing radiation with skin.

transverse waves, with electric and magnetic fields oscillating at right angles to each other and to the direction of propagation. The interaction of the oscillating electric fields with charged matter determines its effect on molecules. In addition to its transverse-wave character, electromagnetic radiation may be described as a stream of discrete packets of energy known as *quanta* or *photons*.

Electromagnetic radiation comprises a continuous spectrum of wavelengths that have been arbitrarily classified into the spectral regions (Fig. 24-2). The portion of the spectrum of direct concern to photobiologists extends from the shortwave ultraviolet C (UVC) through the infrared. Because of atmospheric absorption, largely by ozone, terrestrial sunlight does not include UVC.

Within the ultraviolet and visible light range (Fig. 24-2), a useful wavelength unit is the nanometer (nm); 1 nm equals 10^{-9} m or 10 Å. In the infrared region, the most commonly used unit of wavelength is the micron (μm): 1 μm equals 10^{-6} m or 10^3 nm; older literature used the symbol μ. Radiation of wavelengths shorter than 10 nm generally ionizes molecules (removes electrons) indiscriminately and is therefore known as ionizing radiation.

Radiation in the UVC region causes erythema of normal skin very efficiently and can cause photokeratitis (inflammation of the cornea). UVC is also called germicidal radiation because it kills one-celled organisms.

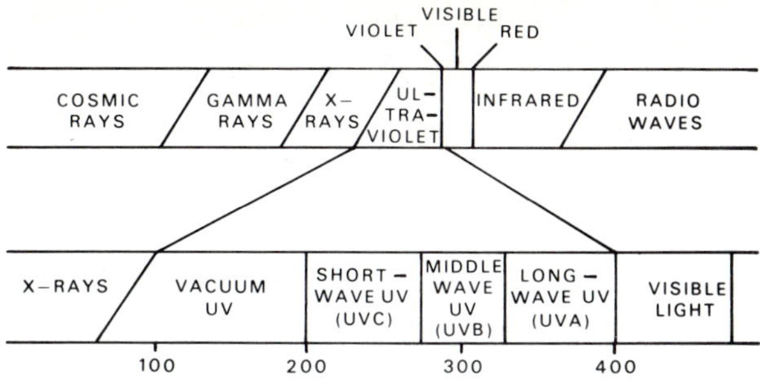

Figure 24-2 The spectrum of electromagnetic radiation. (*From TB Fitzpatrick et al, Dermatology in General Medicine, 3d ed, New York, McGraw-Hill, 1987, p 1443.*)

Solar ultraviolet radiation with wavelengths between 290 and 320 nm (ultraviolet B, UVB) reaches earth in relatively small quantities, but these are sufficient to cause sunburning of human skin. For this reason, UVB is often referred to as the *sunburn spectrum.* UVB induces skin cancer in laboratory animals and mutations in bacteria. Epidemiological evidence strongly suggests that solar UVB causes most skin cancers in humans. Long-term UVB exposure is also the major factor responsible for producing the changes in human skin that are commonly termed *solar aging.*

Longer ultraviolet wavelengths between 320 and 400 nm (ultraviolet A, UVA) are also melanogenic and erythemogenic, but the amount of energy required to produce either effect is much greater than for UVB. This region is frequently responsible for photosensitivity reactions in which chemical photosensitizers and UVA radiation interact to cause biological alterations. Most UVA effects are oxygen dependent and occur through free-radical mechanisms or reactive oxygen species. Cellular targets include lipid membranes and proteins as well as DNA.

UVC and UVB are absorbed by DNA and cause direct photochemical damage, for example, thymine-thymine dimers. Many of the biological effects of UVB are believed to result from such DNA photochemistry, which is independent of oxygen.

Visible and infrared radiation exert predominantly thermal effects on the skin under normal circumstances. However, certain photosensitizing agents such as porphyrins may be activated by visible light.

When photons are absorbed, energy is imparted to the absorbing matter and the photons cease to exist. The energy of electromagnetic radiation is proportional to the frequency ν of oscillation:

$$E = h\nu$$

where E = energy, h = Planck's constant, and ν = frequency. Energy is therefore proportional to wavelength λ, since the product of frequency and wavelength is constant and equal to the speed of light c:

$$\nu\lambda = c$$

$$E = \frac{hc}{\lambda}$$

Shorter wavelengths therefore have greater energy per photon.

INTERACTIONS BETWEEN RADIATION AND MATTER

Only radiation that is absorbed induces photochemical reactions. X-rays, γ rays, and other very high-energy photons affect biological and other material by relatively indiscriminate ionization of molecules, depending on the density of the electrons. The ionized molecules are highly reactive, and bonds may be broken or formed, but since the absorption is relatively nonspecific, the ability to select "target" molecules is limited. In the longer-wavelength regions, in contrast, the most significant biological result of infrared photons and microwaves is a nonselective thermal effect. It is in the intermediate-wavelength regions (ultraviolet and visible) that the energy of photons allows them to selectively cause electronic excitation of biological chromophore molecules, resulting in the photochemistry leading to biological responses. Consequently, this region of the electromagnetic spectrum is of greatest interest; ultraviolet and visible radiation can select from among a wide variety of target molecules and cause specific photochemical reactions. This is important for normal physiology; human color vision is an excellent example of how specific and biologically significant such processes may be. In *disease states,* abnormal photosensitivity to ultraviolet and visible radiation may be present; porphyrias are examples of such conditions. Finally, this region of the electromagnetic spectrum is of value as a *therapeutic tool* whereby photochemical events that are beneficial in treating certain diseases can be intentionally induced.

OPTICAL PROPERTIES OF SKIN AND BLOOD

The complex structures of skin layers and the presence of appendages such as hair follicles, sweat glands, and sebaceous glands make precise modeling of the path of optical radiation within the skin difficult. A schematic representation of the optical pathways of radiation in skin is shown in Fig. 24-3. Within any given layer, four basic optical processes may occur; direct reflection at the boundaries of the layer, due to differences in the index of refraction (greatest at the air–stratum corneum interface); scattering by molecules, particles, fibers, organelles, and cells within the layers; absorption (which may lead to photochemical reactions or dissipation of the absorbed energy via heat, fluorescence, or phosphorescence); and direct transmission through the layer.

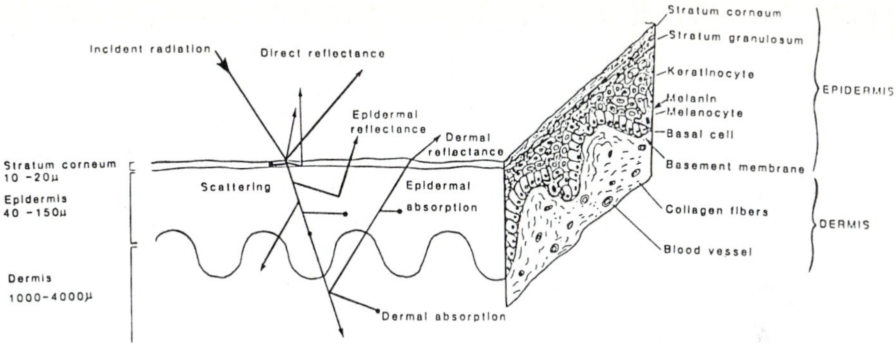

Figure 24-3 Optical pathways in the skin.

When radiation strikes the skin, part is remitted (leaves the skin's surface), part is absorbed in various layers, and part is transmitted inward to successive layers of cells until the energy of the incident beam has been dissipated.[1] A very small fraction of the absorbed radiation is reemitted at longer wavelengths (fluorescence). Between 5 and 7 percent of perpendicularly incident light is reflected by the outer surface of the stratum corneum because of the difference in refractive index between air and skin. This surface reflectance is relatively constant for all visible wavelengths and therefore does not, in general, greatly affect our perception of the color of skin. It does, however, account for the surface textural appearance. Fair Caucasian skin remits about one-half of incident visible and near-infrared radiation, mostly by backward scattering by collagen in the dermis. In passing through the overlying epidermis, visible radiation is absorbed by melanin. Our perception of skin color is, of course, determined by visible remittance, "white" skin remitting more than pigmented skin. Ultraviolet radiation of wavelengths of less than 320 nm is mostly absorbed within the stratum corneum or epidermis. In Caucasians, 35 to 50 percent of incident UVA radiation penetrates to the dermis. In general, in the biologically important range, from 290 nm in the ultraviolet to 1000 nm in the infrared, the longer wavelengths penetrate the skin more deeply. This accounts for the blue color of mongolian blue spots and blue nevi; light reaching and absorbed by melanin present at an abnormally deep location in the dermis is predominantly of longer (red) wavelengths; remitted light therefore contains relatively more of the shorter (blue) wavelengths.

The limited penetration of ultraviolet radiation also allows us to distinguish between dermal and epidermal melanin deposition. Illumination of intact human skin with a UVA source results in autofluorescence of the superficial dermis, and epidermal melanin will markedly reduce this by absorbing both incident and reemitted photons. Dermal melanosis is too deep to alter the autofluorescence and becomes less conspicuous under UVA radiation.

RESPONSES OF NORMAL SKIN TO ULTRAVIOLET RADIATION

Apart from the synthesis of vitamin D,[2] which is the only useful interaction between the skin and ultraviolet radiation so far identified, the acute responses of the skin to ultraviolet radiation may be broadly divided into inflammatory, reparative, and protective types. The initial phase of damage results in inflammation, with the classical signs of redness, swelling, and pain. This is followed by molecular and cellular repair. Adaptive changes such as thickening of the epidermis and stratum corneum and increased melanization also occur, providing increased protection against subsequent radiation.

Erythema

Erythema is the most conspicuous cutaneous response to nonionizing radiation in humans. It indicates an increase in blood in the superficial and deep vascular plexuses of the dermis and in white skin becomes visible when the volume increases by about 38 percent.[3] Detectability of erythema varies according to the degree of pigmentation present.

Erythema may be induced by a single dose of ultraviolet radiation of appropriate wavelengths. The minimal erythema dose (MED) is usually defined as the smallest amount of energy required to produce clearly marginated erythema in the exposed area and is expressed as energy delivered per unit area, usually joules per square meter or millijoules per square centimeter. It does not define the intensity of radiation or the duration of administration.

Most photobiological responses occur in proportion to the total energy or number of photons delivered and not in proportion to the rate of administration; doubling the irradiance and halving the time of irradiation therefore leads to the same magnitude of response. This important reciprocal relationship between intensity and time is called *reciprocity*, and for erythema it holds over a wide range. Reciprocity may break down under some circumstances. For example, when extremely low irradiances are given, repair mechanisms may keep pace with photon-induced damage. At very high irradiances, thermal effects may predominate over the usual photochemistry due to the finite rate at which heat may be dissipated.

In humans, erythema usually begins several hours after UVB irradiation, reaching a maximum between 12 and 24 h later. When intense erythema is induced, for example by administration of 4 to 8 times the MED of UVB, the response begins earlier, takes longer to peak, and is more persistent. The color fades over a period of several days, blending with other, later changes such as delayed tanning or the peeling of the skin, which may follow sufficient damage. The time course of erythema may vary with the wavelength; UVC tends to induce a more rapid response that peaks sooner and is less intense at 24 h than at 8 h. Delayed UVA erythema is maximal at about 6 h.[4]

There are also differences in dose-response relationships in different spectral regions. For example, 10 to 20 times the MED of UVC causes only a slight increase in erythema and scaling, and normal skin can easily tolerate 100 times the MED. In contrast, a relatively modest increase in the dose of UVB or UVA (6 to 8 times the MED) will usually cause intense dusky erythema, sometimes with edema and blistering, taking several weeks to heal. Five times the MED of noonday sun, which consists of polychromatic UVB, UVA, and longer wavelengths, may also cause severe erythema and blistering.

Factors Influencing the Development of Erythema

Many factors determine whether a given dose of ultraviolet radiation will cause erythema. The wavelength of the radiation and the pigmentation of the subject are the most important ones.

Wavelength. For any photobiological response to occur, photons must both penetrate to and be absorbed by the appropriate target molecule (chromophores). Both of these processes are wavelength dependent. Many biomolecules are altered by ultraviolet radiation, but a specific chromophore for the erythema response has not been identified.

The relative effectiveness of different wavelengths in the induction of erythema is expressed as an *erythema action spectrum,* which is obtained by plotting the reciprocal of the lowest exposure dose required to obtain a certain grade of erythema response against wavelength. For minimal erythema, the most erythemogenic wavelengths are in the 250- to 290-nm range of the ultraviolet spectrum, with a rapid decrease in effectiveness as the wavelength increases. Figure 24-4 shows action spectra for erythema and for melanogenesis in fair-skinned humans. The difference between the 8- and 24-h erythema action spectra at shorter wavelengths (UVC) reflects the more rapid time course of erythema induced by this spectral region.

Several pieces of evidence suggest that DNA is the chromophore for erythema induced by UVC and UVB:

1. Up to 334 nm, the shape of the erythema action spectrum resembles the curve obtained if the transmission of the stratum corneum at different wavelengths is multiplied by the absorption spectrum for DNA. This is to be expected if DNA is in fact the major chromophore for erythema induced by photons penetrating the stratum corneum.
2. The action spectrum for ultraviolet-induced pyrimdine dimer formation in epidermal DNA in vivo resembles the erythema action spectrum up to 334 nm.[5]
3. In a marsupial with a very efficient photoenzymatic DNA repair pathway, photo-induced repair of DNA damage (photoreactivation) by exposure to visible light markedly reduces the erythema response.[6]

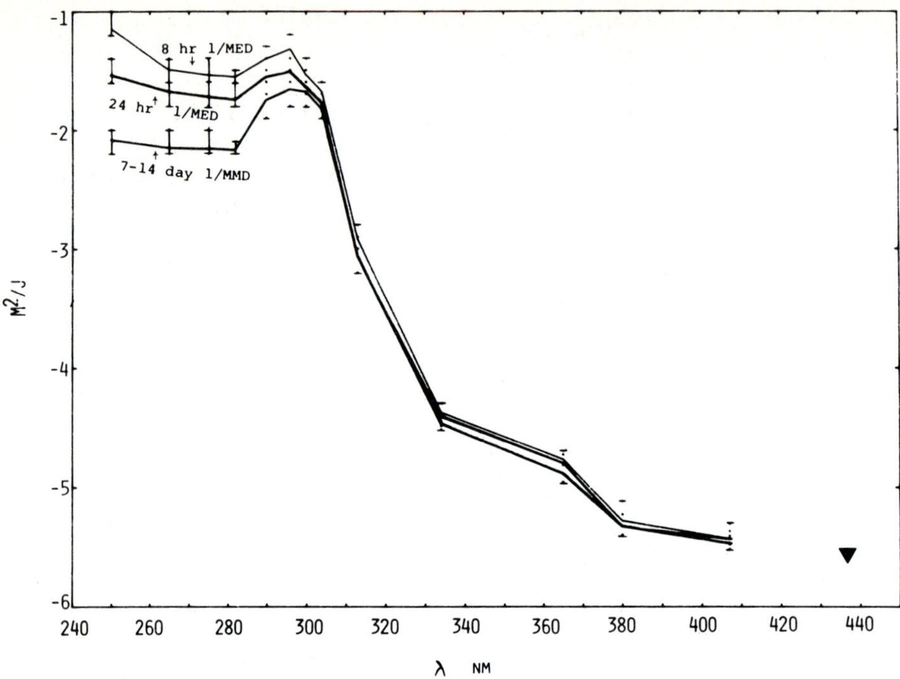

Figure 24-4 Erythema and melanogenesis action spectra in fair-skinned humans. (*From JA Parrish et al, The erythema and melanogenesis action spectra of normal human skin. Photochem Photobiol 36:187, 1982. With permission.*)

Pigmentation. Skin color is another important factor in determining the development of erythema. Resistance to the induction of erythema by ultraviolet radiation is conferred by both racial pigmentation and facultative tanning, but the latter is less photoprotective.

Waveband Interactions

Radiation may interact additively with previously administered doses. Following a single suberythemogenic dose of UVA or UVB, the erythema dose threshold is reduced in the treated area for at least 24 h.[7] Suberythemogenic doses of either UVA or UVB administered repeatedly at 24-h intervals eventually have a cumulative effect resulting in erythema.[8,9]

Solar Erythemogenesis

Although UVA is much less erythemogenic than UVB, the high UVA irradiance present in sunlight means that in practice long wavelengths contribute significantly to the solar erythemogenesis radiation at noon.[10] At other times of the day this proportion may be greater, since with increasing solar zenith angle the atmospheric attenuation of UVB is greater than that of UVA, leading to a relative increase in the contribution of the longer wavelengths. Sunscreens, which absorb UVB more efficiently than UVA, have the same effect.

Release of Inflammatory Mediators in Ultraviolet Erythema

Several mediators have been identified that are believed to be important in the pathogenesis of ultraviolet-induced erythema. Although it is usually assumed that the initial photochemistry occurs in the epidermis, with subsequent diffusion of mediators toward blood vessels, direct injury of dermal cells or blood vessels may also occur.

Prostaglandins can cause vasodilation following intradermal injection and may also potentiate the effects of other mediators. Increased levels of prostaglandins are found in tissue fluid obtained in the first 24 h after UVB,[11–13] UVA,[14,15] and UVC irradiation.[16] Increased levels of 12-hydroxyeicosatetraenoic acid also have been detected after UVB irradiation. The sites of the increased synthesis are not known in ultraviolet-induced inflammation, but most cellular constituents of skin including epidermis, blood cells, and vascular endothelium are known to be capable of prostaglandin synthesis. Indomethacin, a potent inhibitor of the cyclooxygenase pathway and therefore of prostaglandin biosynthesis, inhibits the initial period of UVB-induced delayed erythema.[17,18] After 24 h, however, erythema is usually still present and is unresponsive to inhibitors of prostaglandin synthesis. Presumably in the later phases of delayed erythema, other mediators are more important. Erythema induced by UVA irradiation is unresponsive to topical indomethacin.

Increased histamine levels and mast cell degranulation have both been demonstrated at the onset of UVB-induced erythema.[12] However, antihistamines or histamine depletion do not detectably suppress erythema. Increased serum interleukin (IL)-1 and IL-6 levels have been detected in humans after whole body exposure,[19] which could account in part for the systemic alterations associated with severe sunburn. Increased levels of IL-1 and tumor necrosis factor were detected on epidermal cell membranes in skin biopsy specimens, and the expression of intercellular adhesion molecule-1 (ICAM-1) was induced on human keratinocytes after UVB irradiation.

Histopathologic Changes Associated with Ultraviolet-Induced Erythema

Erythemogenic doses of UVB or UVC cause both epidermal and dermal changes, while longer wavelengths (UVA) cause predominantly dermal changes. Histological changes may be seen in human skin as little as 30 min after ultraviolet irradiation, several hours before erythema develops.[12]

Damaged keratinocytes known as sunburn cells are characteristic of UVB- and UVC-induced epidermal damage. Sunburn cells exhibit either swollen or shrunken cytoplasm that becomes brightly eosinophilic; nuclear alterations also occur, leading to pyknosis and premature disappearance of the nucleus. In humans, sunburn cells occur within 30 min of erythemal radiation[12] and are maximal at 24 h. Irregularly distributed clusters are found mainly in the lower half of the epidermis; neighboring keratinocytes may be normal in appearance.[20] After high ultraviolet doses, sunburn cells may coalesce into a band of necrotic tissue, which is eliminated over a period of 7 days or longer. Since sunburn cell formation may be reduced by antioxidants, a free-radical mechanism has been proposed.[21]

Other acute changes seen in the epidermis include intercellular edema, nuclear alterations, and occasional exocytosis of lymphocytes. Langerhans cells in human skin are reduced in number within 1 h after UVB irradiation[12] and continue to decrease. A normal population density is restored after 15 days.[21]

UVB irradiation also damages blood vessels,[20] leading to partial occlusion of vessels, which may be observed for several days. An infiltrate of mononuclear cells and neutrophils occurs around the more superficial vessels.

In humans, mast cells are reduced in number 1 to 4 h after UVB irradiation[12]; hypogranulated cells are visible, sometimes with extracellular granules in the neighborhood. Twenty-four h later, mast cells regain their normal appearance and density.

The histological changes associated with UVA erythema are quite different. Dermal changes are more pronounced,[20] with a denser mononuclear cell infiltrate with some neutrophils extending to greater depths in the dermis. Vascular damage is severe, with greater degrees of endothelial swelling and red cell extravasation. Ultrastructural studies[22] show wide gaps between endothelial cells, damaged pericytes, platelet aggregation in the lumina, and perivascular fibrin deposition. In the epidermis, sunburn cell formation is very infrequent, but marked intercellular edema may be observed.[14]

The photosensitized response to oral 8-methoxypsoralen plus UVA (PUVA) induces prominent changes in both epidermis and dermis that are more persistent than those seen after ultraviolet radiation alone.[20] Obvious changes are still present 7 days after exposure.

Pigmentation

Ultraviolet radiation also leads to an increase in epidermal melanin pigmentation, which helps to protect the skin against further radiation. The pigmentary response occurs in immediate and delayed phases that have different action spectra. Pigment responses to UVA, but not to UVB, can be abolished by making the skin hypoxic during exposure.[23]

Immediate Tanning

Immediate pigment darkening begins during radiation and is maximal immediately afterward, fading within minutes after exposure to small doses. After larger exposures it is more persistent and blends with delayed tanning. UVA and visible light can both cause immediate pigment darkening, and it may be observed in cadaver skin or in isolated melanosomes. A dose of 2 to 12 J/m^2 of UVA is sufficient to induce immediate pigment darkening in Caucasians who tan readily. Since immediate pigment darkening results from photooxidation of existing melanin, it is most conspicuous in subjects who already have some degree of either constitutive or facultative pigmentation. Immediate pigment darkening does not seem to protect the skin against subsequent ultraviolet radiation.

Delayed Tanning

Delayed tanning, in contrast, is clearly photoprotective, becomes visible after about 72 h, and is due to increased epidermal melanin. The major action spectrum for delayed tanning resembles that for erythema, lying in the UVB region (Fig. 24-4), but UVC, UVA, and visible light also cause delayed tanning. Relative dosage thresholds for erythema and delayed tanning differ with the wavelength; in individuals who tan well, suberythemal doses of UVA are melanogenic, whereas erythemogenic doses of UVB are required to induce delayed tanning. Delayed tanning from either UVA or UVB is associated with similar increases in melanocyte population and activity.[24]

Following irradiation, dendrites are larger and more branched, and tyrosinase activity is enhanced. The size and number of melanocytes increase, and there is accelerated transfer of melanosomes to keratinocytes, resulting in a great increase in the amount of melanin in the epidermis.[24]

The main function of delayed tanning is photoprotection, although the protection conferred by increased melanin alone without stratum corneum thickening, for example, with a UVA tan, is at best moderate. In vitiligo, substantial photoprotection following ultraviolet exposure can occur as a result of stratum corneum thickening alone.[25]

In light-skinned races, skin thickening is probably the more important photoprotective response, whereas in dark-skinned races, constitutive pigmentation is the more important barrier. Although the skin melanin content is much greater in dark-skinned races, the numbers of melanocytes per unit area of skin does not differ significantly among the races. The pathway for ultraviolet-induced activation of melanocytes is not known. Direct or indirect mechanisms are possible, and so far, irradiation of melanocyte cultures has not provided a clear message. The importance of other potential photoprotective mechanisms—for example, endogenous antioxidants such as glutathione or adaptive stress protein responses to ultraviolet exposure[26]—is just beginning to be explored.

Skin Thickening

UVB radiation causes the epidermis to thicken. This response, which is associated with upward transfer of melanin, increases tolerance to subsequent radiation and is the result of increased epidermal mitosis for several days. This is associated with increased synthesis of DNA, RNA, and protein. Preceding these responses, there is a transient depression of mitosis and macromolecular synthetic activity.[26]

The pathway through which stimulation of epidermal proliferation is mediated is not known. Ultraviolet radiation induces a large increase in epidermal ornithine decarboxylase,[27] which is the rate-limiting enzyme in the synthesis of the polyamines putrescine, spermidine, and spermine. These are found in most normal tissues and are increased in amount in proliferative states. UVB and UVC both induce orinithine decarboxylase at doses similar to those causing erythema; induction by UVA has not been demonstrated except in the presence of the photosensitizers anthracene and 8-methoxypsoralen.[28] It is of interest that tumor-promoting compounds such as phorbol esters also induce ornithine decarboxylase[29] and, like ultraviolet radiation, also cause a wave of epidermal proliferation and thickening.[30]

PATHOLOGICAL PHOTOSENSITIVITY

Evaluation of Patients with Photosensitivity

Photosensitivity disorders can be divided into an idiopathic group and those induced by exogenous or endogenous photosensitizers; in addition, patients with defective DNA repair are prone to develop actinically induced carcinomas (Table 24-1). History taking and examination of the morphology and distribution of the skin lesions are important in the evaluation of these patients. A careful history should be obtained to ascertain the causal and temporal relationships between sun exposure and the development of dermatitis, as well as the symptoms of the eruption. In some patients, such as those with solar urticaria and some with erythropoietic protoporphyria, the eruption occurs within minutes of sun exposure. In others, such as those with polymorphous light eruption, phototoxicity, and photoallergy, a latent period of hours to days may be observed between exposure and onset. In disorders with markedly increased photosensitivity, such as persistent light reactivity and actinic reticuloid, even everyday low-level exposure may be sufficient to induce and maintain the response; however, careful questioning usually reveals that the eruptions worsen with exposure to sunlight. In most climates, seasonal variations in prevalence and severity may also suggest the importance of light. Photosensitivity eruptions are frequently seen in spring and early summer. The prevalence of some disorders may decline during the summer; protective responses such as tanning lead to improved sun tolerance.

Examination of the skin is performed to evaluate the morphology and distribution of the eruption. Typically, photodermatitis involves light-exposed areas such as the cheeks, nose, forehead, dorsa of the hands, forearms, V area of the chest, and back of the neck. Areas relatively

Table 24-1

PHOTOSENSITIVITY DISORDERS

1. Idiopathic
   - Polymorphous light eruption
   - Solar urticaria
2. Associated with exogenous photosensitizers
   - Phototoxicity
   - Photoallergy
3. Associated with endogenous photosensitizers
   - Porphyrias
4. Associated with defective DNA repair
   - Xeroderma pigmentosum

protected from sunlight, such as the postauricular area and the area under the chin, are usually spared; in fact, involvement of these areas may suggest that the eruptions are due to exposure to other environmental factors unrelated to sunlight, such as airborne allergens. Both clothing and anatomy are responsible for the relatively straight lines of demarcation between involved and uninvolved skin in photodermatitis.

The MED tests to UVA and UVB are determined in all patients, yielding objective measurements of the sensitivity of the skin to the respective wavelength range. Photopatch testing is performed to exclude the photoallergic reaction. In some patients, determinations of antinuclear antibody and porphyrin profiles are done to rule out the possibility of lupus erythematosus and various forms of porphyria, respectively. Skin biopsy may also be carried out in some patients to establish the diagnosis.

Idiopathic Photosensitivity Disorders

Polymorphous Light Eruption

General Features. Polymorphous light eruption is the most common idiopathic photodermatosis. It usually occurs in young adults and characteristically arises hours or, occasionally, days after sun exposure.[31] The eruption consists of pruritic papules, papulovesicles, nodules, and plaques (Fig. 24-5). However, in a given patient, the eruption is monomorphous. The onset is frequently in the spring in temperate climates, with some resistance being acquired with continued sun exposure; hence the patients become less symptomatic as the summer progresses. The course is chronic and is usually progressive.

Histological changes consist of epidermal spongiosis, dermal edema, and perivascular lymphohistiocytic infiltration. The action spectrum is usually in the UVB range, although patients with sensitivity to UVA or

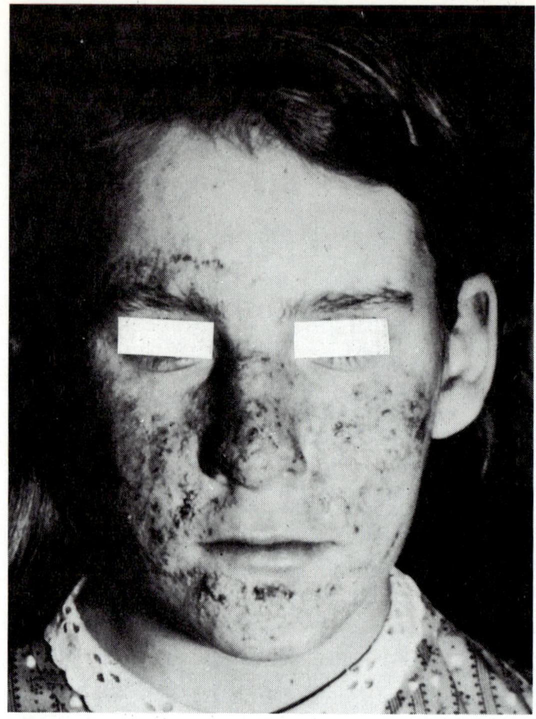

Figure 24-5 Polymorphous light eruption involving light-exposed areas. (*From TB Fitzpatrick et al, Dermatology in General Medicine, 3d ed, New York, McGraw-Hill, 1987, p 1483.*)

visible light have also been described. MED tests are normal, and the result of the photopatch test is negative. Because the eruption usually has resolved by the time the patient sees a physician, the diagnosis is tentatively established by the characteristic history. It can be confirmed by provocative phototesting, performed on sites where eruptions would usually occur. The phototesting can be performed by a single exposure to a 3× to 5× MED or by exposing the site to a gradually increasing doses of UVA or UVB for 4 consecutive days. The appearance of papules or plaques signifies a positive response; the diagnosis can be confirmed by performing a biopsy of the lesion.

Pathophysiology. Studies on the pathophysiology have been unrevealing. Negative direct immunofluorescence examination of lesional skin and insignificant levels of antinuclear antibodies serve to distinguish polymorphous light eruption from lupus erythematosus, which it may resemble both clinically and histologically. Attempts to demonstrate an abnormal response of lymphocytes to ultraviolet light in vitro have not provided useful information.

Solar Urticaria

General Features. This condition occurs most commonly in women in the fourth and fifth decades of life. It develops within seconds to minutes following sun exposure and resolves spontaneously in a few hours. The action spectrum can be in the UVA, UVB, or visible range.

Pathophysiology. Although it has been well established that urticaria can be induced by different wavelengths of light, it is becoming increasingly clear that in some patients a given spectrum of light may induce urticaria while another spectrum may suppress it, suggesting that the urticarial response is the result of these activating and inhibitory spectra.[32,33] A study of six patients with solar urticaria showed that intradermal injection of their own serum or plasma following exposure to visible light in vitro resulted in an urticarial response; a similar result was observed when irradiated normal human serum was used.[34] As determined by gel filtration, the molecular weight of photoallergens generated ranged from 25 to 1×10^3 kd. The fact that photoallergens could be generated from sera of individuals without solar urticaria led the authors to suggest that the chormophores might be endogenous agents that become photoallergens upon exposure to photons; such photoallergens would induce urticaria only in individuals who are "allergic" to them. Another patient was reported to react to eluates of in vitro–irradiated isolated epidermis and irradiated eluates of epidermis, suggesting that the chromophore was present in the skin.[35] Following irradiation in vivo, mast cell degranulation and release of mast cell–derived mediators (histamine, neutrophil and eosinophil chemotactic factors) have been reported.[36,37]

Therefore, it is likely that in patients with solar urticaria, exposure to the appropriate radiation results in the generation of endogenously derived chromophore(s), which induces activation of mast cells. Mast cells may also be involved in psoralens plus UVA (PUVA)- or UVA-induced tolerance observed in these patients,[38] and the inhibitory effect of selected wavebands mentioned above.[32] In vitro, high-dose UVB (100 to 400 mJ/cm^2) has been shown to suppress secretagogue-induced degranulation of purified mast cells, while lower doses (16 to 64 mJ/cm^2) did not.[39,40] Exposure of purified mast cells to PUVA did not suppress the ability of these cells to respond to subsequent stimulation with secretagogues[40]; however, suppression was observed when a mixed cell preparation containing 5 percent mast cells was used.[41] These results suggest that in vivo, interaction of mast cells with electromagnetic radiation may involve other cells in the dermis, although a direct effect can also be observed if mast cells are exposed to sufficiently high doses of radiation.

Photosensitivity Induced by Exogenous Agents

Photosensitivity induced by exogenous agents can be broadly divided into two categories: phototoxicity and photoallergy. Phototoxicity is the equivalent of irritant dermatitis. Theoretically, it can be induced in 100 percent of the individuals exposed to sufficient doses of the phototoxic agents and the appropriate radiation; thiazides, tetracyclines, psoralen, and coal tar are examples of phototoxic agents. In contrast, photoallergy is a delayed hypersensitivity response; it occurs only in individuals who have been previously exposed and sensitized to the photoallergens, and cross-reactivity with antigenically related agents can occur.[42] Halogenated salicylanilides, musk ambrette, para-aminobenzoic acid esters, and chlorpromazine are known photoallergens. Avoidance of the offending agent is the treatment of choice in the management of these patients. Some agents that are not themselves photosensitizers may cause photosensitization indirectly. Porphyria caused by liver damage from the ingestion of the fungicide hexachlorobenzene, added to grain in Turkey in the 1960s, and isoniazid-induced pellagra-like photosensitivity, mediated through alterations of tryptophan metabolism, are examples of this type of response.

Phototoxicity

General Features. The clinical spectrum of phototoxicity is enormous, ranging from erythema, edema, and tenderness of sun-exposed areas following ingestion of systemic medications (thiazides, sulfonamides, tetracyclines, phenothiazines), to onycholysis from tetracycline derivatives, to blistering following contact with furocoumarin-containing plants (phytophotodermatitis), to "tar smarts" (a painful sensation in the skin noted by pitch workers on exposure to light), to pigmentary changes induced by oil of bergamot in perfumes (berloque dermatitis).

Histologically, spongiosis and necrosis of epidermal cells may occur within hours of irradiation, although in the case of psoralens the changes may be delayed for 1 to 2 days. In the dermis, edema may be striking, and evidence of vascular damage and endothelial cell swelling may be observed. Evidence of mast cell degeneration may be seen around blood vessels. There are no specific features that distinguish most phototoxic reactions from sunburn induced by UVB alone.

Pathophysiology. Most phototoxic agents absorb in the UVA region. Since photon absorption is necessary for photochemistry to occur, these are the wavelengths mainly responsible for the induction of phototoxic reactions. Following absorption of a photon, three types of photochemical reactions may take place[43,44]:

1. Reactive oxygen species are generated. Following excitation of the chromophore, energy or an electron is transferred to oxygen, forming singlet oxygen or superoxide anion. These species or their reaction products then react with biological substrates within the cell. Porphyrin-induced phototoxicity is an example of this type of reaction.
2. The chromophore is converted into a photoproduct, which then reacts with a biological substrate. Formation of this photoproduct

may or may not be oxygen dependent. An example of this is phototoxicity induced by chlorpromazine and some of the tetracyclines.

3. The phototoxic compound may bind directly to a substrate as a result of photon absorption. This process is independent of the presence of oxygen. It is the major mechanism of psoralen-induced phototoxicity.

Photochemical reactions requiring oxygen are referred to as *photodynamic processes*. The initial photochemical events described above may lead to damage or functional alterations to nuclear, membrane, or cytoplasmic components of the cell, any of which may be sufficient to disrupt cellular processes. In practice, damage to more than one site occurs frequently.

Nuclear damage. This is an important, but not the only, aspect of phototoxicity due to psoralen compounds. Psoralen phototoxicity is central to PUVA therapy and extracorporeal photopheresis. In addition, phytophotodermatitis can be caused by psoralen-producing plants. Photoaddition of psoralen to DNA results from the absorption of a single photon and is independent of oxygen.[45] Covalent bonding to pyrimidine bases occurs through one of two sites on the psoralen molecule. Formation of this photoproduct probably interferes with transcription and is thought to be mutagenic. Absorption of a second photon may result in the formation of an interstrand cross-link if a suitably aligned second pyrimidine base is present in the opposite DNA strand. This is lethal to the cell if unrepaired.

Membrane damage. Phototoxic damage to cell membranes has been studied extensively, with the erythrocyte as the most commonly used model. Phototoxic injury leads to oxidation of lipids and proteins, impairment of membrane transport mechanisms, and eventual membrane disruption. Protoporphyrin has been shown to mediate photodynamic damage to the cell membrane.[46] Stable chlorpromazine photoproducts cause membrane disruption, perhaps by a detergent-like action.[43] Lysosomal membranes may similarly undergo phototoxic injury; disruption of lysosomal membranes leads to a release of enzymes (acid hydrolases) into the cell, which can induce further damage. Anthracene has been shown to localize in lysosomes in tissue culture[47] and may act in this way. Psoralens have also been shown to induce photodynamic membrane damage.[45,48]

Cytoplasmic components. Psoralens and other agents may undergo oxygen-dependent interactions with cytoplasmic components such as proteins, ribonucleic acids, and enzymes, probably through covalent bonding to aromatic amino acids.[45,48]

Photoallergy

General Features. There are subtle clinical differences between phototoxicity and photoallergy that are helpful in differentiating them, although such a distinction may not always be possible based on cutaneous examination alone. Phototoxicity usually resembles a sunburn reaction.

Photoallergy is a delayed hypersensitivity response; therefore, it resembles contact dermatitis, except that it requires the concomitant presence of photoallergens and electromagnetic radiation. In the acute phase of the photoallergic response, an erythematous, pruritic eruption with vesiculation occurs. Histologically, the changes are both epidermal and dermal, with epidermal spongiosis, intraepidermal vesicle formation, and an inflammatory infiltrate of predominantly mononuclear cells in the dermis. Patients with chronic photoallergy present with marked lichenification of sun-exposed areas, frequently with excoriations and erosions. Histologically, there are epidermal acanthosis and mild spongiosis, a dermal infiltrate consisting of lymphocytes and other mononuclear cells, thickening of the papillary dermis, and vertically streaked collagen bundles in the upper dermis. The diagnosis is confirmed by normal MED tests and a positive photopatch test.

Pathophysiology. A photoallergen, in the presence of the appropriate radiation, binds carrier molecules to form a complete antigen, which initiates a delayed hypersensitivity response.[42] As in allergic contact dermatitis, Langerhans cells and T lymphocytes play important roles in this response. In mice, the photocontact hypersensitivity response was suppressed when the photosensitization site was previously exposed to UVB, which is known to interfere with the antigen-processing function of Langerhans cells.[49] Exposure of the photosensitizing site to low-dose UVB prior to photosensitization in mice resulted in suppression of the photoallergic response, which was associated with the generation of antigen-specific $CD8^+$ (suppressor/cytotoxic) T cells.[50] Systemic immunological tolerance to the photoallergen was induced following exposure to high-dose UVB, which is known to induce generation of $CD8^+$ T cells.[51] Another similarity between contact allergy and photocontact allergy is the participation of mast cells. Prior treatment with reserpine, a mast cell vasoactive amine–depleting agent, suppressed the allergic contact dermatitis response in mice. In the same animal model, elevated serum and urinary histamine levels were reported following the elicitation of allergic contact dermatitis.[52] Similarly, pretreatment of mice with reserpine, which depletes vasoactive amines in mast cells, suppressed the photocontact hypersensitivity response. This response was also suppressed in mast cell–deficient mice, a suppression due to a defect in the induction phase.[53] In contrast to allergic contact hypersensitivity, the photocontact hypersensitivity response in mice was suppressed by treatment with long-acting liposomal superoxide dismutase prior to photosensitization, indicating the role of reactive oxygen species in this process.[54]

Photosensitivity Induced by Endogenous Agents

General Features

Photosensitivity induced by endogenous agents is exemplified by the porphyrias, a group of disorders resulting from heritable or acquired abnormalities of heme synthesis. Heme is synthesized in large quantities to fill the requirements of the body for hemoglobin, cytochrome, catalases, and peroxidases. Under normal circumstances, the intermediate compounds in heme synthesis are present in only small amounts. In patients with the porphyrias, enzyme deficiencies cause the accumulation of the intermediate porphyrinogens, which become oxidized to porphyrins. With the exception of acute intermittent porphyria, all the other types of porphyria are associated with phototoxicity. The phototoxicity is due to the presence of elevated porphyrin levels and exposure to their absorption spectrum, the Soret band (400 ± 10 nm). The lack of photosensitivity in acute intermittent porphyria is due to the fact that its predominant biochemical defect is an elevated excretion of the porphyrin precursors δ-aminolevulinic acid and porphobilinogen; neither is a phototoxic agent.

The two most common types of porphyria are porphyria cutanea tarda and erythropoietic protoporphyria. Patients with porphyria cutanea tarda present with skin fragility, vesicles and erosions on sun-exposed areas (especially the dorsa of the hands), hypertrichosis and mottled hyperpigmentation in the periorbital area, and sclerodermoid changes in sun-exposed as well as non-sun-exposed areas (Fig. 24-6). Most patients do not have subjective discomfort following exposure to sunlight and hence are not aware of the contributory effect of sun exposure to the skin eruption. Porphyria cutanea tarda is inherited in an autosomal dominant fashion in some patients and is often associated with exposure to potential hepatotoxins such as alcohol, estrogen, and chlorinated hydrocarbons. The abnormal porphyrin profile is secondary to defective uroporphyrinogen decarboxylase activity. The predominant porphyrins are 8-carboxyl por-

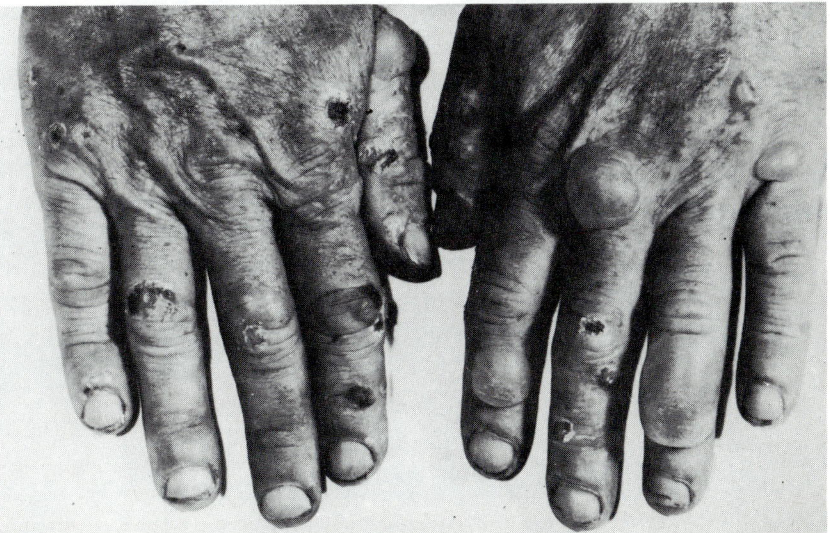

Figure 24-6 Porphyria cutanea tarda showing bullae and erosions on the hands. (*From TB Fitzpatrick et al, Dermatology in General Medicine, 3d ed, New York, McGraw-Hill, 1987, p 1961.*)

phyrin (uroporphyrin) and 7-carboxyl porphyrin in the urine, resulting in the fluorescence of the urine when irradiated with Wood's light. Isocoproporphyrin is the predominant porphyrin in the stool of these patients. Treatment consists of phlebotomy or administration of hydroxychloroquine.

In contrast to patients with porphyria cutanea tarda, patients with erythropoietic protoporphyria complain of a burning and stinging sensation following sun exposure; this is followed by the development of cutaneous erythema, edema, and urticarial lesions (Fig. 24-7). Erythropoietic protoporphyria has an autosomal dominant inheritance and an onset in early childhood. Defective ferrochelatase activity results in the predominant elevation of protoporphyrin in the erythrocytes, plasma, and stool; in contrast to patients with porphyria cutanea tarda, the urine porphyrin profile is normal. β-carotene, taken during the spring and summer months, is the most widely used therapy.

Pathophysiology

The pathophysiology of cutaneous lesions in porphyria cutanea tarda and erythropoietic protoporphyria involves reactive oxygen species and various inflammatory mediators.[55] Several studies in vitro have shown the importance of reactive oxygen species in porphyrin-induced phototoxicity.[46] In vivo, superoxide anions play a significant role in hematophorphyrin derivative–induced phototoxicity in mice.[56] In the presence of porphyrins

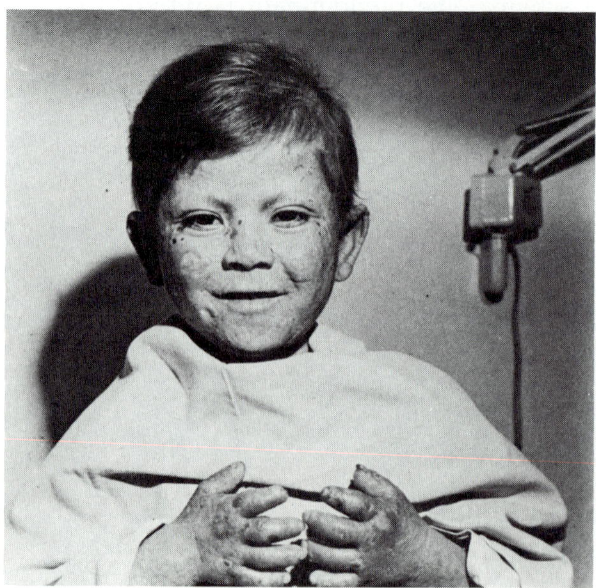

Figure 24-7 Erythropoietic protoporphyria with scars and crusts. (*From TB Fitzpatrick et al, Dermatology in General Medicine, 3d ed, New York, McGraw-Hill, 1987, p 1685.*)

and radiation, activation of the complement system and generation of complement activation products have been demonstrated both in vitro and in vivo.[57] Protoporphyrin, but not uroporphyrin, radiation-induced release of preformed and generated mediators from purified mast cells, and the porphyrin-induced phototoxic response are associated with elevated serum histamine levels and dermal mast cell degranulation.[58] Other studies on the effects of porphyrins on endothelial cells, neutrophils, fibroblasts, and cutaneous eicosanoid-metabolizing enzymes have also contributed to our understanding of their roles in the pathophysiology of porphyrin-induced phototoxicity.

Based on the above data, the following pathogenetic mechanisms for the development of cutaneous phototoxic lesions in porphyrias can be proposed.[55] The discussion will be confined to erythropoietic protoporphyria and porphyria cutanea tarda.

In erythropoietic protoporphyria, exposure of protoporphyrin to 400 to 410 nm of radiation results in complement activation and release of mediators from mast cells (Fig. 24-8). The latter may be enhanced by the presence of anaphylatoxins, generated as a consequence of complement activation. The biological effects of mast cell–derived mediators may account for the development of erythema, edema, urticarial lesions, and pruritus in these patients. Waxy thickening of the skin may be accounted for by the direct effect of protoporphyrin and irradiation on fibroblasts. Furthermore, the results of studies on the interaction of mast cells and fibroblasts suggest that activation of mast cells may also facilitate the development of tissue fibrosis. The inflammatory response may be down-regulated by the above-mentioned effects of protoporphyrin and radiation on endothelial cell and cutaneous eicosanoid metabolism. The fact that reactive oxygen species mediate many of the effects of protoporphyrin and irradiation on cell membranes may explain the therapeutic efficacy of β-carotene in this disorder.

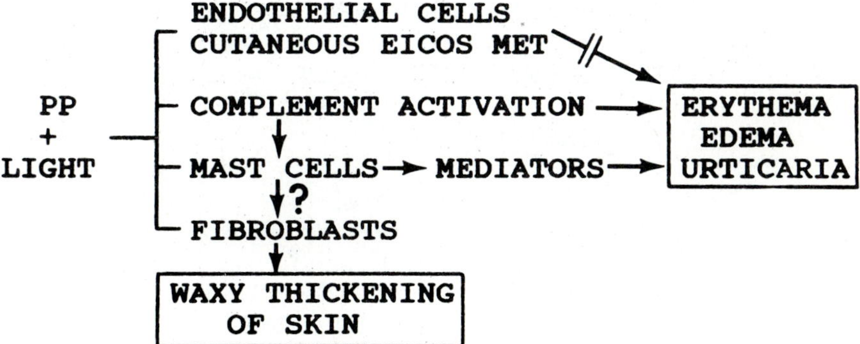

Figure 24-8 Pathophysiology of cutaneous lesions in erythropoietic protoporphyria. PP = protoporphyrin; EICOS = eicosanoids.

The development of vesicles and skin fragility observed in patients with porphyria cutanea tarda may be initiated by activation of the complement system induced by uroporphyrin and radiation (Fig. 24-9). Complement activation products, in turn, may activate mast cells, resulting in the release of their proteinases. It was reported that chymotrypsin-like protease, a normal mast cell constituent, induced dermal-epidermal separation of human skin in vitro; ultrastructurally, this separation occurred at the lamina lucida, the site of separation in four of six blisters examined from patients with porphyria cutanea tarda. It is possible, therefore, that mast cell–derived proteinases may contribute to the development of vesicles and skin fragility. The sclerodermoid skin changes observed in these patients may be accounted for by the light-independent effect of uroporphyrin on collagen biosynthesis by fibroblasts. The possible effect of mast cells on tissue fibrosis may also contribute to these clinical changes. The effects of uroporphyrin on eicosanoid metabolism of endothelial cells and skin may down-regulate the above response.

Defective DNA Repair and Skin Cancer

General Features

Genetic defects in DNA repair resulting in a predisposition to cancer are examplified by xeroderma pigmentosum. Xeroderrma pigmentosum is an autosomal recessive disorder characterized by photosensitivity, a marked predisposition to and early development of actinically induced cutaneous and ocular carcinomas[59] (Fig. 24-10). The prevalence of light-induced skin cancer in xeroderma pigmentosum in white people at the age of 20 years approaches 100 percent—at least 1000 times greater than in the general population; the median age of onset is 8 years. Management of these patients includes total protection of the skin and eyes from sunlight and

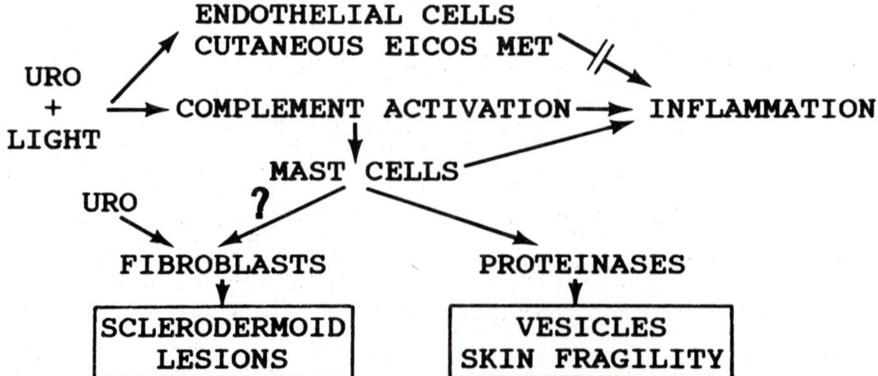

Figure 24-9 Pathophysiology of cutaneous lesions in porphyria cutanea tarda. URO = uroporphyrin; EICOS = eicosanoids.

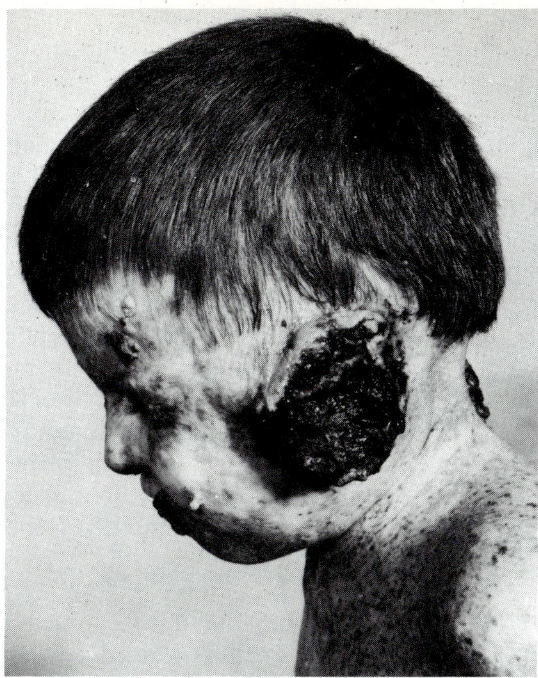

Figure 24-10 Child with xeroderma pigmentosum. Lesion involving ear is invasive squamous cell carcinoma. (*From TB Fitzpatrick et al, Dermatology in General Medicine, 2d ed, New York, McGraw-Hill, 1979, p 392.*)

treatment of the premalignant and malignant lesions as they arise; the use of retinoids as chemopreventive agents should also be considered.

Pathophysiology

Since all patients with xeroderma pigmentosum have deficiencies in DNA repair, it is necessary to review the DNA repair mechanisms in mammalian cells. Although DNA absorbs maximally in the shorter ultraviolet regions (UVC), significant absorption of longer wavelengths present in terrestrial sunlight also occurs. Photochemical reactions between DNA and other endogenous or exogenous molecules may take place, or the DNA itself may become structurally altered; for example, there may be cross-links between strands, covalent bonding between adjacent bases, or, very rarely, strand breaks. The formation of stable cyclobutyl pyrimidine dimers, notably thymine-thymine dimers, is one of the major photochemical consequences of ultraviolet irradiation of DNA.[60] Because of the critical role played by DNA in cell function and reproduction, damage induced by ultraviolet radiation or other agents may have important consequences and, if unrepaired, may lead to disordered cell function, cell death, or genetic damage (mutation) resulting in carcinogenesis. Therefore, it is essential that these DNA damages be repaired. Four DNA repair pathways exist in mammalian cells: excision repair, strand-break repair, postreplication repair, and photoreactivation.

Excision Repair. This pathway involves the removal of a damaged segment of DNA by a series of enzymes; the segment is replaced by the use of the opposite strand as a template. Excision repair is initiated by endonucleases that may be specific for different types of DNA damage. After recognition of the DNA lesion (e.g., a thymine-thymine dimer, alkylating agent–DNA complex, or apurinic site), the endonucleases cause a ''nick'' at an adjacent site in the same strand. The damaged region is then degraded by an exonuclease; a limited number of normal nucleotides are also released. The segment or length removed depends on the type of damage and may be as much as 80 to 100 nucleotides for the area surrounding ultraviolet-induced pyrimidine dimers. The damaged segment is then resynthesized by a DNA repair polymerase. The final step of the excision repair process is the sealing of the newly synthesized segment of the parental DNA strand by a polynucleotide ligase.

Strand-Break Repair. Mammalian cells have the capacity to repair rapidly single-strand breaks in DNA. Most breaks induced by, for example, x-rays are repaired within 10 to 30 min by the enzyme polynucleotide ligase.

Postreplication Repair. Ultraviolet-irradiated cells may have the capacity to divide despite the presence of DNA damage. During the first S phase after ultraviolet irradiation, gaps are present in newly synthesized DNA strands that correspond in position to the ultraviolet-induced damage (e.g., pyrimidine dimers) on the parent strand. These gaps are subsequently filled. This process is known as *postreplication repair* and reflects the cell's ability to replicate past the unrepaired, damaged segments of DNA. Postreplication repair may be error prone and therefore plays a role in mammalian cell mutagenesis.

Photoreactivation. Photoreactivation is the conversion of ultraviolet-induced pyrimidine dimers into monomers by a photoreactivating enzyme. This enzyme binds to the dimer and in the presence of light (300 to 600 nm) converts the dimer to two monomers. While the relative importance of this pathway of DNA repair in the skin is not clear, it has been shown that significant degrees of repair may occur in humans by photoreactivation.[61]

In all patients with xeroderma pigmentosum, at least one DNA repair pathway is defective; in most individuals, it is excision repair that is defective to varying degrees. The defect in excision repair seems to result from a defective excision step, and normal function can be restored by the insertion of endonucleases into the ultraviolet-irradiated xeroderma pigmentosum cells.

Based on the specific molecular defect, patients with xeroderma pigmentosum have been classified into at least 10 complementation groups.[59] Hybridization of excision-defective cells from any two groups leads to a normal excision repair capacity due to the fact that cells from one complementation group have the ability to make up for deficiencies in cells from another group. A tenth group of xeroderma pigmentosum patients is proficient in excision repair but shows defects in both postreplication repair and photoreativation repair. These individuals are known as *xeroderma pigmentosum variants.*

LIGHT AS THERAPY

Sunlight has been used for many years to treat a variety of diseases of the skin and other systems. The mechanisms of response to phototherapy are not always understood, but speculations can be made from our knowledge of the responses of normal skin. Possible mechanisms can be classified as follows: cytotoxicity, stimulation of protective mechanisms, photochemical or immunological alterations, and thermal effects.

Cytotoxicity may be the result of ultraviolet radiation alone or of ultraviolet radiation in combination with a photosensitizer. UVB radiation has been used in the treatment of psoriasis for over 50 years. The dosages of UVB required to cause improvement in this disease are similar to those needed to induce inflammation (erythema), and it seems likely that similar pathways may be involved, with DNA as an important target or chromophore. Since psoriasis is a hyperproliferative disease, ultraviolet-induced inhibition of DNA synthesis, which can be demonstrated in normal skin, is a possible mechanism. This is believed to result from direct damage to nuclear material. Whether the effect of ultraviolet radiation on the immune system plays a role in its therapeutic efficacy remains to be clarified.[62]

PUVA is the name given to the combination of the phototoxic agent 8-methoxypsoralen (8-MOP) with long-wave UVA. The therapeutic mechanism of PUVA for the treatment of psoriasis is not clear. Many psoralens, including 8-MOP, are photobound to DNA in the form of monoadducts to pyrimidine bases and also as cross-links, the psoralen molecule forming a bridge between pyrimidine bases in complementary strands of DNA. Formation of interstrand cross-links is thought to be responsible for the inhibition of DNA synthesis and cell replication, which may be central to the therapeutic effect of PUVA in psoriasis. PUVA has also been used extracorporeally as a treatment of cutaneous T-cell lymphoma; while the mechanism is not completely understood, it may involve "autovaccination" against pathogenic clone(s) of T cells that have been altered by the extracorporeal exposure to PUVA.[63]

PUVA causes aging changes in the skin of many patients, including wrinkling, freckling, and elastosis. Some of these changes are reversible. PUVA is a mutagen in vitro and has been shown to increase the incidence of skin cancer in psoriatic patients. This effect is dose related and is seen particularly in patients with prior exposure to ionizing radiation (an outdated but previously widely used treatment for psoriasis). X-irradiation has been shown to induce a hypermutable state in cells in vitro, and analogous states may exist in vivo. Immune alterations as well as a direct tumor-promoting effect may also be implicated.

Some photodermatoses, for example, polymorphous light eruption, improve with repeated light exposure throughout the summer. This improvement may be due to the activation of protective mechanisms such as tanning and epidermal hyperplasia. This observation has led to the use of UVB and of PUVA for the treatment of light-sensitive disorders in order to stimulate these protective responses.

The symptoms of patients with uremic pruritus are frequently improved by UVB but not UVA phototherapy.[64] The pruritus and, in some patients, the lesions of eosinophilic pustular folliculitis, a dermatosis associated with the acquired immunodeficiency syndrome (AIDS), also improve with UVB phototherapy.[65] The mechanisms are not known. In neonatal hyperbilirubinemia, photoisomerization of unconjugated bilirubin by exposure to blue light leads to the formation of an isomer with increased water solubility, which is more readily excreted in the bile. It is possible that similar photochemical alterations and/or the effect of ultraviolet radiation on mast cells, described previously, are partly responsible for the therapeutic efficacy of ultraviolet radiation in pruritus.

High-intensity radiation produced by lasers can be used to induce local tissue damage by thermal mechanisms. This is used to treat several types of skin lesions, such as telangiectasia, verrucae, and tattoos. The thermal effects induced by the CO_2 laser are nonselective and result in destruction of all tissue components to a certain depth. In the past few years, significant advances have occurred in the use of pulsed laser radiation of specific wavelengths that allows the targeting of a specific chromophore, for example, hemoglobin (to selectively damage blood vessels) or melanin (to alter pigmentation).

ACKNOWLEDGMENTS

Supported in part by grants from the National Institutes of Health (HWL, AR36624, and Skin Disease Research Center grant AR39749) and a grant from the Department of Veterans Affairs, Washington, DC (HWL).

REFERENCES

1. Anderson RR, Parrish JA: The optics of human skin. *J Invest Dermatol* 77:13, 1981.
2. Holick M: The cutaneous photosynthesis of pre-vitamin D_3: a unique photoendocrine system. *J Invest Dermatol* 77:51, 1981.
3. Wan S et al: Quantitative evaluation of ultraviolet-induced erythema. *Photochem Photobiol* 37:643, 1983.
4. Whitman GB et al: Comparative study of erythema response to UVA radiation in guinea pigs and humans. *Photochem Photobiol.* 43:399, 1985.

5. Freeman SE et al: Wavelength dependence of pyrimidine dimer formation in DNA of human skin irradiated in situ with ultraviolet light. *Proc Natl Acad Sci U.S.A.* 86:5605, 1989.
6. Ley RD: Monodelphia domestica: a new animal model for studies in photodermatology. *Photochem Photobiol* 46:207, 1987.
7. Arbabi L et al: Recovery of skin from a single suberythemal dose of ultraviolet radiation. *J Invest Dermatol* 81:78, 1983.
8. Parrish JA et al: Cumulative effects of repeated subthreshold doses of ultraviolet radiation. *J Invest Dermatol* 76:356, 1981.
9. Kaidbey KH, Kligman AM: Cumulative effects from repeated exposure to ultraviolet radiation. *J Invest Dermatol* 76:352, 1981.
10. Parrish JA et al (eds): *UVA. Biological Effects of Ultraviolet Radiation with Emphasis on Human Responses to Longwave Ultraviolet.* New York, Plenum, 1978, p 119.
11. Black AK et al: Time course changes in levels of arachidonic acid and prostaglandins D_2, E_2, $F_{2\alpha}$ in human skin following ultraviolet B radiation. *Br J Clin Pharmacol* 10:453, 1980.
12. Gilchrest BA et al: The human sunburn reaction: histologic and biochemical studies. *J Am Acad Dermatol* 5:411, 1981.
13. Black AK et al: Increased prostaglandins E_2 and $F_2\alpha$ in human skin at 6 and 24 h after ultraviolet B irradiation (290–320 nm). *Br J Clin Pharmacol* 5:431, 1978.
14. Soter NA: Acute effects of ultraviolet radiation in skin. *Semin Dermatol* 9:11, 1990.
15. Hawk JLM et al: Increased concentrations of arachidonic acid, prostaglands E_2, D_2, and 6-oxo-$F_{1\alpha}$, and histamine in human skin following UVA irradiation. *J Invest Dermatol* 80:496, 1983.
16. Camp RD et al: Irradiation of human skin by short wavelength ultraviolet radiation (100–290 nm) (u.v. C): increased concentrations of arachidonic acid and prostaglandins E_2 and $F_2\alpha$. *Br J Clin Pharmacol* 6:145, 1978.
17. Snyder DS, Eaglstein WM: Intradermal antiprostaglandin agents and sunburn. *J Invest Dermatol* 62:47, 1974.
18. Snyder DS, Eaglstein WM: Topical indomethacin and sunburn. *Br J Dermatol* 90:91, 1974.
19. Granstein RD, Sauder DN: Whole-body exposure to ultraviolet radiation results in increased serum interleukin-1 activity in humans. *Lymphokine Res* 6:187, 1987.
20. Rosario R et al: Histological changes produced in the skin by equally erythemogenic doses of UVA, UVB, UVC and UVA with psoralens. *Br J Dermatol* 101:299, 1979.
21. Towes G et al: Epidermal Langerhans cell density determines whether contact sensitivity or unresponsiveness follows skin painting with DNFB. *J Immunol* 124:445, 1980.
22. Kumakiri M et al: Biologic changes due to longwave ultraviolet light upon human skin. *J Invest Dermatol* 69:392, 1977.
23. Kaidbey KH, Kligman AM: The acute effects of longwave ultraviolet light upon human skin. *J Invest Dermatol* 72:253, 1979.
24. Pathak MA et al: Effect of UVA, UVB and psoralen on in vivo melanin pigmentation: cellular and subcellular characterization of delayed tanning reactions induced by single or multiple exposures to UV-A, UV-B, or UV-A and 8-methoxypsoralen, in V Riley (ed), *Pigment Cell.* Basel, Karger, 1976, vol 3, p 291.
25. Everett MA: Protection from sunlight in vitiligo. *Arch Dermatol* 84:997, 1961.
26. Epstein JH et al: Effects of ultraviolet radiation on the mitotic cycle and DNA, RNA and protein synthesis in mammalian epidermis in vivo. *Photochem Photobiol* 12:57, 1970.
27. Verma AK et al: Induction of mouse epidermal ornithine decarboxylase activity and DNA synthesis by ultraviolet light. *Cancer Res* 39:1035, 1979.
28. Gange RW: Epidermal ornithine decarboxylase activity and thymidine incorporation following treatment with ultraviolet A combined with topical 8-methoxypsoralen or anthracene in the hairless mouse. *Br J Dermatol* 105:247, 1981.
29. O'Brien TG: The induction of ornithine decarboxylase as an early possibly obligatory event in mouse skin carcinogenesis. *Cancer Res* 36:2644, 1976.
30. Argyris TS: Epidermal growth following a single application of 12-O-tetradecanoyl phorbol-13-acetate in mice. *Am J Pathol* 98:639, 1980.

31. Epstein JH: Polymorphous light eruption. *Dermatol Clin* 4:243, 1986.
32. Horio T et al: Production and inhibition of solar urticaria by visible light exposure. *J Am Acad Dermatol* 11:1094, 1984.
33. Gange RW: Solar urticaria. *Arch Dermatol* 121:475, 1984.
34. Kojima M et al: Solar urticaria. The relationship of photoallergen and action spectrum. *Arch Dermatol* 122:550, 1986.
35. Leenutaphong U et al: evidence for an epidermal photoallergen in solar urticaria. *J Invest Dermatol* 91:408, 1988.
36. Soter NA et al: Solar urticaria: release of mast cell mediators into the circulation after experimental challenge. *J Invest Dermatol* 72:282, 1979.
37. Hawk JLM et al: Elevated blood histamine levels and mast cell degranulation in solar urticaria. *Br J Clin Pharmacol* 9:183, 1980.
38. Bernhard JD et al: Ultraviolet A phototherapy in the prophylaxis of solar urticaria. *J Am Acad Dermatol* 10:29, 1984.
39. Danno K et al: Suppressed histamine release from rat peritoneal mast cells by ultraviolet B irradiation: decreased diacylglycerol formation as a possible mechanism. *J Invest Dermatol* 90:806, 1988.
40. Mandel MJ et al: Effect of ultraviolet rediation and PUVA on mediator release from purified mast cells. *Photodermatology* 5:211, 1988.
41. Toda K et al: Effect of 8-methoxypsoralen plus long-wave ultraviolet (PUVA) radiation on mast cells. II. In vitro PUVA inhibits degranulation of rat peritoneal mast cells induced by compound 48/80. *J Invest Dermatol* 87:113, 1986.
42. Elmets CA: Drug-induced photoallergy. *Dermatol Clin* 4:231, 1986.
43. Kochevar IE: Phototoxicity mechanisms: chlorpromazine photosensitized damage to DNA and cell membranes. *J Invest Dermatol* 77:59, 1981.
44. Kochevar IE: Mechanisms of drug photosensitization. *Photochem Photobiol* 45:891, 1987.
45. Pathak MA: Mechanisms of psoralen photosensitization reactions. *Natl Cancer Inst Monogr* 66:41, 1984.
46. Goldstein BD, Harber LC: Erythropoietic protoporphyria: lipid oxidation and red cell membrane damage associated with photohemolysis. *J Clin Invest* 51:892, 1972.
47. Allison AC et al: Role of lysosomes and of cell membranes in photosensitization. *Nature* 209:784, 1966.
48. Carraro C, Pathak MA: Studies on the nature of in vitro and in vivo photosensitization reactions by psoralens and porphyrins. *J Invest Dermatol* 90:267, 1988.
49. Miyachi Y, Takigawa M: Mechanisms of contact photosensitivity in mice: II. Langerhans cells are required for successful induction of contact photosensitivity to TCSA. *J Invest Dermatol* 78:363, 1982.
50. Tokura Y et al: Ultraviolet-induced suppressor T cells and factor(s) in murine contact photosensitivity. I. Biological and immunochemical characterization of factor(s) extracted from suppressor T cells. *Cell Immunol* 110:305, 1987.
51. Granstein RD et al: The role of suppressor cells in the induction of murine photoallergic contact dermatitis and its suppression by prior UVB irradiation. *J Immunol* 130:2099, 1983.
52. Kerdel FA et al: Mast cell participation during the elicitation phase of murine allergic contact hypersensitivity. *J Invest Dermatol* 88:686, 1987.
53. Miyachi Y et al: Mechanism of contact hypersensitivity in mice. VII. Diminished elicitation by reserpine and defective expression in mast cell–deficient mice. *J Invest Dermatol* 87:39, 1986.
54. Miyachi Y et al: Mechanisms of contact photosensitivity in mice. VI. Oxygen intermediates are involved in contact photosensitization but not in ordinary contact sensitization. *J Invest Dermatol* 86:26, 1986.
55. Lim HW: Pathophysiology of cutaneous lesions in porphyrias. *Semin Hematol* 26:114, 1989.
56. Athar M et al: A novel mechanism for the generation of superoxide anions in hematoporphyrin derivative–mediated cutaneous photosensitization: activation of the xanthine oxidase pathway. *J Clin Invest* 83:1137, 1989.

57. Lim HW et al: Activation of the complement system and generation of chemotactic activity in vivo in patients with porphyrias. *J Clin Invest* 74:1961, 1984.
58. Kerdel FA et al: In vivo mediator release and degranulation of mast cells in hematoporphyrin derivative–induced phototoxicity. *J Invest Dermatol* 88:277, 1987.
59. Kraemer KH, Slor H: Xeroderma pigmentosum. *Clin Dermatol* 2:33, 1985.
60. Sutherland BM et al: Pyrimidine dimer formation and repair in human skin. *Cancer Res* 40:3181, 1980.
61. D'Ambrosio SM et al: Photorepair of pyrimidine dimers in human skin in vivo. *Photochem Photobiol* 34:461, 1981.
62. Morison W: Effects of ultraviolet radiation on the immune system in humans. *Photochem Photobiol* 50:515, 1989.
63. Edelson R et al: Treatment of cutaneous T-cell lymphoma by extracorporeal photochemotherapy: preliminary results. *N Engl J Med* 316:297, 1987.
64. Gilchrest BA et al: Ultraviolet phototherapy of uremic pruritus. *Ann Intern Med* 91:71, 1979.
65. Buchness MR et al: Eosinophilic pustular folliculitis in the acquired immunodeficiency syndrome: treatment with ultraviolet B phototherapy. *N Engl J Med* 318:1183, 1988.

SECTION TEN

DISORDERS DUE TO MICROBIAL AGENTS

25

Pathophysiology of Certain Bacterial Diseases

James J. Leyden

CUTANEOUS INFECTIONS

Cutaneous infections by bacteria constitute a major form of skin disease. Fortunately, these infections tend to remain relatively superficial and are not a threat of more serious systemic infections. However, systemic signs and symptoms can develop and in certain situations can even be life-threatening. A great deal has been learned in recent years about how various pathogenic organisms colonize skin, proliferate, and induce a host response, which then is manifested clinically as an infection. This chapter includes a brief review of the normal resident flora and its role in protecting the host, the factors known about colonization of the skin by pathogenic bacteria, and the subsequent host response.

Resident Flora

The cutaneous microflora is basically simple and consists of a limited number of species of aerobic and anaerobic bacteria and yeasts of the genus *Pityrosporum;* as such, it stands in contrast to the highly complex flora found in other body areas such as the oral cavity, gastrointestinal tract, and vagina.

Aerobic Cocci

Aerobic cocci are members of the family Micrococcaceae and are found on virtually all body sites. The classification of these organisms has undergone numerous changes in the past 30 years. In the early 1960s, Baird-Parker devised a scheme for dividing the Micrococcaceae into staphylococci and micrococci on the basis of physiological and biochemical characteristics.[1,2] More recent studies, which determined the DNA base composition of these organisms, substantiated Baird-Parker's distinction in that organisms classified as staphylococci by his schemes were shown to have a 30 to 36 percent guanine plus cytosine (G + C) composition, while micrococci had 65 to 75 percent G + C.[3,4] Baird-Parker proposed a less complex system for identification of staphylococci that reduced the predominant species to *Staphylococcus aurus, S. saprophyticus,* and *S. epidermidis.*[5] Micrococci species found in human skin include *Micrococcus luteus, M. roseus,* and *M. varians.* The genus formerly reported as *Sarcina* is now contained in *M. luteus. S. epidermidis* is the most common coccus found on human skin. *S. aureus* is a common transient or contaminant and can be recovered from a high percentage of people who have multiple body sites cultured repeatedly. However, *S. aureus* rarely achieves a true resident status. Exceptions to this rule are intertriginous sites such as the toe web, the axilla, and the perineum, where *S. aureus* occasionally can establish a true residence in the absence of disease. Another noncutaneous site where *S. aureus* can achieve resident status in the absence of disease is the anterior nares.

Aerobic Diphtheroids

The aerobic diphtheroids constitute a large portion of the cutaneous microflora. Recent studies indicate that these organisms belong (on the basis of cell wall constituents) to two genera, *Corynebacterium* and *Brevibacterium.*[6,7] These recent advances have not yet reached the point where generally agreed-upon species exist. As this work progresses important questions should be settled, such as whether the diphtheroids involved in the scaling intertriginous condition known as erythrasma and those involved in interdigital athlete's foot infections are members of the resident flora that act in a pathogenic way under certain circumstances or whether they are inherently more virulent organisms that colonize skin and induce disease.

Anaerobic Diphtheroids

The classification of this group of organisms once included as many as 12 species. The use of cell wall analysis, DNA base composition, and homology demonstrated that these organisms belonged to the genus *Propionibacterium* (not *Corynebacterium,* as was previously thought) and that there were three species, namely, *P. acnes, P. granulosum,* and *P. avidum.*[8] These organisms are normal residents that inhabit sebaceous follicles where the oxygen tension is sufficiently reduced to allow them to thrive. Except in the situation of excessive proliferation, as occurs in acne patients, these organisms are not involved in skin disease.

Yeasts

The only yeast genus found in significant numbers in humans is *Pityrosporum*. The three morphological types, oval, round, and filamentous, gave rise to the delineation of three species, namely, *P. ovale*, *P. orbiculare*, and *Malassezia furfur*. Recent work has demonstrated that the three forms are actually morphological variants of the same species in that they are antigenically similar,[9] have similar nutritional requirements, and are interconvertible.[10] *Pityrosporum* is nonpathogenic except when conditions favor proliferation, which can result in the scaling condition tinea versicolor.[11]

ECOLOGY AND POPULATION DYNAMICS OF RESIDENT FLORA

Different body regions have distinct bacterial populations (Fig. 25-1). The density and the constituent species of a given body site can be interpreted to identify unique cutaneous environments. Three major determinants of cutaneous habitants have been identified: (1) the presence of lipid, (2) the availability of moisture, and (3) the ability to maintain an environment of low oxygen content.

Oily regions, such as the head, upper trunk, and scalp, are rich in sebaceous glands. Sebaceous follicles provide lipid growth substrates and a protected niche that can maintain an anaerobic environment. The

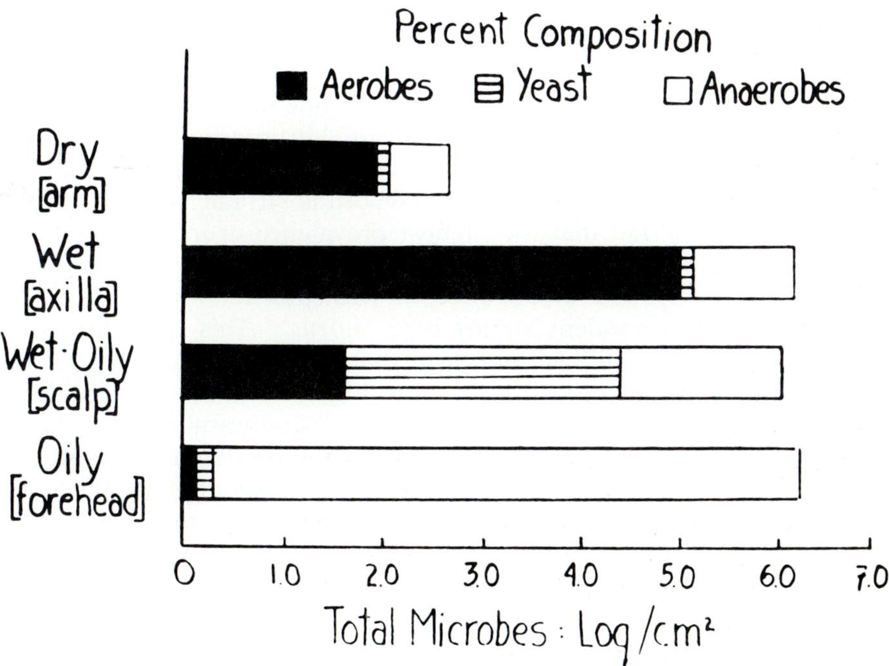

Figure 25-1 Regional variation in the kinds and total number of microorganisms.

dominant bacteria on the face and trunk are the propionibacteria, predominantly *P. acnes.*[12] These anaerobic organisms live in the depths of sebaceous follicles where a reduced or low oxygen level exists. *P. acnes* density correlates well with sebum production, as determined indirectly by quantification of the amount of lipid delivered to the skin surface in a defined time period.[13] The other major inhabitant of body areas rich in sebaceous glands is the yeast *Pityrosporum,* and in a body area extremely rich in sebum such as the scalp (which normally has up to 10 times the amount of lipid per square centimeter found on a similar area of the face), *P. ovale* is the dominant organism. Since both *P. acnes* and *P. ovale* possess potent lipase enzymes,[14] these organisms may utilize glycerol liberated by hydrolysis of sebaceous gland triglycerides as an important growth substrate.

In nonsebaceous regions, the major environmental factor appears to be the availability of water. Areas that are rich in sweat glands and are restricted in airflow, such as the intertriginous regions, have larger populations of bacteria than areas with fewer sweat glands. The axilla, groin, and toe web space support large populations of bacteria including aerobic cocci, diphtheroids, and occasionally low numbers of gram-negative organisms, while areas that are dry, such as the extremities, have mainly cocci in low numbers. The effect of hydration is best appreciated by the effect of applying an occlusive dressing such as impermeable plastic film of adhesive tape to a body area with few bacteria, e.g., the forearm. A rapid expansion from 10^2 to 10^5 or 10^6 organisms per square centimeter occurs within 24 to 48 h.[15]

Resident Flora and Cutaneous Infection

The resident flora appears to provide a first line of defense against one of the most common pathogens involved in skin infection, *S. aureus.* In the case of *S. aureus,* the importance of the resident flora is most strikingly seen in the newborn. The skin of the newborn is virtually sterile at birth. It is during this period that the highest prevalence of infection with *S. aureus* exists.[16] This principle was so firmly established that newborns in nurseries where serious *S. aureus* infection was epidemic were deliberately colonized with less virulent strains of *S. aureus.*[17] This procedure was widely adopted until it became clear that it was not totally free of complications and until the use of strict washing of hands between handling infants and effective antimicrobial cleansers significantly reduced the incidence of *S. aureus* infections. The ability of the resident flora to protect against *S. aureus* infection was also demonstrated in experimental infections in human volunteers. Eradication of the normal flora greatly enhanced both the survival of an *S. aureus* inoculation and subsequent infection.[18] The mechanism(s) by which the resident flora help to ward off *S. aureus* infection has not been clearly established. However, two possible mechanisms have been identified:

1. The resident bacteria produce antibiotics and bacteriocidins that may influence the composition of the flora and inhibit *S. aureus* colonization.[19]

2. Staphylococci must establish adherence to epithelial cells as a primary step in colonization.[20] The presence of *S. epidermidis* on skin may substantially limit the number of available attachment sites and thus interfere with colonization.

Streptococci such as *S. pyogenes* have been shown to be exquisitely sensitive to fatty acids, and since all members of the resident flora possess lipases that can cleave fatty acids from sebaceous gland triglycerides, the resident flora may play an important role in host defense mechanisms against streptococcal infection.[21]

The resident flora does not seem to be an important factor in warding off infection by gram-negative bacteria or *Candida albicans*. In experimentally induced infections in human volunteers, suppression of the resident flora does not enhance either the incidence of colonization or the frequency of infection.[22,23]

OTHER FACTORS INVOLVED IN THE SKIN DEFENSE MECHANISM

Moisture and skin trauma are clearly important factors in the pathophysiology of cutaneous infections. From experimental infection studies in animals and humans, it is clear that survival and subsequent proliferation of an inoculum are significantly enhanced by a warm, humid environment such as provided by an occlusive dressing.[18,23,24] The increased carbon dioxide tension under such a dressing also appears to be important for streptococcal and fungal infections.[25] The stratum corneum also provides a formidable defense against infection by many pathogens, most notably streptococci and gram-negative bacteria.[23,26] Streptococcal infections cannot be induced in either animals or human volunteers without damage to the stratum corneum.[26,27] Likewise, gram-negative bacteria, even *Pseudomonas aeruginosa*, which possess a wide array of proteolytic enzymes, cannot induce a lesion on normal intact skin even when present in extremely high densities.[23] Infections with *S. aureus* are also greatly enhanced by prior damage such as removal of the stratum corneum by cellophane tape stripping.[18] On the other hand, certain organisms can overcome the stratum corneum barrier. *C. albicans, P. ovale, P. orbiculare,* and dermatophytic fungi produce filaments and hyphae that are capable of invading the stratum corneum; thus, prior damage is not essential for development of infection.

COMMON CUTANEOUS INFECTIONS

Primary bacterial infections are those in which there is no underlying chronic abnormality of the skin such as a dermatosis and in which the skin is invaded by a pathogen that proliferates and incites a host reaction, with a resulting clinical disease. Nearly all cutaneous bacterial infections are due to either *S. aureus* or *Streptococcus pyogenes*. For years there was considerable debate over the relative importance of each organism, particularly since both were frequently cultured from pyodermas. Sufficient evidence has now accumulated to indicate that there are definite clinical–microbiological correlations with specific pathophysiological events.

Staphylococcal Infections

S. aureus infections present with an array of clinical findings including pustules, furuncles, blistering lesions, and the scalded skin syndrome.

Folliculitis

This is manifested by pustules and papules with perifollicular areas of slightly infiltrated erythema (Fig. 25-2). Systemic symptoms are rarely present. The pathophysiological events involve *S. aureus* colonization of the skin surface and proliferation with spread into follicular orifices, followed by proliferation within follicles. *S. aureus* chemotactic factors lead to the attraction of polymorphonuclear leukocytes[28] into the follicular lumen. This plus the elaboration of the innumerable enzymes of *S. aureus*, which include hemolysins, leukocidins, enterotoxins, coagulase, and proteases, results in clinical inflammation.

Furuncles

Boils presumably follow the same initial events described above, with the larger area of infiltrated erythema resulting from spread of the organism

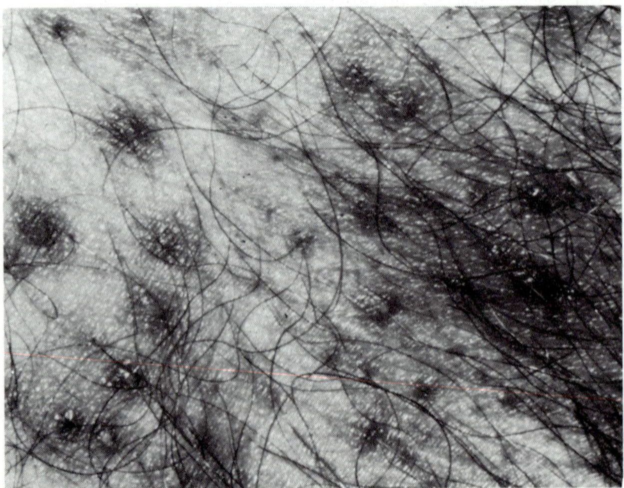

Figure 25-2 *S. aureus* folliculitis due to invasion of follicles followed by the host response of polymorphonuclear leukocytes.

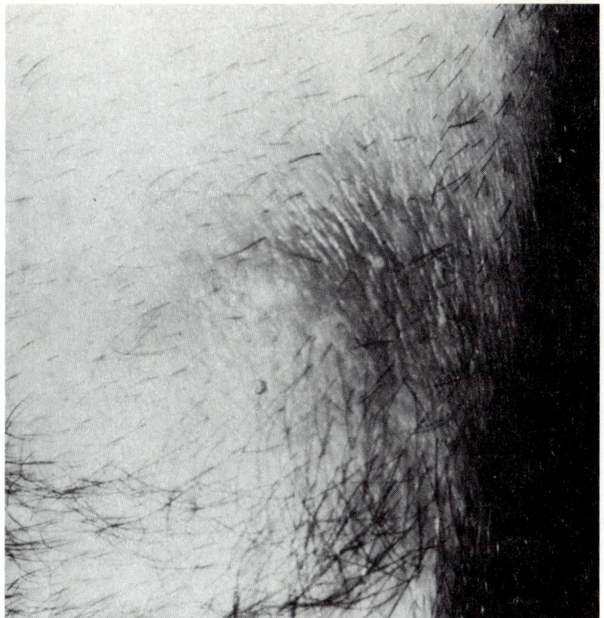

Figure 25-3 Furuncle due to *S. aureus.*

through follicular walls into the dermis (Fig. 25-3). Deep inoculation of *S. aureus* into the dermis through cuts and scratches can be another initial event in the pathogenesis of a furuncle. The quality of a boil can vary enormously and depends on a variety of factors, including the virulence of the infecting strain and the host's reaction. Strains of low virulence produce fairly innocuous lesions that resolve spontaneously or at most require incision and drainage. More virulent strains, such as 52/52A/80/81, produce rapidly enlarging lesions, cellulitis, fever, and lymphadenopathy and are highly contagious. These strains are usually resistant to penicillin because of the production of penicillinase. Some patients may suffer from repeated infections, and such patients are usually, but not invariably, nasal carriers of the infecting strain. The anterior nares can serve as a reservoir for spread onto the skin and subsequent reinfection. There is evidence that staphylococci attach more readily to nasal mucosal cells of carriers than normal, suggesting a fundamental host difference in patients with recurrent infections.[20]

Bullous Impetigo

The characteristic lesions of bullous impetigo are superficial bullae that rapidly rupture and leave behind a 2- to 4-cm area of skin that has a "scalded skin" or second-degree burn appearance (Fig. 25-4). This condition is usually caused by group II phage type 71 strains of *S. aureus,* which produce a toxin known as exfoliatin that causes a subcorneal cleavage.[29]

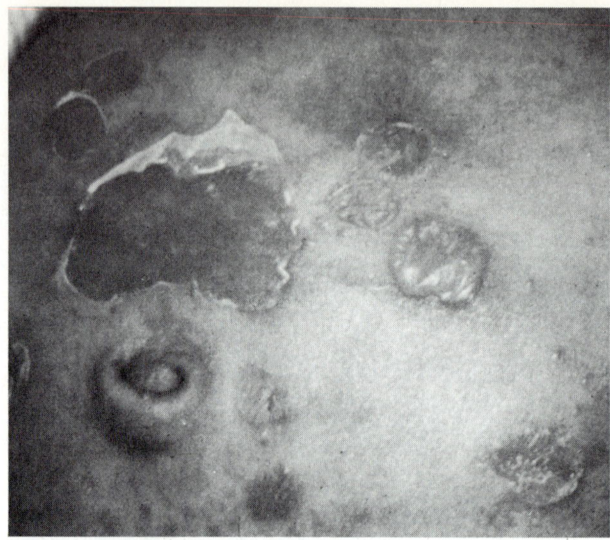

Figure 25-4 Bullous impetigo due to a toxin produced by *S. aureus* resulting in bullae that rupture and leave a scalded skin appearance.

This type of infection thus involves toxin-mediated damage in which cellular adhesion is disrupted, rather than invasion of skin with a host response of recruitment of polymorphonuclear leukocytes. Strains other than group II phage type 71 have been identified, but the majority are due to that particular strain. Since the discovery that genes governing toxin production may be plasmid or chromosomal and that phage group II strains of *S. aureus* may possess both sets of genes, it is clear that two similar but serologically distinct forms of toxin exist.[30] This condition is also fairly contagious, and minor epidemics among schoolchildren are not uncommon. Patients are usually not toxic and do not develop fever until widespread lesions occur. Treatment appears to require systemic antibiotics even when only a few localized lesions are apparent. Treatment failures with topical antibiotics reflect anterior nares colonization and clinically inapparent skin colonization.

Staphylococcal Scalded Skin Syndrome

The most serious staphylococcal skin infection is staphylococcal scalded skin syndrome (SSS), Ritter's disease, or toxic epidermal necrolysis. Most common and devastating in neonates, SSS is the result of an infection with an *S. aureus* strain that produces exfoliative toxin, exfoliatin (ET). Bullous impetigo, conjunctivitis, external otitis, or even asymptomatic nasopharyngeal colonization may lead to SSS. Natural recovery relies on the generation of an antitoxin antibody response and subsequent clearance of the toxin. The greater susceptibility of neonates may relate in some way to a lack of prior immunologic exposure to the toxin.

ET is most frequently produced by phage type 71 staphylococci and is a plasmid-borne toxin. The toxin induces intraepidermal splitting in the stratum granulosum, leading to sloughing of skin. This is in contrast to the necrosis that involves the entire epidermis in the drug-induced toxic epidermal necrolysis.[31]

The precise mechanism by which ET cleaves the stratum granulosum is not understood. Recent work suggests that desmosomes (the point of intercellular attachment) are not the primary target of ET; rather, nondesmosomal intercellular structures are first affected.[32] Experiments demonstrating that protease inhibitors fail to inhibit ET activity suggest that a nonproteinaceous target is involved.

While there is some debate on the relative merits of antibiotic therapy, it appears rational to eliminate the organism producing the offending toxin and thus minimize the amount of toxin to be subsequently neutralized by the host.

Streptococcal Infections

Group A streptococci are not true members of the skin flora, although they may be frequently isolated from normal skin during epidemic episodes of streptococcal impetigo or pyoderma. It has been well documented that the strains that cause skin infections are distinct from those that cause respiratory tract infections, implying a different pathogenic mechanism for skin invasion or differential viability of strains.[33] The finding that throat and skin strains are both highly sensitive to oleic acid and ultraviolet light[21] argues against a role for these germicidal factors as an explanation of why certain strains infect skin. It has been shown that streptococci are not able to survive for more than 24 h on the intact skin of adults and that infection cannot develop without the presence of a break in the skin.[26] Presumably both a break in the integrity of the skin and an inoculum of streptococci do not occur simultaneously with the arrival of streptococci on the skin. While streptococci do not survive for prolonged periods when inoculated on intact human skin, the demonstration that skin strains are better able to survive "starvation" may be an important factor in the pathogenesis of skin infection.[34] An alternative explanation has been suggested by the finding that skin strains preferentially adhere to skin epithelial cells in in vitro tests compared with buccal mucosal cells, while the opposite is true for throat strains.[35] Temporary adherence to skin epithelial cells followed by trauma could then result in cutaneous infection.

Cellulitis

A common form of streptococcal infection is a localized cellulitis. The most frequent area of involvement is the lower leg. Lymphatic ducts are involved, as manifested clinically by red streaking. Fever and lymphadenopathy develop early in the course. A common portal of entry for this infection is an interdigital toe web infection with dermatophytic fungi that produces a break in the stratum corneum. This is particularly true in patients with recurrent attacks of lower leg cellulitis. Erysipelas is a form of streptococcal cellulitis most commonly seen on the face. In children, a similar condition is often due to *Haemophilus influenzae*.[36]

Impetigo–Ecthyma

The most common infectious skin lesion is a localized erosion (impetigo) or ulceration (ecthyma) that becomes covered by a serous crust (Fig. 25-5). This lesion is usually found on the lower part of the leg, primarily in children living in hot, humid climates where hygienic practices are poor. Clinically, this lesion consists of a superficial to deep ulceration covered by a serosanguineous crust that is surrounded by a few millimeters of indurated erythema. Lymphadenopathy and low-grade fever are early signs of ecthyma even with minor lesions.[37] The clinical observation that this infection occurs on the lower legs of young children plus the results of experimentally induced infections makes it clear that minor trauma of the skin is a prerequisite for infection. Group A streptococci do not colonize intact human skin. While they can survive for brief periods, a break in cutaneous integrity is essential for clinical infection to occur.[26]

The crust commonly becomes colonized by *S. aureus*. As many as 59 percent of streptococcal lesions become secondarily colonized.[38] These strains of *S. aureus* are different from those that induce primary *S. aureus* infections, and the evidence from clinical and experimental infection studies

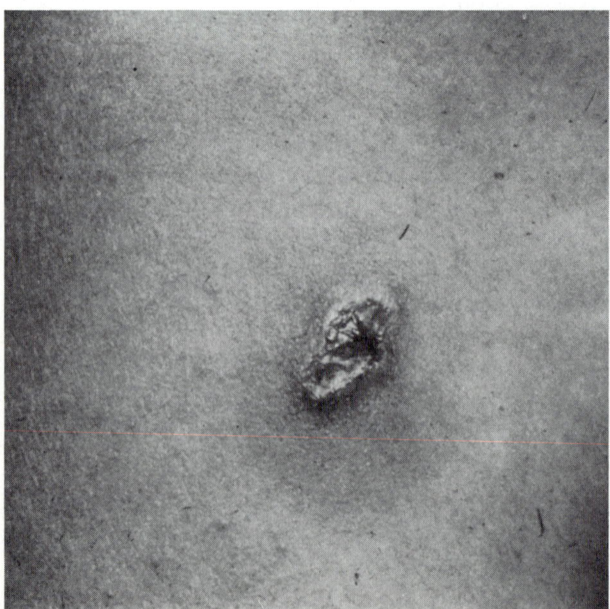

Figure 25-5 Streptococcal pyoderma.

indicates that these strains of *S. aureus* do not significantly influence the course of treatment of streptococcal lesions. For example, penicillin therapy results in prompt clearing of lesions containing penicillin-resistant *S. aureus* organisms.[38]

Treatment of streptococcal impetigo–ecthyma commonly requires systemic antibiotics such as erythromycin or penicillin when lesions are widespread or especially deep and covered by a tenacious crust. More superficial lesions are amenable to compresses that remove the crust and permit delivery of sufficient topical agents to eradicate streptococci.

Recognition of streptococcal forms of pyodermas is important because of the possibility of the complication of postinfection glomerulonephritis.[37] Streptococci of certain M-types can induce glomerulonephritis, particularly in young children.[39] Currently there is no evidence that antibiotic therapy can prevent postinfection nephritis.

The appearance of acute glomerulonephritis following streptococcal pyoderma was in fact accompanied by the discovery of strains with new M-type protein antigens. These strains became known as *nephritogenic* strains. Glomerulonephritis is an immune complex–mediated process and has been experimentally induced in animals with streptococci and streptococcal fractions.[40,41] However, as a practical matter, M-typing is not always feasible, and patterns of M-types tend to change from season to season. A sufficient compromise may reside in the examination of the urine of children found to have streptococcal pyoderma for the presence of red blood cells, red blood cell casts, and protein. If the result of the urinalysis is abnormal, referral to a nephrologist is indicated. Fortunately, glomerulonephritis is usually transient, but chronic nephritis can develop and progress to the point of renal failure.

It is worth noting that antibody responses to streptococci differ markedly between skin and throat infections. In the latter antistreptolysin O (ASO) titers rise, while in skin infections the ASO titer usually does not rise and anti-DNase B titers develop.[37] Cholesterol can suppress the action of streptolysin O and the formation of ASO but will not affect DNase B. Since cholesterol is a major component of human sebum, its presence may account for the lack of ASO response with skin infections.[42]

ROLE OF BACTERIA IN CHRONIC INFLAMMATORY DISORDERS

Dermatitic skin has long been recognized as fertile soil for bacterial colonization and infection, particularly with *S. aureus*. It has also been known for some time that *S. aureus* may be present in eczematous lesions without the classic signs of infection being present. Distinguishing between mere colonization and true infection is important. A lesion cannot be said to be secondarily infected unless it can be shown that bacteria contribute to the intensity or persistence of the underlying dermatitis. Correlation of colony counts from dermatoses with clinical effects during antibiotic therapy demonstrates that counts of *S. aureus* of less than 1×10^6 organisms per square centimeter are harmless and represent colonization without infection.[43] Colony counts in excess of 1×10^6 per square centimeter represent secondary infection. The strains of *S. aureus* that invade eczematous skin appear to be of relatively low virulence. Phage typing reveals either nontypable or group III strains not recognized to be associated with severe primary infections.

The frequency of isolation of *S. aureus* and its density are dependent upon the type of dermatitis. In general, the more exudative the dermatitis, the greater the degree of colonization. For example, *S. aureus* is practically always present in atopic dermatitis, as it is in nummular eczema and neurodermatitis.[44] In psoriasis, *S. aureus* is recovered in low numbers from approximately 50 percent of patients, while only 20 percent of patients with seborrheic dermatitis are colonized by *S. aureus*.[44]

In addition to aggravation of the underlying dermatitis, *S. aureus* colonization of dermatitic skin is occasionally important from a public health viewpoint. Exfoliation of squamae heavily populated with *S. aureus* poses a threat of infection, especially when more vulnerable individuals such as hospitalized patients are exposed. Epidemics of severe wound infections and even deaths have been traced to secondarily infected dermatitic skin.[45,46]

REFERENCES

1. Baird-Parker AC: A classification of micrococci and staphylococci based on physiological and biochemical tests. *J Gen Microbiol* 30:409, 1963.
2. Baird-Parker AC: The classification of staphylococci and micrococci from world-wide sources. *J Gen Microbiol* 38:363, 1965.
3. Silvestri LG, Hill LR: Agreement between deoxyribonucleic acid base composition and taxonomic classification of gram positive cocci. *J Bacteriol* 90:136, 1965.
4. Kloos WE, Schleifer KH: Simplified scheme for routine identification of human staphylococcus species. *J Clin Microbiol* 1:82, 1975.
5. Baird-Parker AC: The basis for the present classification of staphylococci and micrococci. *Ann NY Acad Sci* 28:4, 1974.
6. Pitcher DG: Rapid identification of cell wall components as a guide to the classification of aerobic coryneform bacteria from human skin. *J Gen Microbiol* 10:439, 1977.
7. Pitcher DG: Aerobic cutaneous coryneforms: recent taxonomic findings. *Br J Dermatol* 98:363, 1978.
8. Johnson JL, Cummins CS: Cell wall composition and deoxyribonucleic acid similarities among the anaerobic coryneforms, classical propionibacteria and strains of *Arachnia propionica*. *J Bacteriol* 109:1047, 1972.
9. Tamaka M, Imamura S: Immunological studies on pityrosporum genus and *Malassezia furfur*. *J Invest Dermatol* 73:34, 1979.
10. Salkin IF, Gordon MA: Polymorphism of *Malassezia furfur*. *Can J Microbiol* 23:471, 1977.
11. McGinley KJ et al: Microbiology of tinea versicolor. *Arch Dermatol* 102:168, 1970.
12. McGinley KJ et al: Regional variations of cutaneous proprionibacteria. *Appl Environ Microbiol* 23:471, 1977.
13. McGinley KJ et al: Regional variations in density of cutaneous propionibacteria: correlation of *Propionibacterium acnes* population with sebaceous secretion. *J Clin Microbiol* 12:672, 1980.
14. Marples RR et al: Influence of pityrosporum species in the generation of free fatty acids in human skin surface lipids. *J Invest Dermatol* 58:155, 1972.

15. Marples RR: The effect of hydration on the bacterial flora of the skin, in GH Hildick-Smith, HI Maibach (eds), *Skin Bacteria and Their Role in Infection*. New York, McGraw-Hill, 1965, p 33.
16. Blair EB, Tull AH: Multiple infections among newborns resulting from colonization with *Staphylococcus aureus*. *Am J Clin Pathol* 52:42, 1969.
17. Shinefield HR et al: Interactions of staphylococci colonization. *Am J Dis Child* 111:11, 1966.
18. Singh G et al: Staphylococcus infections in humans. *J Invest Dermatol* 57:149, 1971.
19. Selwyn S, Ellis H: Skin bacteria and skin disinfection reconsidered. *Br Med J* 1:136, 1972.
20. Aly R et al: Bacterial adherance to nasal mucosal cells. *Infect Immun* 17:546, 1977.
21. Speert DP, Wannamaker CW: Susceptibility of group A streptococci to oleic acid and ultraviolet light. *J Lab Clin Med* 96:252, 1980.
22. Rebora A et al: Experimental infection with *Candida albicans*. *Arch Dermatol* 108:69, 1973.
23. Leyden JJ et al: Experimental inoculation of *Pseudomonas aeruginosa* and *Pseudomonas cepaciae* in human skin. *J Soc Cosmet Chem* 31:19, 1980.
24. Maibach H, Kligman AM: The biology of experimental human cutaneous moniliasis (*Candida albicans*) *Arch Dermatol* 85:233, 1962.
25. King RD et al: The effect of occlusion on carbon dioxide emission from human skin. *Acta Dermatol* 58:135, 1978.
26. Leyden et al: Experimental infections with group A streptococci in humans. *J Invest Dermatol* 75:196, 1980.
27. Burnett JW: Trauma in experimental superficial cutaneous infections. *Arch Dermatol* 88:276, 1963.
28. Schmeling DJ et al: Chemotaxigenesis by cell surface components of *Staphylococcus aureus*. *Infect Immun* 26:57, 1979.
29. Dimond RL et al: The staphylococcal scalded skin syndrome: an experimented, histochemical and electron microscope study. *Br J Dermatol* 96:483, 1977.
30. Johnson A et al: Purification and characterization of different types of exfoliative toxin from *Staphylococcus aureus*. *Infect Immun* 24:79, 1979.
31. Amon RB, Dimond RL: Toxic epidermal necrolysis: rapid differentiation between staphylococcal and drug induced disease. *Arch Dermatol* 111:1433, 1975.
32. Elias PM et al: Staphylococcal scalded skin syndrome: clinical features, pathogenesis and recent microbiological and biochemical developments. *Arch Dermatol* 113:207, 1977.
33. Anthony BF et al: The dynamics of streptococcal infections in a defined population of children: serotypes associated with skin and respiratory infections. *Am J Epidemiol* 104:652, 1976.
34. Mortimer GE et al: The survival of "skin" and "throat" streptococci in peptone water-oleic acid and their growth in simple peptone media, in MT Parker (ed), *Pathogenic Streptococci*. Chertsey, Surrey, England, Reedbooks, 1979, p 120.
35. Aly R et al: Bacterial adherence to nasal mucosal cells. *Infect Immunol* 14:549, 1980.
36. Rapkin RH, Bautista G: *Hemophilus influenzae*. *Am J Dis Child* 124:540, 1972.
37. Dillon HC: Impetigo contagiosa, suppurative and non-suppurative complications. *Am J Dis Child* 1115:530, 1968.
38. Dajani AS et al: Natural history of impetigo. II. Etiologic agents and bacterial interaction. *J Clin Invest* 51:2863, 1972.
39. Anthony BF et al: Attack rates of acute nephritis after type 49 streptococcal infection of the skin and respiratory tract. *J Clin Invest* 48:1697, 1969.
40. Markowitz AS et al: Streptococcal related glomerulonephritis. III. Glomerulonephritis in rhesus monkeys immunologically induced both actively and passively with a soluble fraction from nephritogenic streptococcal protoplasmic membranes. *J Immunol* 107:504, 1971.
41. Zabriskie JB: The role of streptococci in human glomerulonephritis. *J Exp Med* 134:180, 1971.
42. Kaplan EL, Wannamaker LW: Suppression of antistreptolysin O response by cholesterol and by lipid extracts of rabbit skin. *J Exp Med* 144:756, 1976.

43. Leyden JJ et al: *Staphylococcus aureus* in the lesions of atopic dermatitis. *Br J Dermatol* 90:525, 1974.
44. Leyden JJ: Antibiotic use in dermatologic practice. *Int J Dermatol* 13:342, 1974.
45. Payne RW: Severe outbreaks of surgical sepsis due to *Staphylococcus aureus* of an unusual type and origin. *Br J Med* 4:17, 1967.
46. Ayliffe GAJ, Collins BJ: Wound infections acquired from a dispenser for an unusual strain of *Staphylococcus aureus*. *J Clin Pathol* 20:195, 1967.

26

Pathophysiology of Cutaneous Viral Infections: Papillomaviruses

Douglas R. Lowy and William D. Ju

In contrast to free-living infectious agents such as bacteria and fungi, which usually replicate outside of cells, viruses express their genes and replicate only when inside the cells they infect. As viruses lack many of the components required for their own reproduction, they have been programmed to obtain these factors from their host's intracellular milieu. Viruses are therefore often called *obligate intracellular parasites* to emphasize their dependence on cellular machinery. In the process of these interactions, viruses may alter normal cellular functions and cause disease in their hosts.

Although the capacity of infectious agents such as viruses to induce severe pathological changes is emphasized, it should also be recognized that most viruses (and other parasites) have coevolved with their natural hosts. Viruses usually exploit a particular biological niche and typically cause only mild disease. More serious disease tends to occur in hosts with impaired defense mechanisms or when the virus is poorly adapted to the host.

The human papillomaviruses (HPVs) and the cutaneous infections they cause exemplify these concepts and are the principal focus of this chapter. Two other groups of viruses, herpesviruses and poxviruses, are also responsible for many viral infections of the integument. HPVs are important to dermatology because they are the causative agents of warts and related conditions.[1,2] Some papillomaviruses have also been associated with malignant tumors of the skin and mucous membranes.[3,4]

Table 26-1

HPV GENOTYPES

Cutaneous (nongenital) lesions
Benign (plantar, common, flat, and "butcher's" warts)—HPVs **1–4,** 7, 28
Potentially malignant—16, 34
Genital-mucosal (genital, oral, and laryngeal) lesions
Mostly benign—**6, 11,** 13, 32, 42–44
Potentially malignant—**16, 18,** 30, 31, 33–35, 39, 45, 51, 52
Epidermodysplasia verruciformis lesions
Mostly benign—**3, 10,** 9, 12, 15, 19, 21–25, 47, 50
Potentially malignant—**5, 8,** 14, 17, 20

The genotypes most commonly found in a given group are in boldface.

More than 60 different HPV genotypes (types) have been described to date[5] (Table 26-1). In the spectrum of HPV infection, a good correlation can often be made between the specific clinical presentation and the presence of a particular HPV type. This chapter discusses some of these correlations and examines the reproductive strategy of HPVs.

STRUCTURE

The Virion

It is useful to consider a virus to be genetic information that has developed the capacity to be replicated inside host cells and to be efficiently transmitted to other potential host cells. This *viral genome* can be DNA or RNA, depending on the specific virus. The strategy adopted by viruses for their transmission to uninfected cells is to surround their nonparticulate viral genome with a proteinaceous coat, forming an infectious particle called a *virion.* This outer protein coat of the virion serves a dual role. First, it protects the viral genome. Second, it fosters the efficient transmission of the viral genome to potential host cells, since it contains determinants that promote enhanced adherence of viral particles to specific receptors located on the host cells; these surface interactions help direct the viral genetic blueprint to its proper target cells. Since the viral genome may exist within a cell in the absence of detectable virus particles, it is convenient to divide a virus life cycle into nonparticulate phases, which occur intracellularly, and particulate phases, which are both intracellular and extracellular.

Virions have a relatively simple structure. The protein shell that surrounds the viral genome is called the *capsid.* Capsid proteins, which are encoded by the virus, are often arranged to form repetitive, multimeric subunits called *capsomeres.* The viral genome and the capsid together are designated the *nucleocapsid.* In some viruses, such as herpesviruses, the capsid may have another outer layer, the *envelope,* which is composed of lipids and proteins. The envelope is acquired as the nucleocapsid buds through the host cell membrane; at least some envelope proteins are encoded by the viral genome. Since the lipoprotein envelope is sensitive to desiccation, herpesviruses and other viruses that use envelopes for adsorption and adherence to host cells lose their infectivity on drying. The virions of poxviruses, such as vaccinia virus, variola virus, and molluscum contagiosum virus, are exceptional in several respects. For example, they have a more complex structure than most other animal viruses and are resistant to drying, although they possess an envelope.

The proteins that contribute to the nucleocapsid and envelope are generally referred to as *structural* viral proteins. The virions of some viruses also contain one or a few virally encoded proteins that serve *nonstructural* functions, such as the reverse transcriptase of retroviruses. Nonstructural virally encoded proteins that do not become incorporated into virions also are generally of great importance to the life cycle of a virus and may be responsible for many of the pathological changes induced by virus infections.

HPV virions are small (about 55 nm in diameter), spherical particles (Fig. 26-1). The capsid of each virion is composed of multiple copies of virally encoded protein subunits. The HPV capsid is "naked" in that it is not surrounded by a lipoprotein envelope, which means that for papillomaviruses the nucleocapsid is the complete virion. Since HPV virions lack an envelope, they are significantly more resistant to drying than are enveloped viruses, so HPV virions tend to retain their infectivity when they are shed along with stratum corneum cells.

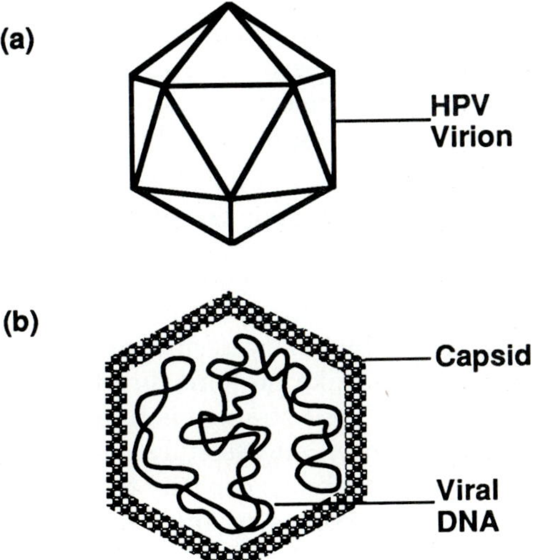

Figure 26-1 (*a*) The HPV virion is an icosahedral (20-sided) particle. (*b*) It is composed of a viral genome surrounded by a proteinaceous capsid.

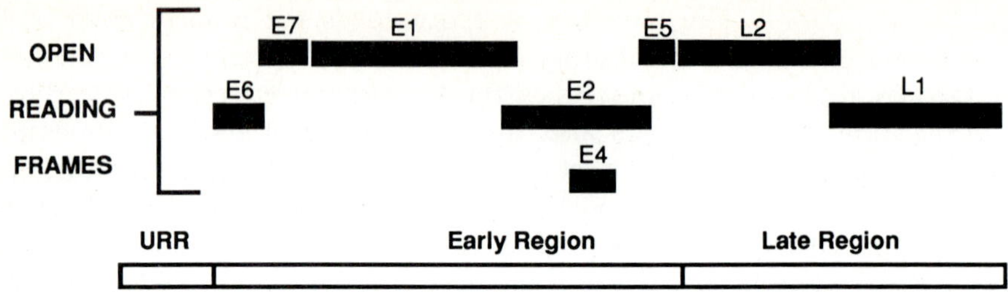

Figure 26-2 The organization of a typical HPV genome. URR = upstream regulatory region.

The Viral Genome

HPV genomes are composed of a single circle of supercoiled, double-stranded DNA that is 7.2 to 8.4 kilobases in length, depending on the particular HPV type.[3,4] The human genome, in contrast, is over 3 million kilobases long. Nucleotide sequence analysis of several HPV genomes has shown that they share a similar, but not identical, overall genetic organization (Fig. 26-2). The HPV genome can be thought of as being composed of three parts: the *early* (*E*) region, which mainly encodes nonstructural proteins important in early phases of the virus life cycle; the *late* (*L*) region, which encodes the structural viral proteins important in late phases of the virus life cycle; and the major *regulatory* region, called the *upstream regulatory region* (*URR*) or *long control region* (*LCR*), which is important in the control of HPV DNA replication and viral gene expression.

HPV genomes have multiple open reading frames. An open reading frame is a stretch of codons (nucleotide triplets), uninterrupted by a translation termination codon, that is long enough potentially to code for a functional protein(s). Typical HPV genomes have eight or nine open reading frames, some of which partially overlap. There are six or seven open reading frames located in the early region of the genome (designated E1, E2, etc.) and two open reading frames in the late region (L1 and L2).

THE VIRUS LIFE CYCLE AND THE MORPHOGENESIS OF WARTS

The life cycle of a virus differs fundamentally from that of free-living infectious agents such as bacteria and fungi. These latter agents are organized as cells that divide by binary fission, as do animal cells. Viruses, in contrast, lack the ability to make proteins directly, which requires them to replicate inside host cells. Their strategy is to make numerous progeny virions in each cell that has been successfully infected by a single virion. The virus accomplishes this feat by its capacity to reprogram the host cell's machinery to make multiple copies of the various virion components, which include the viral genome, structural viral proteins, and, in certain cases, some nonstructural viral proteins. These parts are then assembled into complete virions.

While most viruses successfully infect a variety of cell types, HPVs are *epitheliotropic*, which means that they can only infect epithelial cells. HPV infection is even more restricted in at least three additional ways. First, *productive infection* (the synthesis of progeny virions) by HPVs is restricted to stratified squamous epithelia. This is because virus replication appears to be closely related to the differentiation program of a multilayered epithelium. Second, different HPV types appear to infect distinct cutaneous or mucosal surfaces preferentially, as discussed below in greater detail. Third, HPVs seem incapable of inducing productive infection of nonhuman epithelia, which implies that humans are the only natural hosts for HPV infection. Given the epitheliotropic nature of HPV infection, it is not surprising that the majority of pathological changes induced by these viruses are confined to the epithelium. Subepithelial alterations, such as increased capillary formation, presumably occur as a response to changes in the overlying epithelium.

The life cycle of a virus can be divided into several phases. Many specifics of the HPV life cycle remain unknown because of the inability, thus far, to propagate the virus in tissue culture. Nevertheless, the general principles of viral replication appear to apply to HPVs.

In order for a mature, extracellular virion to produce progeny, it needs to infect a host cell in which its viral replication program can successfully operate. The first steps in this process are designated *adsorption, penetration,* and *uncoating*. The initial event is for the viral capsid to *adsorb* to the plasma membrane of a potential host cell. HPVs appear to infect the skin via direct inoculation rather than by spreading from an internal focus. The virus must adsorb to cells located beneath the stratum corneum, perhaps to basal cells, since cornified cells do not permit the replication of HPV DNA. It is likely that HPVs gain access to deeper keratinocytes through microscopic and visible abrasions, since an intact stratum corneum should serve as a formidable barrier to entry. By analogy with other viruses, HPV adsorption to its target cells is probably significantly and perhaps even critically enhanced by the interaction of certain viral capsid components with specific cell-encoded *receptor* proteins located on the host's membrane.

Following adsorption, the virion *penetrates* the host cell's interior. The details of how HPV gains entry to the cell are not known, but many other viruses, after binding to their receptors, migrate down the shafts of microvilli to special areas of the membrane that are lined on the cytoplasmic side by a protein called *clathrin*. The virions then undergo endocytosis through these clathrin "coated pits." Once inside the host's cytoplasm, the virus-bearing vesicles fuse with endosomes, and here the separation of the viral nucleic acid and capsid begins. This process, known as *uncoating*, enables cell components to interact with the viral genome so that it can be expressed and replicated.

It should be noted that even if virions are able to reach the membranes of their proper host cells, a significant number of the particles will fail at each of the phases of adsorption, penetration, and uncoating. Therefore, the number of infectious units is frequently orders of magnitude smaller than the original number of virions, and the frequency of infection after exposure depends on, among other factors, the size of the inoculum.

After the viral DNA is uncoated, the virus begins its nonparticulate phase. This is the *synthetic phase,* in which the viral genome uses host machinery to manufacture viral components. During the *early synthetic phase,* replication conditions for the viral genome are set in place through the highly ordered expression of viral *early genes.* In addition to regulating the expression of viral proteins, the proteins encoded by the early HPV genes appear to foster replication of the HPV DNA genome by their influence on the expression and function of host cellular proteins. As discussed below, some of these early viral proteins also appear to stimulate cell proliferation, which probably contributes to the increased number of mitotic figures seen in many warts. The successful replication of viral genomes marks the end of the early synthetic phase and the beginning of the *late synthetic phase.* In the case of HPVs, as for viruses in general, viral *late genes* generally code for structural constituents that will make up the capsid.

Once the viral DNA has been replicated and capsid components have been manufactured, progeny virions can be assembled. This *morphogenic* stage returns the virus to its particulate form. Assembly of virions is largely passive and can occur spontaneously because the thermodynamic information embedded in the various viral components is sufficient to arrange individual molecules into proper building blocks, and these, in turn, come together to form complete, mature viral particles. HPV DNA replication and virion assembly occur in the nucleus, as is true for herpesviruses and other DNA-containing viruses except poxviruses, in which replication and assembly occur in the cytoplasm.

When a virus infects a host cell and is able to manufacture progeny virions, the infection is said to be *productive,* and the host cell is termed *permissive* for that specific virus. In contrast, an infection that fails to complete its replication cycle is termed *abortive,* and the infected cell is classified as *nonpermissive.* If a virus is causing no detectable phenotypic changes in its infected host cells, the infection is said to be *latent.*

There are several distinct aspects of HPV infection that are related to the manner in which they infect epithelia (Fig. 26-3). HPVs tend to establish a chronic infection of stratified squamous epithelial cells, whose normal growth and development result in differentiation followed by eventual desquamation. The life cycle of most other viruses, in contrast, is not associated with the differentiation of the host cells, and these infections tend to be acute rather than chronic processes, with the life span of the infected cells frequently being greatly shortened.

HPVs probably induce chronic infection by parasitizing the lower, proliferative layers of the epidermis with their viral DNA (Fig. 26-3). The virus can presumably remain as a nonparticulate viral genome indefinitely in such proliferating cells. HPV DNA and RNA are probably not detected

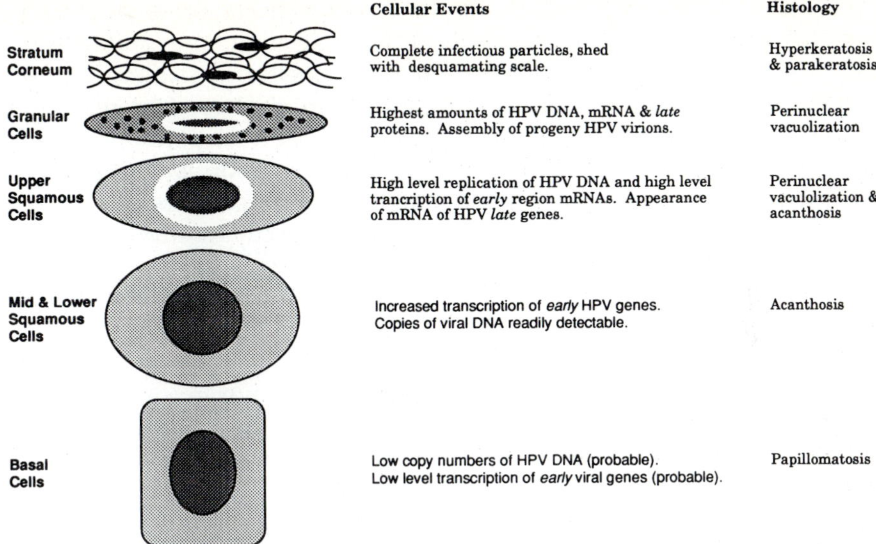

Figure 26-3 Some cellular and molecular events of HPV infection linked to differentiation of the epidermis.

routinely in basal cells because the techniques employed are not sufficiently sensitive to detect viral nucleic acid sequences in the low number of copies believed to be present in these cells. It is not until infected cells reach the stratum spinosum and stratum granulosum that the extensive replication of viral DNA, expression of capsid proteins, and formation of progeny virions become easily apparent.[6]

Many warts contain *koilocytes,* which are large keratinocytes with small, pyknotic nuclei surrounded by a clear cytoplasm. These cells, in which extensive virus replication has taken place, are specific markers of HPV infection. The acanthosis seen in most warts probably results from a combination of delayed desquamation and a variable degree of hyperproliferation. The size of a wart is independent of the number of progeny virions it produces. This has two implications regarding the pathophysiology of HPV lesions. First, it becomes likely that it is the expression of nonstructural viral proteins, rather than of structural viral proteins, that accounts for the size and morphology of a wart. Second, it suggests that the size of an established wart is due primarily to the presence of viral genomes in the proliferative cell layers of the epidermis and not to continuous reinfection of upper-layer keratinocytes with progeny virions. If the latter case were true, one would predict that the growth and size of a wart would correlate directly with the number of HPV virions present, which it does not; similarly, if the latter case were true, one would probably not expect warts to stabilize in size after a period of initial growth. The chronicity and resistance of many warts to treatment is also most consistent with the presence of the viral genome in the lower layers of the epidermis.

In those HPV-infected lesions that become dysplastic or malignant, it is less likely that progeny virions will be present and more probable that early genes will be expressed at detectable levels in proliferating cells. Progeny virions are not produced because both viral genome replication and expression of structural HPV genes probably depend on normal epithelial cell differentiation, and clearly, differentiation is disrupted and abnormal in premalignant and malignant HPV lesions. There is laboratory evidence that expression of early viral genes is directly involved in driving the aberrant proliferation displayed in these lesions.[7]

LESIONS CAUSED BY HPV

It is useful to divide HPV infections into three major groups, since this classification correlates HPV type with the site of infection or a distinct patient population (Table 26-1). The three groups are: nongenital, cutaneous warts in the general population, genital and mucosal lesions in the general population, and HPV lesions in patients with epidermodysplasia verruciformis. Most HPV types are confined to one of these groups, although there is some overlap.

Nongenital cutaneous warts are extremely common, typically occur in children and adolescents, and are usually not associated with malignant changes.[1] Warts vary in appearance and distribution but most commonly appear as raised lesions with a rough, horny surface (Fig. 26-4). They often show punctate bleeding spots. Histologically, there is hyperplasia of all layers of the epidermis, vacuolation of the granular layer, and intranuclear inclusions. The HPV types that induce these lesions are generally

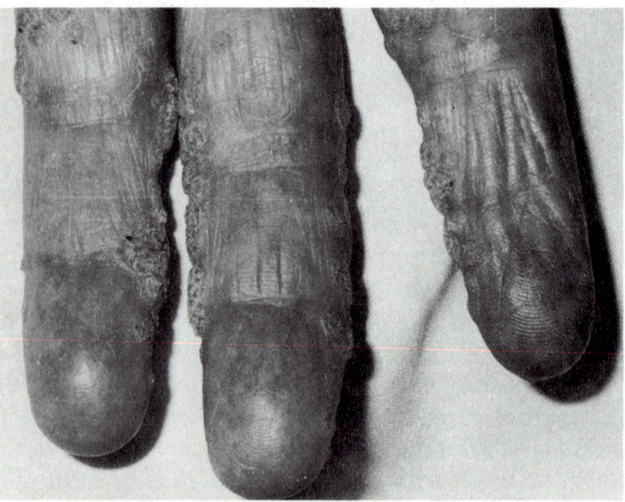

Figure 26-4 Scaly, rough, keratotic papules typical of common warts, confluent on adjacent surfaces of the fingers. *[From TB Fitzpatrick et al (eds), Dermatology in General Medicine, 3d ed, New York, McGraw-Hill, 1987, p 2358.]*

not found in genital or mucosal lesions. However, a minority of genital warts in children may be caused by these HPV types, and HPV2 is sometimes found in the mouth. Most flat warts tend to be caused by HPV3, and certain other HPV types in this group may induce distinct morphological changes.

Epidermodysplasia verruciformis appears to be caused by a genetic defect in which patients possess a unique susceptibility to epidermodysplasia verruciformis–specific HPV types that are not readily found in the general population.[3,4] In patients with epidermodysplasia verruciformis, large areas of the body may be covered with HPV-induced lesions. In contrast to warts in the general population, these lesions almost never remit, even with aggressive treatment. Many patients with epidermodysplasia verruciformis are infected with several HPV types. Some patients have measurable defects in certain cell-mediated immune functions. However, others appear to be normal by these parameters, and the typical patient does not have increased susceptibility to other microbial infections. Most patients with epidermodysplasia verruciformis do not appear to have greater susceptibility to the HPV types that infect the general population. An exception to this rule are those HPV types associated with flat warts, such as HPV3, which may cause extensive lesions in patients with epidermodysplasia verruciformis.

Some patients with epidermodysplasia verruciformis develop multiple cutaneous squamous cell carcinomas (Fig. 26-5). The malignant lesions contain HPV DNA and usually develop in sun-exposed areas and where benign HPV lesions are also present. These observations suggest that the virus represents a necessary, but not sufficient, component in these malignancies and that exposure to ultraviolet light probably represents a carcinogenic cofactor. Despite the large number of epidermodysplasia verruciformis–specific HPV types, malignant lesions usually contain only HPV5 or HPV8, which indicates that these types have greater oncogenic potential than others.

Genital infection by the genital-mucosal HPVs usually represents a sexually transmitted condition. The origin of oral and laryngeal lesions, which are also caused by these HPV types, is often less clear, but in young children these warts may be due to intrapartum exposure to virus in the vaginal tract.

Many epithelial tumors of the genital tract have been found to contain HPV DNA, especially cancers of the uterine cervix.[3,4] As is true of malignancy in epidermodysplasia verruciformis, only a subset of the genital-mucosal HPV types that infect the cervix are highly associated with cervical cancer. A wealth of rapidly accumulating epidemiological and molecular biological evidence has implicated these high-risk HPV types, such as HPV16, 18, 31, and 33, in the pathogenesis of cervical cancer, which is known to behave as a sexually transmitted condition. Another parallel with epidermodysplasia verruciformis is that the development of cervical malignancy apparently requires, in addition to HPV infection, other cofactors, such as cigarette smoking.

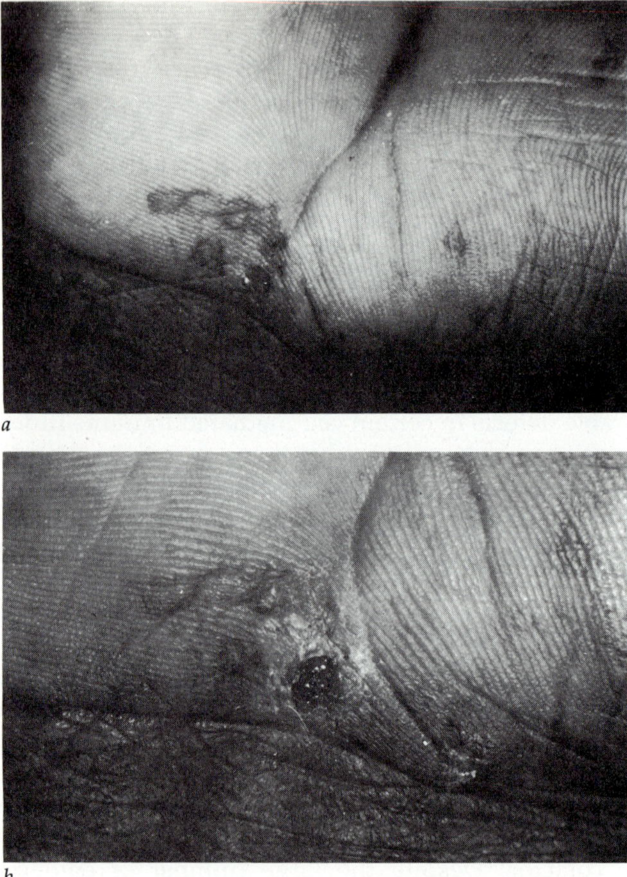

Figure 26-5 (*a*) Portion of the palm exhibiting a number of macular benign epidermodysplasia verruciformis lesions. (*b*) The same area photographed 18 months later, showing that one of the macular lesions has degenerated into a nodular ulcerating lesion, which proved to be an invasive squamous cell carcinoma. *[From TB Fitzpatrick et al (eds), Dermatology in General Medicine, 3d ed, New York, McGraw-Hill, 1987, p 2370.]*

Compared to the genital-mucosal lesions caused by the low-risk HPV types, such as HPV6 and HPV11, cervical infections with the high-risk types are less likely to regress spontaneously and more likely to progress to higher degrees of dysplasia and to carcinoma. In cell culture studies, the high-risk HPV types have been found to be much more efficient in inducing immortalization of primary human keratinocytes, which is an in vitro property associated with malignancy.[7] Furthermore, two viral early genes that are responsible for immortalization and that are selectively retained and expressed in cervical tumors, namely E6 and E7, are more transforming in the high-risk HPV types than in the low-risk types. The viral E2 gene is not usually expressed in tumors; this alteration probably represents a selective advantage for the cancer cells because E2 has been shown to decrease the expression of E6 and E7.

Some caution is required in extending these findings directly to noncervical lesions. While the distinction between high- and low-risk HPV types apparently has considerable relevance for cervical disease, it may not apply as clearly to malignancies of the vagina or the external genitalia, in which low-risk HPV types have been found with some regularity. For example, verrucous carcinoma and giant condyloma acuminatum (Buschke-Lowenstein tumor) usually contain HPV6 or 11. However, HPV16 DNA has been detected in several wart-like, periungual lesions that have the histology of squamous cell carcinoma.

It is not known what accounts for the different regional specificities of the various groups of HPVs, although it seems likely that the HPV types are exploiting putative subtle variations in keratinocytes from different body regions. Along these lines, one could even speculate that the genetic defect in patients with epidermodysplasia verruciformis may somehow render normally nonpermissive keratinocytes permissive to successful infection by epidermodysplasia verruciformis–specific HPV types.

REGRESSION, LATENCY, AND REACTIVATION

Most HPV-induced lesions in the general population persist and then regress after a variable period. The viral and host factors that control persistence and regression are poorly understood.[8] There is considerable evidence of the importance of cell-mediated immune function in many HPV infections. Spontaneous resolution of multiple flat warts often begins with the simultaneous development of erythema around most lesions. This inflammatory response is associated histologically with a perivascular mononuclear cell infiltrate. There is less agreement on the typical histological appearance of regressing common warts. However, patients with various forms of impaired cell-mediated immune function have a higher incidence of HPV infection and are notoriously resistant to treatment. Also, as mentioned previously, many patients with epidermodysplasia verruciformis have impaired cell-mediated immune function parameters. These observations suggest that cell-mediated immune function contributes to the regression of at least some forms of HPV disease and that deficient cell-mediated immune function may allow the persistence of lesions. The lower frequency of common cutaneous warts among adults suggests that they may possess some form of immunological resistance against these nongenital HPV genotypes. In addition, the number of new lesions that develop in most people who already have some warts is usually remarkably small, given that the uninfected skin in these patients presumably is frequently exposed to many infectious virions shed from preexisting lesions. It is therefore reasonable to speculate that host defense factors limit the extent and number of HPV lesions. It is likely, however, that immunity to HPVs tends to be type or group specific. For example, apparent resistance to nongenital HPV types does not seem to protect an individual against infection by genital-mucosal HPV types. The possible viral and/or cell-encoded antigenic determinants and effector mechanisms that may account for immunological responses to HPVs remain to be precisely identified.

When lesions regress, it is often unclear if a clinical cure is associated with a virological cure. The genital-mucosal HPVs can establish latency, and it is likely that other HPVs share this property. Latent infections, by definition, are subclinical. HPV DNA has been found in normal-appearing perilesional tissue in the anogenital tract. Thus, in theory, the reappearance of lesions in the proximity of "successfully" treated primary HPV lesions may be due, at least some of the time, to the activation of latent infections rather than to reinfection. In patients with laryngeal papillomas, there may be long disease-free periods, despite the continued presence of viral DNA in the larynx. This further suggests that host factors may participate in the establishment, maintenance, and reactivation of latent HPV infection. Given the high incidence of clinical HPV infections in patients with acquired impairments of cell-mediated immune function, it is likely that at least some of these lesions represent activation of latent HPV infections that had been previously suppressed by formerly intact host defense mechanisms.

REFERENCES

1. Lowy DR, Androphy EJ: Warts, in TB Fitzpatrick et al, (eds), *Dermatology in General Medicine,* 3d ed. New York, McGraw-Hill, 1987, p 2355.
2. Beutner KR: Human papillomavirus infection. *J Am Acad Dermatol* 20:114, 1989.
3. Salzman NP, Howley PM (eds): *The Papovaviridae,* vol 2: *The Papillomaviruses.* New York, Plenum Press, 1987.
4. Pfister H (ed): *Papillomaviruses and Human Cancer.* Boca Raton, Fla, CRC Press, 1990.
5. De Villiers EM: Heterogeneity of the human papillomavirus group. *J Virol* 63:4898, 1989.
6. Stoler MH et al: Differentiation-linked human papillomavirus types 6 and 11 transcription in genital condylomata revealed by in situ hybridization with message-specific RNA probes. *Virology* 172:331, 1989.
7. Lowy DR, Schiller JT: Transforming genes of bovine and human papillomaviruses, in AL Notkins and MBA Oldstone (eds), *Concepts in Viral Pathogenesis.* New York, Springer-Verlag, 1989, vol III, p 87.
8. Lowry DR: Papillomavirus infection, in RE Jordon (ed), *Immunologic Diseases of the Skin.* Norwalk, CT, Appleton-Century-Crofts, in press.

27

Pathophysiology of Certain Fungal Diseases

Ernesto Gonzalez

Of the more than 100,000 species of fungi that have been described, only approximately 175 are considered to be pathogens to humans. Most of these pathogenic species produce either cutaneous or subcutaneous infections, but only 20 species cause systemic infections.[1] Most of the fungal diseases are produced by exogenous organisms that penetrate the human natural barriers such as the skin or respiratory mucosa. In a few instances, fungal diseases can be produced by endogenous organisms that are part of the normal flora of human beings, such as candidosis and tinea versicolor, which under specific genetic or environmental circumstances allow these endogenous organisms to proliferate abnormally. With the advent of immunosuppressive therapy as well as the recent development of virally induced acquired immunosuppressive states, an increasing list of opportunistic fungi that were previously considered nonpathogens have been added to the above-mentioned list of pathogens.

Fungi are aerobic, nucleated, achlorophyllus organisms that reproduce sexually or asexually.[2,3] An important physiological difference between fungi and humans is the content of the cell membrane. While the major membrane lipid in humans is cholesterol, fungi require ergosterol for biosynthesis of their membrane; this difference has been exploited therapeutically in the past few years to develop antifungal drugs that are not toxic to mammalian cells.[4] The fungal cell wall surrounding the plasma membrane generally contains only 5 to 10 percent protein. About 50 to 60 percent of the cell wall of molds or yeasts, the most primitive forms of fungi, consists of carbohydrate polymers. The cell wall of molds (filamentous fungi), more complex fungal organisms, generally has a very high content of chitin composed of *N*-acetylglucosamine.[5]

Structurally, fungi consist of a variety of reproductive forms associated with sexual and asexual processes in addition to nonreproductive elements that allow the fungi to attach to a substrate. Yeasts are unicellular and reproduce by budding. Molds, on the other hand, are the filamentous forms of a heterogeneous group of fungi. They are more complex and consist of cells that develop from an asexual spore to form a tubular structure called a hypha. Hyphae are usually separated from one another by septa. The hyphae branch out to form a mycelium, which gives these structures a filamentous or cottony appearance in a colony. These molds reproduce by forming spores and/or by fragmentation. The spores are often resistant to environmental conditions. The differentiation of fungi into genera and species is based on the morphology of their reproductive structures.

PATHOPHYSIOLOGY

The fungi that cause disease do so by means of metabolic traits not shared by other taxonomically related species that allow them to survive and grow in human tissue. Dimorphic fungi, for example, which have the ability to convert from yeast-type to mold-type growth, normally grow as saprophytes in the mold form at soil temperature (30°C) but are able to adapt and survive as a yeast at the temperature of the human body (37°C). Many of the pathogenic fungi manifest this dimorphism. Most of the pathogenic fungi, with the exception of a few dermatophytes, are not obligate parasites but rather soil saprophytes. Infectivity and virulence of fungi are controlled by a variety of factors, both of the host and of the parasite.

Two properties of fungi appear to be of paramount importance in the pathogenesis of the diseases they cause.[5] One is tissue tropism, in which the fungus has a predilection to parasitize a particular tissue or organ. *Histoplasm a capsulatum*, for example, has a predilection for cells of the reticuloendothelial system, and *Cryptococcus neoformans* thrives in cells of the central nervous system. The dermatophytes, on the other hand, thrive on keratin and can be so selective as to grow in keratin of one appendage (nail) and not in keratin of another (hair).[5] The second property is their immunogenic characteristics that incite hypersensitivity, primarily cell mediated, which frequently accounts for the pathologic effects produced. The major antigenic determinants of fungi are the cell walls, cytoplasmic constituents, and extracellular products.[6]

TYPES OF INFECTIONS

The most commonly used classification is based on the clinical presentation (Table 27-1). Only certain disorders will be discussed. The superficial

Table 27-1

CLINICAL TYPES OF FUNGAL INFECTIONS

Type of Infection	*Disease*
Superficial	Tinea versicolor Tinea nigra
Cutaneous	Tinea capitis, tinea pedis, onychomycosis, tinea cruris, tinea corporis, tinea barbae; candidosis of skin, mucous membranes, and nails
Subcutaneous	Mycetoma Sporotrichosis Chromomycosis
Systemic	Pathogenic fungi Histoplasmosis Blastomycosis Coccidioidomycosis Paracoccidioidomycosis
	Opportunistic fungi Cryptococcosis Aspergillosis Mucormycosis Candidosis, systemic

infections are those in which the invading pathogen is confined to the stratum corneum, with little or no tissue reaction. In the cutaneous mycoses, all keratinized tissues, i.e., skin, hair, and nails, may be involved. Although the pathogens are generally confined to the nonliving, cornified layers of the skin and its appendages, destruction of tissue is extensive and host immunologic reactions may result. Dermatophytes are the most important causes of this type of infection. Subcutaneous mycoses are caused by implantation of a variety of fungi that involve the cutaneous and subcutaneous tissues after trauma. The systemic mycoses are mainly pulmonary diseases, since the primary site of infection is usually the lungs. Cutaneous and subcutaneous forms of these diseases do occur as the result of dissemination or direct inoculation following injury. The systemic mycoses have been divided into two large groups based on host–parasite interactions. Those produced by pathogenic fungi do not require a compromised host, and those caused by opportunistic fungi become pathogens only in patients debilitated by some other cause and whose normal defense mechanisms are impaired. The use of immunosuppressive and cytotoxic drugs has increased the number and severity of these infections. A similar situation, but more significant, has developed in patients infected with the human immunodeficiency virus who developed the acquired immunodeficiency syndrome (AIDS).

SUPERFICIAL FUNGAL INFECTION

Tinea versicolor is a superficial disease characterized by hypopigmented and hyperpigmented small lesions with fine scales that may coalesce, especially on the trunk and upper neck (Fig. 27-1). Although usually asymptomatic, some patients may experience pruritus. The reported incidence varies from 5 to 50 percent of the population, being higher in hot, humid climates.[7] Since the disease produces minimal discomfort and patients usually do not seek medical attention, the incidence may be higher.

A lipophilic fungus called *Pityrosporum orbiculare* has been incriminated as the cause of tinea versicolor. This organism is part of the normal flora and can be cultured in 90 to 100 percent of healthy individuals. Under the influence of predisposing factors, *P. orbiculare* changes from its saprophytic yeast form to its pathogenic mycelial form.[8] Studies in vitro have shown that *P. orbiculare* produces dicarboxylic acid, which inhibits tyrosinase.[9] This effect may explain the hypopigmentation produced by this organism. Other observers have found aggregates of abnormal small melanosomes in hypopigmented areas compared to large, single melanosomes in hyperpigmented lesions, which also showed an increased turnover rate of the stratum corneum. It is not clear if this difference in the size and distribution of melanosomes is due to a cytotoxic effect in melanocytes by *P. orbiculare* or to an endogenous alteration of the integrity of the epidermal melanin unit during the host–parasite interaction. *P. orbiculare* can be found within cells of the viable epidermis and is associated with an inflammatory infiltrate of granulocytes and lymphocytes.[10,11] Spores are abundant in and near the pilosebaceous follicle, whereas hyphae dominate in the interfollicular areas of the stratum corneum.

Some observers postulate that tinea versicolor is not contagious and that the pathogenic potential of this saprophyte depends on endogenous and exogenous factors. The endogenous factors implicated include a defect in

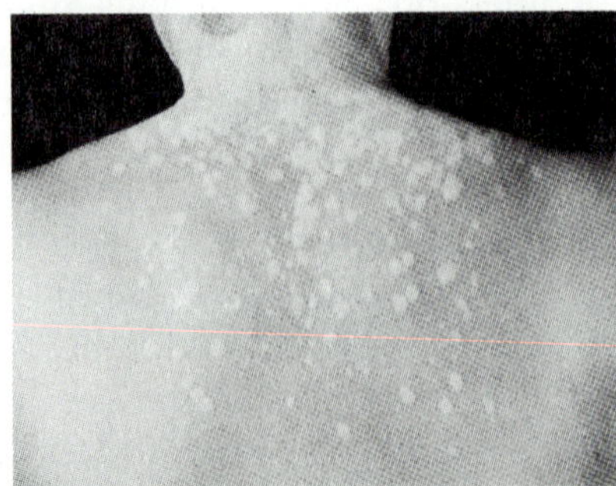

Figure 27-1 Tinea versicolor is a common disorder occurring primarily on the trunk and appearing as scattered, slightly scaling macules or as white macules that may be confused with vitiligo. (*From TB Fitzpatrick et al, Dermatology in General Medicine, 2d ed, New York, McGraw-Hill, 1979, p 1765.*)

the production of lymphokines by the host,[12] genetic factors, and hyperhidrosis; exogenous factors include heat and humidity, the use of ointments that can act as substrate for the fungus, and the administration of therapeutic immunosuppressive agents.

CUTANEOUS MYCOSES

Clinical Features

Classification of infections produced by dermatophytes is based on the anatomic site involved, because the same species may be involved in different diseases, depending on the anatomic site, and because the response to therapy often depends on the site rather than on the species of fungus producing the infection. The dermatophytes are a related group of fungi that cause a variety of clinical conditions, some of which are transmitted from human to human (anthropophilic), others from animal to human (zoophilic), and others from soil to human (geophilic). The invasion of tissue by dermatophytes varies with the species (Table 27-2). The prognosis of certain fungal infections seems to reflect the immune state of the host as well as the species of the organism.

Tinea capitis is an infection of the scalp hair characterized by hair that breaks, leaving scaly, pruritic, bald areas. Certain species can produce an

Table 27-2

CHARACTERISTICS OF SOME DERMATOPHYTES

	Invasion of Tissue	
Hair	Skin	Nail
Microsporum species	*Microsporum* species	*Trichophyton* species
Trichophyton species	*Trichophyton* species	*E. floccosum*
	E. floccosum	
	Source of Fungus	
Geophilic	Zoophilic	Anthropophilic
M. gypseum	*M. canis*	*M. audouini*
	T. mentagrophytes	*E. floccosum*
		T. rubrum
		T. tonsurans
	Fungi That Fluoresce	
Fungus	Fluorescence	Infection
M. canis	Bright yellow-green	Hair
M. audouini	Bright yellow-green	Hair, skin
M. ferrugineum	Bright yellow-green	Hair
T. schoenleinii	Dull green	Hair

Note: *M.* = *Microsporum; T.* = *Trichophyton; E.* = *Epidermophyton* inflammatory disease designated a kerion, which is characterized by an edematous area with numerous follicular pustules that can ulcerate and heal with scar formation. Infections are classified according to the manner in which the fungus invades the hair. *Ectothrix* defines the location of these spores as being outside the cuticle, whereas in *endothrix* infection the spores are within the hair shaft. Certain fungi (e.g., *Microsporum audouini*) affect children, while others (e.g., *Trichophyton tonsurans*) cause disease in adults. Another factor that helps identify the species of fungus is the presence or absence of a brilliant green fluorescence with Wood's lamp. The most common cause of tinea capitis in the United States is *T. tonsurans*, characterized by an endothrix infection in which the hair breaks off sharply at the follicular orifice, leaving a spore-filled stub or black dot.

The feet are infected with dermatophytes more frequently than any other anatomic area, and this infection is referred to as tinea pedis. The infection involves the toe webs, producing interdigital maceration. The soles are also involved, but the presentation varies morphologically depending on the host–parasite interaction. Acute tinea pedis, characterized by inflammatory vesicles and pustules, is associated with pruritus and is an immunologic response to the fungus. Most of these cases are produced by *Trichophyton mentagrophytes*. The diagnosis can be made by scrapings from an intact vesicle for direct microscopic examination with potassium hydroxide or for culture. The chronic, noninflammatory form is characterized by a diffuse, scaly process involving the plantar skin and is usually produced by *Trichophyton rubrum*, an anthropophilic fungus. Scrapings form these scales, particularly of the heels, will demonstrate the organisms. Rarely, a clinicoanatomic entity referred to as two feet–one hand dermatophytosis is seen, which typically shows diffuse scaliness on the soles of both feet and the palm of one hand. The most common dermatophyte producing this entity is *T. rubrum*. This phenomenon has been studied to determine the factors that predispose one hand to be involved, but so far, neither palmar sweating nor handedness has shown any correlation.[13]

Infection of the nails by dermatophytes is characterized by a chalky, dull appearance and the accumulation of yellow to brown debris, usually without inflammation of the nail fold, in the distal part of the nail that crumbles when removed and is known as onychomycosis. The toenails are more frequently involved than the fingernails. Nail infections are usually caused by organisms that belong to the genus *Trichophyton*.

Tinea cruris is characterized by a plaque with a serpiginous border on the glabrous skin of the groin (Fig. 27-2). The process can be asymmetric, but when it is symmetric, both medial aspects of the upper thighs are involved with an advancing, erythematous, scaling border and a quiescent, often pigmented center. Patients with tinea cruris frequently have tinea pedis or onychomycosis. *T. rubrum* and *Epidermophyton floccosum* are the most common fungi affecting this area.

Tinea corporis is an infection of the glabrous skin characterized by a

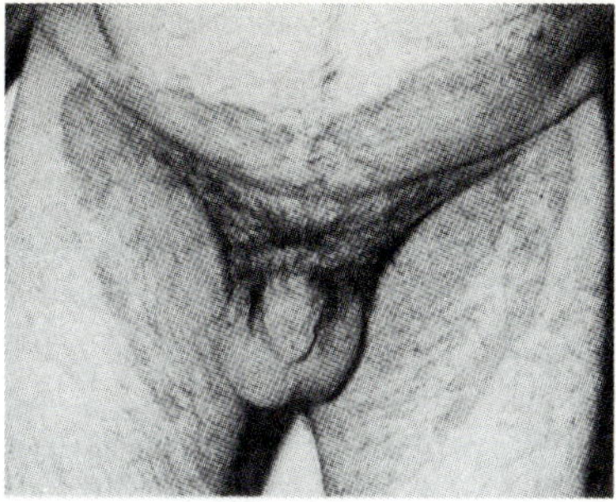

Figure 27-2 Tinea cruris. (*From TB Fitzpatrick et al, Dermatology in General Medicine, 2d ed, New York, McGraw-Hill, 1979, p 1779.*)

ringlike configuration with a serpiginous border consisting of erythematous papules, vesicles, pustules, and scales (Fig. 27-3). Pruritus may be present.

Pathophysiology

Dermatophytes have a minimal capacity to damage skin,[14] and much of the inflammation is a reflection of the host response. The fungi can colonize the stratum corneum, provided that an optimal environment is present in

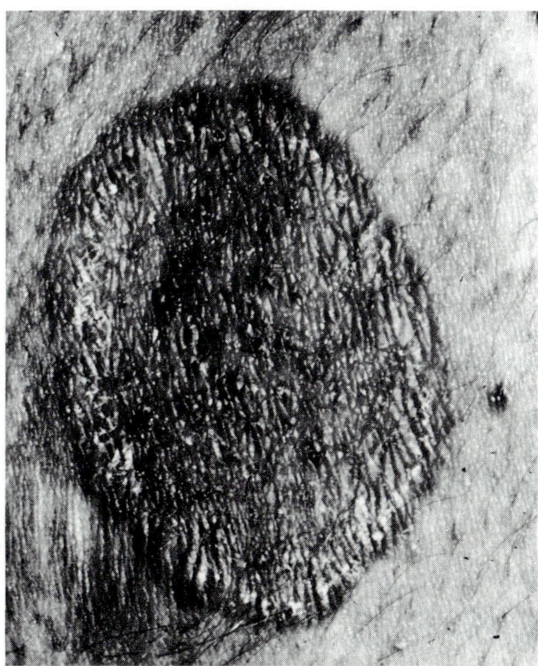

Figure 27-3 Typical lesion of ringworm of the glabrous skin. (*From TB Fitzpatrick et al, Dermatology in General Medicine, 2d ed, New York, McGraw-Hill, 1979, p 1526.*)

which high humidity is the most important factor.[15] Time-dependent adherence of fungal elements (spores) of dermatophytes to keratinocytes has been demonstrated in vitro, with maximum adherence between 3 and 4 h. These elements have more affinity for keratinocytes in the skin of the soles than of the knee.[16] During the colonization phase of the stratum corneum, proteolytic enzymes and other diffusible substances produced by the dermatophytes, as well as the transepidermal leukocyte chemotaxis induced by complement activation, reach the viable layers of the skin and induce an inflammatory response. A delayed hypersensitivity reaction to soluble fungal antigens develops that, in experimental animal infections, is closely associated with increased epidermal proliferation. These host reactions are intended to inhibit growth and facilitate elimination of the fungus from the stratum corneum, and they explain the spontaneous regression of experimentally induced dermatophytosis in the animal model.[17] In human beings, this inflammatory response is not always elicited due to such factors as the impermeability of stratum corneum, the saprophytic adaptability of the fungal species, or the inability of the host to respond to this antigenic stimulus. In such cases, a chronic dermatophytosis can develop. Zoophilic and geophilic fungi usually incite an inflammatory response and produce a more self-limiting disease or are more responsive to therapy, while the anthropophilic dermatophytes establish a symbiotic existence with the skin and induce a minimal inflammatory reaction.

CANDIDOSIS

Clinical Features

Candidosis is defined as an acute or chronic infection caused by species of the genus *Candida.* Although more than a dozen *Candida* species can cause human disease, by far the most common is *Candida albicans.* It can also produce a more generalized mucocutaneous process or a disseminated disease involving almost every organ of the body in patients who are immunologically unresponsive to the organism.

C. albicans is part of the normal flora of the intestinal tract, vagina, and oral mucosa. Some of the factors implicated in establishing this fungus as a pathogen include pregnancy, diabetes mellitus, antibiotic and corticosteroid therapy, cancer, infections such as AIDS, and genetic deficiencies. All these factors seem to depress the immunologic resistance of the host.

Thrush involves the oral mucosa, most commonly the tongue, and is characterized by white patches (Fig. 27-4). Although it is seen in healthy children, in adults it occurs commonly in patients receiving systemic corticosteroids or in those who are immunocompromised. Vulvovaginitis produces a discharge associated with pruritus. It is seen in adults with diabetes mellitus, in pregnancy, and in women taking oral contraceptives. Balanitis occurs especially in uncircumcised men and produces erythematous micropapules that can become confluent.

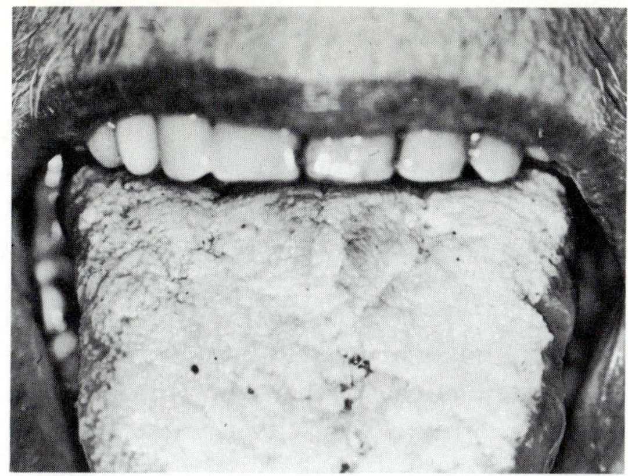

Figure 27-4 Oral candidosis. The tongue is covered with a white, confluent plaque. (*From TB Fitzpatrick et al, Dermatology in General Medicine, 2d ed, New York, McGraw-Hill, 1979, p 1518.*)

Candidosis of the skin in healthy individuals is usually present on flexural or occluded areas. However, immunocompromised hosts can develop lesions of *Candida* in many areas of the skin. Flexural infection is characterized by bilateral involvement with variable but symmetric extension to the adjacent areas of the skin. The lesions are bright red, with fine desquamation at the periphery and satellite pustules outside the affected areas. Frequently, the involved skin is moist and macerated. The groin, inframammary region, axillae, and areas of folding in obese patients are common sites of involvement. Interdigital infection can occur between the toes or between the third and fourth fingers. *Candida* can also produce chronic paronychia in healthy adults and is associated with frequent immersion of the fingers in water. It produces painful swelling and hypertrophy of the proximal nail fold and a seropurulent discharge. The nail eventually becomes dystrophic, with yellow to brown discoloration.

Pathophysiology

Candida species are yeast-like fungi and are considered dimorphic since the mycelial form is observed when the organism is grown at room temperature, while the yeast form is evident at 37°C. Both forms may be seen in the skin lesions, the mycelial one in chronic infection and the yeast one in acute infection. The lesions are apparently produced by nonimmunologic host–parasite interactions that involve complement fixation. As the hyphal tips of the fungus penetrate the viable layer of the epidermis, the alternative complement pathway is activated, resulting in chemotaxis of polymorphonuclear leukocytes with production of the typical pustules.[13] Cell-mediated immunity undoubtedly plays a role in the pathogenesis of the clinical lesions and the host resistance to *Candida*, but specific details remain to be elucidated.[13]

SUBCUTANEOUS FUNGAL INFECTION

Sporotrichosis

Sporotrichosis is a subacute or chronic disease caused by *Sporothrix schenckii,* which is usually limited to the skin and subcutaneous tissue but which, in rare instances, can disseminate to the bone and internal organs.[18] Occasionally, sporotrichosis is manifested as a primary pulmonary infection without skin lesions. The disease is worldwide in distribution, with a high prevalence among horticultural workers. The infection is usually contracted by traumatic cutaneous inoculation with soil or vegetable material from thorns on rose bushes. It is not transmitted from human to human. *S. schenckii* is a dimorphic fungus, and its identification depends on the medium and on the temperature at which it is grown. The cutaneous lymphatic form of sporotrichosis is characterized by a subcutaneous nodule at the inoculation site, commonly the hand or finger, and the successive appearance of nodules in a linear array along the draining lymphatics. The nodules are usually indolent; they may ulcerate and discharge a seropurulent material. In most individuals the disease remains localized but in some it may become systemic, involving bones, joints, and other internal organs.[18,19]

The organisms are usually not seen in histological sections, and culture is the most effective way to identify them. At room temperature on an appropriate medium, a black, tar-like colony is observed; at 37°C a tan-colored yeast colony is observed, and examination under the microscope shows that the cells have a cigar shape.

The host response to this microorganism is both suppurative and granulomatous, with a characteristic stellate microabscess surrounded by epithelioid cells and occasionally Langerhans giant cells. In the center of the microabscess, amorphous, eosinophilic material surrounds a central fungus cell in star-like fashion. This is called an asteroid body and is presumed to be an antigen-antibody reaction around the yeast cell.[19]

SYSTEMIC FUNGAL INFECTION

Histoplasmosis

Histoplasmosis is a systemic fungus infection produced by *Histoplasma capsulatum,* a dimorphic fungus that is acquired by the respiratory route. Although the lungs are the primary focus and the disease is commonly manifested by a self-limited respiratory infection, this fungus can produce a chronic lung disease or a progressive, disseminated form that is usually fatal. Although the disease is of worldwide distribution, it occurs most often in the United States and is considered the most common systemic mycosis in North America. Approximately 40 million people have been infected by the organism in the United States, primarily in the valleys of the Mississippi and Ohio rivers. Bird droppings and bat feces seem to provide an optimal environment for the growth of the fungus.

The yeast form of this dimorphic fungus is observed in tissue as a 3-mm yeast that reproduces by single buds and is generally seen in clusters within histiocytes and in areas of necrosis. The mycelial form, which grows at 30°C, forms tuberculate macroconidia.

Primary cutaneous lesions are occasionally seen in histoplasmosis after direct inoculation of the skin and are manifested as primary skin ulcerations associated with lymphangitis.[20] Other skin lesions that can be seen during the primary infection are erythema nodosum and/or erythema multiforme, nonspecific immunologic hypersensitivity reactions induced by different antigens, which can develop in response to the antigen(s) produced by *H. capsulatum*. The chronic disseminated form of histoplasmosis produces papules, verrucous plaques, and mucocutaneous ulcerations in about 50 percent of the cases.

After inhalation of the spore of *H. capsulatum,* the alveolar macrophages phagocytize the fungal particle, which then dwells inside the histiocytes of the host and persists in the yeast phase either in the lung or in the reticuloendothelial system. It appears that the inability of the macrophage to inhibit intracellular replication of the yeast phase is the first determinant of the outcome of this fungal infection, since humoral defenses do not seem to play an important role in immunity to the disease. The fungus does not elaborate toxins, enzymes, or other substances that play a role in producing lung disease.[21]

FUNGAL DISEASES IN THE IMMUNOCOMPROMISED HOST

The immunologic response by the host to antigens produced by fungi can be profoundly modified by immunosuppressive drugs or disease states such as AIDS, a chronic, severe infection produced by the human immunodeficiency virus (HIV). Patient with AIDS have the most chronic and persistently progressive $CD4^+$ T-cell defect of any group of immunocompromised patients. Clinically, they most closely resemble bone marrow transplant patients during chronic rejection, and both groups manifest severe $CD4^+$ T-cell and B-cell defects. It appears, however, that patients with AIDS respond poorly to opportunistic infections compared to renal transplant patients.[22] Among opportunistic infections, fungal diseases play a major role in the prognosis and outcome of AIDS patients. Therefore, it is important to identify their protean manifestations and implications.

A significantly increased incidence of seborrheic dermatitis, a chronic benign papulosquamous dermatitis of the scalp and face, has been reported in AIDS patients compared with normal subjects. These patients also have a more severe and extensive manifestation of the disease involving the chest, back, and intertriginous areas. A recent study proposed that *P. orbiculare,* the fungal agent causing tinea versicolor, is the cause of seborrheic dermatitis in AIDS patients. This conclusion was based on the quantitative correlation between colonization by the organism and severity of the manifestation, as well as on the response to an antifungal agent.[23]

The prevalence of dermatophyte infection does not seem to be increased when HIV-seropositive homosexual men are compared with their HIV-seronegative counterparts. In patients with advanced HIV infection, however, nail involvement (onychomycosis) is more prevalent and severe than in HIV-negative homosexuals.[24] However, infections with dermatophytes such as *Trichophyton rubrum,* an anthropophilic fungus that maintains a symbiotic existence on the skin of the normal host, have been reported to produce deep local invasion, multivisceral dissemination, and even death in immunocompromised hosts, particularly AIDS patients.[25]

Oral and esophageal candidosis are common manifestations in AIDS patients and are considered two of the early signs of HIV infection. Disseminated infection with *Candida,* however, is rare despite the profound and progressive immunodeficiency that characterizes AIDS. This phenomenon contrasts significantly with disease manifestations in other types of immunocompromised patients, in whom disseminated candidosis is frequent and carries a mortality of approximately 70 percent. To explain this difference, it has been suggested that the cell-mediated immunodeficiency in AIDS patients accounts for their susceptibility to superficial candidosis, while their relatively unimpaired humoral immunity confers protection against dissemination of this opportunistic fungus infection. An antibody against the immunodominant 47kd antigen of *C. albicans* was recently described in patients with chronic mucocutaneous candidosis and AIDS that may be responsible for this protective humoral immunity.[26]

Three systemic mycoses, cryptococcosis, histoplasmosis, and coccidioidomycosis, are considered the most important opportunistic fungal infections affecting AIDS patients because of their frequency and severity and because the response to therapy is very poor. Cryptococcosis is the fourth most common opportunistic infection in patients with AIDS and is usually manifested as meningitis. In approximately 25 percent of these patients, however, the first manifestation can be different. The skin is a frequent target, with atypical lesions that can resemble molluscum contagiosum.[22]

Histoplasmosis has been recognized as an important AIDS-associated opportunistic infection, both by reactivation of a latent focus and by primary infection, and can recur years after the patient has left the endemic region.[27] The lack of a cell-mediated response against *H. capsulatum* in AIDS patients allows the fungus to spread hematogenously, causing either focal or diffuse disseminated disease with a fulminant course. The number of reported cases of disseminated histoplasmosis in AIDS patients is increasing, and its dissemination now constitutes one of the criteria for the diagnosis of AIDS.[27]

The number of severe cases of coccidioidomycosis in AIDS patients is not so large, but this disease is still considered an important opportunistic infection in these patients. The infection primarily involves the lungs.

REFERENCES

1. Rippon JW: *Medical Mycology—The Pathogenic Fungi and the Pathogenic Actinomycetes,* 2d ed. Philadelphia, Saunders, 1982, p 3.

2. Bulmer GS: *Introduction to Medical Mycology.* Chicago, Year Book, 1979, p 1.
3. Eagleson WM, Kane J: *A Synopsis of Mycology for Dermatologists,* 3d ed. Toronto, Eagleson and Kane, 1981, p 7.
4. Jones HE: Current therapies for mycotic disease, in HB Levine (ed), *Ketoconazole in the Management of Fungal Disease.* New York, Adis, 1982, p 14.
5. Bulmer GS: *Introduction to Medical Mycology.* Chicago, Year Book, 1979, p 10.
6. Myrvik QN, Weiser RS: *Fundamentals of Medical Bacteriology and Mycology,* 2d ed. Philadelphia, Lea & Febiger, 1988, p 501.
7. Bulmer GS: *Introduction to Medical Mycology.* Chicago, Year Book, 1979, p 162.
8. Faergemann J, Fredriksson T: Tinea versicolor: some new aspects on etiology, pathogenesis and treatment. *Int J Dermatol* 21:8, 1982.
9. Nazarro Porro M, Passi S: Identification of tyrosine inhibitors in cultures of *Pityrosporum. J Invest Dermatol* 71:205, 1978.
10. Montes LF: Systemic abnormalities and intracellular site of infection of the stratum corneum. *JAMA* 213:1469, 1970.
11. Tosti A et al: The parasitic colonization of the horny layer in tinea versicolor. *J Invest Dermatol* 59:233, 1972.
12. Sohnle PG, Collins-Lech C: Cell-mediated immunity to *Pityrosporum orbiculare* in tinea versicolor. *J Clin Invest* 62:45, 1978.
13. Bender S et al: Correlations between two-feet, one-hand dermatophytosis, palmar sweating, and handedness. *Ann NY Acad Sci* 544:588, 1988.
14. Jones HE, Harrell ER: Superficial fungus infections of the skin, in PD Hoeprich (ed), *Infectious Diseases,* 4th ed. New York, Harper & Row, 1989, p 1034.
15. Knight AG: A review of experimental human infections. *J Invest Dermatol* 59:354, 1972.
16. Zurita J, Hay RJ: Adherence of dermatophyte microconidia and arthroconidia to human keratinocytes in vitro. *J Invest Dermatol* 89:529, 1987.
17. Tagami H: Epidermal cell proliferation in guinea pigs with experimental dermatophytosis. *J Invest Dermatol* 85:153, 1985.
18. Chandler FW et al: Sporotrichosis, in *Color Atlas and Text of the Histopathology of Mycotic Diseases.* Chicago, Year Book, 1980, p 112.
19. Lynch PJ et al: Systemic sporotrichosis. *Ann Intern Med* 73:23, 1970.
20. Tosh FE et al: Primary cutaneous histoplasmosis. *Arch Intern Med* 114:118, 1964.
21. Wheat LJ: Histoplasmosis, in PD Hoeprich (ed), *Infectious Diseases,* 4th ed. New York, Harper & Row, 1989, p 481.
22. Armstrong D: Life threatening opportunistic fungal infections in patients with the acquired immunodeficiency syndrome. *Ann NY Acad Sci* 544:443, 1988.
23. Groissel D et al: Association of *Pityrosporum orbiculare* (*Malassezia furfur*) with seborrheic dermatitis in patients with acquired immunodeficiency syndrome (AIDS). *J Am Acad Dermatol* 20:770, 1989.
24. Torssander J et al: Dermatophytosis and HIV infection: a study in homosexual men. *Acta Derm Venereol (Stockh)* 68:53, 1988.
25. Novick NL et al: Invasive *Trichophyton rubrum* infection in an immunocompromised host. *Am J Med* 82:321, 1987.
26. Mathews R et al: *Candida* and AIDS: evidence for protective antibody. *Lancet* 2:263, 1988.
27. Graybill JR: Histoplasmosis and AIDS. *J Infect Dis* 158:623, 1988.

28

Pathophysiology of Acquired Immunodeficiency Syndrome

Timothy Berger and Marcus A. Conant

Human infection with the human immunodeficiency virus (HIV) may result in a series of clinical disorders of increasing severity, often eventuating in the death of the patient.[1] Certain steps in the progression of the disease have been given specific names—primary HIV infection, progressive generalized lymphadenopathy (PGL), AIDS-related complex (ARC), acquired immunodeficiency syndrome (AIDS). These designations are definitions that are useful in understanding the disease but are not always ideal in classifying the individual patient. It is better to think of infected persons as having a spectrum of manifestations collectively known as HIV disease. Cutaneous disorders occur in a high percentage of persons with HIV disease[2] and frequently are very distressing both symptomatically and cosmetically. While much is known about the causative virus, how infection with this virus leads to skin disease is poorly understood.

Immune deficiency was the aspect of HIV infection that was initially recognized. Immune failure remains the hallmark of the terminal phase of HIV disease—AIDS. Immune failure and the resultant overwhelming opportunistic infection are the usual causes of death. The systemic and cutaneous diseases that appear in HIV infection cannot all, however, be explained by immune deficiency alone. Certain aspects of the immune system appear to be overactive. For example, lymph nodes are enlarged and hyperglobulinemia is frequent. Some of the immune overreactivity may be directed against normal tissues—autoimmunity.[1,3] Thus, *immune*

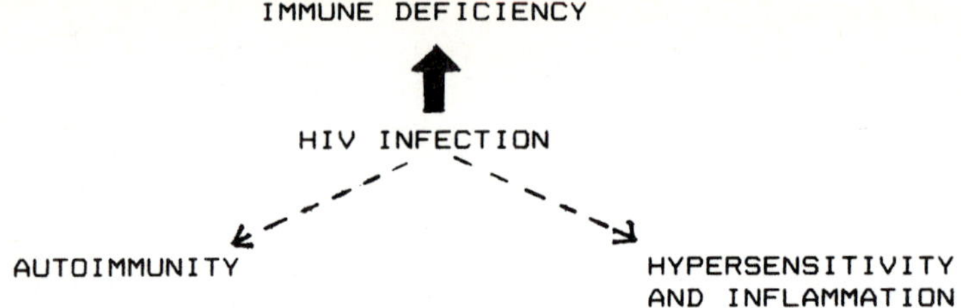

Figure 28-1 The paradox of HIV infection is that while the patient is immunodeficient, he/she may also exhibit hypersensitivity and autoimmunity.

deficiency, hypersensitivity (immune overreactivity), and *autoimmunity* may all occur (Fig. 28-1).

HUMAN IMMUNODEFICIENCY VIRUS

Structure of HIV and Pathogenesis of HIV Disease

HIV is a retrovirus in the lentivirus subfamily and is clearly the cause of HIV disease.[1] Two subtypes have been recovered from humans with AIDS, HIV-1 and HIV-2. The structure of HIV is known (Fig. 28-2). The virus envelope contains two glycoproteins: gp120, the major envelope

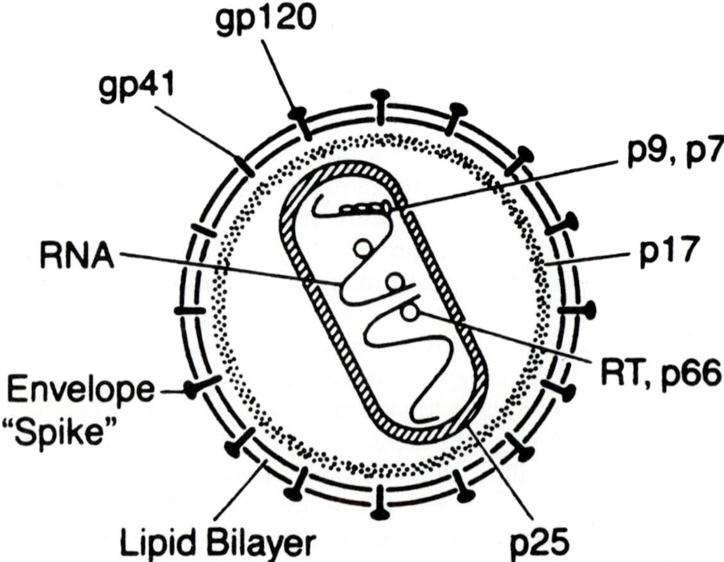

Figure 28-2 The basic structure of HIV. Envelope glycoproteins (gp120 and gp41) and the major viral core proteins (p25, p17, p9, and p7). The core protein, p17, is found outside the viral nucleoid and forms the matrix of the virion. RT indicates reverse transcriptase. (*From JA Levy, Human immunodeficiency viruses and the pathogenesis of AIDS. JAMA* (May 26, 1989) *261:2998, 1989. Copyright 1989, American Medical Association. With permission*).

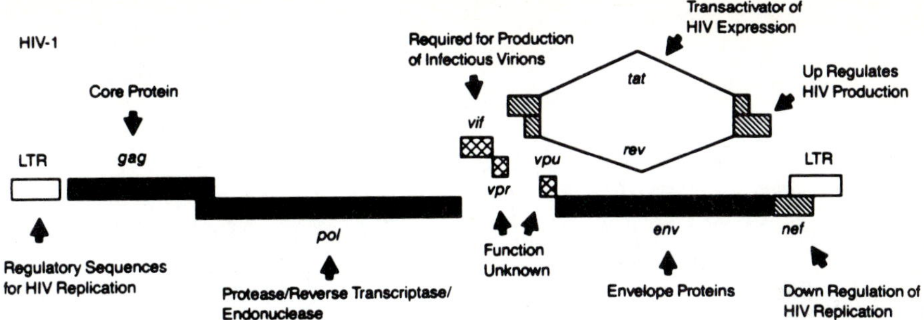

Figure 28-3 Functions of the viral gene products of HIV-1. Structural proteins (*gag, pol,* and *env*) are shown in black. The long terminal repeat (LTR), a major regulatory protein, is shown in white. Regulatory proteins (*tat, rev,* and *nef*) are noted with dashed lines. Genes whose functions are not characterized (*vif, vpr,* and *vpu*) are represented by crosshatching. (*From JA Levy, Human immunodeficiency viruses and the pathogenesis of AIDS, JAMA* (May 26, 1989) *261:2998, 1989. Copyright 1989, American Medical Association. With permission.*)

protein, and gp41, the transmembrane protein, which is the attachment site for gp120. Within the virus are core proteins (p24, etc.), reverse transcriptase, and two identical strands of RNA that constitute the HIV genome.

The virus genome has four regions (Fig. 28-3). The core proteins are encoded by the *gag* region, the two major envelope glycoproteins by the *env* region, the reverse transcriptase by the *pol* region, and a number of regulatory proteins by genes called *tat, rev,* and *nef.*

HIV binds to the CD4 antigen on the surface of cells by gp120 and is taken into the cell by fusion or endocytosis. Inside the cell the viral RNA is transcribed by the reverse transcriptase into double-stranded DNA (dsDNA), which enters the nucleus and integrates into the host chromosome. The infection may remain latent. Productive infection occurs when the viral genome is actively transcribed, producing mRNA coding for viral proteins and the RNA genome. Virions are formed by budding at the cell surface (Fig. 28-4).

While it is clear that HIV is the cause of AIDS, it is not clear how infection leads to disease. There are several possible mechanisms.[3–5] HIV may infect cells directly, causing their death. This may be the way progressive $CD4^+$ (helper) T-cell depletion occurs.[5] Alternatively, HIV may infect cells critical in immune regulation or produce proteins (e.g., gp120) that bind to receptors (CD4) required for normal immune function. These events may lead to a state of immune dysregulation.[3,4] Immune dysfunction and loss of immunocompetent cells may then result from overstimulation of the immune system or from autoimmune destruction of this system.

HIV strains are heterogeneous.[1] When studied in vitro, they have different characteristics associated with differences in their RNA genomes. These strain differences may explain in part the particular disease symptoms

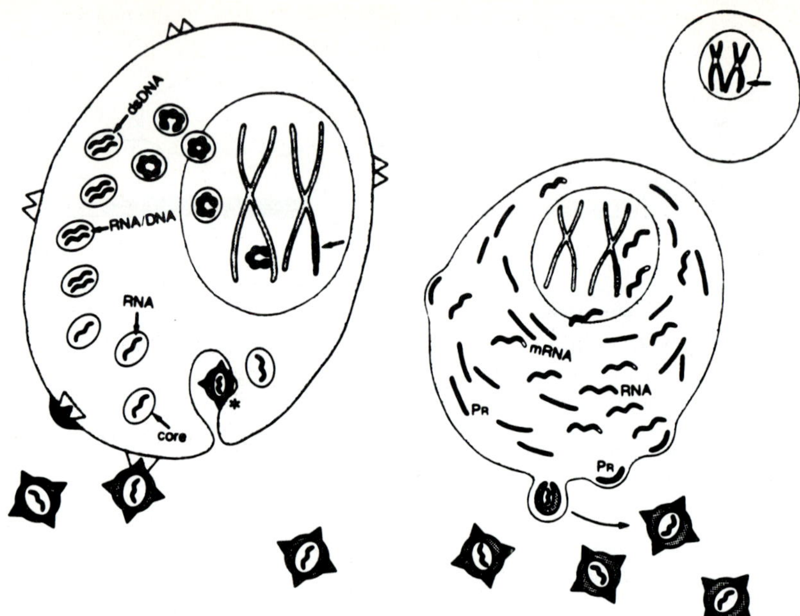

Figure 28-4 Life cycle of HIV. *Left:* the virus attaches to a specific receptor on the cell surface, and entry occurs by fusion of the virus to the cell membrane or by endocytosis (*). In many cells, binding involves the envelope gp120 and the cell surface CD4 molecules. After entry of the viral nucleoid (core) into the cytoplasm, reverse transcriptase within the core begins the events that lead from viral RNA to RNA/DNA hybrids and the dsDNA that is a copy (cDNA) of the viral RNA. Circular cDNA enters the nucleus and integrates into the chromosome (*arrow*). *Right:* after viral infection, the cell may enter a latent (top right) or productive state (bottom right). In the latent state, viral cDNA as an integrated proviral copy (*arrow*) is present in the infected cell; no infectious virions are produced. In the productive state, the proviral DNA produces mRNA and virion RNA. The mRNA codes for the proteins (PR) required for replication of infectious virions. The progeny virus, formed by encapsulation of the virion RNA into a particle, is produced at the cell surface by budding. Maturation of some of the viral proteins takes place at this time. (*From JA Levy, Human immunodeficiency viruses and the pathogenesis of AIDS, JAMA* (May 26, 1989) *261:2998, 1989. Copyright 1989, American Medical Association. With permission.*)

the patient develops. Certain strains of HIV, for instance, appear to be "neurotropic" and are associated with neurologic disease, sometimes without significant immune system impairment. The molecular basis of the heterogeneity may be related in part to the error-prone transcription by the reverse transcriptase.[6] This heterogeneity complicates vaccine development.

Progression of disease may be related to the viral heterogeneity and the interaction of the host with the virus.[1] Viral isolates in patients with advanced disease appear to be more cytopathic than their original isolates. This may be related to mutation of the virus in the host and/or to the predominance of the more pathogenic virus over time. Infected patients have active $CD8^+$ (suppressor/cytotoxic) T cells that prevent virus production by infected cells in vitro. This activity is especially strong in asymptomatic patients and is lost with disease progression. Antibodies against HIV early in the infection suppress infection of cells by HIV. While anti-HIV antibody levels remain high throughout the period of infection, late in the disease the antibodies seem to enhance viral infection. These anti-HIV antibodies may also be responsible for the destruction of $CD4^+$ T cells through autoimmune mechanisms. It seems, therefore, that as HIV disease progresses, both changes in the virus and changes in the host's response to the virus occur. These changes in concert seem to shift the balance from suppression of virus production to enhancement of virus production, and apparently to the appearance of clinical disease.

Phases of HIV Disease

Acute HIV Infection[7–9]

At the time of initial infection with HIV, many persons develop an acute viral syndrome. The incubation period may be as short as 1 week or as long as 2 months, averaging 3 to 6 weeks. The acute syndrome is characteristically a mononucleosis-like illness, with fever, lethargy, anorexia, sore throat, myalgias, headache, arthralgias, retro-orbital pain, lymphadenopathy, a truncal eruption, and occasionally encephalopathy or neuropathy. The illness lasts for about 3 weeks. A cutaneous eruption occurs in approximately 75 percent of patients with this syndrome and usually consists of nonpruritic, diffuse, erythematous macules and papules. An enanthem may accompany the eruption.

During the acute infection the lymphocyte count initially falls, with a reduction in the level of both $CD4^+$ T cells and $CD8^+$ T cells, but a normal $CD4^+/CD8^+$ T-cell ratio is maintained. Subsequently, both the $CD4^+$ and $CD8^+$ T-cell counts rise but the $CD8^+$ T-cell count increases more, resulting in an inverted $CD4^+/CD8^+$ T-cell ratio. This inverted ratio persists despite eventual normalization of both the $CD4^+$ and $CD8^+$ T-cell counts. During the acute infection, HIV antigen (p24) may be detected in the peripheral blood. The disappearance of the HIV antigen from the blood correlates with the increase in the $CD8^+$ T-cell count. Histologically, the acute exanthem shows a superficial mononuclear infiltrate composed predominantly of $CD4^+$ T cells.[10]

Latency (Asymptomatic Infection)

Characteristically, infected individuals recover from the acute syndrome and enter a long period of asymptomatic infection. This may be related to the establishment of HIV latency within the host genome and perhaps to adequate control of HIV replication by host $CD8^+$ T cells. Over time there is a gradual reduction in $CD4^+$ T-cell numbers, and most infected individuals go on to develop symptomatic HIV disease.[11]

Progressive Generalized Lymphadenopathy

Some HIV-infected persons develop unexplained, generalized lymphadenopathy. They may be otherwise asymptomatic.

Symptomatic HIV Disease (ARC and AIDS)[12]

Most infected individuals develop symptoms of HIV infection.[11] Initially, these symptoms may be constitutional—fever, night sweats, weight loss, or diarrhea. They may be primarily neurologic, producing encephalopathy, neuropathy, or dementia. Most commonly, as a result of immunosuppression, opportunistic infections occur. Certain of these opportunistic infections by themselves are diagnostic of AIDS—for example, *Pneumocystis carinii* pneumonia or chronic ulcerative herpes simplex virus persisting for more than 1 month. Other opportunistic infections are diagnostic of AIDS with evidence of HIV seropositivity—disseminated histoplasmosis, for example. Some opportunistic infections are not diagnostic of AIDS but are characteristic of HIV infection—widespread facial molluscum contagiosum or oral candidiasis, for example.[2] Secondary cancers, especially Kaposi's sarcoma and lymphoma, may also appear and are diagnostic of AIDS. The average incubation period (from infection to the development of AIDS) appears to be about 10 years.[13] Except for patients with Kaposi's sarcoma, virtually all persons with symptomatic HIV infection have reduced $CD4^+$ T cell counts and an inverted $CD4^+/CD8^+$ T-cell ratio. At the time symptomatic HIV infection appears, the $CD4^+$ T-cell count is almost always less than 400, and frequently it is less than 200. It is this loss of T-cell activity that accounts for the immune suppression. In addition, viral antigen (p24) may appear in the blood, indicating active HIV replication. A significant proportion of persons with these very low $CD4^+$ T-cell numbers may be asymptomatic, however, indicating that $CD4^+$ T-cell depletion alone does not always lead to AIDS.

SKIN DISEASE IN HIV INFECTION

Bacterial Infections

There are two important cutaneous bacterial pathogens in HIV-infected persons—*Staphylococcus aureus* and the etiologic agent of bacillary angiomatosis. *S. aureus* causes bullous impetigo, folliculitis (with or without pruritus), and secondary infection of dermatoses.[14,15] Staphylococcal infection appears to be increased in HIV-infected persons, due at least in part to their very high nasal carriage rate—about 50 percent.[16,17] Due to the reduction in the number and function of neutrophils in HIV-infected persons, these infections may be difficult to treat and may recur.[18] *S. aureus* is also a major cause of septicemia in HIV-infected persons.[15]

Bacillary angiomatosis (also known as epithelioid angiomatosis and disseminated cat scratch disease) is a systemic bacterial infection with prominent cutaneous manifestations.[19–21] Patients develop vascular skin lesions that may resemble pyogenic granulomas, subcutaneous nodules, or cellulitic plaques. Clinically and histologically, the skin lesions are virtually identical to the lesions seen in the second stage of bartonellosis, or verruga peruana. In addition, bone lesions are seen in about one-third of the patients. The liver, spleen, and respiratory tract may also be involved, resulting in death if the disease is untreated.[21] Once the diagnosis is established by skin biopsy, therapy with erythromycin is curative. With treatment the vascular component of the lesion involutes within 48 to 72 h, suggesting that the bacteria may be producing factors leading to the prominent angiogenesis.

Viral Infections

Three major viral families cause significant cutaneous and sometimes systemic disease in HIV-infected persons—Herpes viruses, papilloma viruses, and molluscum contagiosum. Herpes zoster occurs in approximately 10 percent of HIV-infected persons.[22–24] It is often the initial manifestation of HIV infection, frequently occurring in an at-risk person who is still asymptomatic. The course of the infection is usually typical, but it may be prolonged or severe and frequently causes scars. HIV-infected persons are at greater risk of a second episode of herpes zoster.[24] In patients with AIDS and severe immune suppression, dissemination of herpes zoster may occur, with or without dermatomal infection. It usually involves only the skin.[25] Herpes simplex is very common, and any ulcer, especially in the genital area, in an HIV-infected person should be suspected of being due to herpes simplex virus.[26] The two other members of the herpes virus family, Epstein-Barr virus (the cause of oral hairy leukoplakia) and cytomegalovirus, are also important pathogens in HIV-infected persons. Ulcerative cutaneous infection with cytomegalovirus often manifests as coinfection with herpes simplex virus.[27]

Warts of all types affect HIV-infected persons. Genital warts are particularly common.[2,28,29] There is mounting evidence that cervical, rectal, digital, and penile carcinomas are causally associated with wart virus infection. The immunosuppression of HIV disease may accelerate the progression from wart to carcinoma.[30]

Molluscum contagiosum appears to be much more common in HIV-infected persons than in persons immunosuppressed by other conditions.[2,31] Extensive facial and genital involvement is not uncommon. This may be due to increased sexual exposure to the infectious agent or to some unique feature of the immunosuppression associated with HIV disease.

Syphilis

Syphilis in the HIV-infected person may be unusual in two major ways. First, even patients with secondary syphilis may fail to achieve an immune response, resulting in a false-negative serologic test for syphilis.[32] Examination of a skin biopsy specimen with Warthin-Starry stain may help to establish the diagnosis. Usually this period of seronegativity is less than 3 months; and seroconversion then occurs. Second, clinical infection of the central nervous system (CNS) may occur in HIV-infected persons even after they have been given recommended doses of benzathine penicillin.[33] Invasion of the CNS by the spirochete does not appear to be more common in HIV-infected persons.[33] Standard therapy does not reach therapeutic levels in the cerebrospinal fluid and fails to eradicate the spirochetes in both HIV-seropositive and HIV-seronegative individuals. The reduced cell-mediated immunity in the HIV-infected person, however, more commonly allows progressive infection of the CNS to occur.[33]

Papulosquamous Diseases

Seborrheic dermatitis, psoriasis, and Reiter's syndrome are all more common in HIV-infected persons.[2] The incidence of seborrheic dermatitis may be 50 percent or more in AIDS patients. This may be related to the overgrowth of the normal yeast commensal *Pityrosporum orbiculare*. The addition of an agent effective against this organism, such as an imidazole, appears to enhance therapy. It is interesting to note, however, that while *P. orbiculare* may be associated with the seborrheic dermatitis in HIV disease, the other cutaneous disorder caused by *P. orbiculare*, tinea versicolor, is not seen with increased frequency in this population. This suggests that seborrheic dermatitis in persons with HIV disease is not due solely to the overgrowth of *P. orbiculare*. The known association of seborrheic dermatitis with CNS disorders such as Parkinson's disease supports the speculation that HIV involvement of the CNS may play a role in the pathogenesis of seborrheic dermatitis.[34]

Psoriasis occurs in about 5 percent of HIV-infected persons, two to three times the rate in noninfected individuals.[2,35] In about two-thirds of the HIV-infected, psoriatic patients, psoriasis begins after HIV infection. Compared with patients whose psoriasis began prior to seroconversion, these patients are older and, less commonly, have a family history of psoriasis. This suggests that HIV infection either induces or permits the expression of the cutaneous manifestations of psoriasis. The response of HIV-associated psoriasis to zidovudine, an antiretroviral agent, supports the role of HIV in the pathogenesis of some cases of HIV-associated psoriasis.[36] Intercurrent bacterial, viral, and fungal illnesses may also play an exacerbating role.[35]

Pruritic Eruptions

Many symptomatic, HIV-infected persons have pruritic skin rashes. In Africa and Haiti this is a very common presentation of HIV infection.[37,38] The pathogenesis of many of these conditions is unknown. Drug eruptions are common, especially those due to trimethoprim-sulfamethoxazole.[39] Insect bite reactions are enhanced.[40] Increased levels of antibodies to insect salivary gland antigen may be pathogenically related.[41] Photosensitivity occurs, appearing identical to a polymorphous light eruption.[42] Patients may be sensitive to both ultraviolet A and ultraviolet B.[42]

A significant proportion of patients with pruritic eruptions have folliculitis. About one-half of these patients have staphylococcal folliculitis and respond to appropriate therapy.[14] They do not, in general, have eosinophilia in their blood or tissues and have normal IgE levels.[43] In contrast, some HIV-infected patients with folliculitis do not have bacterial pathogens isolated by routine cultures, have tissue eosinophilia, and occasionally have peripheral eosinophilia and an elevated IgE level. These patients have a condition called eosinophilic pustular folliculitis. The demonstration of degranulating mast cells and eosinophils in the lesions, and the response of these patients to topical cromolyn sodium, suggest that mast cell degranulation is important in the pathogenesis of this disease.[44]

Cutaneous Malignancies in the HIV-Infected Individual

The sudden appearance of Kaposi's sarcoma in 35- to 40-year-old homosexual men in New York and San Francisco and the simultaneous appearance of *P. carinii* pneumonia in the same population in Los Angeles was the first harbinger of the AIDS epidemic.[1,2] Early studies[45,46] showed that while the opportunistic infections associated with AIDS, such as pneumocystis pneumonia and cryptococcal meningitis, generally occurred in individuals with fewer than 200 $CD4^+$ T cells and a $CD4^+/CD8^+$ T-cell ratio of 0.2, Kaposi's sarcoma often occurred when individuals had 400 to 600 $CD4^+$ T cells and a $CD4^+/CD8^+$ T-cell ratio of 0.6.[47] Although this observation has never been explained, it clearly demonstrates that the immune dysfunction that permits the development of Kaposi's sarcoma is not directly related to the $CD4^+$ T-cell number. For this reason, many of us now classify Kaposi's sarcoma as an ARC manifestation of HIV infection and not as AIDS itself.

The lesions of Kaposi's sarcoma can occur anywhere on the body. They appear suddenly and are often symmetric in presentation (Fig. 28-5). The lesions are commonly found on the anterior half of the hard palate and on the plantar surfaces of the feet. A typical lesion of Kaposi's sarcoma may appear at one-half or two-thirds of its final size as a salmon-pink macule surrounded by extravasated biliverdin and bilirubin. The lesion later enlarges and becomes nodular, and the color deepens to a port wine hue. These lesions stabilize over time and often involute. Spontaneous remissions are seen in about 5 percent of all patients. In some instances, particularly on the upper thigh, the lesions coalesce to form large, indurated plaques. On the lower extremities, multiple lesions of Kaposi's sarcoma may result in massive pedal edema with ulceration and profound disability.[48]

The pathophysiology of Kaposi's sarcoma is not understood, but recent research suggests that cytokines released as a consequence of HIV infection

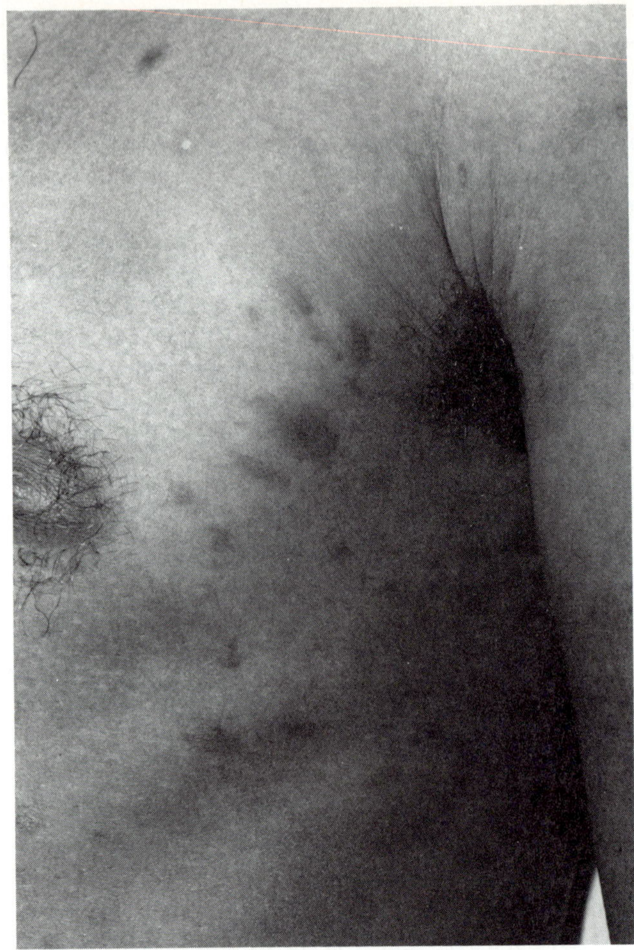

Figure 28-5 Typical lesions of AIDS-associated Kaposi's sarcoma on the trunk. Note the multiplicity of lesions and their tendency to follow skin lines.

may promote or induce the angioneogenesis that leads to the tumor recognized as Kaposi's sarcoma.[49] The major question at this juncture is whether Kaposi's sarcoma is in fact a malignancy or an exuberant vascular hyperplasia that runs rampant because of the HIV infection of the host. Evidence suggesting that Kaposi's sarcoma is not a malignancy is the fact that histologically the lesions usually lack cytologic atypia, are often bilaterally symmetric, and may spontaneously resolve.[50] Kaposi's sarcoma develops in preexisting lesions such as psoriasis, collagen injection sites, graft sites, and edematous legs.

The notion that Kaposi's sarcoma is a vascular hyperplasia caused by an environmental toxin or infectious agent is supported by several observations, the most obvious of which is that this condition occurs almost exclusively in homosexual men. Less than 2 percent of heterosexual individuals infected with HIV as a consequence of blood transfusions, factor VIII, or heterosexual sexual contact develop Kaposi's sarcoma. The number of individuals presenting with Kaposi's sarcoma as their primary diagnosis of AIDS dropped from more than 50 percent in the first 2 years of the epidemic to 15 to 17 percent at the end of 1989.[51] A steady decline in the number of homosexual men presenting with Kaposi's sarcoma has been observed in New York, San Francisco, and Vancouver coincident with a reduction in the rate of sexually transmitted diseases in homosexual men in these communities. A recent report of Kaposi's sarcoma in a small number of HIV-negative homosexual men supports the belief that a sexually transmitted infectious agent is the cause of Kaposi's sarcoma.[52] These men are all alive and well and have normal $CD4^+/CD8^+$ T-cell ratios. Analysis of Kaposi's sarcoma lesions for HIV and the cytomegalovirus genome has been unrewarding.[53]

Cutaneous T-Cell Lymphoma

Cutaneous T-cell lymphoma caused by another retrovirus, human T-cell lymphotropic virus-I (HTLV-I), is common in southern Japan and the Caribbean.[54] This disease has the same epidemiology as HIV infection and is seen in the sexual partners of HTLV-I-infected individuals and intravenous drug users. The incubation period from infection with HTLV-I to disease manifestation may be as long as 30 years and, unlike HIV infection, only a small percentage of infected individuals develop overt disease. HTLV-I has been spread extensively among intravenous drug users in the United States. Recent studies suggest that almost 50 percent of intravenous drug users in some communities are already infected with HTLV-I.

Recent reports suggest that coinfection with HTLV-I and HIV leads to a rapid progression of both diseases.[55–57] This observation may be explained by the fact that the *tat* gene of HIV stimulates the long terminal repeat (LTR) of HTLV-I, and vice versa. Synergism has been demonstrated in vitro; however, synergism in vivo remains speculative.

Of significance to the dermatologist is that patients presenting with adult T-cell lymphoma, Sézary syndrome, and mycosis fungoides should be examined for coinfection with HTLV-I and HIV.

Basal Cell Carcinoma

In HIV-infected men, basal cell carcinomas of the trunk are found with some frequency. These lesions have a typical distribution and morphology. A basal cell carcinoma has metastasized in an HIV-infected individual.[58] These patients are usually white, frequently vacation in tropical climes, and often sunbathe. The question therefore remains of whether truncal basal cell carcinomas are more frequent in the HIV-infected population or whether their appearance is simply the result of sun exposure by the patient or greater scrutiny by the physician.[59]

Immunosuppression and Malignancies

It has been known for two decades that immunosuppression results in a variety of systemic and cutaneous malignancies. Kaposi's sarcoma occurs 400 times more often in the immunosuppressed renal transplant patient than in the general population; T-cell lymphomas occur 360 times more commonly in immunosuppressed patients; squamous cell carcinomas are seen 36 times more commonly; and basal cell carcinomas are seen 3 times more commonly. In individuals immunosuppressed with corticosteroids and antimetabolites, malignancies generally appear 36 months after the initiation of immunosuppression. This observation suggests that as strategies to provide prophylaxis against opportunistic infections improve, and as HIV-infected, immunosuppressed patients live longer, systemic and cutaneous lymphomas and other malignancies will be seen with increasing frequency in the HIV-infected population.

REFERENCES

1. Levy JA: Human immunodeficiency viruses and the pathogenesis of AIDS. *JAMA* 261:2997, 1989.
2. Coldiron BM, Bergstresser PR: Prevalence and clinical spectrum of skin disease in patients infected with human immunodeficiency virus. *Arch Dermatol* 125:357, 1989.
3. Edelman AS, Zolla-Pazner S: AIDS; a syndrome of immune dysregulation, dysfunction, and deficiency. *FASEB J* 3:22, 1989.
4. Ascher MS, Sheppard HW: AIDS as immune system activation. II. The panergic imnesia hypothesis. *J AIDS* 3:177, 1990.
5. Baltimore D, Feinberg MB: HIV revealed: toward a natural history of the infection. *N Engl J Med* 321:1673, 1989.
6. Bradley PD et al: Fidelity of HIV-1 reverse transcriptase. *Science* 242:1168, 1988.
7. Gaines H: Primary HIV infection: clinical and diagnostic aspects. *Scand J Infect Dis* 61(suppl):1, 1989.
8. Tindall B et al: Characterization of the acute clinical illness associated with human immunodeficiency virus infection. *Arch Intern Med* 148:945, 1988.
9. Cooper DA et al: Characterization of T lymphocyte responses during primary infection with human immunodeficiency virus. *J Infect Dis* 157:889, 1988.
10. McMillan A et al: Short communication. Immunohistology of the skin rash associated with acute HIV infection. *AIDS* 3:309, 1989.
11. Lifson AR et al: AIDS commentary. The natural history of human immunodeficiency virus infection. *J Infect Dis* 158:1360, 1988.
12. Centers for Disease Control: Revision of the CDC surveillance case definition for acquired immunodeficiency syndrome. *MMWR* 36(suppl 15):3S, 1987.
13. Bacchetti P, Moss AR: Incubation period of AIDS in San Francisco. *Nature* 338:251, 1989.
14. Duvic M: Staphylococcal infections and the pruritus of AIDS-related complex. *Arch Dermatol* 123:1599, 1987.
15. Rolston KV et al: Bacterial infections in adult patients with the acquired immune deficiency syndrome (AIDS) and AIDS-related complex. *Am J Med* 83:604, 1987.
16. Berger TG et al: Nasal carriage rate of *Staphylococcus aureus* (SA) in AIDS and ARC patients. (abstract 372), in *Program and Abstracts of the Twenty-ninth Interscience Conference on Antimicrobial Agents and Chemotherapy,* Houston, 1989, p 163.
17. Ganesh R et al: Staphylococcal carriage and HIV infection. *Lancet* 2:558, 1989.
18. Ellis M et al: Impaired neutrophil function in patients with AIDS or AIDS-related complex: a comprehensive evaluation. *J Infect Dis* 158:1268, 1988.

19. Koehler JE et al: Cutaneous vascular lesions and disseminated cat-scratch disease in patients with the acquired immunodeficiency syndrome (AIDS) and AIDS-related complex. *Ann Intern Med* 109:449, 1988.
20. Berger TG et al: Bacillary (epithelioid) angiomatosis and concurrent Kaposi's sarcoma in acquired immunodeficiency syndrome. *Arch Dermatol* 125:1543, 1989.
21. Cockerell CJ et al: Epithelioid angiomatosis: a distinct vascular disorder in patients with the acquired immunodeficiency syndrome or AIDS-related complex. *Lancet* 2:654, 1987.
22. Friedman-Kien AE et al: Herpes zoster: a possible early clinical sign for development of acquired immunodeficiency syndrome in high-risk individuals. *J Am Acad Dermatol* 14:1023, 1986.
23. Melbye M et al: Risk of AIDS after herpes zoster. Lancet 1:728, 1987.
24. Colebunders R et al: Herpes zoster in African patients: a clinical predictor of human immunodeficiency virus infection. *J Infect Dis* 157:314, 1988.
25. Cohen PR et al: Disseminated herpes zoster in patients with human immunodeficiency virus infection. *Am J Med* 84:1076, 1988.
26. Siegal FP et al: Severe acquired immunodeficiency in male homosexuals, manifested by chronic perianal ulcerative herpes simplex lesions. *N Engl J Med* 305:1439, 1981.
27. Lee J Y-Y, Peel R: Concurrent cytomegalovirus and herpes simplex virus infections in skin biopsy specimens from two AIDS patients with fatal CMV infection. *Am J Dermatopathol* 11:136, 1989.
28. Milburn PB et al: Disseminated warts and evolving squamous cell carcinoma in a patient with acquired immunodeficiency syndrome. *J Am Acad Dermatol* 19:401, 1988.
29. Rudlinger R et al: Anogenital warts of the condyloma acuminatum type in HIV-positive patients. *Dermatologica* 176:277, 1988.
30. Frazer IH et al: Association between anorectal dysplasia, human papillomavirus, and human immunodeficiency virus infection in homosexual men. *Lancet* 2:657, 1986.
31. Penneys NS, Hicks B. Unusual cutaneous lesions associated with acquired immunodeficiency syndrome. *J Am Acad Dermatol* 13:845, 1985.
32. Hicks CB et al: Seronegative secondary syphilis in a patient infected with the human immunodeficiency virus (HIV) with Kaposi sarcoma. *Ann Intern Med* 107:492, 1987.
33. Lukehart SA et al: Invasion of the central nervous system by *Treponema pallidum:* implications for diagnosis and treatment. *Ann Intern Med* 109:855, 1988.
34. Mathes BM, Douglas MC: Seborrheic dermatitis in patients with acquired immunodeficiency syndrome. *J Am Acad Dermatol* 13:947, 1985.
35. Duvic M et al: Acquired immunodeficiency syndrome-associated psoriasis and Reiter's syndrome. *Arch Dermatol* 123:1622, 1987.
36. Kaplan MH et al: Antipsoriatic effects of zidovudine in human immunodeficiency virus-associated psoriasis. *J Am Acad Dermatol* 20:76, 1989.
37. Colebunders R et al: Generalized papular pruritic eruption in African patients with human immunodeficiency virus infection. *AIDS* 1:117, 1987.
38. Liautaud B et al: Pruritic skin lesions: a common initial presentation of acquired immunodeficiency syndrome. *Arch Dermatol* 125:629, 1989.
39. Gordin FM et al: Adverse reactions to trimethoprim-sulfamethoxazole in patients with the acquired immunodeficiency syndrome. *Ann Intern Med* 100:495, 1984.
40. Diven DG et al: Heightened cutaneous reactions to mosquito bites in patients with acquired immunodeficiency syndrome receiving zidovudine. *Arch Intern Med* 148:2296, 1988.
41. Penneys NS et al: Chronic pruritic eruption in patients with acquired immunodeficiency syndrome associated with increased antibody titers to mosquito salivary gland antigens. *J Am Acad Dermatol* 21:421, 1989.
42. Toback AC et al: Severe chronic photosensitivity in association with acquired immunodeficiency syndrome. *J Am Acad Dermatol* 15:1056, 1986.
43. Scully M, Berger TG: Pruritus, *S. aureus,* and HIV infection. *Arch Dermatol,* in press.
44. Buchness MR et al: The role of mast cells and eosinophils in eosinophilic pustular folliculitis of the acquired immunodeficiency syndrome. *J Invest Dermatol* 92:408, 1989.

45. Gottlieb MS et al: *Pneumocystis carinii* pneumonia and mucosal candidiasis in previously healthy homosexual men. *N Engl J Med* 302:1425, 1981.
46. Friedman-Kien A et al: Disseminated Kaposi's sarcoma in homosexual men. *Ann Intern Med* 96:693, 1981.
47. Ammann A et al: Tumor necrosis factors alpha and beta in acquired immunodeficiency syndrome (AIDS) and AIDS-related complex. *J Clin Immunol* 7:481, 1987.
48. Ziegler JL et al: Kaposi's sarcoma (multiple idiopathic hemorrhagic sarcoma), in TB Fitzpatrick et al (eds), *Dermatology in General Medicine*, 3d ed. New York, McGraw-Hill, 1987, p 1078.
49. Ensoli B et al: AIDS-Kaposi's sarcoma-derived cells express cytokines with autocrine and paracrine growth effects. *Science* 243:223, 1989.
50. Real FX, Krown SE: Spontaneous regression of Kaposi's sarcoma in patients with AIDS. *N Engl J Med* 313:1639, 1985.
51. Beral V et al: Medical science—Kaposi's sarcoma among persons with AIDS: a sexually transmitted infection? *Lancet* 335:123, 1990.
52. Friedman-Kien AE et al: Kaposi's sarcoma in HIV-negative homosexual men. *Lancet* 335:168, 1990.
53. Jahan N et al: Analysis of human KS biopsies and cloned cell lines for cytomegalovirus, HIV-1, and other selected DNA virus sequences. *AIDS Res Human Retroviruses* 5:225, 1989.
54. Dixon A et al: Infection with the human t-lymphotropic virus type I. *West J Med* 151:632, 1989.
55. Harper ME et al: Concomitant infection with HTLV-I and HTLV-III in a patient with T8 lymphoproliferative disease. *N Engl J Med* 315:1073, 1986.
56. Shibata D et al: Human T-cell lymphotropic virus type I (HTLV-I)-associated adult T-cell leukemia-lymphoma in a patient infected with human immunodeficiency virus type 1 (HIV-1). *Ann Intern Med* 111:871, 1989.
57. Baurmann H et al: Adult T-cell leukemia associated with HTLV-I and simultaneous infection by human immunodeficiency virus type 2 and human herpesvirus 6 in an African woman: a clinical, virologic, and familial serologic study. *Am J Med* 85:853, 1988.
58. Sitz KV et al: Metastatic basal cell carcinoma in acquired immunodeficiency syndrome-related complex. *JAMA* 257:340, 1987.
59. Heyer D et al: Changing prevalence of malignancies in men at San Francisco General Hospital during the HIV epidemic. Fifth International Conference on AIDS, abstract W.B.O. 19.

SECTION ELEVEN

NEOPLASMS OF THE SKIN

29

Experimental Skin Carcinogenesis by Ultraviolet Radiation

Honnavara N. Ananthaswamy and Margaret L. Kripke

Skin cancers are the most common type of human cancer. Recent surveys indicate that about 500,000 new cases of skin cancer are diagnosed each year in the United States.[1] Most of these skin cancers are thought to result from repeated exposure to sunlight. The importance of sunlight in the etiology of human skin cancer was recognized as early as 1894.[2] Shortly thereafter, studies with mice and rats confirmed the carcinogenic activity of sunlight and demonstrated that ultraviolet (UV) radiation present in the sunlight was responsible for this effect.[3,4] Since that time, research in this field has focused on three major themes: (1) attempts to define the relationship between exposure to UV radiation and induction of skin cancer in humans and laboratory animals, (2) description of the pathogenesis of skin cancer, and (3) investigation of the mechanism by which UV radiation causes neoplastic transformation. In addition, studies performed in the last 15 years have opened up a new area of research on the immunobiology of UV-induced skin cancers. These studies indicate that UV radiation not only results in the appearance of skin cancers but also interferes with an immune defense mechanism that normally protects against the development of such cancers.[5]

It was noted about 100 years ago that excessive exposure to sunlight was associated with the development of certain types of skin cancer. Epidemiological studies have confirmed this observation by demonstrating that basal and squamous cell carcinomas occur most frequently on skin that receives the most exposure to sunlight. The incidence of skin cancer is directly related to the amount of accumulated sunlight exposure and inversely related to the amount of protective pigment in the skin. Studies using experimental animals have demonstrated that wavelengths in the UV region of the sun's spectrum are responsible for the carcinogenic effect of sunlight. The UV region of the spectrum is divided into three parts—UVA (320 to 400 nm), UVB (280 to 320 nm), and UVC (200 to 280 nm)—based on their different biologic effectiveness (Fig. 29-1). Wavelengths in the UVB region of the solar spectrum are responsible for both tanning and skin cancer induction. These two responses are probably linked because tanning is the skin's response to damage inflicted by UV radiation and serves as a protective response against additional injury to the skin. Wavelengths in the UVA region are known to cause aging and wrinkling of the skin. They have also been shown to cause skin cancer in animals when given in high doses over a long period of time. In contrast, wavelengths in the UVC region are not present in natural sunlight because they are filtered out by the ozone in the atmosphere.

There is a growing concern that the incidence of skin cancer may increase due to the recently reported decrease in stratospheric ozone.[6] Because of increased production and use of chlorofluorocarbon compounds worldwide, the ozone layer in the stratosphere is at risk of diminishing. The major effect of a decrease in the ozone layer would be an increase in

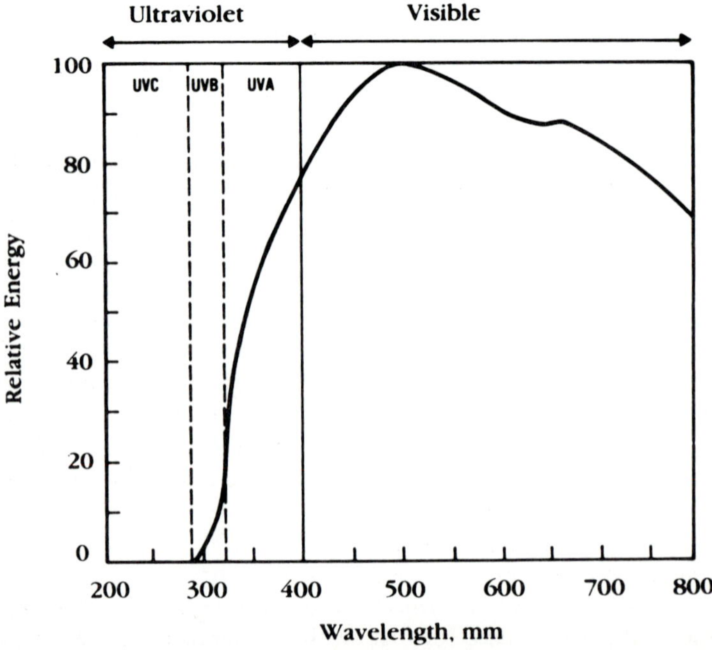

Figure 29-1 Solar spectrum (*From ML Kripke: Sunlight and skin cancer. Tex Med 82:52, 1986.*)

the amount of UV radiation present in natural sunlight. Wavelengths in the UVB region are particularly sensitive to changes in ozone concentration. Although UVA radiation would also be expected to increase if the ozone concentration decreases, the increase would be very small in relation to the amount of UVA already present in sunlight. Even a small increase in the amount of UVB radiation present in sunlight is likely to have important consequences for plant and animal life on earth and will almost certainly affect human health adversely. The most well-defined deleterious effect of UVB radiation on humans is the production of basal and squamous cell carcinomas of the skin. Other possible effects include a contribution to the development of cutaneous melanomas, ocular changes leading to the formation of cataracts, and immunologic perturbations of as yet unknown significance.

This chapter addresses some of the basic concepts of chemical and physical carcinogenesis and summarizes the recent advances in the field of UV carcinogenesis.

CHEMICAL CARCINOGENESIS

Skin cancers can be induced in rats and mice by exposing their skin to chemical or physical carcinogens or by injection of chemical carcinogens. Numerous studies have shown that skin carcinogenesis in mice is a multistep process that involves initiation, promotion, and progression.[7,8] Friedewald and Rous[9] made the initial observation that an agent can exert two kinds of action (initiation and promotion) in the induction of tumors. This led to the concept of a two-stage process of carcinogenesis. Subsequent studies[10,11] provided additional experimental data to support this concept. In this two-stage process, a tumor is first initiated by the application of a subthreshold dose of a carcinogen; subsequently, its development can be accelerated by repetitive treatment with a noncarcinogenic promoter. Complete carcinogenesis protocols involve the application of a single large dose or repeated applications of smaller doses of a carcinogen such as 7,12-dimethylbenz(a)-anthracene (DMBA).[12] Under these experimental conditions, the same carcinogen exerts both the initiating and the promoting actions. In the two-stage carcinogenesis model, the initiation step is achieved by a single topical application of a subcarcinogenic dose of DMBA. In the second stage, repeated topical treatment of the initiated skin with a promoting agent such as croton oil or tetradecanoylphorbol-13-acetate (TPA) results in the formation of many skin tumors. The repetitive application of croton oil or TPA alone on uninitiated skin, in general, does not induce tumor formation.

In two-stage carcinogenesis experiments, the order in which the initiator and the promoter are administered is critical. If repetitive applications of croton oil or TPA are administered before a single subcarcinogenic dose of DMBA, no tumors develop; initiation must precede promotion. An important characteristic of the two-stage carcinogenesis system in mouse skin is that the initiation step is irreversible, whereas the promotion step is initially reversible and is later irreversible.[13] An interval of up to 1 year between the application of the initiator and the beginning of the promoter treatment can still induce skin tumors similar in type and number to those observed when the promoter is given beginning 1 week after initiation.[13]

Besides DMBA and TPA, there are a number of chemical agents that are effective as complete carcinogens and/or initiators or promoters. Some of the chemicals that have skin tumor initiating and/or complete carcinogenic activity on mouse skin are aflatoxin B_1, urethane, *N*-methyl-*N′*-nitro-*N*-nitrosoguanidine, *N*-nitrosourea, 4-nitroquinoline-*N*-oxide, *N*-acetoxy-2-acetamidofluorene, β-propiolactone, and several hundred polycyclic aromatic hydrocarbons.[13] Similarly, a number of chemical agents act as tumor promoters. These include indole alkaloids (teleocidin and lyngbyatoxin), aplysiatoxin, chrysarobin, anthralin, benzo(e)pyrene, and benzoyl peroxide.[13] For more information on the subject of chemical carcinogenesis in general, the reader is referred to Slaga[8] and Hennings.[14]

UV CARCINOGENESIS

UV radiation can act as a complete carcinogen, as well as an initiator and a promoter. Since UV radiation is a potent DNA-damaging and mutagenic agent, it can initiate carcinogenesis by damaging DNA and inducing mutations in one or more genes. The mechanism by which UV radiation acts as a promoter is not well understood. However, UV radiation is known to stimulate DNA synthesis, ornithine decarboxylase activity, prostaglandin synthesis, and epidermal hyperplasia. These responses are similar to those induced by chemical tumor promoters.

Skin cancers can be induced in mice with either a single exposure to a large dose of UV radiation that causes ulceration[15,16] or multiple exposures to smaller doses of UV radiation.[17-21] The most common protocol involves repeated exposure to UV radiation, generally one to seven times per week for many weeks. The time between the first UV treatment and the appearance of a visible skin tumor is generally referred to as the latent period. The results are usually plotted as cumulative tumor incidence, prevalence, or probability of tumor development as a function of time. In order to quantitate the carcinogenesis system, the dose of UV radiation administered must be measured. In mouse carcinogenesis experiments, the UV dose is commonly defined as the amount of radiation integrated over time and measured at the surface of mouse skin. However, the actual amount of UV radiation that is absorbed by the target cells in the skin is difficult to calculate because the upper layers of the epidermis alter the dose absorbed by cells in the basal layer, hair follicle, or dermis. In addition, the first few exposures to UV radiation reduce the transmission properties of the skin due to changes in the epidermis (e.g., thickening and keratinization), which in turn affects the dose absorbed by the target cells during later exposures. Thus, in UV carcinogenesis experiments investigating the effects of dose, dose rate, and dose fractionation on tumor incidence, a correct measurement of the dose absorbed by the target cells is highly desirable but rarely achievable.

The rate of tumor development in three inbred mouse strains following chronic UV irradiation is shown in Fig. 29-2. In this experiment, shaved mice approximately 8 weeks old were exposed to UV radiation from a bank of six Westinghouse FS40 sunlamps for 1 h three times per week (Monday, Wednesday, and Friday). The 6 FS40 sunlamps delivered an average dose rate of about 2.8 $J/m^2/s$ over the wavelength range of 280 to 320 nm. This UV treatment was continued until the animals developed a tumor approximately 10 mm in diameter. The course of tumor development was monitored for several months. The data shown in Fig. 29-2 indicate that all three strains of mice were susceptible to carcinogenesis by UV radiation, although there were several differences in their responses. The most common histological types of tumor observed were fibrosarcomas, followed by squamous cell carcinomas. The tumor types and their frequencies were comparable among the three strains.

Several investigators have also induced tumors in mice by using the two-stage carcinogenesis model. Following exposure of mouse skin to

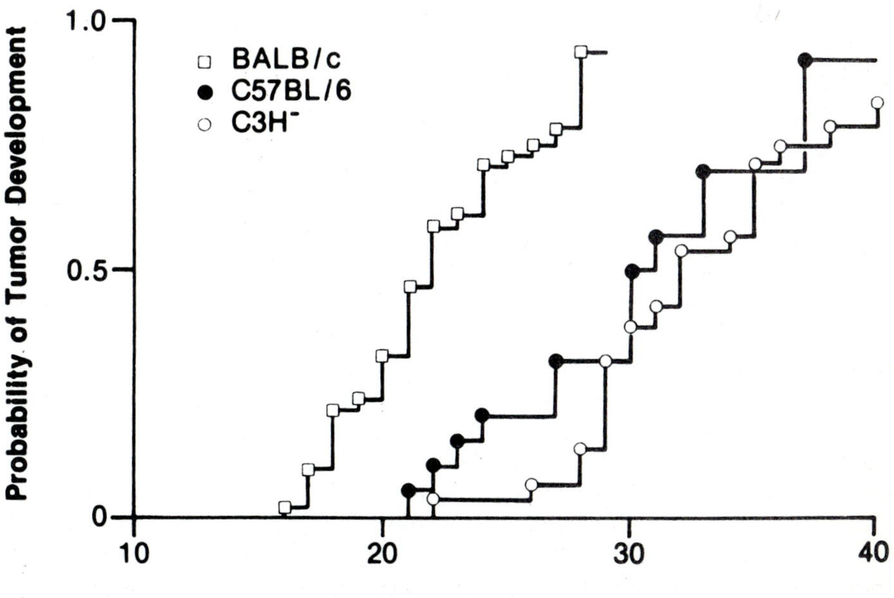

Figure 29-2 Rate of tumor appearance in three strains of mice. Beginning at 8 weeks of age, mice were exposed to UV radiation from a bank of six Westinghouse FS40 sunlamps for 1 h three times per week (Monday, Wednesday, Friday), and their dorsal hair was clipped weekly. This treatment continued until the animals developed a tumor of sufficient size (approximately 10 mm in diameter). Groups consisted of 51 BALB/c females, 19 C57BL/6 males, and 28 C3H females. (*From Kripke.*[19])

Table 29-1

FACTORS THAT INFLUENCE INDUCTION OF SKIN CANCER BY UV RADIATION

Physical	Biologic
Dose response	Genetic background
Dose rate	Age
Dose fractionation	Anatomic site
Radiation quality (wavelength)	

initiating doses of UV radiation, tumor development can be promoted by repeated application of croton oil or TPA. Epstein and Roth[22] first reported that repeated application of croton oil after a single exposure to UV radiation induced tumors in mice. Since then, other investigators have confirmed this observation.[23-26] UV radiation has also been used to promote chemical carcinogenesis. Epstein and Epstein[27] demonstrated that subcarcinogenic doses of UV accelerate tumor induction initiated by a single application of DMBA.

Induction of skin cancers in animals by UV radiation is influenced by various physical and biologic factors. Some of the factors that influence UV carcinogenesis in experimental animals are shown in Table 29-1.

PHYSICAL FACTORS

UV Dose

The pioneering work of Blum and his colleagues in the 1940s provided an invaluable body of information on the quantitative relationship between UV exposure and murine skin cancer.[17] The course of tumor development as a function of UV dose is usually plotted as cumulative tumor incidence or prevalence versus development time.[17] Blum and other investigators used this approach to examine the effect of UV dose, dose rate, and fractionation on tumor development. From these experiments, Blum concluded that the tumorigenic process started with the first dose and that tumor growth was accelerated in proportion to each successive dose. This model suggests that the tumor growth rate depends on the dose per fraction and the number of fractions. However, this model has been challenged by DeGruijl et al.,[28] who have shown that only the initiation of a tumor is dose dependent, whereas the subsequent growth of a tumor is dose independent. The difference between these two models could be attributed to the fact that in Blum's studies the dose–response relationship was measured for tumors of one particular size over a small range of daily UV doses, whereas in DeGruijl's studies the dose–response relationship was ascertained for tumors of different sizes over a wide UV dose range.[28,29]

An important characteristic of experimental UV carcinogenesis is that there is little reciprocity with regard to time and dose. Blum's experiments demonstrated that giving the same total dose of radiation at different dose rates does not necessarily produce the same number of tumors on the ears of strain A mice.[17] Recent studies have demonstrated, in addition, that giving a dose of UV radiation in different patterns of fractionation produces different tumor incidences and induction times.[30] In hairless mice, multiple small doses of radiation are more effective in producing skin cancers than larger, less frequent doses[31] or single acute exposures.[15] These results suggest that induction of tumors in mouse skin requires multiple doses large enough to produce tissue damage. However, in the rat, the opposite result has been reported. Repeated exposures to UV radiation were less effective than an equivalent single exposure for inducing skin tumors in rats, even though the multiple exposures caused more skin damage.[16]

Radiation Quality (Effective Wavelengths)

The UVC region of the solar spectrum is not relevant to human skin cancers because wavelengths below 280 nm are filtered out before they reach the earth's surface. Epidemiological and clinical studies indicate that the carcinogenic effect of sunlight in humans is mediated by the UVB region of the sun's spectrum. In addition, it is well known that patients with the genetic disease xeroderma pigmentosum develop cancers on sun-exposed regions of the skin. However, evidence relating skin cancer to sunlight exposure generally does not distinguish between total spectral irradiance and the UV portion of the spectrum. The involvement of UVB radiation in skin cancer induction is inferred from studies with laboratory animals and from assumptions that the wavelengths inducing an erythemal response are similar to those inducing skin cancer.[32] Although there is some evidence from studies on mice that supports this possibility that erythema-inducing wavelengths are important for carcinogenesis,[33] this remains unsubstantiated for human skin cancer. This problem eventually may be resolved by studies on the long-term effects on skin cancer incidence using sunscreens known to reduce erythema.

In 1934 Roffo[4] reported that skin tumors induced in rats by sunlight and by UV radiation emitted from mercury arc lamps could be prevented by inserting window glass between the source of radiation and the rats. Since the window glass filtered out radiation below 320 nm, this result suggested that wavelengths above 320 nm were not carcinogenic. However, recent studies indicate that UVA radiation can induce tumors in mice if exposure times are long and doses are high.[34-37] Zigman et al.[34] reported that blacklight fluorescent lamps induce skin cancer in laboratory mice. Forbes et al.[38] attributed this effect to the presence of contaminating UVB wavelengths in the unfiltered blacklight lamps. When the blacklight lamps were filtered with window glass, no tumors were induced when the hairless mice were exposed for 8 h/day for several months.[35] However, when the same daily dose was administered at a reduced intensity over a 24-h period for 10 weeks, the hairless mice developed skin tumors. These results indicate that under certain circumstances, UVA radiation can induce tumors in mice, although with reduced efficiency. Similarly, Strickland[37] reported that Mylar-filtered UVA radiation (315 to 400 nm) induced benign papillomas, squamous cell carcinomas, and poorly differentiated (spindle cell) tumors in Sencar mice with a 50 percent probability after 68 weeks of irradiation. Since the Mylar-filtered UVA light source still emitted 0.03 percent of the radiation between 315 and 320 nm, it is possible that these shorter wavelengths contributed significantly to its tumorigenic effectiveness. Thus, additional studies are needed to resolve this issue. A precise quantitation of the tumorigenic effectiveness of UVA radiation will require a comprehensive investigation of both the UVA spectra and the UVA dose rate on tumorigenicity.

Interactions between UVB and UVA Radiation

Even though UVA radiation is reported to be either noncarcinogenic or weakly carcinogenic, it can interact with UVB radiation to modulate skin carcinogenesis. Studies by Willis et al.[39] and Staberg et al.[40] have shown that UVA radiation augments the tumorigenic effectiveness of UVB radiation. On the other hand, Forbes et al.[31] found no effect of UVA radiation on UVB-induced skin carcinogenesis. Clearly, more studies are needed to resolve this issue and to define the possible types of interaction between UVA and UVB in carcinogenesis.

BIOLOGIC FACTORS

Genetic Background

Evidence from human epidemiological studies suggests that genetically determined factors contribute to the susceptibility of individuals to UV-induced skin cancer. In addition to the obvious factor of skin pigmentation, there may be other variables, such as amounts of DNA repair enzymes, production of growth factors, or host immunologic competence, that combine to determine individual susceptibility. Analogous to humans, there are also many differences in UV-induced skin cancer development among various laboratory animals. Susceptibility to tumor induction is quite variable in different rodent species: mice are highly susceptible, and guinea pigs are relatively resistant.[41] Even within various mouse strains, there are wide variations in susceptibility to tumor induction. Kripke[19] compared the carcinogenic effects of UV radiation on three inbred mouse strains with different coat colors and found that albino mice (BALB/cAnN) developed tumors much earlier than did agouti (C3H/HeN) or black (C57BL/6) mice (Fig. 29-2). In addition to differences in tumor incidence, there were differences in the sites of tumor occurrence in different mouse strains. A large proportion of the tumors in the BALB/c mice arose on the ears, in contrast to the other two strains, in which dorsal tumors predominated. Some of these differences could be due to the quantity and distribution of pigment in skin and hair. However, within a strain, hair and pigment distributions do not seem to be the critical factors in the susceptibility of different sites to tumor induction. There is little hair or pigment in the ears of C57BL/6 mice, yet the latency of tumors arising on the ears does not differ from the latency of back tumors.[19] In another study, Rusch and Baumann[42] also found that two strains of albino mice (strains A and C) developed tumors much more rapidly than C57 mice in response to UV radiation. However, these mice were not shaved prior to irradiation; therefore, only ear tumors and a few eye tumors were produced.

UV carcinogenesis experiments have also been performed using Sencar mice, which are extremely susceptible to two-stage skin carcinogenesis by chemical carcinogens.[7,43] Strickland[44] found that Sencar mice were extremely susceptible to UV-induced skin tumors compared to the related stock of CD-1 mice. These results are particularly interesting because Sencar mice were originally selected for susceptibility to skin carcinogenesis by a chemical initiation-promotion protocol.[7,43] Strickland's results indicate that the susceptibility determinants selected for in Sencar mice are not specific for chemical carcinogenesis but are also important in UV carcinogenesis.

Descriptive studies on the development of UV-induced skin cancer have revealed both similarities and differences in its pathogenesis in different strains and species of animals. An important unifying feature of skin cancer induction is its association with precancerous lesions, or actinic keratoses.[45] The existence of such preneoplastic lesions suggests that skin cancer develops by multiple sequential stages rather than as a result of a single infrequent event. A second generalization that emerges from the descriptive studies is that sunlight- or UV-induced skin cancers are among the least aggressive neoplasms. Reports of metastasis of squamous cell carcinoma and basal cell carcinoma in humans are rare, and metastasis appears to be a late occurrence in the evolution of these tumors.[32,46] Metastasis of primary UV-induced skin cancers in mice is also infrequent,[47,48] although many UV-induced fibrosarcomas metastasize after transplantation.[49] However, there is one report that indicates that 40 percent of mice bearing primary UV-induced tumors developed pulmonary metastasis.[50]

Squamous cell carcinoma and fibrosarcoma are the main histological types of tumor produced in mice by UV exposure, but the proportions of these tumors differ in various strains[19] and within a strain under different conditions of UV exposure.[17,48] One important conclusion to be drawn from these studies is that tumors develop only in cells that are exposed directly to UV radiation. This implies that direct interaction between the carcinogen and the target cell is required for carcinogenesis and that cells in tissue layers below the penetration range of the radiation are not at risk for UV carcinogenesis.

Age and Anatomic Site

In experimental UV carcinogenesis using mice, several investigators have reported that young mice are more susceptible to the induction of skin tumors than old mice.[19,51,52] In addition, by performing reciprocal skin graft experiments between young and old mice, Ebbesen and Kripke[53] demonstrated that the difference in susceptibility to UV carcinogenesis between young and old mice was not due to some inherent characteristic of the skin but rather to certain physiological factors in the host that change as a function of age. These results raise the possibility that during the first half of the life span of the animals, the age of the host at the time of first UV exposure may be a determining factor in UV carcinogenesis. However, the nature of these differences in host factors has not been identified, and there are many possible candidates for such an effect. For example, the ability to repair certain types of UV-induced damage in DNA changes with age in BALB/c mice,[54] the proliferative response of epidermal cells to UV radiation differs in animals of different ages,[55] and the activity of various host defense mechanisms changes with age.[56]

As mentioned before, the ear skin of BALB/c mice is more susceptible to tumor induction by UV radiation than the back skin. Skin graft experiments have shown that ear skin grafts on the middorsum of young BALB/c recipients are more susceptible to tumor induction than comparable grafts of back skin.[53] These results suggest that the increased susceptibility of ears to UV carcinogenesis relative to back skin in BALB/c mice does not result from increased exposure of the ears to UV radiation, as might be expected because of their position relative to the back. Instead, this high frequency of tumor development seems to reflect the fact that ear skin is intrinsically more susceptible to the carcinogenic effects of UV radiation than back skin, most likely because of differences in the optical properties of ears and back skin resulting from differences in pelage and in the thickness of the stratum corneum. Thus, although UV dose and genetic background clearly influence carcinogenesis in both humans[18] and experimental animals,[19] other intrinsic properties of the target tissue and age-dependent properties of the host also play a role in the development of UV-induced skin cancers. These findings, coupled with other physical and biologic factors, emphasize the complexity of this tumor model system and illustrate the difficulties underlying calculations of estimated risks of human solar carcinogenesis.

IMMUNE SYSTEM AND UV CARCINOGENESIS

In recent years, immunologic studies using laboratory animals have opened up a new era of research in UV carcinogenesis. Skin cancers induced in mice by UV radiation are highly antigenic, and when they are transplanted into normal, genetically identical mice, most are rejected by the recipient's immune system.[19,57] However, these tumors grow and eventually kill their host when they are transplanted to mice exposed to a short course of UV irradiation. These and other observations led to the conclusion that exposing mice to UV radiation interfered with the ability of their immune system to reject developing skin cancers. This defect can be passively transferred with lymphoid cells and is due, at least in part, to the presence of suppressor T lymphocytes in the lymphoid organs of UV-irradiated animals.[58,59] These suppressor T lymphocytes prevent the rejection of transplanted, UV-induced murine tumors but not the rejection of tumors induced by other carcinogens.

Although the systemic effects of UV radiation were thought to be important for the development of primary UV radiation–induced skin cancers, as well as for the growth of transplanted tumors, this premise was not tested until recently. In 1982, de Gruijl and van der Leun[60] reported that repeated exposure of hairless mice to UV radiation on one side accelerated the subsequent induction of skin cancers by chronic UV irradiation on the opposite side, which had been shielded during the first irradiation period. Their study demonstrated that some systemic effect of UV radiation markedly enhanced the formation of primary UV-induced skin tumors. Experiments by Fisher and Kripke[61] showed, in addition, that UV radiation–induced suppressor lymphocytes could accelerate the development of primary skin cancers induced by chronic UV irradiation. This finding indicated that at least some of the systemic effects of UV radiation on UV carcinogenesis were immunologically mediated and that the immune system played a critical role in cutaneous carcinogenesis.

The systemic effect of UV radiation was also shown to enhance chemical carcinogenesis at a distant site. Roberts and Daynes[62] examined the effects of UV radiation on the formation of skin cancers induced by repeated painting of unirradiated skin with benz(a)pyrene (BP) and found that UV radiation accelerated the development of BP-induced skin tumors at a distant site in UV-irradiated mice relative to unirradiated controls. This enhancement of BP-induced carcinogenesis by UV radiation was also attributed to the immunosuppressive effects of UV radiation, although this was not proved. On the other hand, the induction of melanomas and other skin cancers by DMBA and croton oil was not accelerated by UV irradiation at a distant site.[63]

Studies by Strickland et al.[26] have shown that UV radiation markedly potentiated two-stage skin carcinogenesis resulting from application of UV radiation and TPA at a distant site. Surprisingly, they also found that mice treated with TPA alone on the dorsal skin developed a significant number of dorsal tumors if the mice also had been exposed to UV radiation on the ventral side. These results suggest that a systemic effect of UVB radiation was exerted during the promotion phase of two-stage carcinogenesis. These findings may have broad implications for human cancers. It has long been speculated that UV radiation plays a role in the induction of malignant melanoma.[64] However, these cancers do not necessarily appear on the most heavily sun-exposed parts of the body.[65] The finding that UV radiation can potentiate skin carcinogenesis at a distant body site provides a hypothesis to explain this discrepancy. It also suggests that UV radiation may contribute to the formation of skin cancers and of head and neck cancers that do not occur on heavily sun-exposed sites. More important, these findings imply that a systemic effect of UV radiation interferes with a natural host control mechanism that ordinarily holds skin cancers in check. Contrarily, Romerdahl et al.[63] have reported that induction of melanoma by DMBA and croton oil was not potentiated by UV irradiation at a distant site. However, UV radiation of mice is known to accelerate the growth of transplanted melanomas but not of other types of tumors.[66] Interestingly, this effect is observed when melanoma cells are injected directly into the site of UV irradiation but not when they are injected into an unirradiated site, suggesting that this is a local and not a systemic effect of UV radiation.[66]

An important question that arises from these observations is: how does exposure of the skin to UV radiation bring about systemic changes in host immunity? Recent studies have shown that UV radiation damages Langerhans cells present in the skin.[67] These Langerhans cells are cutaneous macrophages, which take up foreign substances in the skin and present them to T lymphocytes, thereby initiating an immune response. However, Langerhans cells damaged by UV radiation can no longer carry out this antigen-presenting function. When foreign substances are introduced through such UV-damaged skin, the immune response is not initiated. Instead, the suppressive pathway of the immune system is activated, resulting in the production of suppressor T lymphocytes.[68] The suppressor lymphocytes prevent the induction of an immune response against subsequent applications of the same antigen.

MODIFICATION OF UV CARCINOGENESIS

UV radiation can interact with other chemical or physical agents and alter the carcinogenic process. As mentioned before, UVA radiation can enhance UVB-induced carcinogenesis in mice.[39,40] UVB radiation has been shown to enhance x-ray-induced skin carcinogenesis in mice[69] and rats.[70] In addition, it has been reported that tinea capitis patients treated with therapeutic x-rays for scalp infections exhibited a higher incidence of skin tumors in the treated area.[71,72] This high incidence was thought to be caused by exposure to sunlight either prior to or following x-ray therapy. These results imply that humans exposed to both UV and ionizing radiation may be at a higher risk for developing skin tumors than individuals exposed to only one of these agents.

The combination of psoralens and UVA radiation, commonly referred to as PUVA, is widely used in the treatment of psoriasis and other skin disorders.[73] With the increased use of PUVA therapy in humans in the last two decades, considerable attention has focused on understanding the mutagenic and carcinogenic effects of this treatment. Chronic PUVA treatment is known to induce skin tumors in mice.[74] In humans, the carcinogenicity of PUVA treatment has not been firmly established. However, Stern et al.[75] have reported that PUVA therapy is associated with a marked increase in the incidence of skin cancer in patients receiving this treatment for skin disease. In addition, recent studies have shown that PUVA treatment also affects certain immunologic functions in both humans and experimental animals.[76,77] This suggests that the immunologic effect of PUVA might contribute to its carcinogenic effect. In addition to PUVA, a combination of UV radiation and coal tar has been used in the treatment of psoriasis. This treatment is also reported to be carcinogenic in animals. Findlay[78] showed that UV radiation plus tar was much more carcinogenic than tar alone.

Retinoic acid has been shown to inhibit both chemical-induced[79] and ionizing radiation–induced[80] skin carcinogenesis. However, there are conflicting reports on the effect of retinoic acid on UV-induced skin carcinogenesis. Some studies have shown that retinoic acid enhances the development of UV radiation–induced skin tumors in mice,[21,23,81,82] while others have shown that retinoic acid either has no effect[83] or slightly inhibits UV-induced tumorigenesis.[84] In addition to retinoic acid, a variety of other chemical agents, such as butylated hydroxytoluene (an antioxidant),[85] polyunsaturated lipids,[86,87] vitamins,[88] caffeine,[89] and chlorpromazine,[90] have been shown to inhibit UV carcinogenesis in experimental animals. However, the mechanism by which some of these agents inhibit the process of UV carcinogenesis is not well characterized.

IN VITRO UV CARCINOGENESIS

In vitro model systems have also been used to demonstrate the carcinogenic effects of UV radiation. DiPaolo and Donovan[91] first reported that UV radiation can induce morphological transformation of Syrian golden hamster embryonic fibroblasts. Since then several investigators have shown that UV radiation also induces morphological and tumorigenic transformation of the C3H mouse embryo fibroblast cell line 10T1/2.[92-94] In contrast, Mondal and Heidelberger[95] have reported that UV radiation induces transformation of 10T1/2 cells only when followed by repeated treatment with TPA. Morphological transformation of human fibroblasts by in vitro exposure to UV radiation has also been reported.[96,97] However, all of these in vitro transformation studies have used fibroblasts and 254-nm (UVC) radiation. Since UVC radiation is absorbed by ozone in the stratosphere and never reaches the earth, studies using UVC radiation may not be relevant to human skin cancer. Although both UVC and UVB radiation damage DNA, they induce different proportions of various lesions. For example, with increasing wavelength, there is a decrease in thymine dimer formation and an increase in the number of DNA single-strand breaks.[98] In addition, studies using epithelial cells are preferable because most human cancers, including those of the skin, occur in epithelial tissues. In order to address these issues, we used primary epidermal cells from neonatal BALB/c mice to demonstrate the carcinogenic effects of UVB radiation.[99] Our results indicated that exposure of freshly prepared epidermal cells from neonatal BALB/c mouse skin to UVB radiation from a filtered FS40 sunlamp induces foci of morphologically transformed cells. In addition, cells derived from these foci produce tumors when injected subcutaneously into normal and immunosuppressed syngeneic recipients.[99]

In vitro systems have also been employed to demonstrate the carcinogenic effects of UVB[93,99-101] and UVA radiation[93,101] and visible light,[94] and to define an action spectrum for UV carcinogenesis. Because animal models involve lengthy and tedious experiments, an in vivo action spectrum for UV carcinogenesis has not been determined precisely. However, action spectra for in vitro transformation of Syrian hamster embryo fibroblasts[102] and human cells[103] in culture have been established that show a broad maximum around 254 nm. Although these in vitro action spectrum studies reveal the most effective wavelengths and may help to identify the chromophore responsible for the absorption of UV that leads to transformation, their relevance to in vivo carcinogenesis has been questioned. In intact animals, absorption of UV radiation, particularly the shorter wavelengths (below 290 nm), may not be the same as in a monolayer of cells in culture. In addition, in vitro transformation studies do not take into account host factors that may influence the process of carcinogenesis. Therefore, an extrapolation of in vitro data to in vivo conditions without taking into account the transmission properties of the skin and the influence of the host environment on the process of UV carcinogenesis might lead to erroneous conclusions. In spite of these criticisms, in vitro model systems are still valuable in UV carcinogenesis studies.

MECHANISMS OF UV CARCINOGENESIS

Carcinogenesis by UV radiation is a complex process that involves initiation, promotion, and progression. In UV carcinogenesis, as in chemical carcinogenesis, there is a long latent period from the time of first exposure until the appearance of primary skin tumors. The cellular and molecular processes that occur during the initial carcinogen–cell interaction and the onset of tumor growth are largely unknown. Attempts to identify these alterations in vivo have been hampered by the complex nature of the target tissues. In addition, it is presumed that only a minor subpopulation of the cells in the target tissue undergoes changes that lead to the expression of a transformed phenotype.

Several lines of evidence implicate DNA as the target for most of the biologic effects of UV, such as lethality, mutation, and transformation. First, individuals with the genetic disorder xeroderma pigmentosum are extremely sensitive to sunlight and frequently develop skin cancers as a result of exposure to it. In addition, their somatic cells are hypersensitive to killing by UV radiation.[104] This extreme sensitivity of somatic cells to

UV radiation has been attributed to a defect in the repair of UV-induced pyrimidine dimers.[104] Second, the action spectra for cell killing, mutation, and transformation of Syrian golden hamster embryo fibroblasts[102] and human cells[103] are similar to the DNA absorption spectrum as well as to the action spectrum for pyrimidine dimer induction. Third, the reversal of UV-induced pyrimidine dimers in the DNA by enzymatic photorepair reduces the incidence of tumors in the Amazon molly, *Poecilia formosa*,[105] and in the South American opossum, *Monodelphis domestica*,[106] and reduces the frequency of UV-induced transformation of cultured human fibroblasts.[96] These studies also suggest that pyrimidine dimers, the major UV-induced photoproduct in DNA, are responsible for the above-mentioned UV-induced biologic effects.

A number of studies have indicated that there is a causal relationship between induction of pyrimidine dimers and UV carcinogenesis. Hart et al.[105] have shown that injection of UV-irradiated tissue homogenates of *P. formosa* into isogenic recipients resulted in thyroid carcinoma. However, when UV-irradiated tissue homogenates were exposed to photoreactivating light prior to injection, the tumor incidence was reduced significantly, suggesting the involvement of pyrimidine dimers in UV-induced carcinogenesis. Recent studies by Ley et al.[106] have shown that the marsupial, *M. domestica*, which exhibits an efficient enzymatic photoreactivation of UV-induced pyrimidine dimers, is highly susceptible to induction of skin and corneal tumors by UV radiation, and that exposure to photoreactivating light immediately after UV irradiation results in a substantial decrease in the number of UV-induced corneal tumors. Sutherland et al.[96] demonstrated that UV-induced transformation of cells to anchorage-independent growth was susceptible to photoenzymatic repair, again implicating pyrimidine dimers in UV-induced transformation. However, Suzuki et al.[101] reported that although the induction of mutation in V79 Chinese hamster cells and induction of transformation in C3H mouse 10T1/2 cells by a germicidal lamp (254 nm) and an unfiltered sunlamp (290 to 345 nm) matched the DNA absorption spectrum, such was apparently not the case for mutation and transformation induced by a filtered sunlamp (300 to 345 nm). They found that wavelengths greater than 300 nm yielded appreciably more mutation and transformation than can be accounted for by pyrimidine dimer formation. They have suggested that a chromophore other than or in addition to DNA may be involved in induction of mutation and transformation at longer wavelengths.

Recent studies indicate that UV radiation induces, in addition to pyrimidine dimers, other nondimer photoproducts such as [6-4] photoproducts,[107,108] cytosine photohydrates,[109,110] purine photoproducts,[111] and single-strand breaks in the DNA.[112] Various data suggest that [6-4] photoproducts may play a significant role in UV-induced lethality and mutagenesis.[113,114] On the other hand, it is reported that cytosine photohydrates and purine photoproducts, while sparsely formed by UVC radiation, are maximally formed by UVB radiation. However, the role of these nondimer photoproducts in UV carcinogenesis is not known. Recently, Applegate et al.[115] demonstrated that skin fibroblasts from basal cell nevus syndrome patients, who are genetically predisposed to sunlight-induced skin cancers, are hypersensitive to killing by UVB but not by UVC radiation compared to fibroblasts from age- and sex-matched normal individuals. In addition, they found that the increased sensitivity of skin fibroblasts from basal cell nevus syndrome patients to killing by UVB radiation is not due to a defect in the excision repair of UVB-induced pyrimidine dimers. These results suggest that DNA lesions (and repair processes) other than the pyrimidine dimer are also involved in the pathogenesis of sunlight-induced skin cancers in basal cell nevus syndrome patients.

Several lines of evidence support the hypothesis that somatic mutations are involved in the process of neoplasia. Studies utilizing skin fibroblasts from excision repair–deficient human xeroderma pigmentosum patients have shown that they exhibit a higher frequency of UV-induced mutation and transformation than normal human skin fibroblasts.[97,116] These results suggest that defects in DNA repair predisposes xeroderma pigmentosum cells to UV radiation–induced skin cancer because UV radiation induces a much higher frequency of mutation in xeroderma pigmentosum cells than in normal cells, and some of these mutations may be involved in cancer induction.

Since carcinogenesis is considered to be a multistep process, it is possible that genetic changes involving oncogenes may participate in tumor initiation and/or progression. Cellular oncogenes are reported to be activated in a variety of human and rodent tumors. Many normal cells also express these oncogenes (termed proto-oncogenes), which indicates that these genes may play a role in the growth and differentiation of normal embryonic and adult tissues. However, exposure of cells to carcinogenic agents may convert the normal genes into pathological genes by causing them to produce higher levels of their normal gene product or by inducing structurally aberrant gene products. There is evidence that both of these phenomena occur.

Cellular proto-oncogenes can be activated by both point mutations and chromosomal translocations, suggesting that there may be a direct link between exposure to agents that damage DNA and genetic change leading to malignancy.[117–120] Zarbl et al.[119] have shown that in rat tumors induced by nitrosomethylurea, the point mutation (G-A transition) responsible for the activation of the c-Ha-*ras*-1 proto-oncogene was always located at the 12th codon, whereas in rat tumors induced by DMBA, the point mutation was at the 61st codon of the c-Ha-*ras* locus. Similarly, Quintanilla et al.[120] have reported that over 90 percent of tumors, including premalignant papillomas, induced by DMBA and TPA contained a specific A-T transversion at the second nucleotide of codon 61 of the c-Ha-*ras* oncogene. One hypothesis suggested by these observations is that a particular class of carcinogens may activate specific oncogenes during the development of tumors. Since the DNA damage induced by UV radiation is unique and differs from the lesions induced by any other carcinogen, it is possible that UV radiation–induced tumors may contain specific alterations in the oncogene structure.

To address this question, several investigators have analyzed human skin cancers for the presence of activated oncogenes. Ananthaswamy et al.[121] found that genomic DNAs from three of eight human skin cancers occurring on sun-exposed body sites contained activated c-Ha-*ras* oncogenes capable of inducing tumorigenic transformation when introduced into NIH 3T3 cells by DNA-mediated gene transfer. Analysis of six additional human skin cancers revealed that three of them contained an activated N-*ras* oncogene (Ananthaswamy et al., unpublished observations). However, it is not yet known whether the Ha-*ras* and N-*ras* oncogenes detected in human skin cancers contain specific mutations or whether these mutations are located at codons containing two or more pyrimidine bases. The presence of mutations at specific pyrimidine sites would support the possibility that these sites are the targets for UV-induced mutagenic lesions such as pyrimidine dimers and/or [6-4] photoproducts.

In fact, recent studies have provided experimental evidence to support this hypothesis. Suarez et al.[122] have reported that two of eight nonmelanoma skin tumors from xeroderma pigmentosum patients contained A-T point mutations at the 61 codon of the N-*ras* oncogene and that this mutation occurred in a T-T sequence. Keijzer et al.[123] have reported that a melanoma cell line from a xeroderma pigmentosum patient also contained a mutated N-*ras* oncogene and that this mutation occurred within a short stretch of pyrimidine bases. Similarly, Van't Veer et al.[124] have reported that 7 of 37 cutaneous melanomas from sun-exposed body sites contained mutations in the N-*ras* oncogene and that these mutations were all at or near dipyrimidine sites. These results suggest that UV radiation is actively involved in the induction of mutations in the N-*ras* oncogene of both nonmelanoma and melanoma human skin cancers. In addition, these results imply that UV-induced pyrimidine dimers, but not [6-4] photoproducts, are likely candidates for causing activation of the N-*ras* oncogene in these tumors. The involvement of pyrimidine dimers in the activation of the N-*ras* oncogene has also been demonstrated by in vitro irradiation experiments. Van der Lubbe et al.[125] have shown that in vitro UV-irradiated N-*ras* proto-oncogene DNA, but not unirradiated DNA, induced transformed foci upon transfection into Rat-2 cells. Interestingly, most of these transformants contained mutations at the 61st codon similar to those found in skin tumors induced in vivo. In addition, these investigators found that treatment of the UV-irradiated N-*ras* proto-oncogene DNA prior to transfection with photoreactivating enzyme, which specifically repairs pyrimidine dimers but not other photoproducts, reduced the transformation frequency severalfold. These results suggest that UV radiation is capable of activating the N-*ras* proto-oncogene in vitro, probably through the formation of pyrimidine dimers. In addition to the activation of the N-*ras* proto-oncogene by in vitro UV irradiation, activation of the human c-Ha-*ras* proto-oncogene by in vitro UV irradiation has also been demonstrated by Pierceall et al.[126] These in vitro studies may help to identify the UV-induced lesions responsible for the activation of specific oncogenes.

Specific mutations at the 61st codon of the c-Ha-*ras* oncogene are also known to occur in human skin cancers. Corominas et al.[127] reported that 30 percent of human keratoacanthomas and 13 percent of squamous cell carcinomas contained specific mutations (A:T to T:A transversion) in the second position of codon 61 of the c-Ha-*ras* oncogene. The discovery that a relatively high percentage of c-Ha-*ras* mutations was found in keratoacanthomas as compared to squamous cell carcinomas suggests that activated c-Ha-*ras* genes may play a role in the early stages of carcinogenesis but not in the later stages of tumor progression. It is assumed that oncogenesis involves more than a simple activation of a single oncogene. Indeed, in some human tumors including skin tumors, quantitative or qualitative alterations involving more than one oncogene have been reported. For example, Suarez et al.[128] found that two skin tumors from the same xeroderma pigmentosum patients contained an amplified c-*myc* gene and an amplified and rearranged c-Ha-*ras* gene, in addition to an activated N-*ras* oncogene. These observations lend credence to the hypothesis that a number of genetic and epigenetic alterations must occur for normal cells to become cancerous and ultimately invasive and metastatic. In addition to the activation of oncogenes, loss of certain genes may play a role in carcinogenesis. Numerous studies have shown that allelic loss of *ras* and other genes occurs frequently in tumors such as retinoblastoma, Wilms' tumor, bladder cancer, breast cancer, lung cancer, colorectal cancer, and ovarian cancers. Studies by Ananthaswamy et al.[129] have also shown that loss of the c-Ha-*ras*-1 allele occurs frequently in human basal cell and squamous cell carcinomas developing on sun-exposed body sites. The deletion of specific alleles is thought to unmask recessive mutations. Thus, these molecular approaches are beginning to provide new insights into the mechanisms involved in UV carcinogenesis.

REFERENCES

1. Scotto J et al: Incidence of nonmelanoma skin cancer in the United States. NIH Publication No. 83-2433, 1983.
2. Unna PG: *Die Histopathologic der Hautkrankheiten.* Berlin, A Hirschwald, 1894.
3. Findlay GM: Ultraviolet light and skin cancer. *Lancet* 215:1070, 1928.
4. Roffo AH: Cancer et soleil: carcinomes et sarcomes provoquées par l'action du soleil in toto. *Bull Cancer (Paris)* 23:590, 1934.
5. Kripke ML: Immunology and photocarcinogenesis: new light on an old problem. *J Am Acad Dermatol* 14:149, 1986.
6. Report of the Ozone Trends Panel. NASA, March 1988.
7. Boutwell RK: Some biological aspects of skin carcinogenesis. *Prog Exp Tumor Res* 4:207, 1964.
8. Slaga TJ: *Mechanisms of Tumor Promotion: Tumor Promotion and Skin Carcinogenesis.* Boca Raton, FL, CRC, 1984, vol 2, p 189.
9. Friedewald WF, Rous P: The initiating and promoting elements in tumor production. *J Exp Med* 80:101, 1944.

10. Mottram JC: A developing factor in experimental blastogenesis. *J Pathol Bacteriol* 56:181, 1944.
11. Berenblum I, Shubik P: A new, quantitative approach to the study of the stages of chemical carcinogenesis in the mouse's skin. *Br J Cancer* 1:383, 1947.
12. Slaga TJ: Cellular and molecular mechanisms involved in multistage skin carcinogenesis, in CJ Conti et al. (eds), *Carcinogenesis—A Comprehensive Survey: Skin Tumors, Experimental and Clinical Aspects.* New York, Raven, 1989, vol 11, p 1.
13. Slaga TJ et al: Studies on the mechanisms involved in multistage carcinogenesis. *J Cell Biochem* 18:99, 1982.
14. Hennings H: Experimental skin carcinogenesis, in NA Soter, HP Baden (eds), *Pathophysiology of Dermatologic Diseases,* New York, McGraw-Hill, 1984, p 389.
15. Hsu J et al: Induction of skin tumors in hairless mice by a single exposure to UV radiation. *Photochem Photobiol* 21:185, 1975.
16. Strickland PT et al: Induction of skin tumors in the rat by a single exposure to ultraviolet radiation. *Photochem Photobiol* 30:683, 1979.
17. Blum HF: *Carcinogenesis by Ultraviolet Light.* Princeton, NJ, Princeton University Press, 1959.
18. Urbach F: *The Biologic Effects of Ultraviolet Radiation.* New York, Pergamon, 1969.
19. Kripke ML: Latency, histology, and antigenicity of tumors induced by ultraviolet light in three inbred mouse strains. *Cancer Res* 37:1395, 1977.
20. Epstein JH: Photocarcinogenesis: a review. *Natl Cancer Inst Monogr* 50:13, 1978.
21. Forbes PD: Experimental ultraviolet light photocarcinogenesis: an overview. *J Invest Dermatol* 77:139, 1981.
22. Epstein JH, Roth HL: Experimental ultraviolet light carcinogenesis: a study of croton oil promoting effects. *J Invest Dermatol* 50:387, 1968.
23. Pound AW: Induced cell proliferation of skin tumor formation in mice by ultraviolet light. *Pathology* 2:269, 1970.
24. Stenback F: Ultraviolet irradiation as initiating agent in skin tumor formation by the two-stage method. *Eur J Cancer* 11:241, 1975.
25. Fry RJ, Ley RD: Ultraviolet radiation carcinogenesis, in TJ Slaga (ed), *Mechanisms of Tumor Promotion.* Boca Raton, FL, CRC, 1984, vol 2, p 73.
26. Strickland PT et al: Enhancement of two-stage skin carcinogenesis by exposure of distant skin to UV radiation. *J Natl Cancer Inst* 74:1129, 1985.
27. Epstein JH, Epstein WL: Cocarcinogenic effect of ultraviolet light on DMBA tumor initiation in albino mice. *J Invest Dermatol* 39:455, 1962.
28. DeGruijl FR et al: Dose-time dependency of tumor formation by chronic UV exposure. *Photochem Photobiol* 37:53, 1983.
29. DeGruijl FR: The dose–response relationship for UV-tumorigenesis. Ph.D. thesis, University of Utrecht, The Netherlands, 1982.
30. Forbes PD et al: Photocarcinogenesis in hairless mice: dose–response and the influence of dose-delivery. *Photochem Photobiol* 34:361, 1981.
31. Forbes PD et al: Experimental ultraviolet photocarcinogenesis: wavelength interactions and time–dose relationships. *Natl Cancer Inst Monogr* 50:31, 1978.
32. *Environmental Impact of Stratospheric Flight.* Appendix C: Estimates of increases in skin cancer due to increases in ultraviolet radiation caused by reducing stratospheric ozone. Washington, DC, National Academy of Science, 1975, p 177.
33. Freeman RC: Data on the action spectrum for ultraviolet carcinogenesis. *J Natl Cancer Inst* 55:1119, 1975.
34. Zigman S et al: Black light induction of skin tumors in mice. *J Invest Dermatol* 67:723, 1976.
35. Forbes PD et al: Photocarcinogenesis by UV-A alone. Tenth Annual Meeting of the American Society for Photobiology, 1982, p 66.
36. Van Weelden H et al: Tumors induced by UV-A in mice (abstr). *Photochem Photobiol* 37:S79, 1983.
37. Strickland P: Photocarcinogenesis by near-ultraviolet (UVA) radiation in Sencar mice. *J Invest Dermatol* 87:272, 1986.

38. Forbes PD et al: Emission spectrum differences in fluorescent blacklight lamps. *Photochem Photobiol* 24:613, 1976.
39. Willis I et al: The rapid induction of cancers in the hairless mouse utilizing the principle of photoaugmentation. *J Invest Dermatol* 76:404, 1981.
40. Staberg B et al: The carcinogenic effect of UVA radiation. *J Invest Dermatol* 81:517, 1983.
41. Stenbach F: Species-specific neoplastic progression by ultraviolet light. *Oncology* 31:209, 1975.
42. Rusch HP, Baumann CA: Tumor production in mice with ultraviolet radiation. *Am J Cancer* 35:55, 1939.
43. DiGiovanni J et al: Comparison of the tumor-initiating activity of 7,12-dimethylbenz[a]anthracene and benzo[a]pyrene in female Sencar and CD-1 mice. *Carcinogenesis* 1:381, 1980.
44. Strickland PT: Tumor induction in Sencar mice in response to ultraviolet radiation. *Carcinogenesis* 3:1487, 1982.
45. Epstein JH: Ultraviolet carcinogenesis. *Photophysiology* 5:235, 1970.
46. Mikhail GR et al: Metastatic basal cell carcinoma. *Arch Dermatol* 113:1261, 1977.
47. Grady HG et al: Pathology of tumors of the external ear in mice induced by ultraviolet radiation. *J Natl Cancer Inst* 2:269, 1941.
48. Spikes JD et al: Time of appearance and histology of tumors induced in the dorsal skin of C3H mice by ultraviolet radiation from a mercury arc lamp. *J Natl Cancer Inst* 59:1637, 1977.
49. Kripke ML et al: Metastatic heterogeneity of cells from an ultraviolet light-induced murine fibrosarcoma of recent origin. *Cancer Res* 38:2962, 1978.
50. Talmadge JE et al: Therapy of autochthonous skin cancers in mice with intravenously injected liposomes containing muramyltripeptide. *Cancer Res* 46:1160, 1986.
51. Blum HF et al: Relationship between dosage and rate of tumor induction by ultraviolet light. *J Natl Cancer Inst* 3:91, 1942.
52. Forbes PD et al: Aging, environmental influences, and photocarcinogenesis. *J Invest Dermatol* 73:131, 1979.
53. Ebbesen P, Kripke ML: Influence of age and anatomical site on ultraviolet carcinogenesis in BALB/c mice. *J Natl Cancer Inst* 68:691, 1982.
54. Ananthaswamy HN, Fisher MS: Photoreactivation of ultraviolet radiation-induced pyrimidine dimers in neonatal BALB/c mouse skin. *Cancer Res* 41:1829, 1981.
55. Grekin DA, Epstein JH: Effects of age on acute UVB-induced skin responses. *Proc Am Soc Photobiol* 9:75, 1981.
56. Makinodon T: Mechanism, prevention and restoration of immunologic aging. *Birth Defects* 14:197, 1978.
57. Kripke ML: Antigenicity of murine skin tumors induced by ultraviolet light. *J Natl Cancer Inst* 53:1333, 1974.
58. Fisher MS, Kripke ML: Nature of a systemic alteration induced in mice by ultraviolet irradiation and its relationship to ultraviolet carcinogenesis. *Proc Natl Acad Sci USA* 74:1688, 1977.
59. Daynes RA, Spellman CW: Evidence for the generation of suppressor cells by ultraviolet radiation. *Cell Immunol* 31:182, 1977.
60. de Gruijl FR, van der Leun JC: Systemic influence of pre-irradiation of a limited skin area on UV-tumorigenesis. *Photochem Photobiol* 35:379, 1982.
61. Fisher MS, Kripke ML: Suppressor lymphocytes control the development of primary skin cancers in ultraviolet-irradiated mice. *Science* 216:1133, 1982.
62. Roberts LK, Daynes RA: Modification of the immunogenic properties of chemically induced tumors arising in hosts treated concomitantly with ultraviolet light. *J Immunol* 125:438, 1980.
63. Romerdahl CA et al: The role of ultraviolet radiation in the induction of melanocytic skin tumors in inbred mice. *Cancer Commun* 1:209, 1989.
64. Scotto J et al: Measurements of ultraviolet radiation in the United States and comparisons with skin cancer data. DHEW Publication No. (NIH)76-1029. Bethesda, MD, National Institutes of Health, 1976.

65. Crombie IK: Distribution of malignant melanoma on the body surface. *Br J Cancer* 43:842, 1981.
66. Romerdahl CA et al: Effect of ultraviolet-B radiation on the in vivo growth of murine melanoma cells. *Cancer Res* 48:4007, 1988.
67. Toews GB et al: Epidermal Langerhans cell density determines whether contact hypersensitivity or unresponsiveness follows skin painting with DNFB. *J Immunol* 124:445, 1980.
68. Elmets CA et al: Analysis of the mechanism of unresponsiveness produced by haptens painted on skin exposed to low dose of ultraviolet radiation. *J Exp Med* 158:781, 1983.
69. Fry RJM et al: Radiation induction of cancer of the skin. *Br J Radiol* 19(Suppl):58, 1986.
70. Strickland PT et al: Induction of skin tumors in the rat by single exposure to ultraviolet radiation. *Photochem Photobiol* 30:683, 1979.
71. Boden B et al: Radiation-induced head and neck tumors. *Lancet* 1:277, 1974.
72. Shore RE et al: Follow-up study of patients treated by x-ray epilation for tinea capitis. *Arch Environ Health* 31:21, 1976.
73. Parrish JA et al: Photochemotherapy of psoriasis with oral methoxalen and longwave ultraviolet light. *N Engl J Med* 291:1207, 1974.
74. Stern RS: PUVA and the induction of skin cancer, in CJ Conti et al. (eds), *Carcinogenesis—A Comprehensive Survey: Skin Tumors, Experimental and Clinical Aspects.* New York, Raven, 1989, vol 11, p 85.
75. Stern RS et al: Risk of cutaneous carcinoma in patients treated with oral methoxalen photochemotherapy for psoriasis. *N Engl J Med* 300:809, 1979.
76. Kripke ML: Immunosuppressive effects of ultraviolet (280–320 nm) radiation and psoralen plus ultraviolet (320–400 nm) radiation in mice. *J Natl Cancer Inst* 69:171, 1982.
77. Kripke ML et al: Systemic suppression of contact hypersensitivity in mice by psoralen plus UVA radiation (PUVA). *J Invest Dermatol* 81:87, 1983.
78. Findlay GM: Ultraviolet light and skin cancer. *Lancet* 215:1070, 1928.
79. Sporn MB et al: Prevention of chemical carcinogenesis by vitamin A and its synthetic analogs. *Fed Proc* 35:1332, 1976.
80. Burns FJ et al: Radiation-induced cancer in rat ski, in CJ Conti et al. (eds), *Carcinogenesis—A Comprehensive Survey: Skin Tumors, Experimental and Clinical Aspects.* New York, Raven, 1989, vol 11, p 293.
81. Forbes PD et al: Enhancement of experimental photocarcinogenesis by topical retinoic acid. *Cancer Lett* 7:85, 1979.
82. Epstein JH: Comparison of the carcinogenic and cocarcinogenic effects of UV light on hairless mice. *J Natl Cancer Inst* 34:741, 1965.
83. Kligman LH, Kligman AM: Lack of enhancement of experimental photocarcinogenesis by retinoic acid, in Orfanos CE (ed), *Retinoids—Advances in Basic Research and Therapy.* Berlin, Springer-Verlag, 1981, p 411.
84. Epstein JH: Inhibition of ultraviolet-induced carcinogenesis by all-trans retinoic acid. *J Invest Dermatol* 76:178, 1981.
85. Black HS, Tigges J: Evaluation of structurally-related phenols for anti-photocarcinogenic and photoprotective properties. *Photochem Photobiol* 43:403, 1986.
86. Orengo IF et al: Influence of dietary menhaden oil upon carcinogenesis and various cutaneous responses to ultraviolet radiation. *Photochem Photobiol* 49:71, 1989.
87. Black HS et al: Relation of antioxidants and level of dietary lipid to epidermal lipid peroxidation and ultraviolet carcinogenesis. *Cancer Res* 45:6254, 1985.
88. Pauling L et al: Incidence of squamous cell carcinoma in hairless mice irradiated with UV light in relation to intake of ascorbic acid (vitamin C) and of D,h-*a*-tocopheryl acetate (vitamin E). *Third International Symposium on Vitamin C.* Publication No. 150. Palo Alto, CA, Linus Pauling Institute of Science and Medicine, 1980.
89. Zajdela F, Laterjet R: Inhibition of skin carcinogenesis in vivo by caffeine and other agents. *Natl Cancer Inst Monogr* 50:133, 1978.
90. Peak MJ et al: Chlorpromazine ingestion inhibits UV-induced skin carcinogenesis. *Photochem Photobiol* 46:1, 1987.
91. DiPaolo JA, Donovan PJ: In vitro morphologic transformation of Syrian hamster cells

by UV radiation is enhanced by X-irradiation and unaffected by chemical carcinogens. *Int J Radiat Biol* 30:41, 1976.

92. Chan GL, Little JB: Induction of oncogenic transformation in vitro by ultraviolet light. *Nature* 264:442, 1976.
93. Kennedy AR et al: Fluorescent light induces malignant transformation in mouse embryo cell cultures. *Science* 207:1209, 1980.
94. Ananthaswamy HN: Lethality and transformation of 10T1/2 mouse embryo fibroblast cell line by various wavelengths of ultraviolet radiation. *Photodermatology* 1:265, 1984.
95. Mondal S, Heidelberger C: Transformation of C3H/10T1/2CL8 mouse embryo fibroblasts by ultraviolet radiation and a phorbol ester. *Nature* 260:710, 1976.
96. Sutherland BM et al: Ultraviolet light-induced transformation of human cells to anchorage-independent growth. *Cancer Res* 40:1934, 1980.
97. Maher VM et al: Frequency of UV-induced neoplastic transformation of human diploid fibroblasts is higher in xeroderma pigmentosum cells than in normal cells. *Proc Natl Acad Sci USA* 79:2613, 1982.
98. Webb RB: Lethal and mutagenic effects of near-ultraviolet radiation, in KC Smith (ed), *Photochemical and Photobiological Reviews*. New York, Plenum, 1977, vol 2, p 169.
99. Ananthaswamy HN, Kripke ML: In vitro transformation of primary cultures of neonatal BALB/c mouse epidermal cells with ultraviolet radiation. *Cancer Res* 41:2882, 1981.
100. Withrow TJ et al: Transformation of BALB 3T3 cells exposed to a germicidal UV lamp and a sunlamp. *Photochem Photobiol* 31:135, 1980.
101. Suzuki F et al: Spectral dependencies of killing, mutation and transformation in mammalian cells and their relevance to hazards caused by solar ultraviolet radiation. *Cancer Res* 41:4916, 1981.
102. Doniger J et al: Ultraviolet light action spectra for neoplastic transformation and lethality of Syrian hamster embryo cells correlate with spectrum for pyrimidine dimer formation in cellular DNA. *Proc Natl Acad Sci USA* 78:2378, 1981.
103. Sutherland BM et al: Action spectra for ultraviolet light-induced transformation of human cells to anchorage-independent growth. *Cancer Res* 41:2211, 1981.
104. Cleaver JE, Bootsma D: Xeroderma pigmentosum—biochemical and genetic characteristics. *Annu Rev Genet* 9:19, 1975.
105. Hart RW et al: Evidence that pyrimidine dimers in DNA can give rise to tumors. *Proc Natl Acad Sci USA* 75:5574, 1977.
106. Ley RD et al: UVA/visible light suppression of ultraviolet radiation–induced skin and eye tumors of the marsupial *Monodelphis domestica*. *Photochem Photobiol* 47:45S, 1988.
107. Haseltine WA: Ultraviolet light repair and mutagenesis revisited. *Cell* 33:13, 1983.
108. Mitchell DL, Nairn RS: The biology of the (6-4) photoproduct. *Photochem Photobiol* 47:805, 1989.
109. Weiss RB, Duker NJ: Endonucleolytic incision of UV-B-irradiated DNA. *Photochem Photobiol* 45:763, 1987.
110. Doetsch PW et al: Wavelength dependence for human redoxyendonuclease-mediated DNA cleavage at sites of UV-induced photoproducts. *Radiat Res* 113:543, 1988.
111. Gallagher PE, Duker NJ: Formation of purine photoproducts in a defined human DNA sequence. *Photochem Photobiol* 49:599, 1989.
112. Peak MJ et al: Induction of direct and indirect single-strand breaks in human cell DNA by far- and near-ultraviolet radiations: action spectrum and mechanisms. *Photochem Photobiol* 45:381, 1987.
113. Brash DE, Haseltine WA: UV-induced mutation hotspots occur at DNA damage hotspots. *Nature* 298:189, 1982.
114. Brash DE: UV mutagenic photoproducts in *Escherichia coli* and human cells: a molecular genetics perspective on human skin cancer. *Photochem Photobiol* 48:59, 1988.
115. Applegate LA et al: Hypersensitivity of skin fibroblasts from basal cell nevus syndrome patients to killing by ultraviolet B but not ultraviolet C radiation. *Cancer Res* 50:637, 1990.
116. Maher VM et al: Frequency of ultraviolet light–induced mutation is higher in xeroderma pigmentosum variant cells than in normal human cells. *Nature* 261:593, 1976.

117. Land H et al: Cellular oncogenes and multistep carcinogenesis. *Science* 222:771, 1983.
118. Bishop MJ: Cellular oncogenes and retroviruses. *Annu Rev Biochem* 52:301, 1983.
119. Zarbl H et al: Direct mutagenesis of Ha-*ras*-1 oncogenes by *N*-nitroso-*N*-methylurea during initiation of mammary carcinogenesis in rats. *Nature* 315:382, 1985.
120. Quintanilla M et al: Carcinogen-specific mutation and amplification of Ha-*ras* during skin carcinogenesis. *Nature* 322:78, 1986.
121. Ananthaswamy HN et al: Detection and identification of activated oncogenes in human skin cancers occurring on sun-exposed body sites. *Cancer Res* 48:3341, 1988.
122. Suarez HG et al: Activated oncogenes in human skin tumors from a repair-deficient syndrome, xeroderma pigmentosum. *Cancer Res* 49:1223, 1989.
123. Keijzer W et al: Establishment and characterization of a melanoma cell line from a xeroderma pigmentosum patient: activation of N-*ras* at a potential pyrimidine dimer site. *Cancer Res* 49:1229, 1989.
124. Van't Veer LJ et al: N-*ras* mutations in human cutaneous melanoma from sun-exposed body sites. *Mol Cell Biol* 9:3114, 1989.
125. Van der Lubbe JLM et al: Activation of N-*ras* induced by ultraviolet irradiation in vitro. *Oncogene Res* 3:9, 1988.
126. Pierceall WE et al: Activation of the human c-Ha-*ras*-1 proto-oncogene by in vitro UV-irradiation. *Proc Am Assoc Cancer Res* 30:188, 1989.
127. Corominas M et al: Oncogene activation in human benign tumors of the skin (kerato-acanthomas): is HRAS involved in differentiation as well as proliferation? *Proc Natl Acad Sci USA* 86:6372, 1989.
128. Suarez HG et al: Multiple activated oncogenes in human tumors. *Oncogene Res* 1:201, 1987.
129. Ananthaswamy HN et al: Deletion of the c-Ha-*ras*-1 allele in human skin cancers. *Mol Carcinogen* 2:298, 1989.

30

Pathophysiology of Epidermal Malignant Disorders

Harley A. Haynes

PATHOGENESIS

Basal and squamous cell carcinoma are commonly grouped together and referred to as nonmelanoma skin cancer. It is estimated that the present annual incidence of nonmelanoma skin cancer in whites in the United States is 165 per 100,000 population. This translates into about 300,000 cases of skin cancer in whites in the United States each year. Both carcinomas share an origin from the epidermal cell and many common features of epidemiology and carcinogenesis, and the prognosis in both is excellent in most cases. Although basal cell carcinoma almost never metastasizes, squamous cell carcinoma has a low incidence of metastatic disease.

There are several proven causes of nonmelanoma skin cancer, including chemical carcinogenesis, ultraviolet light, ionizing radiation, immunologic suppression, and genetic defects. Viral carcinogenesis is known principally in the genetic immunodeficiency disease epidermodysplasia verruciformis but probably plays a role in chronically immunosuppressed allograft recipients as well. In both instances, oncogenic human papilloma virus

This chapter was excerpted and modified from HA Haynes et al: Cancers of the skin, in VT DeVita Jr et al (eds), *Cancer: Principles and Practice of Oncology*, Philadelphia, Lippincott, 1985, p 1343.

appears to be responsible. Scars, including burn scars, and chronic inflammation are also associated with carcinomas, although the operant stimuli are unknown.[1] However, the most important carcinogenic stimulus for skin is clearly ultraviolet radiation.

The experiment of nature in which different intensities of ultraviolet radiation occur at different global latitudes has provided the opportunity for epidemiologic studies to show a greater incidence of nonmelanoma skin cancer in the white population compared with the black and Asiatic peoples, as well as an increased incidence at latitudes closer to the equator compared with latitudes farther from the equator. There is an unequivocal inverse relationship between latitude and nonmelanoma skin cancer.[2,3] For example, the incidence of nonmelanoma skin cancer is 379 per 100,000 persons in the Dallas/Fort Worth, Texas, area (32.8° north latitude) but only 124 per 100,000 persons in Iowa (42° north latitude). On this scale of geographic relationship to skin cancer, individual phenotypes are noted to be more susceptible to skin cancer within any given geographic area. The susceptible persons tend to have poor tanning ability with easy sunburning and, in addition, often have fair skin, light hair, and blue eyes.[4] In addition to this general phenotype susceptibility, it has been observed that Celtic ancestry tends to predispose to the development of nonmelanoma skin cancer.[5] Two major effects of ultraviolet radiation on the skin that seem likely to be responsible for the carcinogenic effects are photochemical alteration of DNA and alterations in immunity. The inability to repair DNA damage from ultraviolet radiation in patients with xeroderma pigmentosum results in a dramatic and early onset of numerous skin cancers and melanoma. Immunosuppressive therapy in renal or cardiac allograft recipients is well documented to increase greatly the incidence of basal and squamous cell carcinomas of the skin. These cancers also generally occur in sun-exposed skin.

While chemical carcinogenesis of skin does not seem to be nearly as frequent a cause of cancer of the skin as ultraviolet radiation, it was described over a century earlier. Sir Percival Pott noted occupational chemical carcinogenesis when he described the high incidence of carcinoma of the scrotal and penile skin in chimney sweeps. He attributed this to soot and chronic irritation. Approximately 100 years later, the observation was made of the increased frequency of skin cancer in workers exposed to paraffin, pitch, and shale oil tar. In 1915, Yamagiwa and Ichikawa first produced skin cancer experimentally by the prolonged and repeated application of tar to the skin of the ears of rabbits. Systemic chemical carcinogenesis occurs in individuals exposed to chronic ingestion of inorganic arsenic. In the skin, both basal and squamous cell carcinomas occur. Carcinomas of multiple other organ systems occur in increased incidence as well. Photochemotherapy with oral psoralen and topical UVA (PUVA) also causes a small increase in squamous cell carcinoma of the skin.

The most important step the average person can take to reduce the risk of skin cancer is to reduce exposure to ultraviolet radiation by the use of clothing and topical sunscreen agents and by the avoidance, when possible, of the most intense radiation close to solar noon.

NATURAL HISTORY AND CLINICAL PRESENTATION

Basal Cell Carcinoma

Basal cell carcinoma is the most common form of skin cancer, representing at least 75 percent of cases in the southern United States and over 90 percent of cases in the northern United States.[6–8] It is believed by many to arise from cells in the basal layer of the epidermis, but some dispute this, regarding the cells of the dermal adnexa as the site of origin. A nodular, or nodular ulcerative, lesion is the most frequent (Fig. 30-1). Basal cell carcinoma is seen most often on the skin of the head and neck and only 10 percent of the time on the trunk. It is much less frequent on the upper extremities, quite uncommon on the lower extremities, and rare on skin surfaces never exposed to the sun. This kind of lesion is usually slow growing and relatively asymptomatic, except for possible crusting or bleeding with minor trauma. The lesion is generally smooth, shiny, and translucent in appearance, with telangiectatic vessels commonly seen just beneath the surface. There is generally no tenderness or pain noted, even if ulceration occurs. The overall color of the lesion is not very different from normal skin color and is usually a bit lighter. However, some lesions have melanin pigment, which appears as scattered tattoo-like dots that can become confluent, causing the whole lesion to have brown, black, or even blue pigmentation. Occasionally, this may cause confusion with melanoma, but the correct diagnosis is established by biopsy.

The next most frequent type of basal cell carcinoma is the superficial type, usually found on the skin of the chest or back; in contrast to the

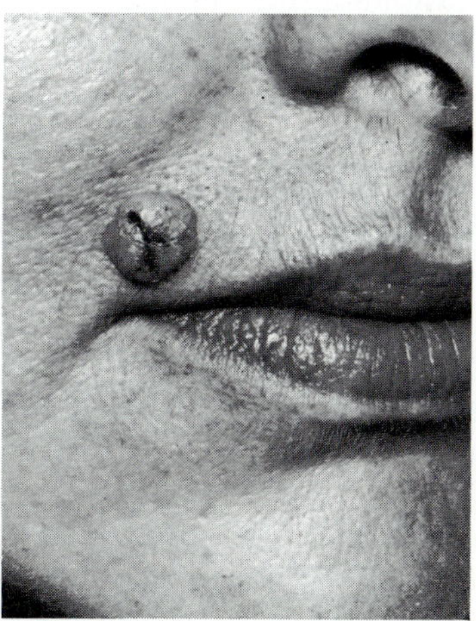

Figure 30-1 Basal cell tumor on skin otherwise appearing normal. (*From TB Fitzpatrick et al, Dermatology in General Medicine, 3d ed, New York, McGraw-Hill, 1987, p 761.*)

nodular lesions, it is erythematous. It starts as a very subtle erythematous plaque, almost flat and very difficult to palpate. The surface of the lesion may be scaly, with scattered fine crusts, and is sometimes smooth and shiny. When a lesion is more mature, tiny translucent papules in a string-of-pearls–like configuration are seen at the margin. The lesion is frequently mistaken for some other dermatologic problem or mild irritation. Therefore, patients with a history of basal cell carcinoma should have such lesions biopsied. These lesions may have pigment dots scattered throughout them but rarely are confused with melanomas.

A morphea-like basal cell carcinoma is an uncommon type, often masquerading as a scar. It presents as a smooth, fibrotic patch without evident telangiectasia, ulceration, or raised, pearly papules at the edge. The margins of this kind of lesion are often quite indistinct. It may grow to a great width and depth before its true nature is recognized.

Less commonly, basal cell carcinoma is seen in the basal cell nevus syndrome, chronic radiation dermatitis from ionizing radiation, and scars from vaccination.

Basal cell carcinomas of any type rarely metastasize. However, they are capable of invading widely and deeply, extending through the subcutaneous tissue to involve neurovascular structures, and occasionally invading bone. When located on the head, they may erode through the skull and into the brain.

Morphea-like basal cell carcinomas show defects in the basal lamina and basement membrane immunoreactivity for laminin and type IV collagen, with increased levels of type IV collagenase activity in their cytoplasm.[9] Other demonstrated abnormalities include a defect in the expression of G71 antigen in the lamina lucida of the basement membrane[10] and the suprabasilar intercellular localization of α_3/β_1 integrins when the basement membrane is fragmented.[11] These abnormalities of the extracellular matrix component suggest alterations in the cell growth and invasiveness of this tumor cell.

Squamous Cell Carcinoma

The clinical presentation of squamous cell carcinoma makes clinical diagnosis much more difficult than it is in basal cell carcinoma.[8,12] Squamous cell carcinomas are erythematous lesions with varying degrees of scaling and crusting (Fig. 30-2). In sun-exposed areas of the body they tend to occur on the most highly irradiated portions of skin, such as the top of the nose, forehead, tips of the helixes of the ears, lower lip, and backs of the hands. These lesions on the skin surface generally have about the same biologic malignancy as basal cell carcinomas, only rarely showing metastatic disease. An exception to this occurs in immunosuppressed patients who develop metastases more frequently. When squamous cell carcinoma arises on mucous membranes or mucocutaneous junctions, it also tends to metastasize more frequently. Squamous cell carcinomas

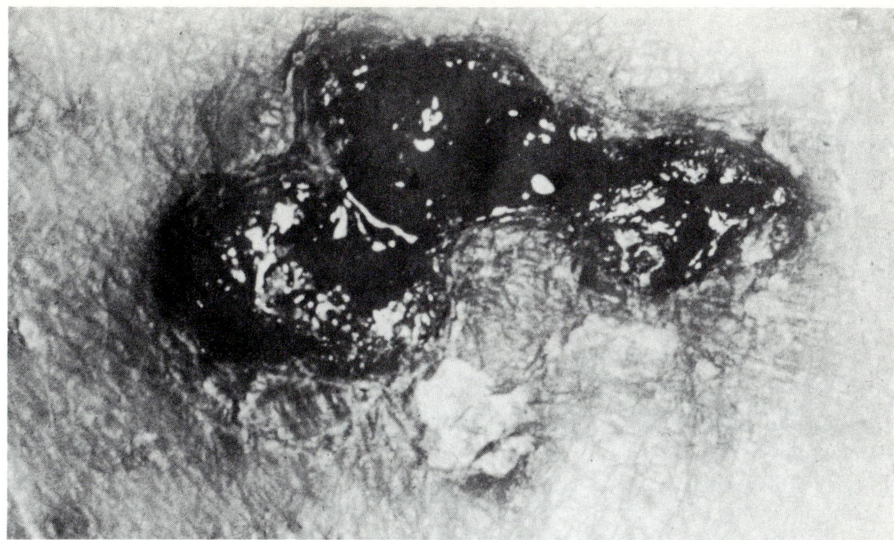

Figure 30-2 Squamous cell carcinoma: multinodular tumor with surface loss due to the absence of normal epidermis.

arising on skin unexposed to the sun have much greater biologic malignancy, with a higher frequency of metastatic disease.

There is a premalignant stage of squamous cell carcinoma known as *actinic keratosis*. These lesions are always found on sun-exposed skin and present as rough, red plaques only barely raised from the skin's surface. Patients with actinic keratosis are more prone to develop skin cancers. An in situ stage of squamous cell carcinoma known as *Bowen's disease* exists in which the lesion presents as a well-demarcated, slightly raised, erythematous, scaling plaque with more substance than an actinic keratosis.

Nodular or nodular-ulcerative squamous cell carcinoma generally appears as a red, firm tumor elevated from the surrounding skin, with the surface showing a scale, a hornlike elevation, or an ulceration with a crust. On the external genitalia, erythematous plaques with an exudative surface or verrucous nodules with ulceration are the usual presentations in squamous cell carcinoma. When cutaneous squamous cell carcinoma metastasizes, it usually spreads first to local lymph nodes, but hematogenous spread can occur, with lung lesions being a frequent manifestation.

Keratoacanthoma

Keratoacanthoma generally appears very rapidly over a 2- to 3-week period on a sun-exposed site without a preexisting lesion. It is a smooth, red nodule with a central keratinous plug that at times has been lost, leaving an erosion with a verrucous base in the center. The red rim of the tumor nodule is often a bit smoother than that of the usual squamous cell carcinoma, and telangiectatic vessels may be seen. At times, keratoacanthomas may grow to substantial size, particularly on the face, producing a great deal of disfigurement before they regress and resulting in considerable scarring and disfigurement after regression. These lesions never metastasize, but the clinical problem is differentiating them from squamous cell carcinoma, which, of course, can metastasize. A biopsy should be done. In a case of any questionable pathology, the lesion should be treated as though it were a squamous cell carcinoma.

PATHOLOGY OF EPIDERMAL SKIN CANCER

Histologically, basal cell carcinomas occur in a variety of patterns, but the tumor cell usually has a large oval nucleus with fine chromatin and stains deeply basophilic (Fig. 30-3). There is little cytoplasm, and mitoses are scarce. The peripheral cells of individual tumor clusters line up in a highly characteristic palisade formation. The tumor cells form small nodular clusters or lacelike strands and may show a glandular or cystic structure. Frequently what appears to be the point of origin in the basal layer of the epidermis is noted, with nests of tumor cells extending down from this point into the dermis. In the superficial type there may be multiple such points of origin, with tumor cells extending into the dermis only to a depth equal to about twice the thickness of the epidermis. In infiltrating carcinoma, the stroma of the tumor predominates. It consists of dense connective tissue composed of both elastin and collagen fibers running throughout, within which are strands and small nests of tumor cells presenting the appearance of basal cells with oval basophilic nuclei.

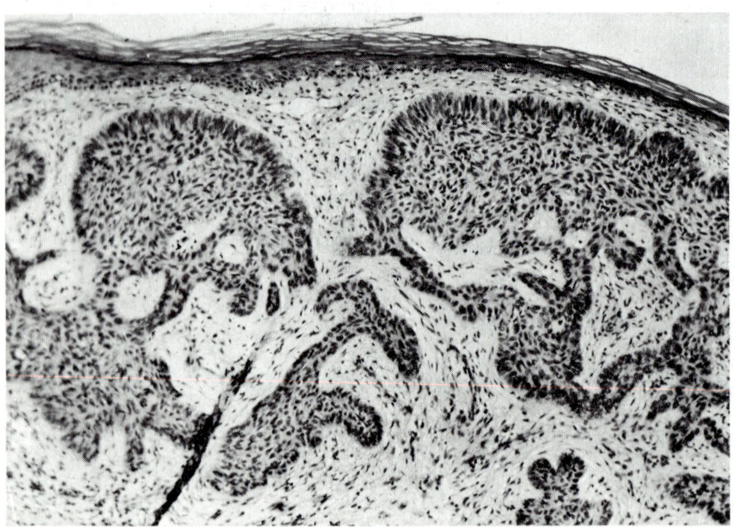

Figure 30-3 Basal cell tumor. Cell nests show no signs of keratinization. (*From TB Fitzpatrick et al, Dermatology in General Medicine, 3d ed, New York, McGraw-Hill, 1987, p 763.*)

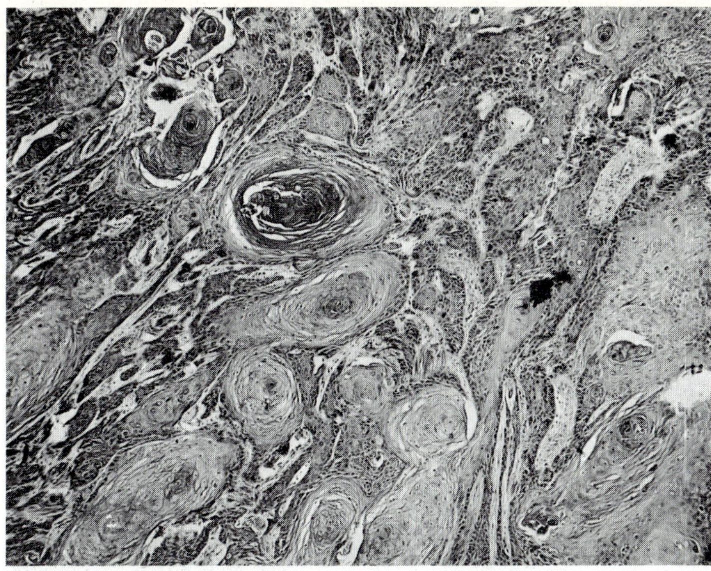

Figure 30-4 Well-differentiated invasive squamous cell carcinoma showing multiple areas of keratinization. ×60 in the original magnification. (*From TB Fitzpatrick et al, Dermatology in General Medicine, 3d ed, New York, McGraw-Hill, 1987, p 754.*)

Squamous cell carcinoma of the skin histologically resembles neoplasms arising from stratified squamous epithelium in other organ sites. In a well-differentiated tumor, the cellular appearance is similar to that seen in normal squamous epithelium, with a large, polygonal outline, intercellular bridges, pale-staining eosinophilic cytoplasm, and round nuclei (Fig. 30-4). Keratinization of individual cells and formation of keratin pearls are common. As the tumors become less well differentiated, keratinization and keratin pearls diminish, and nuclei become more bizarre in shape and mitoses more numerous. The cells tend to lose their polygonal shape and become more elongated; in very undifferentiated tumors they may be fusiform in appearance, resembling sarcoma cells. As might be expected, the more differentiated tumors tend to be relatively slow growing and show little aggressiveness in invading other tissues. On the other hand, highly undifferentiated tumors may be expected to invade relatively early, becoming readily fixed to underlying structures. Fortunately, the majority of squamous cell carcinomas of the skin are of the lower-grade varieties.

Histologically, three stages of keratoacanthoma are described. Initially there is marked proliferation of the epithelial cells with rapid extension into the dermis of tumor cell nests. Atypism may be noted in the advancing rim of these nests. In the second stage, continued proliferation of the squamous cells with keratinization and formation of the characteristic keratin plug exists. In the third stage, involution occurs with dissolution of the nests; these cells are then surrounded by an inflammatory infiltrate of lymphocytes and macrophages. The involution of the tumor cells is followed by scarring of the dermis. Many of the features (e.g., cellular atypism and perforation of the basement membrane) are histologically indistinguishable from those of squamous cell carcinoma.

REFERENCES

1. Kaplan RP: Cancer complicating chronic ulcerative and scarifying mucocutaneous disorders, in JP Callen et al (eds), *Advances in Dermatology,* vol. 2. Chicago, Year Book, 1987, p 19.
2. Macdonald EJ: Epidemiology of skin cancer, 1975, in W Malkinson (ed), *Neoplasms of the Skin and Malignant Melanoma.* Chicago, Year Book, 1976, p 27.
3. Scotto J et al: Nonmelanoma skin cancer among Caucasians in four areas of the United States. *Cancer* 34:1333, 1974.
4. Urbach F et al: Ultraviolet carcinogenesis: experimental, global, and genetic aspects, in TB Fitzpatrick (ed), *Sunlight and Man.* Tokyo, University of Tokyo Press, 1974, p 259.
5. Lane-Brown MM, Melia DF: A genetic diathesis to skin cancer. J Invest Dermatol 61:39, 1973.
6. Popkin GL, DeFeo CP Jr: Basal cell epithelioma, in R Andrade et al (eds), *Cancer of the Skin, Biology—Diagnosis—Management.* Philadelphia, Saunders, 1976, p 821.
7. Carter DM: Basal cell carcinoma, in TB Fitzpatrick et al (eds), *Dermatology in General Medicine,* 3d ed. New York, McGraw-Hill, 1987, p 759.
8. MacKie RM: Tumours of the skin, in A Rook et al (eds), *Textbook of Dermatology,* 4th ed. Oxford, Blackwell Scientific, 1986, p 2375.
9. Barsky SH et al: Desmoplastic basal cell carcinomas possess unique basement membrane–degrading properties. *J Invest Dermatol* 88:324, 1987.
10. Tidman MJ et al: Abnormal expression of G71 antibody at the epidermal basement membrane in basal cell carcinoma. *Cancer* 65:1955, 1990.
11. Peltonen J et.al: Localization of integrin receptors for fibronectin, collagen, and laminin in human skin: variable expression in basal and squamous cell carcinomas. *J Clin Invest* 84:1916, 1989.
12. Stoll HL Jr, Schwartz RA: Squamous cell carcinoma, in TB Fitzpatrick et al (eds), *Dermatology in General Medicine,* 3d ed. New York, McGraw-Hill, 1987, p 746.

31

Biology of Malignant Melanoma

Arthur J. Sober

Melanoma is a malignant neoplasm of the melanocyte and originates at the dermal-epidermal junction (except for those that arise in some giant congenital nevi, in which a deep dermal or subcutaneous origin may occur). The current incidence of melanoma in the United States is approximately 28,000 per year (which makes it one-fifth as common as breast cancer and one-sixth as common as lung cancer). Melanoma is responsible for 6000 deaths each year. The deaths in the United States have doubled over the past decade. Although melanomas occur spontaneously in many animals (e.g., salamanders, mice, swine, dogs, horses), no satisfactory animal model exists that mimics the evolution of human melanoma. Recently an ultraviolet light–induced melanoma model in the South American opossum has been proposed that may mimic more closely the developmental biology of human melanoma.[1]

EPIDEMIOLOGY IN HUMANS

Incidence rates show no sex preference in the United States, Canada, and Australia (the ratio in Britain and West Germany is 2:1 female:male), although in nearly all studies, women have higher survival rates. Tumors have been noted rarely in newborns, both from transplacental metastases and from spontaneous degeneration of congenital nevi. Melanoma is rare in infancy and childhood (1 per 10^6 per year) but becomes more common with each subsequent decade (age-adjusted incidence rates rise with age). The mean age for development of melanomas is in the early to mid-forties and is falling. When the distribution by age and tumor type is examined, it is apparent that melanoma frequently affects individuals from the middle to the late teenage years on, in marked contrast to the other forms of skin cancer, which affect primarily older individuals. The cause of skin cancer other than melanoma fits a cumulative solar exposure model, whereas an intermittent traumatic exposure model may play a role in the development of melanoma. Lentigo maligna melanoma (which comprises 5 percent of all melanomas) also fits a cumulative solar exposure model in that it occurs on chronically sun-damaged skin of the head and neck in older individuals. Shorter induction and latency periods for melanoma in contrast to those of the nonmelanoma skin cancers are obvious. Additionally, a cohort effect is observed for melanoma similar to that noted for carcinomas of the lung. Since about 1900, each successive generation has had higher age-specific incidence rates, suggesting that some environmental change (exposure or behavior alteration) is affecting younger groups to a greater degree than individuals born in earlier decades. Also, within certain countries, there exists a latitude gradient in incidence and death rates. Higher rates are noted at latitudes closer to the equator. Additionally, higher rates are noted for individuals who have lived for longer periods in sunny climates (e.g., natives of Israel and Australia have higher age-specific rates than immigrants to these countries). The rate of melanoma formation is much lower in blacks (one-sixth to one-seventh of the rate in whites) and the sites of most frequent occurrence (palms, soles, nail beds, mucous membranes) are different from those in whites. The explanation for these locations in blacks is not clear, but lighter skin in these areas, the presence of more nevi, and trauma have been offered as possibilities. The sites of occurrence in whites show an intriguing sparing of completely covered areas (i.e., breasts in women, buttocks in both sexes) and a pronounced sex difference, with the lower leg noted as a frequent site in women. The sex difference suggests that different exposure resulting from clothing patterns may be a factor. The back is the most frequent site in men and one of the most frequent sites in women. All of these observations have been used to implicate solar exposure indirectly as an etiologic factor. Table 31-1 summarizes the weight of evidence for solar and other causes.

The evidence of a solar cause of melanoma is by no means as strong as that relating sun exposure to the other forms of skin cancer. At present, sunlight interacting with some other factor (e.g., a precursor lesion) is a current prominent etiologic hypothesis.

PRECURSOR LESIONS

Specific lesions that are prone to develop into melanoma have been described. These include lentigo maligna,[2,3] congenital nevus,[4–7] and dysplastic nevus.[8–12]

Table 31-1

ETIOLOGIC FACTORS FOR CUTANEOUS MELANOMA

Ultraviolet Light	
Age (cumulative exposure)	Strong relationship for lentigo maligna melanoma but not for other types (mid-age peak)
	Individuals at the same age born in successively more recent decades have higher age-specific rates
Cohort	Strong cohort effect since 1900–1920
Sex	Equal incidence in the United States and Australia; 2:1 female:male ratio in Britain and West Germany
Latitude gradient	Strong within countries
Occupation	Indoor white-collar workers at higher risk
	Highly educated, high-income men and women at higher risk
Lifestyle	Intermittent high-intensity exposure may be a factor
Common sites	Light-skinned whites: back of both sexes; anterior torso of males, legs of females
	Blacks, Orientals, and dark-skinned whites: palms, soles, nail beds, mucous membranes
Skin color	Melanoma increased in light-skinned whites, especially Australians, Celtics, and Scandinavians.
	Albinos: few melanomas reported; tumors are nonpigmented, and many need electron microscopic examination for recognition
	Rare in blacks, Orientals, and dark-skinned whites
Skin reaction type	Types I and II at highest risk
Abnormal DNA repair	Xeroderma pigmentosum
	Defect in repair in leukocytes of melanoma patients
Artificial ultraviolet	Increased risk reported from ultraviolet sunlamps
Precursor Lesions	
Genetic	Familial melanoma/dysplastic nevi
Acquired	Nonfamilial acquired dysplastic nevi
Congenital	Congenital melanocytic nevi
Chemical Exposure	Oral contraceptives? Levodopa? Polychlorinated biphenyls?

Lentigo Maligna

Lentigo maligna (Fig. 31-1) provides the most clear-cut evidence of melanoma produced by chronic solar exposure.[2,3] These lesions occur almost exclusively in elderly individuals on chronically sun-damaged, sun-exposed skin (head and neck, extremities). Clinically, these lesions appear as hyperpigmented tan to brown macules that have irregular borders and contain dark brown or black flecks. Within the lentigo maligna, increased numbers of bizarre-shaped, irregularly sized melanocytes are seen at the dermal-epidermal junction extending down hair follicles and sweat ducts. The melanocytes of lentigo maligna are confined to the epidermis by the basement membrane. Once melanocytes have invaded the dermis, the lesion is termed lentigo maligna melanoma. The lentigo maligna may slowly evolve for 5 to 50 years before invasion occurs. This evolution has been estimated to occur in 5 to 33 percent of lentigo maligna.[13]

Congenital Nevi

The giant forms of congenital nevi (Fig. 31-2) were the first type of congenital nevus clearly associated with the risk of malignancy.[4,5] The lifetime risk of melanoma development in a giant congenital nevus is thought to be about 6 to 7 percent. The risk appears to be greatest in the first decade of life. More recently, the risk associated with the smaller, more common forms of congenital nevi (present in 1 percent of the population) has been discerned.[6] Depending on the histopathologic criteria used, between 2 and 6 percent of melanomas arise in association with small congenital nevi.[6] A recent study that employed photographs of patients has adequately documented cases of cutaneous melanoma arising in small congenital nevi.[7] The available data have led some groups to recommend prophylactic removal of congenital nevi.

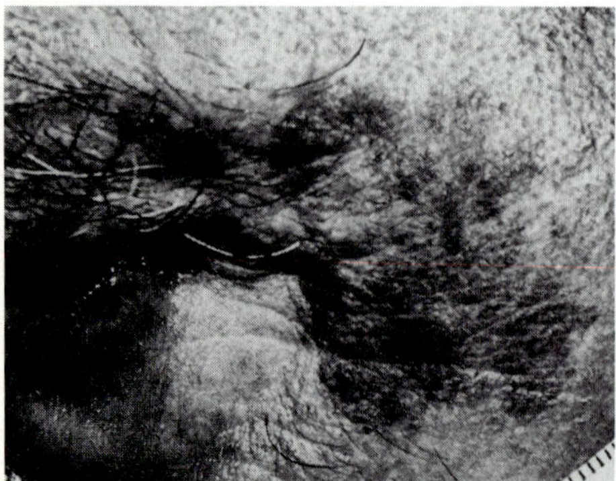

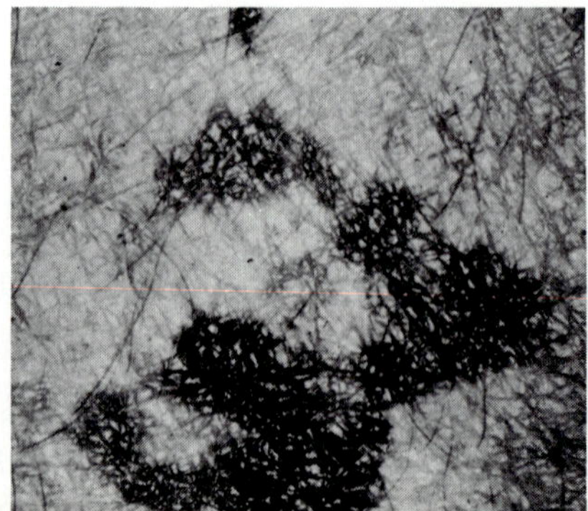

Figure 31-1 Lentigo maligna displaying irregular borders and an irregular pigment pattern. (*From TB Fitzpatrick et al, Dermatology in General Medicine, 3d ed, New York, McGraw-Hill, 1987, p 950.*)

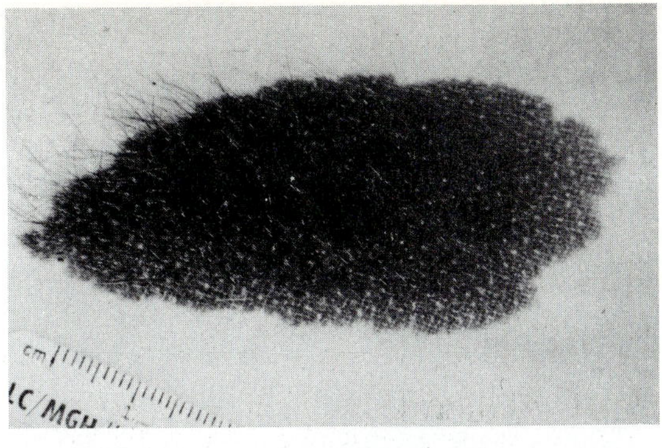

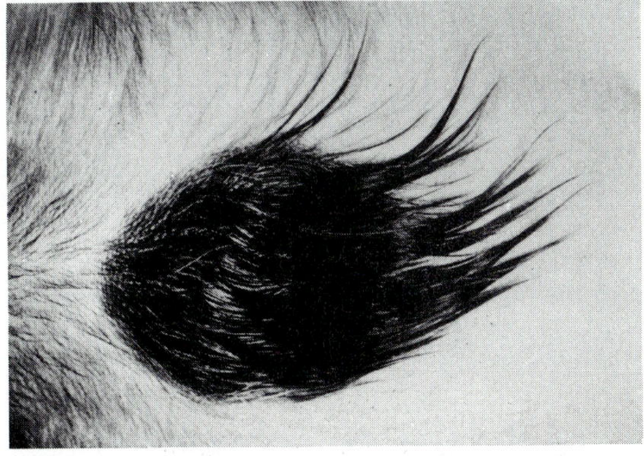

Figure 31-2 Congenital melanocytic nevi. (*From TB Fitzpatrick et al, Dermatology in General Medicine, 3d ed, New York, McGraw-Hill, 1987, p 952.*)

Dysplastic Nevi

The dysplastic nevus is perhaps the most fascinating of the precursor lesions, since it demonstrates the genetic transmission of a pigmented lesion that can develop into melanoma. This lesion appears to be transmitted in some families in an autosomal dominant pattern,[8,9] although polygenetic inheritance has been suggested.[14] Localization of the melanoma trait to chromosome 1 has been recently reported.[15] Hypersensitivity to G_2 chromatid radiation damage has been reported in skin fibroblasts in patients with the familial form of dysplastic nevi and melanoma.[16] This study noted more chromatid breaks and gaps after x irradiation in comparison to an unaffected control group. While familial melanoma represents only about 10 percent of melanomas, the dysplastic nevus has been seen in association with sporadic melanoma in perhaps another 30 to 40 percent of tumors. Thus dysplastic nevi may be the precursor responsible for approximately one-half of all melanomas. In addition to being a genetically determined *precursor* lesion, the dysplastic nevus can serve as a *marker* of increased risk. Individuals who bear dysplastic nevi may develop cutaneous melanoma de novo in apparently normal skin. Clinically, these lesions are

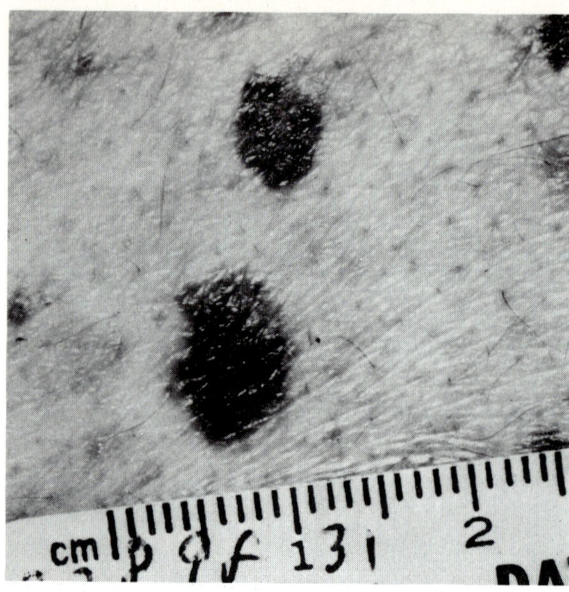

Figure 31-3 Dysplastic nevi. Note the irregularity of the borders and pigment pattern. (*From TB Fitzpatrick et al, Dermatology in General Medicine, New York, McGraw-Hill, 3d ed, 1987, p 953.*)

usually larger than 5 mm and exhibit a variegated pigment pattern and indistinct borders (Fig. 31-3). Most often, patients have several to a few hundred nevi, but occasionally only one may be present. See Table 31-2 for the clinical characteristics that distinguish dysplastic nevi from benign acquired nevi. The dysplastic nevus has a larger number of melanocytes of increased cell size at the dermal-epidermal junction compared with solar lentigines and normal nevi.[10] An increase in abnormal melanosomes has also been noted.[17] Since lesions with the phenotypic appearance of dysplastic nevi occur in approximately 5 percent of the "normal" population, these individuals must be studied to determine whether there exist benign phenotypic "look-alikes" or whether these "normal" individuals bear an increased risk of developing melanoma. In some centers, all patients with dysplastic nevi are considered to be at increased risk, and individuals having the familial melanoma syndrome to be at greatly increased risk (150 fold increase).[18] A recent paper suggesting a much higher prevalence of dysplastic nevi has added to the controversy about the significance of the presence of sporadic dysplastic nevi in the population at large.[19] Resolution of this issue awaits the establishment of universally reproducible and agreed-upon characteristics for the clinical/histopathologic definition of the dysplastic nevus followed by careful population-based surveys to establish its frequency and its relationship to the development of melanoma. In the study by Rigel et al., who prospectively

Table 31-2

CLINICAL FEATURES DISTINGUISHING DYSPLASTIC NEVI FROM BENIGN ACQUIRED NEVI

Clinical Feature	Dysplastic Nevi	Benign Acquired Nevi
Color	Variable mixtures of tan, brown, black, or red/pink within a single nevus; nevi may look very different from each other	Uniformly tan or brown.
Shape	Irregular borders; pigment may fade off into surrounding skin; macular portion at the edge of the nevus	Round; sharp, clear-cut borders between the nevus and the surrounding skin; may be flat or elevated.
Size	Usually more than 6 mm; may be more than 10 mm; occasionally smaller than 6 mm	Usually less than 6 mm in diameter.
Number	Often very many (more than 100), but occasionally may be only one	In a typical adult: 10 to 40 are scattered over the body; perhaps 15% of patients have no nevi.
Location	Sun-exposed areas; the back is the most common site, but dysplastic nevi may also be seen on the scalp, breasts, and buttocks	Generally on the sun-exposed surfaces of the skin above the waist; the scalp, breasts, and buttocks are rarely involved.

Source: Modified from RJ Friedman et al: Early detection of malignant melanoma: the role of physical examination and self-examination of the skin. *CA* 35:130, 1985.

followed 452 patients with dysplastic nevi, 16 patients developed 18 melanomas during an average follow-up period of 27 months.[12] For a recent review of these and other risk factors, see Rhodes et al.[20]

DEVELOPMENTAL BIOLOGY AND NATURAL HISTORY[3,13]

There are at least four clear-cut forms of melanoma[21,22] (Table 31-3). Three of these types [superficial spreading melanoma (Fig. 31-4), lentigo maligna melanoma, acral lentiginous melanoma] exhibit a radial (lateral) growth phase within the epidermis and/or upper dermis for substantial periods of time (months to years) before developing deep invasion and the capacity for metastasis. During this period of radial growth, a prominent

Table 31-3

CLINICAL FEATURES OF MALIGNANT MELANOMA

Type	Site	Average Age at Diagnosis, Years	Duration of Known Existence, Years	Color
Lentigo maligna melanoma	Usually on exposed surfaces, particularly malar region of cheek and temple; uncommonly on unexposed surfaces	70	5–20* or longer	In flat portions, shades of brown and tan predominant, but whitish-gray occasionally present; in nodules, shades of reddish brown, bluish gray, bluish black
Superficial spreading melanoma	Any site (more common on upper back in both sexes and on lower legs in women)	40–50	1–7	Shades of brown mixed with bluish red (violaceous), bluish black, reddish brown, and often whitish pink; border of lesion is at least in part visibly and/or palpably elevated
Nodular melanoma	Any site	40–50	Months to less than 5 years	Reddish blue (purple) or bluish black; either uniform in color of mixed with brown or black
Acral lentiginous melanoma	Palm, sole, nail bed, mucous membrane	60	1–10	In flat portions, dark brown predominantly; in raised lesions (plaques), brown-black or blue-black predominantly

* During much of this time, the precursor stage, lentigo maligna, is actively confined to the epidermis.

Source: Modified from RG Petersdorf et al (eds), *Harrison's Principles of Internal Medicine*, 10th ed, New York, McGraw-Hill, 1983, p 836.

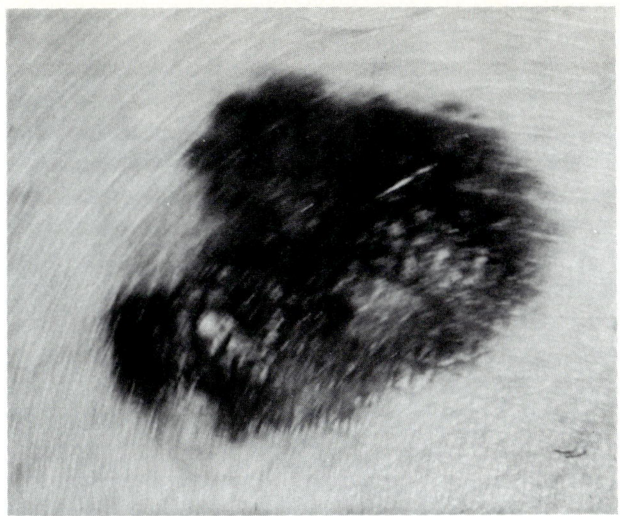

Figure 31-4 Superficial spreading melanoma. Note the irregular borders.

mononuclear cell–host response is present beneath the tumor. A dynamic interaction exists between the host response and the tumor that keeps the tumor in check and may result in partial or complete regression of the primary tumor. The combination of radial growth and regression results in the characteristic features clinically diagnostic of melanoma[23,24]: irregularity of the border (irregular growth and regression), irregularity in pigment pattern (variable pigment production by different tumor cell clones, pigment in dermal macrophages of the host response), and variation in color (pinks and reds from inflammation, grays and whites from regression, blue from melanin deep in the dermis).

Appreciable height of the tumor is associated with vertical growth and the capacity to metastasize. At this time, the host response at the base of the tumor is usually sparse or absent, and multiple clones of cells can be noted in the tumor. The prognosis (likelihood of metastasis) can be directly correlated with the thickness of tumor[25–28] (Table 31-4).

Table 31-4

PROGNOSIS BASED ON THICKNESS OF THE PRIMARY TUMOR

Thickness, mm	Prognosis, Percent Survival at 5 Years
<0.85	99
0.85–1.69	94
1.70–3.64	78
>3.65	42

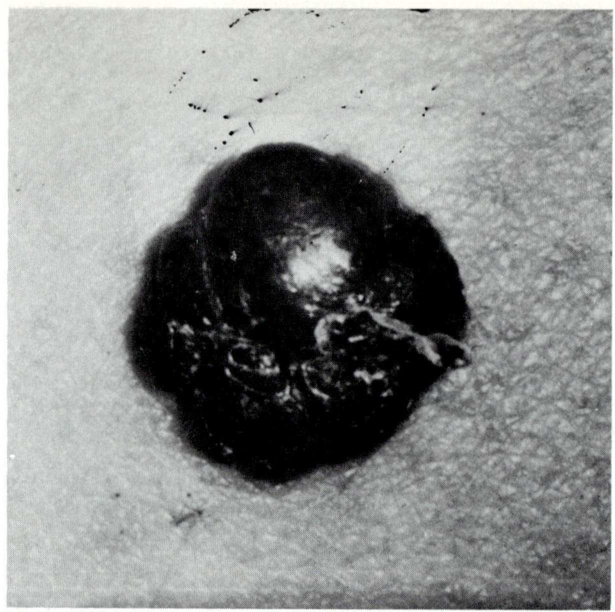

Figure 31-5 Nodular melanoma.

The fourth tumor type, nodular melanoma (Fig. 31-5), lacks the radial growth phase and appears in the vertical growth phase from the onset. These tumors are consequently thicker at first detection and are associated, on average, with the worst prognosis.

The factors that cause alteration in the host response or development of multiple clones in the tumor are not understood.

SPREAD OF TUMOR

Malignant melanocytes are well adapted to live in relative harmony in the human host. Patients can function quite well while carrying kilograms of tumor deposits in their bodies. Melanoma spreads via two routes: (1) the cutaneous lymphatics, with intracutaneous metastasis noted and involvement of the regional lymph nodes, and (2) the venous system, in which virtually any organ can be involved. Common sites of metastasis are the liver, lung, bone, and brain. With production of sufficient melanin precursors, the tumor burden of melanoma may be so great that melanosis may develop, with diffuse blue-gray skin and brownish blood and urine. In patients with diffuse melanosis, single malignant melanocytes may be seen in the dermis at times; however, more often, melanin in dermal melanophages and melanin metabolites in the circulation are responsible for the color change noted clinically.

PROGNOSIS

The likelihood of metastasis and/or death has been correlated with the volume of the primary tumor. A simple estimate of this volume can be determined by measuring the vertical tumor thickness.[25] When this is done, both low-risk and high-risk groups can be defined (Table 31-4). Estimations of the prognosis are important in tailoring therapy to the severity of the disease. Anatomic location of the primary tumor is also a factor, with palms and soles, mucous membranes, and scalp being relatively unfavorable sites.[28] Conversely, the lower leg and the forearm are especially favorable sites.[28] The frequency of lower-leg location in women, with its attendant favorable prognosis, has been one explanation for the higher survival of women. In addition, there is a direct correlation between the thickness of the primary tumor and the likelihood of spread to the regional nodes.[27]

HOST FACTORS

A substantial literature demonstrating humoral and cellular immunologic interactions between host and tumor exists. Spontaneous disappearance of all or part of the primary tumor is a clinical example of this interaction. At times, a halo of depigmentation may develop around the primary tumor or around nevi. Hypopigmentation at distant sites, uveitis (inflammation of the pigment cells of the eye), and poliosis (graying of hair) may also be noted. Cytotoxic circulating antibodies and mononuclear cells directed against cultured melanoma cells have also been observed. The lack of a well-characterized melanoma antigen has limited the research in this area. Several laboratories using various techniques have found conflicting results. Nonetheless, taken in aggregate, a strong case can be made for a dynamic interaction between patient and tumor, leading immunologically oriented oncologists to attempt to influence the outcome of the disease by immune manipulation of the patient.

Two developments that may increase the understanding of the progression from melanocyte to melanoma are advances in cell culture techniques and the availability of monoclonal antibody panels directed against a variety of melanocyte/melanoma cell surface antigens. Cell culture techniques were developed that first supported the growth of metastatic melanoma cells (the easiest to grow). Refinements subsequently allowed the growth of radial growth phase primary melanoma, and further refinements led to the culture of normal melanocytes and nevi. The ability to grow substantial quantities of these cells has permitted investigations impossible with in vivo material alone.

The monoclonal antibodies that recognize different antigens expressed on the cell surface at various developmental phases are classified into two types. Monoclonal antibody to *differentiation antigens* distinguishes melanocytes of fetal origin from those present in adults. Monoclonal antibody to *progression antigens* distinguishes the gradient from normal melanocytes to nevus cells to dysplastic nevus cells to primary radial growth phase melanoma cells to vertical growth phase melanoma cells to metastatic melanoma cells. None of these monoclonal antibodies is 100 percent specific for any one phase (overlap is noted), but some recognize early phases of progression and others late phases. Tumor progression of melanocytic cells is accompanied by quantitative differences in antigen expression.[29] In general, monoclonal antibodies have shown similar profiles for atypical dysplastic nevus cells and radial growth phase primary melanoma cells, and similar profiles for vertical growth phase primary melanoma cells and metastatic melanoma cells.[29] Studies can be performed on fresh frozen tissue as well as on paraffin block material with some of the newer monoclonal antibodies.

Some of the observations that appear to be immunologic may actually have a molecular biologic explanation devolving from the primary characterstics of the tumor itself and relatively unrelated to host factors. This situation should be clarified when the results of molecular biologic studies in progress become available.

TREATMENT

The primary treatment for cutaneous melanoma is surgical excision. Standard chemotherapies have been of only modest value in the treatment of disseminated tumor. Rational strategies for treatment are possible based on the biology and chemistry of the melanocyte. The melanocyte-stimulating hormone (MSH) receptor on the cell surface could be exploited by attaching a chemotherapeutic agent to MSH. Cell surface antigens might be a point of attack by using monoclonal antibodies as a carrier for an active agent. Recently, a polyvalent melanoma antigen vaccine has been produced by preparing melanoma antigenic material from substances shed from multiple human melanoma cell lines grown in serum-free medium.[30] This vaccine is currently being evaluated for its efficacy in reducing melanoma recurrence in patients at high risk of recurrent disease. Other strategies include using agents that bind to melanin, such as chlorpromazine, as carriers. The melanin synthesis pathway might be exploited; for example, the differential uptake of dopa or its congeners could be used to poison the melanocyte.[31] Dihydroxybenzylamine, a congener of dopa, has recently been approved for clinical trials in disseminated melanoma.[32] Depigmenting agents that destroy pigment cells and generate an immunologic response might be of use. Manipulation of the host's immune system, with an increase in tumoricidal factors, might be helpful. Present investigations with biologic response modifiers such as interleukin-2 and tumor-infiltrating lymphocytes bear watching.[33,34]

REFERENCES

1. Ley RD et al: Ultraviolet radiation–induced malignant melanoma in *Monodelphis domestica*. *Photochem Photobiol* 50:1, 1989.
2. Clark WH Jr, Mihm MC Jr: Lentigo maligna and lentigo maligna melanoma. *Am J Pathol* 55:39, 1969.
3. Clark WH Jr et al: The histogenesis and biologic behavior of primary human malignant melanoma of the skin. *Cancer Res* 29:705, 1969.
4. Kaplan EN: The risk of malignancy in large congenital nevi. *Plast Reconstr Surg* 53:421, 1974.
5. Trozak DJ et al: Metastatic malignant melanoma in prepubertal children. *Pediatrics* 55:191, 1974.
6. Rhodes AR, Melski JW: Small congenital nevocellular nevi: risk of cutaneous melanoma. *J Pediatr* 100:219, 1982.
7. Illig L et al: Congenital nevi ≤10 cm as precursors to melanoma. *Arch Dermatol* 121:1274, 1985.
8. Reimer RR et al: Precursor lesions in familial melanoma. *JAMA* 239:744, 1978.
9. Elder DE et al: Dysplastic nevus syndrome: a phenotypic association of sporadic cutaneous melanoma. *Cancer* 46:1787, 1980.
10. Rhodes AR et al: Increased intraepidermal melanocyte frequency and size in dysplastic melanocytic nevi and cutaneous melanoma: a comparative quantitative study of dysplastic melanocytic nevi, superficial spreading melanoma, nevocellular nevi, and solar lentigines. *J Invest Dermatol* 80:452, 1983.
11. Rhodes AR et al: Dysplastic melanocytic nevi in histologic association with 234 cutaneous melanomas. *J Am Acad Dermatol*, 9:563, 1983.
12. Rigel DS et al: Dysplastic nevi: markers for increased risk for melanoma. *Cancer* 63:386, 1989.
13. Weinstock MA, Sober AJ: The risk of progression of lentigo maligna to lentigo maligna melanoma. *Br J Dermatol* 116:303, 1987.
14. Happle R et al: Arguments in favor of a polygenic inheritance of precursor nevi. *J Am Acad Dermatol* 6:540, 1982.
15. Bale SJ et al: Mapping the gene for hereditary cutaneous malignant melanoma-dysplastic nevus to chromosome 1p. *N Engl J Med* 320:1367, 1989.
16. Sanford KK et al: Hypersensitivity to G_2 chromatid radiation damage in familial dysplastic nevus syndrome. *Lancet* 2:1111, 1987.
17. Rhodes AR et al: Melanosomal alterations in dysplastic melanocytic nevi. *Cancer* 61:358, 1988.
18. Kraemer KH et al: Risk of cutaneous melanoma in dysplastic nevus syndrome types A and B. *N Engl J Med* 315:1615, 1986.
19. Piepkorn M et al: The dysplastic melanocytic nevus: a prevalent lesion that correlates poorly with clinical phenotype. *J Am Acad Dermatol* 20:407, 1989.
20. Rhodes AR et al: Risk factors for cutaneous melanoma. *JAMA* 258:3146, 1987.
21. Sober AJ et al: Primary melanoma of the skin: recognition and management. *J Am Acad Dermatol* 2:179, 1980.
22. Mihm MC Jr et al: The clinical diagnosis, classification, and histogenetic concepts of the early stages of cutaneous malignant melanoma. *N Engl J Med* 284:1078, 1971.
23. Mihm MC Jr et al: Early detection of primary cutaneous malignant melanoma: a color atlas. *N Engl J Med* 289:989 1973.
24. Sober AJ et al: Early recognition of cutaneous melanoma. *JAMA* 242:2795, 1979.
25. Breslow A: Tumor thickness, level of invasion and node dissection in stage I cutaneous melanoma. *Ann Surg* 182:572, 1975.
26. Balch CM et al: A multifunctional analysis of melanoma: prognostic histopathological features comparing Clark's and Breslow's staging methods. *Ann Surg* 188:732, 1978.
27. Day CL Jr et al: Malignant melanoma patients with positive nodes and relatively good prognosis: microstaging retains prognostic significance in clinical stage I melanoma patients with metastases to regional nodes. *Cancer* 47:955, 1981.

28. Sober AJ et al: Primary melanoma of the skin: recognition of precursor lesions and estimation of prognosis in stage I, in TB Fitzpatrick et al (eds), *Update: Dermatology in General Medicine.* New York, McGraw-Hill, 1983, p 98.
29. Elder DE et al: Antigenic profile of tumor progression stages in human melanocytic nevi and melanomas. *Cancer Res* 49:5091, 1989.
30. Bystryn JC et al: Immunogenicity of a polyvalent melanoma antigen vaccine in humans. *Cancer* 61:1065, 1988.
31. Wick MM: Experimental approach to chemotherapy of melanoma. *J Invest Dermatol* 74:63, 1980.
32. FitzGerald G, Wick MM: 3,4-Dihydroxybenzylamine: an improved dopamine analog cytotoxic for melanoma cells in part through oxidation products inhibitory to DNA polymerase. *J Invest Dermatol* 80:119, 1983.
33. Lotze MT et al: High-dose recombinant interleukin 2 in the treatment of patients with disseminated cancer: responses, treatment-related morbidity, and histologic findings. *JAMA* 256:3117, 1986.
34. Rosenberg SA et al: Use of tumor-infiltrating lymphocytes and interleukin-2 in the immunotherapy of patients with metastatic melanoma: a preliminary report. *N Engl J Med* 319:1676, 1988.

32

Pathophysiology of Cutaneous T-Cell Lymphomas

Peter W. Heald and Richard L. Edelson

As discussed in the chapters on the skin as an immunologic organ (Chap. 7), allergic contact dermatitis (Chap. 10), and atopic dermatitis (Chap. 11), the skin has an integral role in the life and function of lymphocytes. The varied activities of T cells all have clinical relevance in the pathophysiology of the cutaneous T-cell lymphomas (CTCL).

T CELLS AND THE SKIN

A curious feature of CTCL is that a tumor of mesenchymal origin develops a symbiosis with an ectodermally derived tissue. The affinity of T cells for ectodermal tissue begins prenatally with the programming of T cells in close proximity to thymic keratinocytes (these internalized keratinocytes are termed thymic epithelium). When mature T cells leave the thymus, they exhibit distinctive characteristics, as described by cell surface analysis and molecular biologic techniques. These techniques have enabled clinicians to further identify the components of T-cell lymphomas seen by dermatologists.

In their contribution to the symbiosis with the skin, T cells can organize an effective defense against many non-self invaders—biologic or chemical. Mature T cells are defined by the presence of a T-cell receptor complex. One component of this complex is a protein that binds to foreign antigen and activates the T cell to direct the immune response. T-cell receptors for

Table 32-1

CELL SURFACE MARKERS THAT PLAY PATHOPHYSIOLOGIC ROLES IN CUTANEOUS T-CELL LYMPHOMAS

Marker	Cells	Description
CD2	T cells	Adhesion, mediates rosetting
CD3	T cells	Transduces the activation signal from the antigen receptor
CD4	Helper T cells	Class II MHC binding
CD8	Suppressor T cells	Class I MHC binding
CD30	Abnormal T cells	Ki-1 marker, Hodgkin's disease
CD25	Activated (early) cells	High-affinity interleukin-2 receptor, in HTLV-1
BE2	CTCL cells Activated (late) cells	Sézary cell protein
LFA-1	Activated lymphocytes	Binds ICAM-1 on target cells such as thymic epithelia and keratinocytes
LFA-3	All tissues	Binds CD2
ICAM-1	Keratinocytes, activated cells	Binds LFA-1 on lymphocytes

antigen are derived from proteins rearranged in immunoglobulin-like permutations of α-β chains (90 percent) or γ-δ chains (10 percent). Other lymphocyte surface proteins that play a role are described in Table 32-1. Cell surface markers are now standardized in the cluster designation (CD) system. Many of the surface proteins provide valuable insights for staging, following, and understanding the disease. Those most frequently utilized are CD3, which transduces the signal from antigen receptor to cell activation; CD4, which binds major histocompatibility complex (MHC) class II antigens; CD1, which binds MHC class I; CD8, which binds class I MHC; CD25, the interleukin-2 receptor that increases with activation; and BE-2, which is present on malignant cells and occurs in normal cells under conditions of T-cell growth.

Immunochemical methods for studying cell surface markers include immunoperoxidase staining of tissue[1] and flow cytometry of peripheral blood cells.[2] The major molecular biologic technique utilized in the study of CTCL patients is Southern blotting of the T-cell receptor gene.[3] This technique is most sensitive in detecting whether an expanded T-cell clone is present in skin, blood, or lymph nodes. Since each T cell has an immunoglobin-like surface protein for its antigen receptor, each T cell contains a unique gene sequence derived from an immunoglobin-like rearrangement of T-cell receptor genes. Thus each T cell and its progeny contain a unique T-cell receptor gene sequence that can be used to distinguish one T cell and its progeny from another. The method that accomplishes this is called Southern blotting. After DNA is isolated from lymphocytes and digested, the fragments are separated by size. If there is one particular clone that has expanded, the fragments unique to this clone will appear on the Southern blot. Thus this test can determine whether there is a clonal expansion of T cells, but it cannot easily quantify it.

GROWTH OF T CELLS IN THE SKIN

An early stage of disease development is the localization of T-cell collections to the skin. In general, T cells always predominate in an infiltrate.[4] Thus it is extremely difficult to know when this predominance is pathological. Yet out of nonspecific lymphocytic and inflammatory infiltrates, the histopathologic features of lymphoma appear as the malignant T-cell clone expands in that location.

The T-cell trophic microenvironment of the skin has soluble and surface components. The similarity of keratinocytes and thymic epithelia extends to the types of keratins they produce, surface markers that are shared, and cytokines that they produce. Surface proteins involved in the attractions of lymphocytes, particularly T cells, are intercellular adhesion molecule-1 (ICAM-1) and class II MHC. Both of these can be demonstrated in lesional but not in nonlesional skin in CTCL.[5] Class II MHC bind to the CD4 protein of $CD4^+$ (helper/inducer) T cells and ICAM-1 binds to lymphocyte adhesion molecule-1 (LFA-1) on lymphocytes (Fig. 32-1*a*). Keratinocytes constitutively produce immunologically active cytokines, many of which are membrane associated as if to provide an instant reserve when keratinocytes are activated or damaged. The first cytokine was termed *e*pidermal derived *T*-cell *a*ctivating *f*actor (ETAF). Subsequently, it was shown that there is a family of ETAFs[6] (Fig. 32-1*b*): interleukin-1, granulocyte-monocyte colony-stimulating factor, and interleukin-6. These factors activate T cells in proximity to the epidermis. In addition, several ETAFs stimulate T-cell growth and maturation. Thus, T-cell surface proteins that mediate adhesion and cytokine interaction are at the forefront of the pathophysiology of this disease. The CTCL tumor-associated antigen BE-2 has unknown functions, but it appears in normal T cells under conditions of T-cell growth. Its appearance in the peripheral blood of CTCL patients reflects extension of disease into this compartment.

Once the malignant cells have localized to the skin, there appear to be two components of disease spread—local growth and hematogenous spread. Local growth generates plaques and, in its extreme form, tumors. The local effectors that limit this process are probably Langerhans cells, along with $CD8^+$ (suppressor/cytotoxic) T lymphocytes. The observation

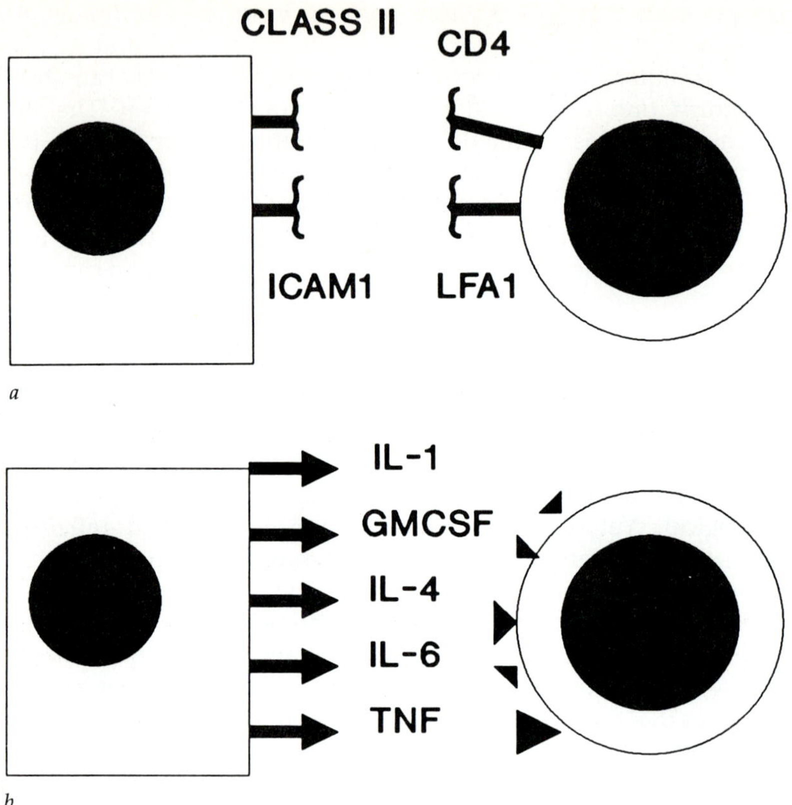

Figure 32-1 Components of keratinocyte. (*a*) T-cell interactions include surface proteins. ICAM1 = intercellular adhesion molecule-1; LFA1 = lymphocyte adhesion molecule-1. (*b*) Cytokines. IL-1 = interleukin-1; GMCSF = granulocyte macrophage colony stimulating factor; IL-4 = interleukin-4; IL-6 = interleukin-6; TNF = tumor necrosis factor.

that a given plaque can remain stable for years suggests that there is effective local growth control on the periphery of the lesion. Progression of the local growth phase of CTCL to the tumor stage is not just the failure of local control measures. There are distinct morphologic features such as nucleolar prominence, paler cytoplasm, and a tendency to not express mature cell markers.[7]

The checks on systemic spread of disease involve local lymph nodes and the reticuloendothelial system. Circulating abnormal cells in CTCL tend to generate diffuse erythema, but there is no tendency for plaque or tumor formation. One proposed step in the achievement of the leukemic state is a decrease in ICAM-1 expression by the epidermis, thus providing less attraction for epidermotropism.[8] Another feature that may well contribute to the loss of epidermotropism is that circulating abnormal cells constitutively produce their own interleukin-6, which may explain the ability of these cells to flourish in the absence of keratinocytes.[9]

CLINICAL PATTERNS OF CTCL

The clinicians' views of CTCL differ according to the varying degrees of epidermal infiltration, inflammatory response, systemic spread, and local growth of the abnormal cells. A partial list of recognized syndromes is presented. All of these conditions have two features: clonal T-cell proliferation in the skin (as defined by Southern blots) and the fact that patients with CTCL can exhibit any variety of these patterns.

SPECTRUM OF CUTANEOUS T-CELL DYSCRASIAS

Parapsoriasis There are many subsets of this general syndrome. Cells are mature, inflammation and atrophy are prominent, and there is infrequent progression to more malignant behavior.

Alopecia Mucinosa There is a pronounced perifollicular infiltration. A benign subtype occurs in younger age groups, whereas it tends to be associated with more severe CTCL in adults.

Poikiloderma Vasculare Atrophicans Cell-poor infiltrates occur with pronounced atrophy. This form tends to be benign in behavior.

Pityriasis Lichenoides et Varioliformis Acuta Mature-appearing cells, which are clonal, are accompanied by a scarring inflammatory response. Lesions tend to appear in crops and to be self-limited. Occasional cases are associated with mycosis fungoides.

Lymphomatoid Papulosis Although this form resembles pityriasis lichenoides et varioliformis acuta, the cells are malignant in appearance and progression to lymphoma is much more common. It is still striking that most of the lesions in this condition are self-limited, implying that the inflammatory response adequately protected the host from the malignant clone. CTCL is the most frequent lymphoma associated with lymphomatoid papulosis.

Sézary Syndrome This is an erythrodermic form with circulating abnormal cells (Sézary cells with hyperconvoluted nuclei). The diffuse inflammation of the skin is not always associated with epidermotropism.

HTLV-1 Lymphoma/Leukemia The retrovirus known as human T-cell lymphotropic virus-1 (HTLV-1) transforms $CD4^+$ T cells, and a rapidly growing clone develops. This form mimics mycosis fungoides and Sézary syndrome. Circulating cells bear the Tac receptor, which distinguishes them from other lymphomas and reflects the proliferative nature of these cells. Skin infiltration occurs early in the disease but becomes less marked later, probably reflecting greater autonomy of the more malignant subclones.

Mycosis Fungoides The early stages of involvement clinically present as flat, erythematous patches or indurated plaques, both of which tend to develop scales. The clinical findings are often confused with those of atopic dermatitis, contact dermatitis, and psoriasis. In the early phases of mycosis fungoides, there often is a considerable degree of inflammation that not only is associated with pruritus and excoriations but also may obscure the diagnosis. Epidermotropism of mature malignant cells is the hallmark (Fig.

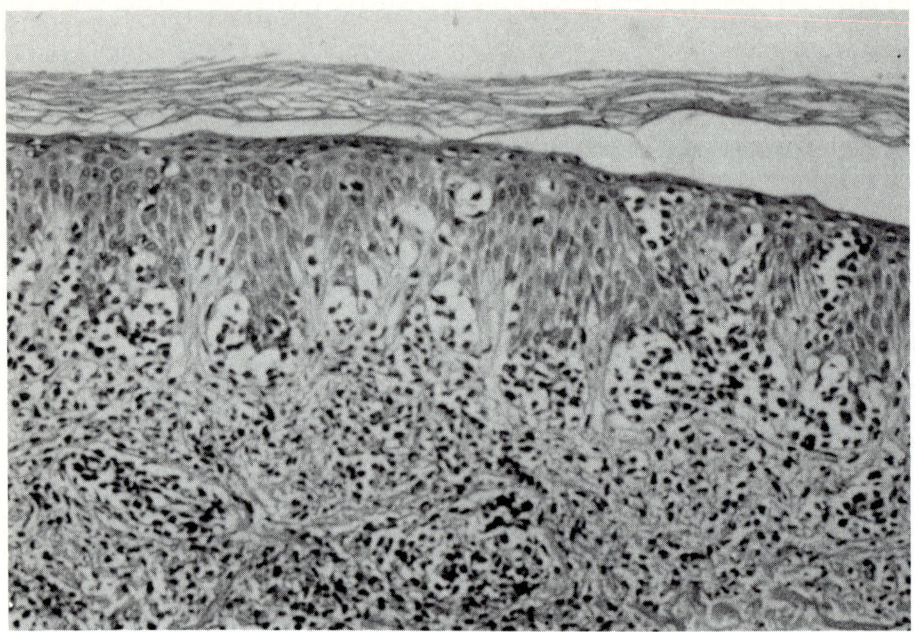

Figure 32-2 CTCL shows the epidermotropism and dermal infiltrate of malignant cells. ×400 in the original magnification.

32-2). A Pautrier microabscess (Fig. 32-3) composed of malignant lymphocytes characterizes the patch and plaque stages (Fig. 32-4). The further progression of the disease to erythroderma or the tumor stage is erratic. The median survival for mycosis fungoides in general appears to be greater than 8 years.[10] Overall survival is considerably shortened by the development of tumor, lymph node involvement, or erythroderma.[11] It is of interest that the development of these stages is associated with a loss of the epidermotropism characteristic of the early stages. Mycosis fungoides is the most common form of CTCL.

PARANEOPLASTIC PHENOMENA

Additional clinical findings in CTCL are created by the variety of paraneoplastic phenomena that appear as a result of $CD4^+$ T cell functions. Cutaneous infections that are dependent on T cells for their control are more common. In fact, disseminated herpetic eruptions are favored not only by the disruption of the T-cell compartment but also by the diffuse skin involvement in some patients.[12] $CD4^+$ T cells are required for antibody production by B cells. The immunoglobulin abnormalities in CTCL include monoclonal gammopathies,[13] increased autoantibodies,[14] and increased IgA and IgE levels.[15] Antitumor immunity is mediated by T cells, and there is an appreciable appearance of second malignancies in this popu-

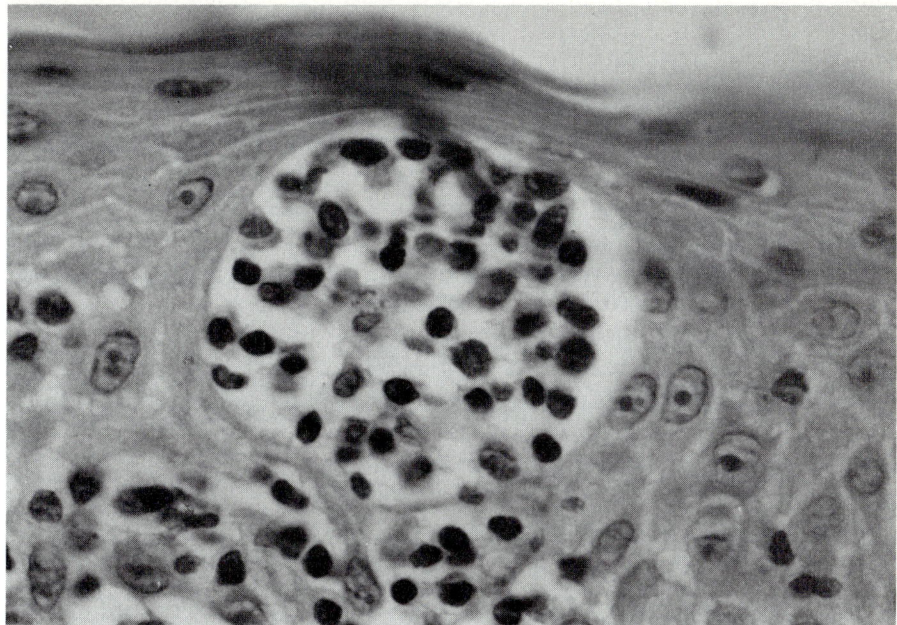

Figure 32-3 A Pautrier microabscess results from a collection of epidermotropic malignant cells in the skin. ×1000 in the original magnification.

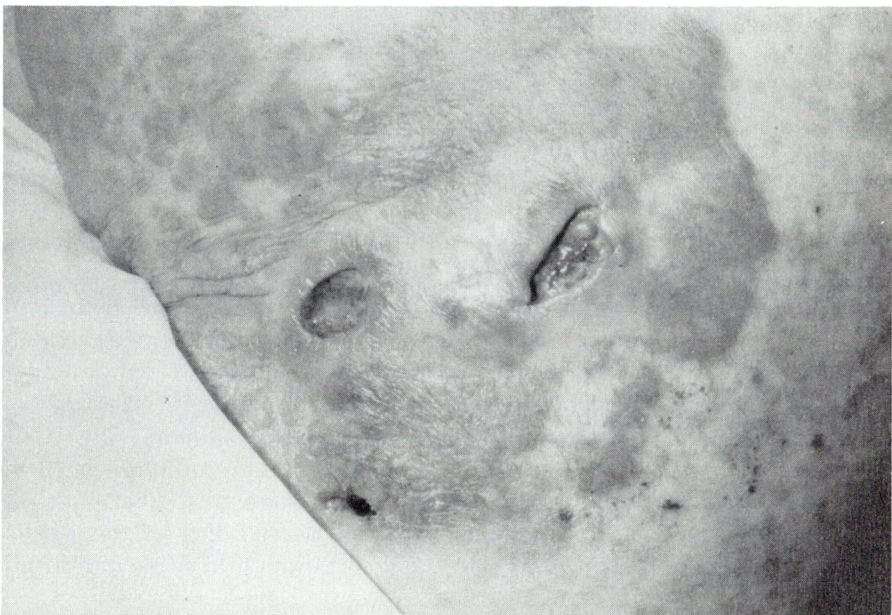

Figure 32-4 Clinical lesions of the plaque stage of CTCL.

lation.[16] As with many other pruritic skin eruptions and lymphomas, there may be eosinophilia associated with CTCL. It is even possible that some of the severe pruritus associated with CTCL is a systemic effect of lymphoma similar to the severe pruritus of Hodgkin's disease.

THERAPY

The goals of therapy are to match the modality with the stage of disease. In the most common plaque and patch stage of the disease, the major emphasis is on treatment of the skin with topical nitrogen mustard,[17] psoralens plus ultraviolet A (PUVA) photochemotherapy,[18] electron beam[19] or ultraviolet B phototherapy.[20] The outcome of nitrogen mustard therapy indicates that the best results are obtained if the entire skin is treated, not just the perilesional and lesional areas. This conclusion suggests that this treatment (and the same could be said for PUVA therapy) may be treating the keratinocyte contribution to the malignancy. With nitrogen mustard and PUVA, treatments can be decreased in frequency once remission is attained. With electron beam therapy, follow-up chemotherapy is advised to prolong the disease-free interval. Relapses or persistent disease often prompt the addition of a second cutaneous modality or adjunctive therapy such as an oral retinoid.

When the cutaneous growth phase excessively dominates the clinical picture, resulting in thick plaques and tumors, the best ablative therapy is radiotherapy to eliminate the lesion. When the disease has entered the tumor phase, it is aggressive, and postradiotherapy adjunctive treatments must be given in an attempt to prevent relapse. These adjuncts include chemotherapy, photopheresis, PUVA, and nitrogen mustard.

When the circulating phase of the disease dominates the clinical picture, as detected by peripheral blood studies and/or the presence of erythroderma, the treatment of choice is photopheresis. An autologous "vaccine" of white blood cells is prepared by photoinactivating a portion of the circulating lymphocytes. This appears to stimulate a host response against these circulating cells.[21] When white blood cell counts are over 50,000/mm^3, large numbers of circulating cells can be removed by leukapheresis as a symptomatic adjunct to this therapy.

Thus, a knowledge of the disease components (Fig. 32-5) is helpful in designing the overall treatment regimen.[22] For example, a patient with tumors and circulating cells would be best treated with radiotherapy followed by photopheresis.

Protocol studies are currently being developed following the basic research on T cells and keratinocytes. Biologic response modifiers such as interferon, cytokines, and antibodies have demonstrated their usefulness in preliminary studies. Clearly, the further understanding of the T-cell–keratinocyte relationship will lead to the incorporation of these entities in multimodality lymphoma regimens.

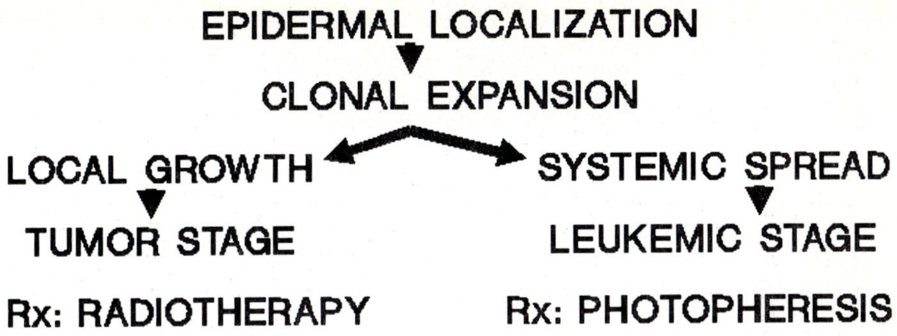

EPIDERMAL LOCALIZATION
▼
CLONAL EXPANSION

LOCAL GROWTH ⟷ SYSTEMIC SPREAD
▼ ▼
TUMOR STAGE LEUKEMIC STAGE

Rx: RADIOTHERAPY Rx: PHOTOPHERESIS

Figure 32-5 A model for the biology of CTCL.

REFERENCES

1. Chu A et al: In situ study of T-cell subpopulations in cutaneous T-cell lymphoma, diagnostic criteria. *Cancer* 54:2414, 1984.
2. Kung PC et al: Monoclonal antibodies defining distinctive human T cell surface antigens. *Science* 206:347, 1979.
3. Weiss LM et al: Clonal rearrangements of T-cell receptor genes in mycosis fungoides and dermatopathic lymphadenopathy. *N Engl J Med* 313: 539, 1985.
4. Vonderheid EC et al: Clinical implications of immunologic phenotyping in cutaneous T cell lymphoma. *J Am Acad Dermatol* 17:40, 1987.
5. Nickoloff BJ: Role of interferon gamma in cutaneous trafficking of lymphocytes with emphasis on molecular and cellular adhesion events. *Arch Dermatol* 124:1835, 1988.
6. Kupper TS: Interleukin 1 and other human keratinocyte cytokines: molecular and functional characterization. *Adv Dermatol* 3:293, 1988.
7. Salhany KE et al: Transformation of cutaneous T cell lymphoma to large cell lymphoma. *Am J Pathol* 132:265, 1988.
8. Nickoloff BJ et al: Markedly diminished epidermal keratinocyte expression of intercellular adhesion molecule-1 (ICAM-1) in Sézary syndrome. *JAMA* 261:2217, 1989.
9. McNamara J, Bottomley K: personal communication.
10. Weinstock MA, Horm JW: Mycosis fungoides in the United States: increasing incidence and descriptive epidemiology. *JAMA* 260:42, 1988.
11. Sausville EA et al: Histopathologic staging at initial diagnosis of mycosis fungoides and the Sézary syndrome: definition of three distinctive prognostic groups. *Ann Intern Med* 109:372, 1988.
12. Gahlen-Shulte S et al: Generalized cutaneous herpes infection in mycosis fungoides (Kaposi's varicelliform eruption) *Z Hautkr* 57:1737, 1982.
13. Venencie PY et al: Monoclonal gammopathy and mycosis fungoides: report of four cases and review of the literature. *J Am Acad Dermatol* 11:576, 1984.
14. Schocket AL et al: Humoral immunity in Stage I mycosis fungoides: an increased incidence of lymphocytotoxic antibodies. *Br J Dermatol* 107:285, 1982.
15. Cooperrider PA, Roenigk H: Selective immunologic evaluation of mycosis fungoides. *Arch Dermatol* 114:207, 1978.
16. Olsen EA et al: Second malignancies in cutaneous T-cell lymphoma. *J Am Acad Dermatol* 10:197, 1984.
17. Vonderheid EC et al: Long term efficacy, curative potential, and carcinogenicity of topical mechlorethamine chemotherapy and cutaneous T-cell lymphoma. *J Am Acad Dermatol* 20:416, 1989.

18. Hönigsmann H et al: Photochemotherapy for cutaneous T cell lymphoma: a follow-up study. *J Am Acad Dermatol* 10:238, 1984.
19. Braverman IM et al: Combined total body electron beam irradiation and chemotherapy for mycosis fungoides. *J Am Acad Dermatol* 17:40, 1987.
20. Milstein HJ et al: Home ultraviolet phototherapy of early mycosis fungoides: preliminary observations. *J Am Acad Dermatol* 6:355, 1982.
21. Edelson RL et al: Treatment of cutaneous T cell lymphoma by extracorporeal photochemotherapy. *N Engl J Med* 316:297, 1987.
22. Kaye FJ et al: A randomized trial comparing combination electron beam radiation and chemotherapy with topical therapy in the initial treatment of mycosis fungoides. *N Engl J Med* 321:1784, 1989.

SECTION TWELVE

PSYCHIATRIC CONSIDERATIONS IN SKIN DISEASE

33

Psyche and Skin

Richard Masters

In the middle of this century, the word "psychosomatic" was used to describe the concept of relationships between states of mind and bodily disease.[1] How such relationships were effected was unknown, although some physiological observations of autonomic function, such as the effect of stress on heart rate, intestinal motility, and sweating, were made. It is reasonable to separate mind and brain; they are not synonymous. Mind arises from the functioning of the brain, but it is not the same, any more than the motion of a limb is the same as its muscles, bones, and nerves. The workings of the mind have their own distinct language and set of operational explanations, which are found in the various schools of psychiatry and psychology. The working of the brain, with its neural connections and networking of astronomical proportions, is best described by electrical biochemical, molecular biological, and electron microscopic studies. In psychiatry, one speaks of love, hate, anger, sadness, memory, interpersonal relationships, perception, consciousness, the unconscious, and self-consciousness in contrast to membranes, voltage, gating, influxes, neurotransmitters, peptides, and receptors. It is inappropriate today to describe the mechanisms producing organic disease states solely by metaphysical or psychoanalytic terminology. Application of psychiatric investigations may uncover sources of intrapsychic conflict (stress) and maladaptive perceptions that cause stress and may lead to organic disease, but it has not been particularly productive to try to relate specific personality types or sets of emotions to a particular cutaneous disease.

An overview of comparative evolutionary development[2] shows that the nervous system has developed from a nerve net in the first multicellular organisms to a central nervous system as multiple differentiated organ systems developed to help coordinate and control their activities. The largest organ, the skin, is responsible in part for maintaining the internal milieu by resisting fluid, electrolyte, and metabolite loss, by maintaining temperature control, by protecting the body from harmful solar radiation, and by informing the brain about proximate objects in its capacity as a sensory organ. Continuation of the evolutionary process led to a phenomenal development of the neocortex, and a new dimension was added to a central nervous system that had acted largely reflexly to control and integrate organ function in a variable environment. This new dimension allowed the central nervous system to function somewhat independently of its sensory input; it could store and re-create time past and project into time future (planning, anticipation of the consequences of action or thought, creative and abstract thinking). The new evolutionary development may have partially eclipsed one evolutionary force (considering environmental change to be a stimulus to evolution) by now comprehending enough to change the environment (purposefully or inadvertently). Additionally, neocortical function gave birth to self-consciousness and to a capacity for self-surveillance (a sixth sensory input) and comparative surveillance.[3] The skin and its appendages then acquired a new role; they became that portion of the physical self that is presented for evaluation in interpersonal relations.

Much twentieth-century psychiatric thinking, beginning with the studies of Freud (*das Ich*—the ego or the I, and presumably the self) and following with the studies of Fairbairn, Horney, Kernberg, Kohut, and Sullivan, among others, explored the normal and pathological development and expression of the self. It is likely that the skin, which contains the receptors for touch, plays a very significant role in this process of development of the psychological self. The postulated importance of the skin dates back to the Abbe de Condillac, whose theory was summarized by Brazier as follows: "For the initial sensation, Condillac's model relies on the tactile sense; the act of touch was held by him to be our only source of information about objects in the external world. The other senses learned to recognize external objects only by conjunction of their impressions with the factual evidence of touch."[4] It has become increasingly clear that the sense of touch is crucial to early childhood development.[5] It is partly through the skin and the sense of touch that the affectional mother–child bond is established and maintained.[6] One may infer the degree of importance of cutaneous sensory modalities to early development by the disproportionate representation of the hand and mouth in the sensory cortex, and by the neuroanatomic connections of the neocortex including the sensory cortex to the limbic system, which is related to emotional states and their physiological, as well as affectional, expression.[7,8] "The limbic system can be viewed as a neural mechanism that not only monitors the sensory processes of the cerebral cortex, but also can reach out to intervene in these processes. It could then be suspected . . . that the functional set of the limbic system affects not only the organism's visceral and endocrine functions and its motivational state, but also the sensory and associative mechanisms involved in its perceptions and ideational processes."[9]

Studies on the biochemical and physiological effects of maternal separation suggest that separation of a neonate from its mother produces psychological (behavioral) distress in whatever animals have been studied—rat, cat, dog, monkey, and human.[10] Biochemically, separated infant rats were found to have reduced levels of ornithine decarboxylase in the brain and decreased growth hormone levels in the plasma.[11] In humans, maternal deprivation was associated with patterns of abnormal withdrawal behavior in isolated children (anaclitic depression).[12–14] Maternal (or parental) deprivation is thought to be responsible for the syndrome of deprivation dwarfism or psychosocial dwarfism, in which there is a failure of growth hormone secretion despite apparently adequate nutrition.[15–19] Monkeys that survive separation from their mothers remain socially and biologically inept and aloof compared to normally raised offspring.[20] Bowlby has written extensively on the maternal–child bond, which develops partly through the sense of touch and which is necessary for the development of subsequent separation and individuation of the child.[6]

The survival and well-being of the offspring of most animals depend on maternal licking and physical contact (as well, of course, as on warmth and feeding).[21] Much of what is considered grooming behavior in animals is probably less related to cleanliness than to the cutaneous stimulation necessary for proper functioning. Without perineal stimulation from material licking, newborn rats and cats will not develop proper gastrointestinal and genitourinary functions and will succumb to obstructive disease. Maternal self-licking is a necessary stimulus for proper breast development, nest-building, and nursing behavior in rats—consistent with hormonal effects secondary to cutaneous stimulation. Captive rats that are frequently handled ("gentled") have a greater ability to withstand stress, gain weight faster, respond to immunization with higher antibody titers, and show increased activity generally compared with rats that are not handled.

In the course of normal brain development, there are "critical periods"—a term referring to a very limited time period during which a specific chemical (hormonal) or environmental stimulus must be presented to the brain or its maturation and functioning with respect to that kind of stimulus will be faulty.[22] Failure to present visual stimuli to one eye of a young monkey during a given time period will result in permanent failure of development of part of the occipital cortex and cortical blindness in that eye.[23] Sexual differentiation of the brain, at least in lower mammals, occurs only at a specific early time (the neonatal period in rats). Failure to present the appropriate hormonal (estrogenic) stimulation to the brain at that time results in permanent failure to develop appropriate adult sexual behavior—mating, nest building, rearing of young—despite normal hormone levels.[24]

Using the concept of critical periods and the analogy with the studies of Hubel and Wiesel on the development of the occipital cortex cited above, as well as the situation with regard to sexual development, one may indeed wonder whether the absence or failure of adequate cutaneous sensory stimulation in early life leads to inadequate development of the sensory cortex and/or the sensory cortical-limbic pathways, with decreased cortical control of the limbic centers for emotion (anger, rage, frustration anxiety). If so, one might begin to understand itching and chronic rubbing of the skin in the absence of a pathological state as attempts at self-soothing (or limbic control) in periods of tension or emotional stress—akin to increasing the voltage or current in the presence of inadequate wiring to get enough current across from cortex to limbic system.

Cutaneous sensation in general, and especially the sense of touch, participates in at least three processes: (1) survival, (2) stimulation of the endocrine system to support growth, and (3) the formation of the mother–child bond that supports psychological growth and ultimately leads to individuation and separation.[25,26] Touch is a very early form of communication. It allows the infant to define the limits of its own body, as well as to establish a sense of belonging, without which the processes of separation and individuation would be impaired. The skin, then, early on, becomes established as the interface between the physical "me" and the rest of the world. The importance of touch is reflected linguistically in the very extensive, meaningful, and emotionally descriptive use of the word. One has a happy touch, or is a soft touch, or is touchy, or touched, or tactful, or tactless. An obvious core of truth about an object, a situation, or an idea is tangibly true (or false). Under conditions of stress or surprise, one pinches oneself to know that one is awake or alive.

The enormous growth of the neocortex in the course of evolution is associated with the development of a sense of self and a capacity for self-consciousness. One might consider self-consciousness as a sixth sense, a surveying sense, born out of awareness of or influence of all the sensory inputs (environmental input), molded by learning, memory and experience, partially freed from automaticity by the capacity for abstract and creative thought and imagination, and yet tied to the governing functions of the brain over all other body systems. While the brain is the conductor of the human orchestra, with the score written in DNA (hard wiring), the sensory inputs and capacity for learning and memory influence its growth, development, and function (soft wiring, plasticity, epigenetic phenomena). The mechanisms of learning and memory are poorly understood.[27–34] Learning is a reflection of the plasticity of the brain and probably involves aspects of facilitated synoptic transmission and/or the development or selective use of neural networks. The sense of self, while partly genetically determined, is probably largely learned. It is likely, in the course of normal childhood social development, that events occur and perceptions and misperceptions are made that establish networks of thought or memory, some of which are incorrect or maladaptive. Distortions in the perceptions of the reality of ourselves, the world, and others constitute a major concern of psychiatry, but since such distortions are a source of intrapsychic stress, they also play a significant role in clinical medicine.

Some misconceptions remain conscious, while others join a repository of emotions, thoughts, feelings, and drives that have been termed the "unconscious mind." Although there is no known specific anatomic localization for unconscious processes, the often charged emotional content suggests that they may be related to the functioning of the limbic system and its hypothalamic, thalamic, and autonomic connections. The neural mechanisms that permit the neocortex to keep aggression, hostility, rage, hatred, and fear adequately suppressed are largely unknown, though the possible involvement of the sensory cortex has been alluded to above. If much effort, time, and networking are chronically required to keep strong or unpleasant emotions subdued, it is reasonable to suppose that other neocortical functions may be diminished. Hubel, in commenting on sensory receptors and their response to stimulation, stated: "We need above all to know about changes; no one wants or needs to be reminded sixteen hours a day that his shoes are on."[23] When primitive emotions chronically intrude on conscious thought, we are, by analogy, in the position of being reminded that our shoes are on sixteen hours a day. The energy required to keep this useless turmoil from usurping a good part of our conscious lives probably detracts from the creative and adaptive functions of the neocortex.

Stress has been implicated as a major precipitating factor in the psychosomatic diseases. Stress is an inherent facet of normal life. It may originate in a perceived external threat to one's equilibrium or safety (realistic or not), in intrapsychic conflict, or in the perceived (or misperceived) absence of affirmation or positive denigration of the self. Some events are universally perceived as stressful, such as an automobile accident. Many situations are stressful to some people but not to others, depending on their past history and experiences. An important facet of taking a history is to try to fathom the degree, sources, and significance of stress in the patient's life. Whatever the source of stress may be, it is translated into physiological or biochemical terms by the three major semiautonomous and partially related effector systems the brain has at its disposal. These are the autonomic (and peripheral) nervous system, the endocrine system, and, as is now being increasingly recognized, the immune system.

The immune system has some properties similar to those of the nervous system. It must learn to recognize and discriminate between self and nonself; it has a molecular memory that produces a heightened response to a previously encountered antigen; it utilizes cell-to-cell communication.[35] Nervous system–immune system interrelations have been reviewed by Ader,[36] Besedovsky,[37] Stein et al,[38] and Locke.[39] Among notable recent reviews of the interrelations between the nervous system, endocrine system and the immune system are those of Weigert and Blalock,[40] Dunn,[41,42] Saphier,[43] Jankovic,[44] Ader and Cohen,[45] Ader et al.,[46] and Bateman et al.[47] Extensive reviews of brain–endocrine system–immune system relationships have been included in the fifth edition of *Comprehensive Psychiatry* by Kaplan and Sadock.[15] In addition, the immunology of the skin has been reviewed by Longley et al.[48] and Dezutter-Dambuant.[49] Neuropeptides in skin have been reviewed by Brain and Williams[50] and by Weike and Hartschuh.[51] To sample a few examples of nervous system–endocrine system–immune system relationships, it has been observed that the peripheral nervous system may modify immune and hypersensitivity reactions and inflammation by the release of neuropeptides—substance P, somatostatin, and vasoactive intestinal peptide—for which lymphocytes have receptors.[52,53] Basophils and tissue mast cells may be affected by neuropeptides, which may stimulate or inhibit histamine release.[54] Increased T- and B-cell β-adrenergic receptor density and altered immune responsiveness follow ablation of the sympathetic nervous system.[55] Pert et al. conclude that "neuropeptides and their receptors thus join the brain, glands, and immune system in a network of communication between brain and body, probably representing the biochemical substrate of emotion."[56]

CLINICAL DISCUSSION[57,58]

As mentioned at the outset, a search for point-for-point correlations among a state of mind, an emotional disturbance, a personality or character type, and a specific skin disease is not a reliable approach to psychosomatics. From general medicine, we know that we do not all respond to or tolerate a given drug in the same way, and we don't heal identically after surgery. Every patient must be evaluated on his or her own terms. To start with, we should regard the patient as a whole, literally. Punctuality should be noted; apprehensive or compulsive patients may present as much as an hour early, and constantly late patients may be testing to see if they are acceptable. One should note the patient's general dress and demeanor; it is a measure not only of how the patient regards himself or herself, but also of how the patient wishes you to regard him or her. All outer garments, as well as skin and hair, are meant to be communicative, as well as protective and decorative. A quick glance at the cosmetic cover may give some inkling to what is being hidden (often a sensitivity). Never underestimate the importance of hair. Culturally and symbolically, it is one of the most meaning-laden parts of the body.[59] Complaints of hair loss in the absence of visible thinning may represent mild anxiety, relievable in part by explanation and reassurance, or more severe depression. One needs to try to get a sense of how much decorative behavior is simply cultural expression, how important it is in a sexual sense, how devastated and sexually unattractive cutaneous flaws and hair changes or loss make a patient feel, how invested the "ego" is in particular aspects of appearance that the patient now sees as failing ("I've always been known for my hair"), and, not least, in an older patient, how important it is to maintain the illusion of youth or at least minimize the changes of age. The skin is in part an organ of communication both psychologically and physiologically. In sexual relationships, not only touch but also psychological factors are as important as hormonal preconditioning as determinants of sexual behavior.[60] In addition, skin is a mirror of emotions, as reflected in sweating, flushing, and pallor, as well as in the decorative arts.

In addition to a visual scan, one should pay attention not only to what the patient says, but how it is said—the tone of voice (whining, complaining, impatient, imperious), the choice of expression, the intensity of seriousness of the complaint, the pressure of speech (rapidity, decibel level, can you get a word in edgewise?)—all the affective cues of vocal communication. Even before the patient is formally examined, a disparity between the intensity of the complaint and the visual findings may be evident, and should prompt further inquiry about the general state of satisfactions and/or dissatisfactions with life—at home, at school, at work, and with personal relationships. Morphologic dermatology is in a sense the clinical study of gross pathology. A disparity between what is described by the patient and what is seen by the physician signifies that there may be more meaning to what is said than what is seen. That meaning lies elsewhere than on the skin. It may reflect a displacement to the skin of other emotional baggage (e.g., excessive anxiety) or, alternatively, as with the princess who could feel a pea under 10 mattresses, an overly sensitive and overly narcissistic self-image.

In the course of the first two decades of life, we develop a sense of self and a self-image as part of the process of individuation. It is the rock on which we all stand to take on the world. Chips or cracks in the rock unsteady the whole structure. Narcissism is a normal human quality that endows us with a reasonable degree of pride and confidence and a realistic sense of self and self-image; it is a kind of mental glue or cement that fills the chips and cracks and holds the rock together.[61] Pathological narcissism reflects a defective perception of oneself; it is the substitution of glue for sections of rock. It bespeaks a deficiency of real substance, and therefore entails a fragility that has little sense of give-and-take and tolerates criticism poorly. It entails a fanciful sense of self-importance (occasionally bordering on omnipotence), with a disregard for others, and a sense of entitlement—a right to be well, often immediately, which the physician is expected to implement promptly. Pathological narcissism is found abundantly in psychiatry and plastic surgery, and may be seen in dermatology as an insistent demand for cure of relatively minor problems and difficulty in adjusting to more serious ones.

All illness damages one's self-image and self-esteem. This is particularly true in skin disease, where the problem is often evident for all to see. The adolescent, still in the formative years of development, is particularly vulnerable and may need sympathetic and encouraging assistance to deal with the manifest psychic trauma. The older patient, who more often than not has suffered a collection of "slings and arrows of outrageous fortune" and is beset not only with unfulfilled dreams and expectations and fading hopes of ever realizing them, but also with taunting physical reminders of the aging process such as real hair loss, facial hair growth, wrinkles, discolorations, and assorted cutaneous growths, also needs sympathetic and reassuring assistance. A reasonable perspective, a sense of humor, and a sympathetic awareness of the human condition are usually adequate to deal helpfully with most situations. We cannot decrease entropy, but we can help patients accept inevitable change. The catalog of skin diseases that potentially threaten self-esteem can serve as the index of a textbook of dermatology. When diseases affect exposed parts of the body, everyone can see them, as the patient is actively aware. When they affect covered areas, public embarrassment is spared but self-awareness of the pathology remains, as well as concerns about defectiveness.

The human mind constantly seeks to establish meaning in events. If reasonable explanations are not readily at hand, it creates them. A person who has not been trained scientifically to think about disease in a logical framework based on previous verifiable experience will think or fantasize about it and explain it in terms with which he or she is familiar. These explanations may reflect old childhood fears and notions. All diseases have meaning to a patient. A major illness arouses concerns about life itself, the welfare of one's family, the security of one's job and home, and one's ability to cope with the exigencies of life. In short, it arouses fears about losses. The concerns are usually significant and realistic, as the illness may make considerable demands on the patient's capacity to adapt and, if necessary, alter his or her lifestyle. Most skin diseases are not life-threatening but have varying degrees of chronicity. The meanings that may be attached to skin diseases are less likely to be the serious realistic concerns associated with life-threatening illnesses, but are more likely to consist of disturbances of self-image and concerns about interpersonal relationships (am I dirty, am I contagious, will people avoid me or stare at me?). Whether or not these concerns are unrealistic, they are a source of worry and concern to the patient.

We have all been taught to think in logical or experiential terms about disease. The patient comes to you for an explanation of a problem and for cure or helpful treatment. We can be helpful if we can explain to the patient, in his or her own terms, what the problem is. We can be more helpful if, in addition, we can discover what the patient's fears, worries, and understanding of the disease are so that we can try to neutralize undue anxiety and inject a reasonable amount of reality into his or her field of thought. If we wish to find out what the patient thinks and how the patient understands (or misunderstands) the problem, then we must listen. The patient's notions are in no book, on no list of differential diagnoses, on no computer printout. They are only in the patient's mind. If we listen patiently, ask clarifying questions, and bear the anxiety, we may find out. Then we may be able to help restore a modicum of ease of the dis-ease.

There are several clues that may serve as a basis for additional history taking in relation to the search for intrapsychic conflict or psychosocial stress. One is a long delay between onset of illness and presentation for medical attention. Why does the patient present at this particular time? What external factors have recently come into play (e.g., family illness, newspaper or television coverage of some illness or environmental threat)? And why the delay?

Another clue to the presence of significant emotional factors is the question, could the disease be due to "nerves?" This may be the patient's way of introducing the issue of emotional stress and should be followed up promptly by inquiring what the patient is nervous about. There are three broad areas in anyone's life that may be easily inquired into—family, work, and friends. Deaths, conflicts, job insecurity or loss, economic problems, emotional problems, alcohol or other substance abuse, problems with parents or children, disappointments, or other emotionally laden issues will often be included in those three areas. If no answers are forthcoming on the first inquiry, the patient is at least aware that the physician is interested in him or her as a person, and a later inquiry may prove useful.

Additional clues to sources of conflict may be gleaned by observing who accompanies the patient and who answers the questions. A young adult accompanied by a parent, usually the mother, who repeatedly answers questions before the patient, who contradicts the patient's answers, or who supplements or modifies each of the patient's statements indicates an inappropriate dependency problem (in both). The implication here is that parental resistance may take the form of diminished patient compliance with the therapeutic program.

Many examples of physician–patient interactions in dermatologic practice, as well as a list of character types known to every physician, may be found in a review by Waisman.[62] Another approach to the complexities of the doctor–patient relationship is described by Cotterill in terms of game theory.[63]

Somatization, the displacement of affective symptoms, particularly in states of anxiety and depression, to physical complaints, is a general medical problem.[64] Katon et al. point out that somatization may be culturally determined in groups that frown on direct emotional expression, may be learned in childhood as a way of coping with emotional distress or of getting attention, may be used as the most effective way to get relief from sources of anxiety (e.g., work-related problems), and may inadvertently be reinforced by extensive medical investigation. One clue to somatization, as mentioned above, is the discrepancy between the complaints and the physical findings. In other branches of medicine, physical complaints require a considerable workup to define or exclude organic pathology, whereas in skin disease the pathology is usually immediately visible, and so is the discrepancy.

Whitlock reviewed extensively and critically the psychophysiological aspects of skin disease.[65] He concluded, first, that it is likely invalid to read into a psychosomatic symptom (e.g., pruritus, especially pruritus ani or vulvae) a universal symbolic meaning. Whatever symbolic meaning there is in any cutaneous symptom will likely vary from patient to patient and will depend on that patient's particular life history, experience, genetic determinants, and integrative capacities. Second, a symptom may well be tinged with affect such as guilt, anxiety, envy, or rage, but it would be hazardous to make more extended etiologic interpretations. Third, the proximity on one occasion between an emotional upset and a physical change does not necessarily establish a causal relationship at all times. Fourth, Whitlock indicates, in the area of skin disease, an emotional state accompanied by a physiological response (e.g., flushing) does not necessarily produce permanent organic change, as in acne rosacea. Finally, he points out that the apparent improvement in or cure of a disorder by psychological treatment does not ipso facto prove psychogenesis. In addition to the placebo effect, long-term psychotherapy leaves room for many other changes to occur coincidentally.

The classification of skin diseases with a psychological component is at best inexact. Medansky and Handler have suggested three broad categories that appear adequately inclusive without being too restrictive: (1) primary psychological disturbance with secondary cutaneous lesions produced or fantasized by the patient; (2) organic skin disease with secondary psychological effects; and (3) the largest group, in which there may be an interplay between psychological and physical factors.[66]

In the first group, lesions are imposed on essentially normal skin and skin appendages by an external force. These types of cutaneous lesions are excoriations of various geometric (not usually naturally occurring) forms, chemical and thermal burns, bruises, swellings induced by rubber bands or other ligatures, genital and perianal ulcerations, hemorrhage from various orifices, and discolorations.[67] The lesions are located on the extremities and parts of the trunk within easy reach. There may be an asymmetric distribution on the back related to the handedness of the patient. Across the shoulders, upper back, and upper arms, one may find partially depigmented, small, flat, discrete scars consonant with old healed excoriations. Black eschars reflect a greater depth of tissue damage, possibly induced by heat (cigarette burns) or chemical injury (silver nitrate). Sneddon[67] recommends that unexplained ulcers be tested with litmus paper to evaluate the possible presence of strong acids or alkalis. Patient interference should be kept in mind when operative incisions or skin grafts fail to heal as expected. Injection of foreign material may cause painful, erythematous nodules and possibly an associated factitial fever. It has been estimated that 10 percent of prolonged fevers of unknown origin may be factitial.[68] Health care personnel may be especially difficult patients in this regard because of their familiarity with medical procedures. One may also include in this first group those with essentially trivial lesions who present with cancerophobia or syphilophobia (and now fear of the acquired immunodeficiency syndrome, AIDS). Schizophrenia or depression may present this way.

While factitial disease may at times be a substitute for a direct request for help, attempts to provide help, particularly psychiatric consultation, are often rejected.[69] Rather than direct confrontation, which is often not helpful, Lyell has recommended that it be indicated to the patient that the problem is understood and sympathized with.[70] Relaxation exercises supervised by a clinical psychologist have been recommended by Sneddon as more acceptable to the patient while providing opportunities for therapeutic discussion. For some people, illness is a preferred way of life.[71] The assumption that everyone wants to get better may be erroneous. In a 12-year follow-up of 33 patients, Sneddon and Sneddon found that one-third continued to produce lesions.[72] Improvement was better correlated with changes in life circumstances and environment than with medical intervention. Therapeutic intervention in illness that is financially well compensated for may be ineffective.

Trichotillomania is a mechanically induced hair loss consequent to twisting hair about one or more fingers forcefully and repeatedly, resulting in irregular patches of scalp hair loss with a scattering of broken hairs in the affected area. It may be done unconsciously and assumes the proportions of obsessive-compulsive behavior. Alopecia areata, in contrast, is a spontaneous, rapid hair loss, usually completely, in discrete oval or circular patches, sometimes temporally related to emotional shock or stress. The mechanism of hair loss may involve an immune process as judged by its association with other "autoimmune" processes, such as pernicious anemia, thyroiditis, and Addison's disease.

Delusions of parasitism (monosymptomatic hypochondriacal psychosis) most commonly affect elderly unmarried women with the unshakable conviction that the skin is infested.[73] The ensuing excoriations are readily acknowledged as an attempt to remove the offending agent. Characteristically, patients present a small box containing lint, dried skin scales, or other small objects, allegedly removed from the skin, as evidence of the infestation. It is important to examine these to avoid embarrassment in the occasional case where parasites may be present. Except for this specific delusion, patients may carry on a very reasonable conversation. Unfortunately, the delusion may create considerable havoc in that extensive attempts—fumigation of homes, changing furniture or even houses, vigorous complaints to civic authorities, etc.—may be made to destroy the offending agent. Diseases that may cause altered cutaneous sensation—contact dermatitis, diabetes, peripheral neuritis, liver or kidney disorders, pellagra, intoxications, drug reactions, lymphoproliferative disorders, and possible environmental causes—should be ruled out.[74] Consultation with a psychiatrist is indicated for possible use of antipsychotic drugs.

The psychogenic purpuras constitute a set of most unusual disorders including self-induced bruising, self-induced anticoagulation (usually with coumadin), stigmata, the autoerythrocyte sensitization or Gardner-Diamond syndrome, and possibly DNA sensitivity on skin testing. Ratnoff has reviewed the subject in detail.[75] Emotional pathology appears to be the outstanding feature in a majority of patients, most of whom are young women.

The main complaint of a group of patients described by Cotterill with dermatologic non-disease was burning, particularly involving the face, scalp, and perineum.[76] Preoccupation with the nose may be a psychotic symptom necessitating prompt psychiatric referral.

The second group proposed by Medansky and Handler comprises illnesses that are primarily cutaneous or systemic, such as large nevi, hemangiomas, neurofibromatosis, ichthyotic states, ectodermal dysplasia, and burns. These may produce secondary emotional changes, depending on the extent of the distortion of the body image, the age of onset of the problem, and the reactions of the parents or other caretakers to the problem.

The third group of diseases in which there is an interplay between psyche and skin includes urticaria, atopic dermatitis, seborrheic dermatitis, psoriasis, acne vulgaris, acne rosacea, alopecia areata, warts, hyperhidrosis and dyshidrosis, lichen planus, and Raynaud's disease, among others. There is no convincing etiologic relationship between specific emotional states or personality types and the onset of the skin disorder. Nor is psychotherapeutic intervention a reliable cure. Stress and other emotional factors may aggravate these diseases, and it is here that the interplay among endocrine, nervous, vascular, and immune systems comes to the fore. The psychiatric mechanisms proposed for these disorders have been thoroughly reviewed by Panconesi[77] and Koblenzer.[57] The sudden hair loss in alopecia areata has been interpreted as related to sudden emotional trauma associated with losses (e.g., death of a family member). The mechanism remains obscure, but the association of alopecia areata and the immune system, as well as the recent studies on neuroimmunomodulation, suggest that the immune system may be the effective pathway for this disorder.

In atopic dermatitis, a hereditary disorder, there is an alteration of immune function, as evidenced by elevated IgE levels in some 70 percent of patients, and by increased susceptibility to cutaneous infections, especially herpes simplex viral infections. Itching is the most prominent and disturbing feature of atopic dermatitis. Emotional disturbances increase itching by causing vasodilatation, increased perspiration, and increased sensitivity to minor stimuli. Psychotherapy may be helpful in general in atopics, but it is not specifically helpful for that disease.

CONCLUSION

In conclusion, it is important to bear in mind that in the final analysis we are dealing with one subject—the individual, who is an expression of the complex interrelationships and reciprocal relationships of all the systems of the body. For purposes of study and research in psychosomatics, we may tentatively consider three areas of function:

1. The mind—the psychological level, consisting of the perceptual, cognitive, emotional, learned, and recalled ways of regarding ourselves, others, and our environment. Classic psychiatric and psychological literature deals with this level of understanding and does not, in terms of mechanism, engage the other two levels in drawing conclusions about the effects of psychic factors on disease. Modern psychiatry, with the advent of psychopharmacological methods of treatment, now is concerned with brain function and its relation to thought processes.
2. The area of brain function proper, which requires a functional understanding of the interconnections and reciprocal influences of neocortical and subcortical processes, as well as of the biologic processes that constitute learning, perception, memory, and abstract thought on the one hand, and the range of emotions on the other.
3. The effector systems—the peripheral and autonomic nervous systems, the endocrine, immune, and vascular systems—by which brain and body communicate with and influence each other.

The search to understand these three areas in humans is comparable to the search for a unified field theory in physics.

REFERENCES

1. Dunbar F: A survey of literature on psychosomatic interrelationships, in *Emotions and Bodily Changes*, 4th ed. New York, Columbia University Press, 1954, p 1910.
2. Delbruck M: *Mind from Matter*. Oxford, Blackwell Scientific, 1986.
3. Masters R: The psyche and the skin. *Neurol Clin* 5:483, 1987.
4. Brazier MAB: Challenges from the philosophers ot the neuroscientists, in *Brain and Mind*. Amsterdam, Ciba Foundation Symposium 69 (new series), 1979, p 5.
5. Ackerman D: *A Natural History of the Senses*. New York, Random House, in press.
6. Bowlby J: *Attachment and Loss*, vol 1: *Attachment*. New York, Basic Books, 1969.
7. Sinclair D: *Mechanisms of Cutaneous Sensation*, 2d ed. New York, Oxford University Press, 1981.
8. Darian-Smith I: Touch in primates. *Annu Rev Psychol* 33:155, 1982.
9. Nanta WJH, Domesick VB: Ramifications of the limbic system in psychiatry and the biology of the human brain, in S Matthysse (ed), *A Symposium Dedicated to Seymour S. Kety*. New York, Elsevier North-Holland, 1981, p 165.
10. Hofer MA: Toward a developmental basis for disease predisposition: the effects of early maternal separation on brain, behavior, and cardiovascular system, in H Weiner et al (eds), *Brain and Bodily Disease*. New York, Raven Press, 1981, p 209.
11. Kuhn CM et al: Selective depression of serum growth hormone during maternal deprivation in rat pups. *Science* 201:1034, 1978.

12. Spitz RA: Hospitalism: an inquiry into the genesis of psychiatric conditions in early childhood in *The Psychoanalytic Study of the Child.* New York, International Universities Press, 1945, vol 1, p 53.
13. Spitz RA: Hospitalism: a follow-up report in *The Psychoanalytic Study of the Child.* New York, International Universities Press, 1946, vol 2, p 113.
14. Spitz RA: Analytic depression in *The Psychoanalytic Study of the Child.* New York, International Universities Press, 1946, vol 2, p 313.
15. Kaplan HI, Sadock BJ: *Comprehensive Textbook of Psychiatry,* 5th ed., 1989, Baltimore, Williams & Wilkins, 1989, p 1897.
16. Powell GF et al: Emotional deprivation and growth retardation simulating idiopathic hypopituitarism. *N Engl J Med* 276: 1271, 1279, 1967.
17. Rose RM, Sachar E: Psychoendocrinology, in RH Williams (ed), *Textbook of Endocrinology,* 6th ed. Philadelphia, Saunders, 1981, p 646.
18. Green WH et al: Psychosocial dwarfism, infantile autism and attention deficit disorder, in CB Nemeroff, PT Loosen (eds), *Handbook of Clinical Psychoneuroendocrinology.* New York, Guilford Press, 1987, p 109.
19. Frasier SD: Abnormalities in growth, in R Collu et al (eds), *Pediatric Endocrinology.* New York, Raven Press, 1981, p 167.
20. Harlow HF: The nature of love. *Am Psychol* 13:673, 1958.
21. Montagu A: *Touching: the Human Significance of the Skin.* New York, Columbia University Press, 1971.
22. Kandel ER: Environmental determinants of brain architecture and of behavior. Early experience and learning, in ER Kandell, JH Schwartz (eds), *Principles of Neural Science.* New York, Elsevier North-Holland, 1981, p 620.
23. Hubel DH: The brain. *Sci Am* 241(No. 3):44, 1979.
24. Gorski RA: Sexual differentiation of the brain: mechanisms and implications for neuroscience, in SS Easter Jr., et al (eds), *From Message to Mind.* Sunderland, Mass., Sinauer Associates.
25. McDonald M: The psychoanalytic concept of the self. *Psychiatr Clin, N Amer* 4:429, 1981.
26. Ornstein A: Self-pathology in childhood: developmental and clinical considerations. *Psychiatr Clin North Am.* 4:435, 1981.
27. Kandel ER: Cellular insights into behavior and learning. *The Harvey Lectures,* Series 73, 1977–1978. New York, Academic Press, 1979, p 19.
28. Kandel ER, Castellucci VF: Cellular approaches to short- and long-term memory and to nonassociative and associative learning, in S. Matthysse (ed), *Psychiatry and the Biology of the Human Brain.* New York, Elsevier North-Holland, 1981, p 103.
29. Walters ET et al: Habituation, sensitization and associative learning in aplysia, in AL Beackman (ed), *The Neural Basis of Behavior.* New York, Spectrum, 1982.
30. Lynch G, Lee K: Some capacities for structural growth and functional change in the neuronal circuitries of the adult hippocampus, in AL Beackman (ed), *The Neural Basis of Behavior.* New York, Spectrum, 1982, p 103.
31. Warburton DM: Neurochemistry of behavior. *Br Med Bull* 37:121, 1981.
32. Squire LR: *Memory and Brain.* New York, Oxford University Press, 1987.
33. Kandel ER et al: Cell-biological interrelationships between short-term and long-term memory, in *Molecular Neurobiology in Neurology and Psychiatry,* 1987, vol 65, p 111.
34. Shepherd GM: *Neurobiology,* 2d ed. New York, Oxford University Press, 1988.
35. Janeway CA Jr. et al: Modes of cell: cell communication in the immune system. *J Immunol* 135:739s, 1985.
36. Ader R: *Psychoneuroimmunology.* New York, Academic Press, 1981.
37. Besedovsky HO et al: Immune-neuroendocrine interactions. *J Immunol* 135:750s, 1985.
38. Stein M et al: Stress and immunomodulation: the role of depression and neuroendocrine function. *J Immunol* 135:827s, 1985.
39. Locke S et al: *Foundations of Psychoneuroimmunology.* New York, Aldine, 1985.
40. Weigent DA, Blalock JE: Interactions between the neuroendocrine and immune systems: common hormones and receptors. *Immunol Rev* 100:79, 1987.

41. Dunn AJ: Nervous system–immune system interactions: an overview. *J Receptr Res* 8:589, 1988.
42. Dunn AJ Psychoneuroimmunology for the psychoneuroendocrinologist: a review of animal studies of nervous system–immune interactions. *Psychoneuroendocrinology* 14:251, 1989.
43. Saphier D: Neurophysiological and endocrine consequences of immune activity. *Psychoneuroendocrinology* 14:63, 1989.
44. Jankovic BD: Neuroimmunomodulation: facts and dilemmas. *Immunol Lett* 21:101, 1989.
45. Ader R, Cohen N: CNS–immune system interactions: conditioning phenomena. *Behav Brain Sci* 8:379, 1985.
46. Ader R et al: Brain, behavior and immunity. *Brain Behav Immunity* 1:1, 1987.
47. Bateman A et al: The immune-hypothalamic-pituitary-adrenal axis. *Endocrine Rev* 10:92, 1989.
48. Longley BJ et al: Immunology and the skin: current concepts. *Ann NY Acad Sci* 548:225, 1988.
49. Dezutter-Dambuant C: Role of Langerhans cells in cutaneous immunologic processes. *Semin Dermatol* 7:163, 1988.
50. Brain SD, Williams TJ: Neuropharmacology of peptides in skin. *Semin Dermatol* 7:278, 1988.
51. Weihe E, Hartschuh W: Multiple peptides in cutaneous nerves: regulators under physiological conditions and a pathogenetic role in skin disease? *Semin Dermatol*, 7:284, 1988.
52. O'Dorisio MS et al: Vasoactive intestinal peptide and neuropeptide modulation of the immune response. *J Immunol* 135:792s, 1985.
53. Payan DG, Goetzl EJ: Modulation of lymphocyte function by sensory neuropeptides. *Immunology* 135:783s, 1985.
54. Goetzl EJ et al: Neuropeptide regulation of the expression of immediate hypersensitivity. *J Immunol* 135:802s, 1985.
55. Miles K et al: sympathetic ablation alters lymphocyte membrane properties. *J Immunol* 135:797s, 1985.
56. Pert CB et al: Neuropeptides and their receptors: a psychosomatic network. *J Immunol* 135:820s, 1985.
57. Koblenzer CS: *Psychocutaneous Disease*. Orlando, Fla, Grune & Stratton, 1987.
58. Gupta MA, Vorhees JJ: Psychosomatic dermatology: is it relevant? *Arch Dermatol* 126:90, 1990.
59. Leach ER: Magical hair, in J Middleton (ed), *Myth and Cosmos: Reading in Mythology and Symbolism*. Garden City, NY, Natural History Press, 1967.
60. Larsson K, Beyer C: Some aspects of the neuroendocrine regulation of mammalian sexual behavior, in PB Hrdina, RL Singha (eds), *Neuroendocrine Regulation and Altered Behavior*. New York, Plenum, 1981, p 95.
61. Cooper A: Narcissism, in S Arrieti (ed), *American Handbook of Psychiatry*, 2d ed. New York, Basic Books, 1981, vol 7, p 297.
62. Waisman M: Patient encounters—patterns, perceptions, perplexities, precautions. *J Am Acad Dermatol* 1:134, 1979.
63. Cotterill JA: Dermatological games. *Br J Dermatol* 105:311, 1981.
64. Katon W et al: Depression and somatization: a review: part 1. *Am J Med* 72:127, 1982.
65. Whitlock FA: *Major Problems in Dermatology*, vol 1: *Psychophysiological Aspects of Skin Disease*. Philadelphia, Saunders, 1976.
66. Medansky, RS, Handler RM: Dermatopsychosomatics: classification, physiology, and therapeutic approaches. *J Am Acad Dermatol* 5:125, 1981.
67. Sneddon IB: Simulated disease and hypochondriasis in the dermatology clinic. *Semin Dermatol* 2:177, 1983.
68. Adnon RP et al: Factitious fever and self-induced infection. *Ann Intern Med* 90:230, 1979.
69. Fabisch W: Psychiatric aspects of dermatitis artefacta. *Br J Dermatol* 102:29, 1980.
70. Lyell A: Dermatitis artifacts in relation to the syndrome of contrived disease. *Clin Exp Dermatol* 1:109, 1976.

71. Sneddon J: Patients who do not want to get better. *Semin Dermatol* 2:183, 1983.
72. Sneddon I, Sneddon J: Self-inflicted injury: a follow-up study of 43 patients. *Br Med J* 3:527, 1975.
73. Munro A: Delusional parasitosis: a form of monosymptomatic hypochondriacal psychosis. *Semin Dermatol* 2:197, 1983.
74. Lyell A: Delusions of parasitosis. *Semin Dermatol* 2:189, 1983.
75. Ratnoff O: The psychogenic purpuras: a review of autoerythrocyte sensitization, autosensitization to DNA, "hysterical" and factitial bleeding, and the religious stigmata. *Semin Hematol* 17:192, 1980.
76. Cotterill JA: Psychodermatology. *Semin Dermatol* 2:171, 1983.
77. Panconesi E: Psychosomatic dermatology. *Clin Dermatol* 2:94, 1984.

Index

Page numbers in *italics* indicate illustrations or tables.